OXFORD MEDICAL PUBLICATIONS

Oxford Handbook of Clinical Haematology

Third edition

[redacted]

Published and forthcoming Oxford Handbooks

Oxford Handbook for the Foundation Programme 2/e
Oxford Handbook of Acute Medicine 3/e
Oxford Handbook of Anaesthesia 2/e
Oxford Handbook of Applied Dental Sciences
Oxford Handbook of Cardiology
Oxford Handbook of Clinical and Laboratory Investigation 2/e
Oxford Handbook of Clinical Dentistry 4/e
Oxford Handbook of Clinical Diagnosis 2/e
Oxford Handbook of Clinical Examination and Practical Skills
Oxford Handbook of Clinical Haematology 3/e
Oxford Handbook of Clinical Immunology and Allergy 2/e
Oxford Handbook of Clinical Medicine – Mini Edition 7/e
Oxford Handbook of Clinical Medicine 7/e
Oxford Handbook of Clinical Pharmacy
Oxford Handbook of Clinical Rehabilitation 2/e
Oxford Handbook of Clinical Specialties 8e
Oxford Handbook of Clinical Surgery 3/e
Oxford Handbook of Complementary Medicine
Oxford Handbook of Critical Care 3/e
Oxford Handbook of Dental Patient Care 2/e
Oxford Handbook of Dialysis 3/e
Oxford Handbook of Emergency Medicine 3/e
Oxford Handbook of Endocrinology and Diabetes 2/e
Oxford Handbook of ENT and Head and Neck Surgery
Oxford Handbook of Epidemiology for Clinicians
Oxford Handbook of Expedition and Wilderness Medicine
Oxford Handbook of Gastroenterology and Hepatology
Oxford Handbook of General Practice 3/e
Oxford Handbook of Genitourinary Medicine, HIV and AIDS
Oxford Handbook of Geriatric Medicine
Oxford Handbook of Infectious Diseases and Microbiology
Oxford Handbook of Key Clinical Evidence
Oxford Handbook of Medical Sciences
Oxford Handbook of Nephrology and Hypertension
Oxford Handbook of Neurology
Oxford Handbook of Nutrition and Dietetics
Oxford Handbook of Obstetrics and Gynaecology 2/e
Oxford Handbook of Occupational Health
Oxford Handbook of Oncology 2/e
Oxford Handbook of Ophthalmology
Oxford Handbook of Paediatrics
Oxford Handbook of Palliative Care 2/e
Oxford Handbook of Practical Drug Therapy
Oxford Handbook of Pre-Hospital Care
Oxford Handbook of Psychiatry 2/e
Oxford Handbook of Public Health Practice 2/e
Oxford Handbook of Reproductive Medicine and Family Planning
Oxford Handbook of Respiratory Medicine 2/e
Oxford Handbook of Rheumatology 2/e
Oxford Handbook of Sport and Exercise Medicine
Oxford Handbook of Tropical Medicine 3/e
Oxford Handbook of Urology 2/e

Oxford Handbook of Clinical Haematology

THIRD EDITION

Drew Provan

Senior Lecturer in Haematology
Barts and The London School of Medicine and Dentistry
University of London, UK

Charles R.J. Singer

Consultant Haematologist
Royal United Hospital
Bath, UK

Trevor Baglin

Consultant Haematologist
Addenbrookes NHS Trust
Cambridge, UK

Inderjeet Dokal

Professor of Paediatrics
Barts and The London School of Medicine and Dentistry
University of London, UK

OXFORD
UNIVERSITY PRESS

OXFORD
UNIVERSITY PRESS

Great Clarendon Street, Oxford OX2 6DP

Oxford University Press is a department of the University of Oxford. It furthers the University's objective of excellence in research, scholarship, and education by publishing worldwide in

Oxford New York

Auckland Cape Town Dar es Salaam Hong Kong Karachi Kuala Lumpur Madrid Melbourne Mexico City Nairobi New Delhi Shanghai Taipei Toronto

With offices in

Argentina Austria Brazil Chile Czech Republic France Greece Guatemala Hungary Italy Japan Poland Portugal Singapore South Korea Switzerland Thailand Turkey Ukraine Vietnam

Oxford is a registered trade mark of Oxford University Press in the UK and in certain other countries

Published in the United States by Oxford University Press Inc., New York

First edition published 1998
Second edition published 2004
Third edition published 2009

British Library Cataloguing in Publication Data
Data available

Library of Congress Cataloging-in-Publication-Data
Data available

Typeset by Cepha Imaging Private Ltd., Bangalore, India
Printed in China
on acid-free paper by
Asia Pacific Offset

ISBN 978–0–19–922739–6

10 9 8 7 6 5 4 3 2 1

Preface to the third edition

It is hard to believe that at least three years have passed since the second edition of the handbook. As with all medical specialties, Haematology has seen major inroads with new diagnostic tests, treatments and a plethora of guidelines. In fact, Haematology has the largest collection of guidelines covering all aspects of haematology care (http://www.bcshguidelines.com) and was the first specialty to design guidelines in the 1980s.

The book underwent a major revision with the second edition, most notably the sections dealing with malignant disease. For the new edition these have been brought right up to date by Charles Singer. Coagulation has been entirely rewritten by Trevor Baglin and now truly reflects the current investigation and management of coagulation disorders. Following the retirement of Professor Sir John Lilleyman we needed to find a new author for the Paediatric Haematology component of the book. Thankfully, we were able to persuade Professor Inderjeet Dokal to take on this mantle and he has revised this section thoroughly.

In addition to these significant changes, we have gone through the entire book and attempted to ensure that obsolete tests have been removed and that the Handbook, in its entirety, reflects contemporary haematology practice.

As ever, we are very keen to hear about errors or omissions, for which we are entirely responsible! We would also very much like readers to contact us if there are topics or subject areas which they would like to see included in the fourth edition (email a.provan@virgin.net). We also need more trainee input so if there are any volunteer proof-readers or accuracy checkers among the haematology trainee community we would very much like to hear from you.

DP
CRJS
TB
ISD
2008

Preface to the second edition

Haematology has seen many changes since 1998 when the first edition of this small book was written. Most notably, there are major advances in the treatments of malignant blood disorders with the discovery of tyrosine kinase inhibitors which have transformed the outlook for patients with CML, the rediscovery of arsenic for AML, and many other new therapies. Progress has been slower in the non-malignant arena since there is still limited evidence on which to base decisions. We have attempted to update each section in the book in order to ensure that it reflects current practice. Although molecular diagnostics have seen huge changes through the Human Genome Project and other methodological developments, we have not included these in great detail here because of lack of space. We have attempted to focus more on clinical aspects of patient care.

This edition welcomes two new authors: Professor Sir John Lilleyman, immediate Past-President of the Royal College of Pathologists, is a Paediatric Oncologist at Barts and The London, Queen Mary's School of Medicine and Dentistry, University of London. John is a leading figure in the world of paediatric haematology with an interest in both malignant and non-malignant disease affecting children. He has extensively revised the Paediatric section of the book, in addition to Immunodeficiency. Dr Trevor Baglin, Consultant Haematologist at Addenbrookes Hospital, Cambridge is Secretary of the British Committee for Standards in Haematology Haemostasis and Thrombosis Task Force. Trevor is the author of many evidence-based guidelines and peer-reviewed scientific papers. He has rewritten the Haemostasis section of the book and brought this in line with modern management.

Other features of this edition include the greater use of illustrations such as blood films, marrows, and radiological images which we hope will enhance the text and improve readers' understanding of the subject. We have increased the number of references and provided URLs for key websites providing easy access to organisations and publications.

There will doubtless be omissions and errors and we take full responsibility for these. We are very keen to receive feedback (good or otherwise!) since this helps shape future editions. If there is something you feel we have left out please complete the Readers comment card.

DP
CRJS
TB
JL
2004

Preface to the first edition

This small volume is intended to provide the essential core knowledge required to assess patients with possible disorders of the blood, organize relevant investigations and initiate therapy where necessary. By reducing extraneous information as much as possible, and presenting key information for each topic, a basic understanding of the pathophysiology is provided and this, we hope, will stimulate readers to follow this up by consulting the larger haematology textbooks.

We have provided both a patient-centred and disease-centred approach to haematological disease, in an attempt to provide a form of 'surgical sieve', hopefully enabling doctors in training to formulate a differential diagnosis before consulting the relevant disease-orientated section.

We have provided a full review of haematological investigations and their interpretation, handling emergency situations, and included the commonly used protocols in current use on Haematology Units, hopefully providing a unified approach to patient management.

There are additional sections relating to patient support organizations and Internet resources for further exploration by those wishing to delve deeper into the subject of blood and its diseases.

Obviously with a subject as large as clinical haematology we have been selective about the information we chose to include in the handbook. We would be interested to hear of diseases or situations not covered in this handbook. If there are inaccuracies within the text we accept full responsibility and welcome comments relating to this.

DP
MC
ASD
CRJS
AGS
1998

Foreword to the first edition

The Concise Oxford Dictionary defines a handbook as 'a short manual or guide'. Modern haematology is a vast field which involves almost every other medical speciality and which, more than most, straddles the worlds of the basic biomedical sciences and clinical practice. Since the rapidly proliferating numbers of textbooks on this topic are becoming denser and heavier with each new edition, the medical student and young doctor in training are presented with a daunting problem, particularly as they try to put these fields into perspective. And those who try to teach them are not much better placed; on the one hand they are being told to decongest the curriculum, while on the other they are expected to introduce large slices of molecular biology, social science, ethics, and communication skills, not to mention a liberal sprinkling of poetry, music, and art.

In this over-heated educational scene the much maligned 'handbook' could well stage a come-back and gain new respectability, particularly in the role of a friendly guide. In the past this genre has often been viewed as having little intellectual standing, of no use to anybody except the panicstricken student who wishes to try to make up for months of misspent time in a vain, one-night sitting before their final examination. But given the plethora of rapidly changing information that has to be assimilated, the carefully prepared précis is likely to play an increasingly important role in medical education. Perhaps even that ruination of the decent paragraph and linchpin of the pronouncements of medical bureaucrats, the 'bullet-point', may become acceptable, albeit in small doses, as attempts are made to highlight what is really important in a scientific or clinical field of enormous complexity and not a little uncertainty.

In this short account of blood diseases the editors have done an excellent service to medical students, as well as doctors who are not specialists in blood diseases, by summarizing in simple terms the major features and approaches to diagnosis and management of most of the blood diseases that they will meet in routine clinical practice or in the tedious examinations that face them. And in condensing this rapidly expanding field they have, remarkably, managed to avoid one of the great difficulties and pitfalls of this type of teaching; in trying to reduce complex issues down to their bare bones, it is all too easy to introduce inaccuracies.

One word of warning from a battle-scarred clinician however. A précis of this type suffers from the same problem as a set of multiple-choice questions. Human beings are enormously complex organisms, and sick ones are even more complicated; during a clinical lifetime the self-critical doctor will probably never encounter a 'typical case' of anything. Thus the outlines of the diseases that are presented in this book must be used as approximate guides, and no more. But provided they bear this in mind, students will find that it is a very valuable summary of modern haematology; the addition of the Internet sources is a genuine and timely bonus.

D. J. Weatherall

April 1998

Contents

Detailed contents

Acknowledgements

We are indebted to many of our colleagues for providing helpful suggestions and for proofreading the text. In particular we wish to thank Dr Helen McCarthy, Specialist Registrar in Haematology; Dr Jo Piercy, Specialist Registrar in Haematology; Dr Tanay Sheth, SHO in Haematology, Southampton; Sisters Clare Heather and Ann Jackson, Haematology Day Unit, Southampton General Hospital; Dr Mike Williams, Specialist Registrar in Anaesthetics; Dr Frank Boulton, Wessex Blood Transfusion Service, Southampton; Dr Paul Spargo, Consultant Anaesthetist, Southampton University Hospitals; Dr Sheila Bevin, Staff Grade Paediatrician; Dr Mike Hall, Consultant Neonatologist; Dr Judith Marsh, Consultant Haematologist, St George's Hospital, London; Joan Newman, Haematology Transplant Coordinator, Southampton; Professor Sally Davies, Consultant Haematologist, Imperial College School of Medicine, Central Middlesex Hospital, London; Dr Denise O'Shaughnessy, Consultant Haematologist, Southampton University Hospitals NHS Trust; Dr Kornelia Cinkotai, Consultant Haematologist, Barts and The London NHS Trust; Dr Mansel Haeney, Consultant Immunologist, Hope Hospital, Salford; Dr Adam Mead, Specialist Registrar Barts and The London; Dr Chris Knechtli, Consultant Haematologist, Royal United Hospital, Bath; Dr Toby Hall, Consultant Radiologist, Royal United Hospital Bath, Craig Lewis, Senior Biomedical Scientist, Royal United Hospital Bath, Bob Maynard, Senior Biomedical Scientist, Royal United Hospital Bath and Rosie Simpson, Senior Pharmacist, Royal United Hospital Bath. We would like to thank Alastair Smith, Morag Chisholm and Andrew Duncombe for their contributions to the first edition of the handbook. Three Barts & The London SpRs helped edit some of the sections of 3e, namely Drs John de Vos, Tom Butler and Jay Pandya. Dr Jim Murray, Queen Elizabeth Hospital, Birmingham, corrected the Haematological Emergencies section, though he did this in error since he was supposed to be proof-reading something completely different but he was too polite to say anything (bless).

We would like to acknowledge the patience and forbearance of our wives and families for the months of neglect imposed by the work on this edition. Warm thanks, as ever, are extended to Oxford University Press, and in particular Catherine Barnes, Senior Commissioning Editor for Medicine, Elizabeth Reeve, Commissioning Editor, Beth Womack, Managing Editor, and Kate Wilson, Production Manager. We fell behind schedule with this edition and are grateful to the whole OUP team for bearing with us so patiently and not harassing us! We apologize for anyone omitted but this is entirely unintentional.

Contributors

Tom Butler
Specialist Registrar in Haematology, Barts and the London NHS Trust, London, UK

Johannes de Vos
Specialist Registrar in Haematology, Barts and the London NHS Trust, London, UK

Symbols and abbreviations

🕮	cross-reference
↓	decreased
↑	increased
►	important
►►	very important
↔	normal
🖰	websites
♀	female
♂	male
1°	primary
2°	secondary
2,3 DPG	2,3 diphosphoglycerate
2-CDA	2-chlorodeoxyadenosine
A2-M	alpha$_2$ microglobulin
6-MP	6-mercaptopurine
99mTc-MIBI	^{99m}Tc methoxyisobutyl-isonitride or ^{99m}Tc-MIBI scintigraphy
AA	aplastic anaemia or reactive amyloidosis
Ab	antibody
ABVD	adriamycin (doxorubicin), bleomycin, vinblastine,
ACD	acid-citrate-dextrose *or* anaemia of chronic disease
ACE	angiotensin converting enzyme
ACL	anticardiolipin antibody
ACML	atypical chronic myeloid leukaemia
ADA	adenosine deaminase
ADE	cytosine arabinoside (Ara-C) daunorubicin etoposide
ADP	adenosine 5-diphosphate
AFB	acid fast bacilli
Ag	antigen
AIDS	acquired immunodeficiency syndrome
AIHA	autoimmune haemolytic anaemia
AIN	autoimmune neutropenia
AITL	angio-immunoblastic T-cell lymphoma
AL	(1°) amyloidosis
ALB	serum albumin
ALCL	anaplastic large cell lymphoma

ALG	anti-lymphocyte globulin
ALIPs	abnormal localization of immature myeloid precursors
ALL	acute lymphoblastic leukaemia
ALS	advanced life support
ALT	alanine aminotransferase
AML	acute myeloid leukaemia
AMP	adenosine monophosphate
ANA	antinuclear antibodies
ANAE	alpha naphthyl acetate esterase
ANCA	anti-neutrophilic cytoplasmic antibody
ANH	acute normovolaemic haemodilution
APC	activated protein C
APCR	activated protein C resistance
APL	antiphospholipid antibody
APML	acute promyelocytic leukaemia
APS	antiphospholipid syndrome
APTR	activated partial thromboplastin ratio
APTT	activated partial thromboplastin time
ARDS	adult respiratory distress syndrome
ARF	acute renal failure
ARMS	amplification refractory mutation system
ASCT	autologous stem cell transplantation
AST	aspartate aminotranferase
AT (ATIII)	antithrombin III
ATCML	adult-type chronic myeloid (granulocytic) leukaemia
ATG	anti-thymocyte globulin
ATLL	adult T-cell leukaemia/lymphoma
ATP	adenosine triphosphate
ATRA	all-trans retinoic acid
A-V	arteriovenous
AvWS	acquired von Willebrand syndrome
β2-M	beta-2-microglobuline
BAL	broncho-alveolar lavage
B-CLL	B-cell chronic lymphocytic leukaemia
bd	bis die (twice daily)
BEAC	BCNU, etoposide, cytosine, cyclophosphamide
BEAM	BCNU, etoposide, cytarabine (ara-C), melphalan
BFU-E	burst-forming unit-erythroid
BJP	Bence Jones protein
BL	Burkitt lymphoma

BM	bone marrow
BMJ	*British Medical Journal*
BMM	bone marrow mastocytosis
BMT	bone marrow transplantation
BNF	*British National Formulary*
BP	blood pressure
BPL	BioProducts Laboratory
BSS	Bernard–Soulier syndrome
BTG	B-thromboglobulin
BU	Bethesda Units
C/I	consolidation/intensification
Ca	carcinoma
Ca^{2+}	calcium
CABG	coronary artery by pass graft
cALL	common acute lymphoblastic leukaemia
CAMT	congenital amegakaryocytic thrombocytopenia
CaPO4	calcium phosphate
CBA	collagen binding activity
CBV	cyclophosphamide, carmustine (BCNU), etoposide
CCF	congestive cardiac failure
CCR	complete cytogenetic response
CD	cluster differentiation or designation
CDA	congenital dyserythropoietic anaemia
cDNA	complementary DNA
CEL	chronic eosinophilic leukaemia
CGL	chronic granulocytic leukaemia
CHAD	cold haemagglutinin disease
CHOP	cyclophosphamide, adriamycin, vincristine, prednisolone
CJD	Creutzfeldt–Jakob disease (v = variant)
Cl^-	chloride
CLD	chronic liver disease
CLL	chronic lymphocytic ('lymphatic') leukaemia
CM	cutaneous mastocytosis
CMC	chronic mucocutaneous candidiasis
CML	chronic myeloid leukaemia
CMML	chronic myelomonocytic leukaemia
CMV	cytomegalovirus
CNS	central nervous system
COAD	chronic obstructive airways disease
COC	combined oral contraceptive

COMP	cyclophosphamide, vincristine, methotrexate,
CR	complete remission
CRF	chronic renal failure
CRP	C-reactive protein
CRVT	central retinal renous thrombosis
CSF	cerebrospinal fluid
CT	computed tomography
CTLp	cytotoxic T-lymphocyte precursor assays
CTZ	chemoreceptor trigger zone
CVA	cerebrovascular accident
CVP	cyclophosphamide, vincristine, prednisolone; central
CVS	chorionic villus sampling
CVS	cardiovascular system
CXR	chest x-ray
CyA	ciclosporin A
CytaBOM	cytarabine, bleomycin, vincristine, methotrexate
d	day
DAGT	direct antiglobulin test
DAT	direct antiglobulin test daunorubicin, cytosine (Ara-C),
dATP	deoxy ATP
DBA	Diamond–Blackfan anaemia
DC	dyskeratosis congenita
DCS	dendritic cell system
DCT	direct Coombs' test
DDAVP	desamino D-arginyl vasopressin
DEAFF	detection of early antigen fluorescent foci
DEB	diepoxy butane
DFS	disease-free survival
DHAP	dexamethasone, cytarabine, cisplatin
DI	delayed intensification
DIC	disseminated intravascular coagulation
dL	decilitre
DLBCL	diffuse large B-cell lymphoma
DLI	donor leucocyte/lymphocyte infusion
DMSO	dimethyl sulphoxide
DNA	deoxyribonucleic acid
DOB	date of birth
DPG	diphosphoglycerate
DRVVT	dilute Russell's viper venom time/test
DTT	dilute thromboplastin time

DVT	deep vein thrombosis
DXT	radiotherapy
EACA	epsilon aminocaproic acid
EBV	Epstein–Barr virus
EBVP	etoposide, bleomycin, vinblastine, prednisolone
ECG	electrocardiograph
ECOG	European Co-operative Oncology Group
EDTA	ethylenediamine tetraacetic acid
EEC	endogenous erythroid colonies
EFS	event-free survival
EGF	epidermal growth factor
ELISA	enzyme-linked immunosorbent assay
EMEA	European Medicines Agency
EMH	extramedullary haemopoietic
EMU	early morning urine
EPO	erythropoietin
EPOCH	etoposide, vincristine, doxorubicin, cyclophosphamide, prednisone
EPS	electrophoresis
ESHAP	etoposide, methylprednisolone, cytarabine, platinum
ESR	erythrocyte sedimentation rate
ET	essential thrombocythaemia or exchange transfusion
ETTL	enteropathy type T-cell lymphoma
FAB	French–American–British
FACS	fluorescence-activated cell sorter
FBC	full blood count
FCM	fludarabine, cyclophosphamide, melphalan
FDG-PET	^{18} fluoro–D–2–deoxyglucose positron emission tomography
FDP	fibrin degradation products
Fe	iron
FEIBA	factor eight inhibitor bypassing activity
FEL	familial erythrophagocytic lymphohistiocytosis
FeSO4	ferrous sulphate
FFP	fresh frozen plasma
FFS	failure-free survival
Fgn	fibrinogen
FH	family history
FISH	fluorescence in situ hybridisation
FITC	fluorescein isothiocyanate
FIX	factor IX

fL	femtolitre
FL	follicular lymphoma
FNA	fine needle aspirate
FOB	faecal occult blood
FVIII	factor VIII
FVL	factor V Leiden
g	gram
G&S	group, screen, and save
G6PD	glucose-6-phosphate dehydrogenase
GA	general anaesthetic
GCS	graded compression stockings
G-CSF	granulocyte colony stimulating factor
GIT	gastrointestinal tract
GM-CSF	granulocyte macrophage colony stimulating factor
GP	glycoprotein
GPI	glycosylphosphatidylinositol
GPS	gray platelet syndrome
GT	Glanzmann's thrombasthenia
GvHD	graft versus host disease
GvL	graft versus leukaemia
h	hour
H/LMW	high/low molecular weight
HAART	highly active antiretroviral therapy
HAV	hepatitis A virus
Hb	haemoglobin
HbA	haemoglobin A
HbA_2	haemoglobin A_2
HbF	haemoglobin F (fetal Hb)
HbH	haemoglobin H
HBsAg	hepatitis B surface antigen
HBV	hepatitis B virus
HC	hydroxycarbamide *or* heavy chain
HCD	heavy chain disease
HCG	human chorionic gonadotrophin
HCII	heparin cofactor II
HCL	hairy cell leukaemia
HCO_3	bicarbonate
Hct	haematocrit
HCV	hepatitis C virus
HD	haemodialysis

HDM	high dose melphalan
HDN	haemolytic disease of the newborn
HDT	high dose therapy
HE	hereditary elliptocytosis
HELLP	haemolysis, elevated liver enzymes and low platelets
HES	hypereosinophilic syndrome
HHT	hereditary haemorrhagic telangiectasia
HI	haematological improvement
HIT(T)	heparin-induced thrombocytopenia (with thrombosis)
HIV	human immunodeficiency virus
HL	Hodgkin's lymphoma (Hodgkin's disease)
HLA	human leucocyte antigen
HLH	haemophagocytic lymphohistiocytosis
HMP	hexose monophosphate shunt
HMWK	high molecular weight kininogen
HPA	human platelet antigen
HPF	high power field
HPFH	hereditary persistence of fetal haemoglobin
HPLC	high performance liquid chromatography
HPP	hereditary pyropoikilocytosis
HRT	hormone replacement therapy
HS	hereditary spherocytosis
HTLV-1	human T-lymphotropic virus type 1
HTO	high titre antibodies
HUMARA	human androgen receptor gene assay
HUS	haemolytic uraemic syndrome
IAGT	indirect antiglobulin test
IAHS	infection-associated haemophagocytic syndrome
ICE	ifosfamide, carboplatin, etoposide
ICH	intracranial haemorrhage
ICUS	idiopathic cytopenia of uncertain (undetermined) significance
IDA	iron deficiency anaemia
IF	involved field (radiotherapy)
IFA	intrinsic factor antibody
IFN-α	interferon alpha
Ig	immunoglobulin
IgA	immunoglobulin A
IgD	immunoglobulin D
IgE	immunoglobulin E
IgG	immunoglobulin G

IgM	immunoglobulin M
IL-1	interleukin-1
IM	intramuscular
IMF	idiopathic myelofibrosis
INR	International normalized ratio
inv	chromosomal inversion
IPC	intermittent pneumatic compression devices
IPF	immature platelet fraction
IPI	International Prognostic Index
IPSS	International Prognostic Scoring System
ISM	Indolent systemic mastocytosis
ISS	International Sensitivity Index
IT	intrathecal
ITP	idiopathic thrombocytopenic purpura
ITU	Intensive Therapy Unit
IU	international units
IUGR	intrauterine growth retardation
IUT	intrauterine transfusion
IV	intravenous
IVI	intravenous infusion
IVIg	intravenous immunoglobulin
JCMML	juvenile chronic myelomonocytic leukaemia
JML	juvenile myelomonocytic leukaemia
JVP	jugular venous pressure
KCT	Kaolin clotting time
kg	kilogram
L	litre
LA	lupus anticoagulant
LAP	leucocyte alkaline phosphatase (score)
LC	light chain
LCH	Langerhans cell histiocytosis
LDH	lactate dehydrogenase
LDHL	lymphocyte depleted HL
LFS	leukaemia free survival
LFTs	liver function tests
LGL	large granular lymphocyte
LLN	lower limit of normal
LMWH	low molecular weight heparin
LN	lymph node(s)
LP	lumbar puncture

LPD	lymphoproliferative disorder
LRCHL	lymphocyte rich classical HL
LSCS	lower segment Caesarian section
LTC	large transformed cells
M&P	melphalan and prednisolone
MACOP-B	methotrexate, doxorubicin, cyclophosphamide, vincristine, bleomycin, prednisolone
MAHA	microangiopathic haemolytic anaemia
MALT	mucosa-associated lymphoid tissue
m-BACOD	methotrexate, bleomycin, adriamycin (doxorubicin), cyclophosphamide, vincristine, dexamethasone
mc	micro
MC	mast cell(s)
MCH	mean cell haemoglobin
MCHC	mean corpuscular haemoglobin concentration
MCHL	mixed cellularity HL
MCL	mast cell leukaemia *or* mantle cell lymphoma
MCP	mitoxantrone, chlorambucil, prednisolone
MCR	major cytogenetic response
MCS	mast cell sarcoma
M-CSF	macrophage colony stimulating factor
MCV	mean cell volume
MDS	myelodysplastic syndrome
MetHb	methaemoglobin
MF	myelofibrosis
mg	milligram
MGUS	monoclonal gammopathy of undetermined significance
MHC	major histocompatibility complex
MI	myocardial infarction
min	minute(s)
mL	millilitre
MLC	mixed lymphocyte culture
MM	multiple myeloma
MMC	mitomycin C
MNC	mononuclear cell(s)
MoAb	monoclonal antibody
MP	melphalan and prednisolone
MPCM	maculopapular cutaneous mastocytosis
MPD	myeloproliferative disease
MPO	myeloperoxidase
MPS	mononuclear phagocytic system

MPT	melphalan, prednisolone, and thalidomide
MPV	mean platelet volume
MRD	minimal residual disease
MRI	magnetic resonance imaging
mRNA	messenger ribonucleic acid
MRSA	meticillin-resistant *Staphylococcus aureus*
MSBOS	maximum surgical blood ordering schedule
MSU	midstream urine
MT	mass: thoracic
MTX	methotrexate
MUD	matched unrelated donor (transplant)
MZL	mantle zone lymphoma
Na^+	sodium
NaCl	sodium chloride
NADP	nicotinamide adenine diphosphate
NADPH	nicotinamide adenine diphosphate (reduced)
NAIT	neonatal alloimmune thrombocytopenia
NAP	neutrophil alkaline phosphatase
NBT	nitro blue tetrazolium
NEJM	*New England Journal of Medicine*
NHL	non-Hodgkin's lymphoma
NLPHL	nodular lymphocyte predominant HL
NRBC	nucleated red blood cells
NS	nodular sclerosing
NS	non-secretory (myeloma)
NSAIDs	non-steroidal antiinflammatory drugs
NSE	non-specific esterase
NSHL	nodular sclerosing HL
OAF	OC-activating factor
OB	osteoblast
OC	osteoclast
OCP	oral contraceptive pill
od	*omni die* (once daily)
OPG	osteoprotogerin
OPG	orthopantomogram
OR	overall response
OS	overall survival
OWR	Osler–Weber–Rendu
PA	pernicious anaemia
PAI	plasminogen activator inhibitor

PaO_2	partial pressure of O_2 in arterial blood
PAS	periodic acid–Schiff
PB	peripheral blood
PBSC	peripheral blood stem cell
PC	protein C
PCC	prothrombin complex concentrate
PCH	paroxysmal cold haemoglobinuria
PCL	plasma cell leukaemia
PCP	*Pneumocystis carinii* pneumonia
PCR	polymerase chain reaction
PCV	packed cell volume
PD	peritoneal dialysis
PDGF	platelet-derived growth factor
PDW	platelet distribution width
PE	pulmonary embolism
PEP	post-expoure prophylaxis
PET	pre-eclamptic toxaemia or position emission tomography
PF	platelet factor
PFA	platelet function analysis
PFK	phosphofructokinase
PFS	progression-free survival
PGD2	prostaglandin D2
PGE1	prostaglandin E1
PGK	phosphoglycerate kinase
Ph	Philadelphia chromosome
PIG	phosphatidylinositol glycoproteins
PIVKA	protein induced by vitamin K absence
PK	pyruvate kinase
PLL	prolymphocytic leukaemia
PML	promyelocytic leukaemia
PNET	primitive neuroectodermal tumour
PO	per os (by mouth)
PPH	post-partum haomorrhage
PPI	proton pump inhibitor
PPP	primary proliferative polycythaemia
PRCA	pure red cell aplasia
PRN	as required
ProMACE	prednisolone, doxorubicin, cyclophosphamide, etoposide
PRV	polycythaemia rubra vera
PS	protein S

PSA	pure sideroblastic anaemia *or* prostate-specific antigen
PT	prothrombin time
PTCL	peripheral T-cell lymphomas
PTP	pretest probability *or* post-transfusion purpura
PUVA	phototherapy with psoralen plus UV-A
PV	polycythaemia vera
PVO	pyrexia of unknown origin
qds	*quater die sumendus* (to be taken 4 times a day)
QoL	quality of life
RA	refractory anaemia
RAEB	refractory anaemia with excess blasts
RAEB-t	refractory anaemia with excess blasts in transformation
RAR	retinoic acid receptor
RARS	refractory anaemia with ring sideroblasts
RBC	red blood cell
RCC	red blood cell count
RCM	red cell mass
RCMD	refractory cytopenia with multilineage dysplasia
RDS	respiratory distress syndrome
RDW	red cell distribution width
RE	relative erythrocytosis; reticuloendothelial
REAL	Revised European American Lymphoma
RES	reticuloendothelial system
RFLP	restriction fragment length polymorphism
Rh	Rhesus
rhAPC	recombinant human activated protein C
rhG-CSF	recombinant human granulocyte colony stimulating factor
rHuEPO	recombinant human erythropoietin
RI	remission induction
RIA	radioimmunoassay
RIC	reduced-intensity conditioning
RiCoF	ristocetin cofactor
RIPA	ristocetin-induced platelet agglutination
RS	Reed–Sternberg or ringed sideroblasts
RT	reptilase time
RT-PCR	reverse transcriptase polymerase chain reaction
s	second(s)
SAA	serum amyloid A protein
SAGM	saline adenine glucose mannitol
SaO_2	arterial oxygen saturation

VMP	melphalan, prednisolone, bortezomib
VOD	veno-occlusive disease
VTE	venous thromboembolism
vWD	von Willebrand disease
vWF	von Willebrand factor
vWFAg	von Willebrand factor antigen
WAS	Wiskott–Aldrich syndrome
WBC	white blood cell
WBRT	whole brain radiotherapy
WCC	white cell count
WM	Waldenström macroglobulinaemia
X match	cross-match
XDPs	cross-linked fibrin degradation products

Chapter 1

Clinical approach

History taking in patients with haematological disease

Approach to patient with suspected haematological disease

An accurate history combined with a careful physical examination are fundamental parts of clinical assessment. Although the likely haematological diagnosis may be apparent from tests carried out before the patient has been referred, it is nevertheless essential to assess the clinical background fully—this may influence the eventual plan of management, especially in older patients.

It is important to find out early on in the consultation what the patient may already have been told prior to referral, or what he/she thinks the diagnosis may be. There is often fear and anxiety about diagnoses such as leukaemia, haemophilia, or HIV infection.

Presenting symptoms and their duration

A full medical history needs to be taken to which is added direct questioning on relevant features associated with presenting symptoms:

- *Non-specific symptoms* such as fatigue, fevers, weight loss.
- *Symptoms relating to anaemia* e.g. reduced exercise capacity, recent onset of breathlessness and nature of its onset, or worsening of angina, presence of ankle oedema.
- *Symptoms relating to neutropenia* e.g. recurrent oral ulceration, skin infections, oral sepsis.
- *Evidence of compromised immunity* e.g. recurrent oropharyngeal infection.
- *Details of potential haemostatic problems* e.g. easy bruising, bleeding episodes, rashes.
- *Anatomical symptoms* e.g. abdominal discomfort (splenic enlargement or pressure from enlarged lymph nodes), CNS symptoms (from spinal compression).
- *Past medical history* i.e. detail on past illnesses, information on previous surgical procedures which may suggest previous haematological problems (e.g. may suggest an underlying bleeding diathesis) or be associated with haematological or other sequelae e.g. splenectomy.
- *Drug history*: ask about prescribed and non-prescribed medications.
- *Allergies*: since some haematological disorders may relate to chemicals or other environmental hazards specific questions should be asked about occupational factors and hobbies.
- *Transfusion history*: ask about whether the patient has been a blood donor and how much he/she has donated. May occasionally be a factor in iron (Fe) deficiency anaemia. History of previous transfusion(s) and their timing is also critical in some cases e.g. post-transfusion purpura.
- *Tobacco and alcohol consumption* is essential; both may produce significant haematological morbidity.
- *Travel*: clearly important in the case of suspected malaria but also relevant in considering other causes of haematological abnormality, including HIV infection.

- *Family history* is also important, especially in the context of inherited haematological disorders.

A complete history for a patient with a haematological disorder should provide all the relevant medical information to aid diagnosis and clinical assessment, as well as helping the haematologist to have a working assessment of the patient's social situation. A well taken history also provides a basis for good communication which will often prove very important once it comes to discussion of the diagnosis.

Physical examination

This forms part of the clinical assessment of the haematology patient. Pay specific attention to:

General examination—e.g. evidence of weight loss, pyrexia, pallor (the latter is not a reliable clinical measure of anaemia), jaundice, cyanosis or abnormal pigmentation or skin rashes.

The mouth—ulceration, purpura, gum bleeding, or infiltration, and the state of the patient's teeth. Hands and nails may show features associated with haematological abnormalities e.g. koilonychia in chronic Fe deficiency (rarely seen today).

Record—weight, height, T°, pulse, and blood pressure; height and weight give important baseline data against which sequential measurements can subsequently be compared. In myelofibrosis, for example, evidence of significant weight loss in the absence of symptoms may be an indication of clinical progression.

Examination—of chest and abdomen should focus on detecting the presence of lymphadenopathy, hepatic and/or splenic enlargement. Node sizes and the extent of organ enlargement should be carefully recorded.

Lymph node enlargement—often recorded in centimetres e.g. 3cm × 3cm × 4cm; sometimes more helpful to compare the degree of enlargement with familiar objects e.g. pea. Record extent of liver or spleen enlargement as maximum distance palpable from the lower costal margin.

Erythematous margins of infected skin lesions—mark these to monitor treatment effects.

Bones and joints—recording of joint swelling and ranges of movement are standard aspects of haemophilia care. In myeloma, areas of bony tenderness and deformity are commonly present.

Optic fundi—examination is a key clinical assessment in the haematology patient. May yield the only objective evidence of hyperviscosity in paraproteinaemias (📖 Hyperviscosity, p.640) or hyperleucocytosis (📖 p.655) such as in e.g. CML. Regular examination for haemorrhages should form part of routine observations in the severely myelosuppressed patient; rarely changes of opportunistic infection such as candidiasis can be seen in the optic fundi.

Neurological examination—fluctuations of conscious level and confusion are clinical presentations of hyperviscosity. Isolated nerve palsies in a patient with acute leukaemia are highly suspicious of neurological involvement or disease relapse. Peripheral neuropathy and long tract signs are well recognized complications of B_{12} deficiency.

Splenomegaly

Many causes. Clinical approach depends on whether splenic enlargement is present as an isolated finding or with other clinical abnormalities e.g. jaundice or lymphadenopathy. Mild-to-moderate splenomegaly has a much greater number of causes than massive splenomegaly.

Table 1.1 Causes of splenomegaly

Infection	Viral	EBV, CMV, hepatitis
	Bacterial	SBE, miliary tuberculosis, *Salmonella*, *Brucella*
	Protozoal	Malaria, toxoplasmosis, leishmaniasis
Haemolytic	Congenital	Hereditary spherocytosis, hereditary elliptocytosis, sickle cell disease (infants), thalassaemia, pyruvate kinase deficiency, G6PD deficiency
	Acquired	AIHA (idiopathic or 2°)
Myeloproliferative and leukaemic		Myelofibrosis, CML, polycythaemia rubra vera, essential thrombocythaemia, acute leukaemias
Lymphoproliferative		CLL, hairy cell leukaemia, Waldenström's, SLVL, other NHL, Hodgkin lymphoma, ALL and lymphoblastic NHL
Autoimmune disorders and storage disorders		Rheumatoid arthritis, SLE, hepatic cirrhosis, Gaucher's disease, histiocytosis X, Niemann–Pick disease
Miscellaneous		Metastatic cancer, cysts, amyloid, portal hypertension, portal vein thrombosis, tropical splenomegaly

Clinical approach essentially involves a working knowledge of the possible causes of splenic enlargement and determining the more likely causes in the given clinical circumstances by appropriate further investigation. There are fewer causes of massive splenic enlargement, i.e. the spleen tip palpable below the level of the umbilicus.

Massive splenomegaly

- Myelofibrosis.
- CML.
- Lymphoproliferative disease—CLL and variants including SLVL, HCL, and marginal zone lymphoma.
- Tropical splenomegaly.
- Leishmaniasis.
- Gaucher's disease.
- Thalassaemia major.

Lymphadenopathy

Occurs in a range of infective or neoplastic conditions; less frequently enlargement occurs in active collagen disorders. May be isolated, affecting a single node, localized, involving several nodes in an anatomical lymph node grouping, or generalized, where nodes are enlarged at different sites. As well as enlargement in the easily palpable areas (cervical, axillary, and iliac) node enlargement may be hilar or retroperitoneal and identifiable only by imaging. Isolated/localized lymphadenopathy usually results from local infection or neoplasm. Generalized lymphadenopathy may result from systemic causes, especially when symmetrical, as well as infection or neoplasm. Rarely drug-associated (e.g. phenytoin).

Table 1.2 Causes of lymphadenopathy

Infective	Bacterial	Tonsillitis, cellulitis, tuberculous infections, and 1° syphilis usually produce isolated or localized node enlargement
	Viral	EBV, CMV, rubella, HIV, HBV, HCV
	Other	Toxoplasma, histoplasmosis, chlamydia, cat-scratch
Neoplastic		Hodgkin lymphoma (typically isolated or localized lymphadenopathy), NHL isolated, generalized or localized, CLL, metastatic carcinoma, acute leukaemia (ALL especially, but occasionally AML)
Collagen and other systemic disorders		E.g. rheumatoid arthritis, SLE, sarcoidosis

History and examination—points to elicit

- Age.
- Onset of symptoms, whether progressing or not.
- Systemic symptoms, weight loss (>10% body weight loss in <6 months).
- Night sweats.
- Risk factors for HIV infection.
- Local or systemic evidence of infection.
- Evidence of systemic disorder such as rheumatoid arthritis.
- Evidence of malignancy; if splenic enlargement present then lymphoreticular neoplasm is more likely.
- Specific disease-related features e.g. pruritus and alcohol-induced lymph node pain associated with Hodgkin's disease.
- Determine the duration of enlargement ± associated symptoms, whether nodes are continuing to enlarge, and whether tender or not. Distribution of node enlargement should be recorded as well as size of node.

Investigations

- FBC and peripheral blood film examination.
- ESR or plasma viscosity.
- Screening test for infectious mononucleosis and serological testing for other viruses.

- Imaging—e.g. chest radiography; chest abdominal ± pelvic CT scanning may also be helpful to define hilar, retroperitoneal, and para-aortic nodes.
- Microbiology—e.g. blood cultures, indirect testing for TB, and culture of biopsied or aspirated lymph node material.
- Lymph node biopsy for definitive diagnosis especially if a neoplastic cause suspected. Aspiration of enlarged lymph nodes is generally unsatisfactory in providing effective diagnostic material. Avoid biopsy of groin nodes since these often show only non-specific features.
- BM examination should be reserved for staging in confirmed lymphoma or leukaemia cases—it is not commonly a useful 1° investigation of lymphadenopathy.

Unexplained anaemia

Evaluate with the combined information from clinical history, physical examination, and results of investigations.

History—focus on

- Duration of symptoms of anaemia—short duration of dyspnoea and fatigue etc. suggests recent bleeding or haemolysis. Gradual anaemia of longer duration often associated with adaptation and fewer symptoms.
- Specific questioning on blood loss—include system-related questions e.g. GIT and gynaecological sources, ask about blood donation.
- Family history—e.g. in relation to hereditary problems such as HS or ethnic Hb disorders such as thalassaemia or HbSS.
- Past history—e.g. association of gastrectomy with later occurrence of Fe and/or B_{12} deficiency.
- Drug history—including prescribed and non-prescribed medication.
- Dietary factors—mainly relates to folate and Fe deficiency, rarely B_{12} in vegans. Fe deficiency always occurs because Fe losses exceed intake (*it is extremely rare in developed countries for diet to be the sole cause of Fe deficiency*).

Examination

- May identify indirectly helpful signs e.g. koilonychia in chronic Fe deficiency (rare), jaundice in haemolytic disorders.
- Lymphadenopathy suggesting lymphoreticular disease or viral infection.
- Hepatosplenomegaly in lymphoproliferative or myeloproliferative disorders.

Full blood count

📖 Laboratory investigation of anaemia is discussed fully in Chapter 2.
Anaemia in adult ♂ if Hb <13.0g/dL and in adult ♀ if Hb <11.5g/dL.

Table 1.3 MCV useful for initial anaemia evaluation

↓ MCV (<76fL)	Fe deficiency
	α & β thalassaemia, HbE, HbC
	Anaemia of chronic disorders
Normal MCV (78–98fL)	Recent bleeding
	Anaemia of chronic disorders
	Most non-haematinic deficiency causes
	Combined Fe + B_{12}/folate deficiency
↑ MCV (>100fL)	Folate or B_{12} deficiency
	Haemolytic anaemia
	Liver disease
	Marrow dysplasia and failure syndromes including aplastic anaemia
	2° to antimetabolite drug therapy e.g. hydroxyurea (now called hydroxcarbamide)

The need for film examination, reticulocyte counting, and additional tests on the FBC sample such as checking for Heinz bodies is based on the initial clinical and FBC findings. The findings from the initial FBC examination have a major influence in determining the nature and urgency of further clinical investigation.

Serum ferritin level will identify Fe deficiency and focus on the need for detailed investigation for blood loss which, for adult males and postmenopausal females, will frequently require large bowel examination with colonoscopy or barium enema, and gastroscopy. BM examination may occasionally be required.

Anaemia is not a diagnosis—it is an abnormal clinical finding requiring an explanation for its cause. There is no place for empirical use of Fe therapy for management and treatment of 'anaemia' in modern medical practice.

Patient with elevated haemoglobin

Finding a raised Hb concentration requires a systematic clinical approach for differential diagnosis and further investigation. Initially it is essential to check whether the result ties in with the known clinical findings—if unexpected the FBC should be re-checked to exclude a mix-up over samples or a sampling artefact. Dehydration and diuretic therapy may ↑ the Hct and these should be excluded in the initial phase of assessment.

Having determined that the ↑ Hb concentration is genuine the issue is whether there is a genuine ↑ in red cell mass or not, and the explanation for the elevated Hb.

Anoxia is a major stimulus to RBC production and will result in an increase in erythropoietin with consequent erythrocytosis.

History and examination should assess:

- Recent travel and residence at high altitude (>3000m).
- COAD, other hypoxic respiratory conditions, cyanotic congenital heart disease, other cardiac problems causing hypoxia.
- Smoking—heavy cigarette smoking causes ↑ carboxyHb levels leading to ↑ RBC mass to compensate for loss of O_2 carrying capacity.
- Ventilatory impairment 2° to gross obesity, alveolar hypoventilation (Pickwickian syndrome).
- Possibility of high-affinity Hb abnormalities arises if there is a FH of polycythaemia, otherwise requires assessment through Hb analysis.
- If obvious secondary causes excluded possibilities include:
  - ***Spurious polycythaemia***—pseudopolycythaemia or Gaisbock's syndrome, associated features can include cigarette smoking, obesity, hypertension, and excess alcohol consumption; sometimes described as 'stress polycythaemia'.
  - ***Primary proliferative polycythaemia (polycythaemia rubra vera)***—plethoric facies, history of pruritus after bathing or on change of environmental temperature, and presence of splenomegaly are helpful clinical findings to suggest this diagnosis.
  - ***Inappropriate erythropoietin excess***—occurs in a variety of benign and malignant renal disorders. Rare complication of some tumours including hepatoma, uterine fibroids, and cerebellar haemangioblastoma.

Part of clinical assessment must also include an evaluation of thrombotic risk; previous thrombosis or a family history of such problems ↑ the urgency of investigation and appropriate treatment (📖 see also Chapter 7, pp.260–274).

1. McMullin, M.F., *et al.* (2005) Guidelines for the diagnosis, investigation and management of polycythaemia/erythrocytosis. *Br J Haematol*, **130**, 174–95.

Anaemia and hypoxia are detected by the renal sensors. This leads to ↑ production of Epo which drives the marrow (through BFU-E and CFU-E) to produce RBCs. Other factors may also drive red cell production, including androgens and growth hormone as shown in Fig. 1.1.

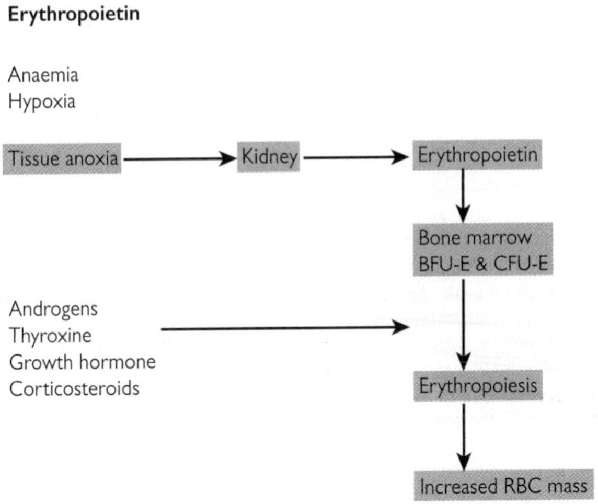

Fig. 1.1

Elevated WBC

Leucocytosis is defined as elevation of the WCC >2 SD above the mean. The detection of leucocytosis should prompt immediate scrutiny of the automated WBC differential (generally accurate except in leukaemia) and the other FBC parameters. Blood film should be examined and a manual differential count performed. Important to evaluate leucocytosis in terms of the age-related absolute normal ranges for neutrophils, lymphocytes, monocytes, eosinophils, and basophils (📖 Normal ranges (adult), p.808; Paediatric normal ranges, p.810) and the presence of abnormal cells: immature granulocytes, blasts, nucleated red cells, and 'atypical cells'.

Leukaemoid reaction—leucocytosis >50 × 10^9/L defines a neutrophilia with marked 'left shift' (band forms, metamyelocytes, myelocytes, and occasionally promyelocytes and myeloblasts in the blood film). Differential diagnosis is CGL and in children, juvenile CML. Primitive granulocyte precursors are also frequently seen in the blood film of the infected or stressed neonate, and any seriously ill patient e.g. on ITU.

Leucoerythroblastic blood film—contains myelocytes, other primitive granulocytes, nucleated red cells, and often tear drop red cells, is due to BM invasion by tumour, fibrosis, or granuloma formation and is an indication for a BM biopsy. Other causes include anorexia and haemolysis.

Leucocytosis due to blasts—suggests diagnosis of acute leukaemia and is an indication for cell typing studies and BM examination.

FBC, blood film, white cell differential count, and the clinical context in which the leucocytosis is detected will usually indicate whether this is due to a 1° haematological abnormality or reflects a 2° response.

► It is clearly important to seek a history of symptoms of infection and examine the patient for signs of infection or an underlying haematological disorder.

Neutrophilia

- 2° to acute infection is most common cause of leucocytosis.
- Usually modest (uncommonly >30 × 10^9/L), associated with a left shift and occasionally toxic granulation or vacuolation of neutrophils.
- Chronic inflammation causes less marked neutrophilia often associated with monocytosis.
- Moderate neutrophilia may occur following steroid therapy, heatstroke, and in patients with solid tumours.
- Mild neutrophilia may be induced by stress (e.g. immediate postoperative period) and exercise.
- May be seen following a myocardial infarction or major seizure.
- Frequently found in states of chronic BM stimulation (e.g. chronic haemolysis, ITP) and asplenia.
- Primary haematological causes of neutrophilia are less common. CML is often the cause of extremely high leucocyte counts (>200 × 10^9/L), predominantly neutrophils with marked left shift, basophilia and occasional myeloblasts. A low LAP score (seldom used now) and the presence of the Ph chromosome on karyotype analysis are usually helpful to differentiate CGL from a leukaemoid reaction.

- Less common are juvenile CML, transient leukaemoid reaction in Down syndrome, hereditary neutrophilia, and chronic idiopathic neutrophilia.

BM examination is rarely necessary in the investigation of a patient with isolated neutrophilia. Investigation of a leukaemoid reaction, leucoerythroblastic blood film, and possible CGL or juvenile CML are firm indications for a BM aspirate and trephine biopsy. BM culture, including culture for atypical mycobacteria and fungi, may be useful in patients with persistent pyrexia or leucocytosis.

Lymphocytosis

- Lymphocytosis $>4.0 \times 10^9/L$.
- Normal infants and young children <5 years have a higher proportion and concentration of lymphocytes than adults.
- Rare in acute bacterial infection except in pertussis (may be $>50 \times 10^9/L$).
- Acute infectious lymphocytosis also seen in children, usually associated with transient lymphocytosis and a mild constitutional reaction.
- Characteristic of infectious mononucleosis but these lymphocytes are often large and atypical and the diagnosis may be confirmed with a heterophil agglutination test (Monospot®; Paul–Bunnell).
- Similar atypical cells may be seen in patients with CMV and hepatitis A infection.
- Chronic infection with brucellosis, tuberculosis, 2° syphilis, and congenital syphilis may cause lymphocytosis.
- Lymphocytosis is characteristic of CLL, ALL, and occasionally NHL.

Where a 1° haematological cause is suspected, immunophenotypic analysis of the peripheral blood lymphocytes will often confirm or exclude a neoplastic diagnosis. BM examination is indicated if neoplasia is strongly suspected and in any patient with concomitant neutropenia, anaemia, or thrombocytopenia, or if there are constitutional symptoms e.g. sweats, weight loss.

Reduced WBC

It is uncommon for absolute leucopenia (WBC <4.0 × 10^9/L) to be due to isolated deficiency of any cell other than the neutrophil though in marked leucopenia several cell lines are often affected.

► Neutropenia

Defined as a neutrophil count <2.0 × 10^9/L. The risk of infective complications is closely related to the absolute neutrophil count. More severe when neutropenia is due to impaired production from chemotherapy or marrow failure rather than to peripheral destruction or maturation arrest where there is often a cellular marrow with early neutrophil precursors and normal monocyte counts. Type of infection determined by the degree and duration of neutropenia. Ongoing chemotherapy further ↑ the risk of serious bacterial and fungal opportunistic infection and the presence of an indwelling IV catheter ↑ the incidence of infection with coagulase-negative staphylococci and other skin commensals. Patients with chronic immune neutropenia may develop recurrent stomatitis, gingivitis, oral ulceration, sinusitis, and peri-anal infection.

Table 1.4 Clinical significance of neutropenia

Neutrophil count	Risk of infection
1.0–1.5 x 10^9/L	No significant ↑ risk of infection
0.5–1.0 x 10^9/L	Some ↑ in risk; some fevers can be treated as an outpatient
<0.5 x 10^9/L	Major ↑ in risk; treat all fevers with broad spectrum IV antibiotics as an inpatient

History and physical examination provide a guide to the subsequent management of a patient with neutropenia. Simple observation is appropriate initially for an asymptomatic patient with isolated mild neutropenia who has an unremarkable history and examination. If there has been a recent viral illness or the patient can discontinue a drug which may be the cause, follow-up over a few weeks may see resolution of the abnormality.

Investigations

BM examination—if there is concomitant anaemia or thrombocytopenia, history of significant infection, or if lymphadenopathy or organomegaly on examination. Usually unhelpful in patients with an isolated neutropenia >0.5 × 10^9/L. However, if neutropenia persists, perform BM aspiration, biopsy and cytogenetics, and check serology for collagen diseases, anti-neutrophil antibodies, HIV, and immunoglobulins.

Differential diagnoses

Isolated neutropenia may be the presenting feature of myelodysplasia, aplastic anaemia, Fanconi anaemia, or acute leukaemia but these conditions will usually be associated with other haematological abnormalities.

Post-infectious (most usually post-viral) neutropenia may last several weeks and may be followed by prolonged immune neutropenia.

Severe sepsis—particularly at the extremes of life.

Drugs—cytotoxic agents and many others, e.g. phenothiazines, many antibiotics, NSAIDs, anti-thyroid agents, and psychotropic drugs. Neutrophil recovery starts ~a few days of stopping offending drug.

Autoimmune neutropenia due to anti-neutrophil antibodies may occur in isolation or in association with haemolytic anaemia, ITP, or SLE.

Felty's syndrome neutropenia is accompanied by seropositive rheumatoid arthritis and splenomegaly.

Chronic benign neutropenia of infancy and childhood is associated with fever and infection; resolves by age 4 years, probably has immune basis.

Benign familial or racial neutropenia is a feature of rare families and of certain racial groups, notably negroes, is associated with mild neutropenia but no propensity to infection.

Chronic idiopathic neutropenia is a diagnosis of exclusion, associated with severe neutropenia but often a benign course.

Cyclical neutropenia is a condition usually of childhood onset and dominant inheritance characterized by severe neutropenia, fever, stomatitis, and other infections occurring at 4-week intervals.

Hereditary causes (less common) include Kostmann syndrome (📖 p.593), Shwachman–Diamond–Oski syndrome (📖 p.593), Chediak–Higashi syndrome (📖 p.599), reticular dysgenesis, and dyskeratosis congenita.

Management

Febrile episodes should be managed according to the severity of the neutropenia (Table 1.4) and the underlying cause (BM failure is associated with more life-threatening infections). Broad spectrum IV antibiotics may be required and empirical systemic antifungal therapy may be required in those who fail to respond to antibiotics. Prophylactic antibiotic and antifungal therapy may be helpful in some patients with chronic neutropenia as may G-CSF. Antiseptic mouthwash is of value and regular dental care is important.

► Lymphopenia

Lymphopenia ($<1.5 \times 10^9$/L) may be seen in acute infections, cardiac failure, pancreatitis, tuberculosis, uraemia, lymphoma, carcinoma, SLE and other collagen diseases and after corticosteroid therapy, radiation, chemotherapy, and anti-lymphocyte globulin therapy. Most common cause of chronic severe lymphopenia in recent years is HIV infection (📖 HIV infection and AIDS, p.548).

Chronic severe lymphopenia ($<0.5 \times 10^9$/L) is associated both with opportunistic infections notably *Candida species*, *Pneumocystis jerovicii*, CMV, Herpes zoster, *Mycoplasma* spp., *Cryptosporidium*, and toxoplasmosis and with an ↑ incidence of neoplasia particularly NHL, Kaposi's sarcoma and skin and gastric carcinoma.

1. Palmblad, J.E., *et al.* (2002) Idiopathic, immune, infectious, and idiosyncratic neutropenias. *Semin Hematol*, **39**, 113–20.

Elevated platelet count

Thrombocytosis is defined as a platelet count >400 × 10^9/L. May be due to a *primary* myeloproliferative neoplasm (MPN) or a *secondary* reactive feature. If the platelet count is markedly elevated a patient with a MPN has a risk of haemorrhage (due to the production of dysfunctional platelets), or thrombosis, or both. The patient's history may reveal features of the condition to which the elevated platelet count is secondary. Clinical examination may provide similar clues or reveal splenomegaly which suggests a MPN. FBC may provide useful information: marked leucocytosis with left shift (in the absence of a history of infection), basophilia, or an elevated haematocrit and red cell count are highly suggestive of a MPN when associated with thrombocytosis. Unusual for reactive thrombocytosis to cause a platelet count >1000 × 10^9/L. *Note*: platelet counts below this may occur in MPNs.

Differential diagnosis

Table 1.5 Differetial Diagnosis of Thrombocytosis

Myeloproliferative neoplasms	Disorders associated with ↑ platelets
1° thrombocythaemia	Haemorrhage
Polycythaemia vera	Trauma
Chronic granulocytic leukaemia	Surgery
Idiopathic myelofibrosis	Fe deficiency anaemia
	Malignancy (Ca lung, Ca breast, Hodgkin's disease)
	Acute and chronic infection
	Inflammatory disease e.g. rheumatoid arthritis, UC
	Post-splenectomy

Investigation

- BM aspirate may show megakaryocyte abnormalities in MPN.
- BM trephine biopsy may show marked myeloid hyperplasia, clusters of abnormal megakaryocytes, and ↑ reticulin or fibrosis in MPN.

Management

- In reactive thrombocytosis treat the underlying condition.
- Unusual to require treatment to ↓ the platelet count in a patient with reactive thrombocytosis.
- Consider low dose aspirin (or if contraindicated, dipyridamole).
- Reactive thrombocytosis is generally transient.
- If secondary to Fe deficiency—review FBC after Fe therapy: the platelet count normalizes if thrombocytosis was due to Fe deficiency.
- Fe deficiency may have masked PRV—this will be revealed by Fe therapy.
- If impossible to define the cause of thrombocytosis then a watch-and-wait policy should be followed in an asymptomatic patient.
- If MPN is suspected—📖 see Essential thrombocythaemia, p.276.

Reduced platelet count

Thrombocytopenia is defined as a platelet count <150 × 10^9/L. Although there is no precise platelet count at which a patient will or will not bleed, most patients with a count >30 × 10^9/L are asymptomatic. The risk of spontaneous haemorrhage ↑ significantly <10 × 10^9/L. Purpura is the most common presenting symptom usually found on the lower limbs and areas subject to pressure. May be followed by bleeding gums, epistaxis, or more serious life-threatening haemorrhage. A patient with newly diagnosed severe thrombocytopenia with or without purpura is a medical emergency and may require admission for further investigation and treatment.

Confirm low platelet count by examination of the blood sample for clots (artefactual low platelets) and the blood film for platelet aggregates (causing pseudothrombocytopenia). History and examination will determine the clinical severity of the thrombocytopenia and should also reveal the duration of symptoms, presence of any prodromal illness, causative medication, or underlying disease.

Determine whether the cause of thrombocytopenia is failure of production or ↑ consumption. FBC may be helpful as the MPV is often elevated in the latter group (large platelets may also be seen on the blood film). May also reveal additional haematological abnormalities (normocytic anaemia or neutropenia) suggestive of a BM disorder. A coagulation screen should also be performed. Examination of the BM is the definitive investigation in all patients with moderate or severe thrombocytopenia—may reveal normal megakaryocytes or compensatory hyperplasia in peripheral destruction syndromes or marrow hypoplasia or infiltration. Tests for platelet antibodies are unreliable but an autoimmune screen may be helpful to exclude lupus.

Management

Treat underlying condition. Most patients with a platelet count >30 × 10^9/L require no specific therapy. Avoid aspirin. In the event of life-threatening haemorrhage platelet transfusion should be administered to thrombocytopenic patients *with the exception of those with HITT and TTP.*

1. Spencer, F.A. (2000). Heparin-induced thrombocytopenia: patient profiles and clinical manifestations. *J Thromb Thrombolysis*, **10**, Suppl **1**, 21–5.

Table 1.6 Differential diagnosis of thrombocytopenia

Failure of production	**Increased consumption**
Drugs and chemicals (📖 p.484)	ITP (📖 p.486)
Viral infection	Drugs (📖 p.484)
Radiation	DIC (📖 p.488)
Aplastic anaemia (📖 p.98)	Infection
Leukaemia	Massive haemorrhage and transfusion (📖 p.502)
Marrow infiltration (📖 pp.484)	SLE
Megaloblastic anaemia (📖 pp.46)	CLL and lymphoma (📖 pp.150, 484)
HIV (📖 p.548)	Heparin (📖 p.508)
	TTP (📖 p.534)
	Hypersplenism (📖 p.486)
	Post-transfusion purpura (📖 p.486)
	HIV (📖 p.548)

Easy bruising

Evaluation of a patient who complains of easy bruising involves a detailed history, physical examination with particular attention to any current haemorrhagic lesions, and the performance of basic haemostatic investigations. More common in ♀ and often difficult to evaluate. Also a frequent complaint in the elderly.

History

Careful attention to the history is essential to the diagnosis of all the haemorrhagic disorders and one must attempt to define the nature of the bruising in a patient with this complaint. *Note*: many normal healthy people believe that they have excessive bleeding or bruising. Conversely some people with haemorrhagic disorders and abnormal bleeding histories will not volunteer the information unless asked directly or indeed may consider their bleeding to be normal. Remember that excessive bruising may be a manifestation of a blood vessel disorder rather than a coagulopathy or platelet disorder.

Ask about

Presenting complaint—how long and how frequently has easy bruising occurred? Is it ecchymoses or purpura? How extensive are bruises? Are they located in areas subject to trauma (e.g. limbs) or pressure (e.g. waist band)? Do petechiae occur? Are bruises painful? How long to resolution? How many currently?

Associated symptoms

Has there been gum bleeding? Has the patient experienced prolonged bleeding after skin trauma, dental extraction, childbirth, or surgery? Has there been any other form of haemorrhage e.g. epistaxis, menorrhagia, joint or soft tissue haematoma, haematemesis, melaena, haemoptysis, or haematuria? Is there a history of poor wound healing?

Family history

Has any other family member a history of excessive bleeding or bruising?

Drug history

Is the patient on any medication (remember self-medication of vitamins and food supplements), most notably aspirin, anticoagulant therapy?

Systematic enquiry

Is there evidence of a disorder associated with a haemorrhagic tendency e.g. hepatic or renal failure, malabsorption, leukaemia, connective tissue disorder, or amyloid?

Physical examination

Haemorrhagic skin lesions are likely to be present in a patient with a serious problem and their distribution will often indicate the extent to which they are likely to be related to trauma. Senile purpura is almost invariably on the hands and forearms. True purpura is easily differentiated from erythema and telangiectasis by pressure. Petechiae are highly suggestive of a platelet or vascular disorder whilst palpable purpura is associated with anaphylactoid purpura. In addition there may be other physical findings which may indicate an underlying disorder e.g. splenomegaly or lymphadenopathy in leukaemia, signs of hepatic failure, telangiectasia in Osler–Rendu–Weber syndrome or hyperextensible joints and paper-thin scars in Ehlers–Danlos syndrome.

Basic haemostatic investigations

All patients should be investigated except those in whom history and examination has given strong grounds for believing that they are normal and in whom there is a history of a normal response to a haemostatic challenge e.g. surgery or dental extraction.

Screening tests

- FBC and blood film.
- APTT.
- PT.
- Thrombin clotting time and/or fibrinogen.
- Bleeding time (a largely obsolete investigation, of dubious value).

If these investigations are normal there is no indication for further haemostatic investigations unless the history provides strong grounds for believing that there is indeed a haemostatic disorder. The appropriate further investigation of the haemostatic mechanism is discussed in Chapter 10 (📖 Haemostasis and thrombosis, p.448).

Differential diagnoses

- Common diagnoses:
  - Simple easy bruising (purpura simplex).
  - Trauma (including non-accidental injury in children).
  - Senile purpura.
- Haemostatic defects:
  - Thrombocytopenia.
  - Platelet function defects.
  - Coagulation abnormalities (rarely).
- Vascular defects:
  - Corticosteroid excess.
  - Collagen diseases.
  - Uraemia.
  - Dysproteinaemias.
  - Anaphylactoid purpura.
  - Ehlers–Danlos syndrome.
  - Scurvy.
  - Vasculitis.

Recurrent thromboembolism

A hypercoagulable state should be suspected in all patients with recurrent thromboembolic disease, family history of thrombosis, thrombosis at a young age or at an unusual site (in addition to recurrent thromboembolism) associated with inherited thrombophilia. Further important aspects of the history are precipitating factors at the time of thrombosis and lifestyle considerations e.g. smoking, exercise, and obesity. Clinical examination may reveal signs suggestive of an associated underlying condition.

Table 1.7 Hypercoagulable states

Inherited	Activated protein C resistance (factor V Leiden)
	Protein C deficiency
	Protein S deficiency
	Prothrombin gene mutation
	Hyperhomocysteinaemia
	Sickle cell disease
	Antithrombin deficiency and some very rare abnormalities of fibrinogen, plasminogen, and plasminogen activator
Acquired	Immobilization
	Oral contraceptive or oestrogen therapy
	Postpartum
	Old age
	Postoperative
	Malignancy (notably Ca pancreas)
	Nephrotic syndrome
	Myeloproliferative disorders
	Hyperhomocysteinaemia
	Antiphospholipid syndrome (lupus anticoagulant)
	Hyperviscosity
	Paroxysmal nocturnal haemoglobinuria
	Thrombotic thrombocytopenic purpura
	Heparin-induced thrombocytopenia

Laboratory investigation

📖 see Thrombophilia, p.530.

1. Kyrle, P.A., *et al.* (2004.) The risk of recurrent venous thromboembolism in men and women. *N Engl J Med*, **350**, 2558–63.

Pathological fracture

Fracture in a bone compromised by the presence of a pathological process resulting in fracture following relatively minor trauma. Most commonly due to local neoplastic involvement or osteoporosis.

Haematological causes

- Local bony damage.
- Myelomatous deposits.
- Lymphoma.
- Metastatic carcinoma (± marrow infiltration); breast, prostate, and lung are commoner 1° sites.
- Gaucher's disease.
- Sickle cell anaemia.
- Homozygous thalassaemia.
- Osteoporosis from prolonged corticosteroid therapy e.g. for autoimmune disease.

Clinically

Presentation as local pain, discomfort, and restriction of mobility.

Diagnosis

Confirmed by x-ray or other imaging.

Management

- Awareness of risk/possibility and early diagnosis.
- Analgesia.
- Orthopaedic—immobilization and support as appropriate for nature and site of injury, surgical intervention including pinning or other fixation.
- Radiotherapy—local management of fracture 2° to local malignancy.
- Mobilization—physiotherapy.
- Treatment of underlying condition predisposing to fracture.

Raised ESR

The ESR remains an established, empirical test clinically useful as a method for identifying and monitoring the acute phase response. It is influenced by changes in fibrinogen, α-macroglobulins, and immunoglobulins which enhance red cell aggregation *in vitro*.

Plasma viscosity is also an effective measure of acute phase reactants and can be used as an alternative to the ESR in clinical practice; ↑ in ESR and plasma viscosity generally parallel each other.

Normal ranges

- 0–10mm/h for ♂ 18–65 years.
- 1–20mm/h for ♀ 18–65 years.
- Upper limits of normal ↑ by 5–10mm/h for patients >65 years.
- Other factors e.g. Hct influences the ESR.
- Should be regarded as semiquantitative.
- Marked elevations are clinically significant.
- Modest elevations can be more problematic to interpret.

The main advantages to the ESR are its low cost and technical simplicity allied to the absence of a more accurate, inexpensive, and technically simple alternative.

Table 1.8 Causes of raised ESR

Pregnancy	↑ in pregnancy; maximal in 3rd trimester
Infections	Acute and chronic infections, including TB *Note:* ↑ ESR also occurs in HIV infection
Collagen disorders	Rheumatoid, SLE, polymyalgia rheumatica, vasculitides etc. (including temporal arteritis); ESR useful as non-specific monitor of disease activity
Other inflammatory processes	Inflammatory bowel disease, sarcoidosis, post-MI
Neoplastic conditions	Carcinomatosis, NHL, Hodgkin lymphoma and paraproteinaemias (benign and malignant)

Investigations

Given the wide range of situations in which a raised ESR can arise, further investigation depends on a carefully conducted history and examination. In the absence of likely causes from these, simple initial laboratory and radiology assessments to include urinalysis, FBC and blood film examination, urea, electrolytes, plasma protein electrophoresis, an autoimmune profile, and CXR should represent a practical and pragmatic primary diagnostic screen.

📖 See Haematological investigations, p.747.

1. Gabay, C., *et al.* (1999). Acute-phase proteins and other systemic responses to inflammation. *N Engl J Med*, **340**, 448–54.

Serum or urine paraprotein

Differential diagnosis

Common

- Monoclonal gammopathy of undetermined significance (MGUS).
- Smouldering myeloma.
- Multiple myeloma.
- Solitary plasmacytoma.
- Lymphoproliferative disorders e.g. CLL, NHL, Waldenström's.

Less common

- Autoimmune disorders e.g. rheumatoid arthritis, SLE.
- Polymyalgia rheumatica.

Rare

- AL amyloid (1° amyloid).
- Plasma cell leukaemia.
- Heavy chain disease.

Discriminating clinical features

MGUS—no symptoms or signs of end-organ damage, normal FBC and biochemical profile, paraprotein level <30g/L and *stable*, immuneparesis (rarely present), BM plasma cells <10%, no lytic lesions.
Smouldering myeloma—as for MGUS but higher stable paraprotein level >30g/L or BM plasma cells >10% without end-organ damage.

Plasmacytoma—localized bone pain, low paraprotein level, isolated bony lesion.

Myeloma—symptoms and signs of anaemia or hyperviscosity (📖 see Hyperviscosity, p.640); bone pain or tenderness, raised Ca^{2+}, creatinine, urate; high β-2 micro-globulin and low albumin; immuneparesis; *paraprotein >30g/L of IgG or >20g/L of IgA or heavy Bence Jones proteinuria; BM >10% plasma cells; lytic bone lesions on x-ray*. Minimum diagnostic criteria are at least 2 of italicized items.

Plasma cell leukaemia—as myeloma but fulminant history. Plasma cells seen on blood film.

Heavy chain disease—rare, characterized by a single heavy chain only in serum or urine electrophoresis. Presence of any light chain excludes.

Amyloid—myriad clinical features. Diagnosis on biopsy of affected site or, if inaccessible, by BM or rectal biopsy—characteristic fibrils stain with Congo Red and show green birefringence in polarized light.

CLL and NHL—systemic symptoms e.g. fever, night sweats, weight loss. Lymphadenopathy or hepatosplenomegaly likely. Confirm on BM or node biopsy.

Waldenström's—as for CLL but with symptoms or signs of hyperviscosity (📖 Waldenström's macroglobulinaemia, p366).

Autoimmune disorders—suggested by joint pain, skin rashes, multisystem disease. Confirm on autoimmune profile including rheumatoid factor, ANA, ANCA.

📖 See Multiple myeloma, p.330.

Anaemia in pregnancy

Physiological changes in red cell and plasma volume occur during pregnancy.

- Red cell mass ↑ by ≤30%.
- Plasma volume ↑ ≤60%.
- Net effect to ↑ blood volume by ≤50% with lowering of the normal
- Hb concentration to 10.0–11.0g/dL during pregnancy. MCV ↑ during pregnancy.
- Fe deficiency is a common problem and cause of anaemia in pregnancy.

Table 1.9 Iron utilization in pregnancy

Cause of ↑ requirements	Amount of additional Fe
↑ Red cell mass	~500mg
Fetal requirements	~300mg
Placental requirements	~5mg
Basal losses over pregnancy (1.0–1.5mg/d)	~250mg

These result in a total requirement of ≤1000mg Fe requiring an average daily intake of 3.5–4.0mg/d. Average Western diet provides <4.0mg Fe/d so that balance is marginal during pregnancy. Diets with Fe mainly in non-haem form (e.g. vegetables) provide less Fe available for absorption. Thus a high risk of developing Fe deficiency anaemia which is exacerbated if preconception Fe stores are reduced.

Folate requirements are ↑ during pregnancy because of ↑ cellular demands; folate levels tend to drop during pregnancy.

Prophylaxis recommendation to give 40–60mg elemental Fe/d which will ↑ availability of dietary absorbable Fe and protect against chronic Fe deficiency; debated whether supplements required by all pregnant women or only for those in at-risk socio-economic and nutritionally deficient groups. Folate supplementation is recommended for all and also appears to reduce incidence of neural tube defects.

- Dilutional anaemia—Hb seldom <10.0g/dL (requires no therapy).
- Fe deficiency—may occur with normal MCV because of ↑ MCV associated with pregnancy; check serum ferritin and give Fe replacement; assess and treat the underlying cause.
- Blood loss—sudden ↓ in Hb may signify fetomaternal bleeding or other forms of concealed obstetric bleeding.
- Folate deficiency—macrocytic anaemia in pregnancy almost invariably will be due to folate deficiency (B_{12} deficiency is extremely rare during pregnancy).
- Microangiopathic haemolysis/DIC may be seen in eclampsia or following placental abruption or intrauterine death. HELLP syndrome (📖 p.92) is a rare but serious cause of anaemia.
- Anaemia may also arise during pregnancy from other unrelated causes and should be investigated.

Thrombocytopenia in pregnancy

A normal uncomplicated pregnancy is associated with a platelet count in the normal range though up to 10% of normal deliveries may be associated with mild thrombocytopenia (>100 × 10^9/L). Detection of thrombocytopenia in a pregnant patient requires consideration not only of the diagnoses listed in the previous section but also the conditions associated with pregnancy which cause thrombocytopenia. An additional important consideration is the possible effect on the fetus and its delivery.

If thrombocytopenia is detected late in pregnancy, most women will have a platelet count result from the booking visit (at 10–12 weeks) for comparison. Mild thrombocytopenia (100–150 × 10^9/L) detected for the first time during an uncomplicated pregnancy is not associated with any risk to the fetus nor does it require special obstetric intervention other than hospital delivery.

Non-immune thrombocytopenia

- Thrombocytopenia may develop in association with pregnancy-induced hypertension, pre-eclampsia, or eclampsia. Successful treatment of hypertension may be associated with improvement in thrombocytopenia which is believed to be due to consumption. Treatment of hypertension, pre-eclampsia, or eclampsia may necessitate delivery of the fetus who is not at risk of thrombocytopenia. HELLP syndrome (haemolysis, elevated liver enzymes, and low platelets) may occur in pregnancy.
- A number of obstetric complications, notably retention of a dead fetus, abruptio placentae, and amniotic fluid embolism, are associated with DIC (📖 Disseminated intravascular coagulation, p.488).

Immune thrombocytopenia may occur in pregnancy and women with chronic ITP may become pregnant. Therapeutic considerations must include an assessment of the risk to the fetus of transplacental passage of antiplatelet antibody causing fetal thrombocytopenia and a risk of haemorrhage before or during delivery. There is no reliable parameter for the assessment of fetal risk which, although relatively low, is most significant in women with pre-existing chronic ITP. *Note*: the severity of the mother's ITP has no bearing on the fetal platelet count.

Women with a platelet count <20 × 10^9/L due to ITP should receive standard prednisolone therapy or IVIg (📖 Immune thrombocytopenia, p.486). If prednisolone fails or is contraindicated, IVIg should be administered and may need to be repeated at 3-week intervals. Splenectomy should be avoided (high rate of fetal loss). Enthusiasm has waned for assessing the fetal platelet count during pregnancy by cordocentesis followed by platelet transfusion. Fetal scalp sampling in early labour is unreliable and hazardous. Delivery should occur in an obstetric unit with paediatric support and the neonate's platelet count should be monitored for several days as delayed falls in the platelet count occur.

1. BCSH Guidelines (2003). Guidelines for the investigation and management of idiopathic thrombocytopenic purpura in adults, children and in pregnancy. *Br J Haematol*, **120**, 574–96.

Prolonged bleeding after surgery

Prolonged bleeding following surgery often requires urgent haematological opinion and investigation. The cause of the bleeding is usually surgical, rather than due to any underlying systemic bleeding disorder.

History and clinical assessment

- Past history in relation to previous haemostatic challenges e.g. previous surgery, dental extractions. Ask specific questions about whether blood transfusion was required.
- Presence of specific clinical problems e.g. impaired liver or renal function.
- Recent drug history—especially aspirin or NSAIDs which can affect platelet function. Also enquire about cytotoxic drugs and anticoagulants.
- Family history of bleeding problems especially after surgery.
- Nature of the surgery and intrinsic haemorrhagic risks of procedure.
- Whether surgery was elective or emergency (in emergency surgery known risk factors are less likely to have been corrected).
- Check case record or ask surgeon/anaesthetist for information on intraoperative bleeding, technical problems etc.
- Whether surgery involves a high risk of triggering DIC e.g. pancreatic or major hepatobiliary surgery.
- Detailed physical examination is not usually practical but bruising, ecchymoses, or purpura should be assessed especially if remote from the site of surgery.
- What blood products have been used and over how long? Transfusion of several units of RBCs over a short period of time will dilute available clotting factors.
- Review preoperative investigation results and other information available in the record on past procedures and/or investigations.

Investigations

- Ensure samples not taken from heparinized line.
- FBC with platelet count and blood film examination.
- PT, APTT, and fibrinogen.

With normal platelets and coagulation screen bleeding is usually surgical and the patient should be supported with blood and urgent surgical re-exploration undertaken. Platelet function abnormalities may occur with aspirin/NSAIDs, uraemia, or extracorporeal circuits. Prolongation of both PT and APTT suggests massive bleeding and inadequate replacement, DIC, underlying liver disease, or oral anticoagulants. Disproportionate, isolated ↑ in either PT or APTR are more likely to indicate previously undiagnosed clotting factor deficiencies. A low platelet count may reflect dilution and consumption from bleeding or DIC if platelets were known to be normal preoperatively.

Treatment

- Low platelets or platelet function abnormalities: give 1–2 adult doses of platelets stat.
- DIC—give 2 adult doses of platelets and 4 units FFP (10–20 units of cryoprecipitate if fibrinogen low) and recheck PT, APTT, and FBC.

- Anticoagulant effect:
  - Heparin—reverse with protamine sulphate.
  - Warfarin—reverse with FFP or PCC.
- Empirical tranexamic acid or aprotinin may be tried if bleeding continues despite the above.

1. Michel, M., *et al.* (2003). Intravenous anti-D as a treatment for immune thrombocytopenic purpura (ITP) during pregnancy. *Br J Haematol*, **123**, 142–6.

Positive sickle test (HbS solubility test)

The $\downarrow$ solubility of deoxyHbS forms the basis of this test. Blood is added to a buffered solution of a reducing agent e.g. sodium dithionate. HbS is precipitated by the solution and produces a turbid appearance. *Note*: does not discriminate between sickle cell *trait* and *homozygous disease*.

Use

This is a quick screening test (takes ~20min), often used preoperatively to detect HbS.

Action if sickle test +ve

- Delay elective operation until established whether disease or trait.
- Ask about family history of sickle cell anaemia or symptoms of SCA.
- FBC and film (Table 1.10).
- Hb electrophoresis, or more commonly HPLC.
- Group and antibody screen serum.

False +ve results

- Low Hb.
- Severe leucocytosis.
- Hyperproteinaemia.
- Unstable Hb.

False –ve results

- Infants <6 months.
- HbS <20% (e.g. following exchange blood transfusion).

Sickle test not recommended as a screening test in pregnancy as it will not detect other Hb variants that interact with HbS e.g. β thalassaemia trait. Standard Hb electrophoresis of at-risk groups should be performed (and of all pregnant women if a high local ethnic population).

Table 1.10 FBC and film features of sickle trait vs. disease

Sickle cell trait	FBC—normal or $\downarrow$ MCV and MCH, no anaemia Film normal (may be microcytosis or target cells)
Sickle cell disease	FBC—Hb ~7–8g/dL (range ~4–11g/dL)
	Film—sickled RBCs, target cells, polychromasia, basophilic stippling, NRBC (hyposplenic features in adults)

1. Balasubramaniam, J., *et al.* (2001) Evaluation of a new screening test for sickle cell haemoglobin. *Clin Lab Haematol*, **23**, 379–83.

Chapter 2

Red cell disorders

The peripheral blood film in anaemias

Table 2.1 Morphological abnormalities and variants

Microcytic RBCs	Fe deficiency, thalassaemia trait and syndromes, congenital sideroblastic anaemia, anaemia of chronic disorders
Macrocytic RBCs	Alcohol/liver disease (round macrocytes), MDS, pregnancy and newborn, haemolysis, B_{12} or folate deficiency, hydroxyurea and antimetabolites (oval macrocytes), acquired sideroblastic anaemia, hypothyroidism, chronic respiratory failure, aplastic anaemia
Dimorphic RBCs	Fe deficiency responding to Fe, mixed Fe and B_{12}/folate deficiency, sideroblastic anaemia, post-transfusion
Polychromatic RBCs	Response to bleeding or haematinic Rx, haemolysis, BM infiltration
Spherocytes	HS, haemolysis e.g. warm AIHA, delayed transfusion reaction, ABO HDN, DIC and MAHA, post-splenectomy
Pencil/rod cells	Fe deficiency anaemia, thalassaemia trait and syndromes, PK deficiency
Elliptocytes	Hereditary elliptocytosis, MPD, and MDS
Fragmented RBCs	MAHA, DIC, renal failure, HUS, TTP
Teardrop RBCs	Myelofibrosis, metastatic marrow infiltration, MDS
Sickle cells	Sickle cell anaemia, other sickle syndromes (not sickle trait)
Target cells	Liver disease, Fe deficiency, thalassaemia, HbC syndromes
Crenated red cells	Usually storage or EDTA artifact. Genuine RBC crenation may be seen post-splenectomy and in renal failure
Burr cells	Renal failure
Acanthocytes	Hereditary acanthocytosis, a-β-lipoproteinaemia, McLeod red cell phenotype, PK deficiency, chronic liver disease (esp. Zieve's)
Bite cells	G6PD deficiency, oxidative haemolysis
Basophilic stippling	Megaloblastic anaemia, lead poisoning, MDS, haemoglobinopathies
Rouleaux	Chronic inflammation, paraproteinaemia, myeloma
↑ reticulocytes	Bleeding, haemolysis, marrow infiltration, severe hypoxia, response to haematinic therapy
Heinz bodies	Not seen in normals (removed by spleen), small numbers seen post-splenectomy, oxidant drugs, G6PD deficiency, sulphonamides, unstable Hb (Hb Zurich, Köln)
Howell–Jolly bodies	Made of DNA, generally removed by the spleen, dyserythropoietic states e.g. B_{12} deficiency, MDS, post-splenectomy, hyposplenism
H bodies	HbH inclusions, denatured HbH (β_4 tetramer), stain with methylene blue, seen in HbH disease (– –/– α), less prominent in α thalassaemia trait, not present in normals
Hyposplenic blood film	Howell–Jolly bodies, target cells, occasional nucleated RBCs, lymphocytosis, macrocytosis, acanthocytes

Anaemia in renal disease

Anaemia is consistently found in the presence of chronic renal failure since the kidneys are the main source of erythropoietin. Severity generally relates to the degree of renal impairment although anaemia may occur even if modest renal impairment. The dominant mechanism is inadequate production of erythropoietin (Epo). Other contributory factors include (i) suppressive effects of uraemia and (ii) ↓ in RBC survival. Uraemia impairs platelet function leading to blood loss and Fe deficiency. Small amounts of blood are inevitably left in the tubing following dialysis so that blood loss and Fe deficiency are further contributory factors in dialysis patients. Folate is lost in dialysis and supplementation is required to avoid deficiency. Aluminium toxicity (from trace amounts in dialysis fluids) and osteitis fibrosa from hyperparathyroidism are rare contributory factors.

Laboratory features

- Hb typically 5.0–10.0g/dL.
- MCV ↔
- Blood film—mostly normochromic RBCs; schistocytes and acanthocytes present. No specific abnormalities in WBC or platelets.
- Microangiopathic haemolytic changes present in vasculitic collagen disorders with renal failure and classically in HUS and TTP.

Management

- Short term treatment with RBC transfusion, based on symptoms (*not Hb concentration*).
- Correction of Fe and folic acid deficiencies.
- Epo will correct anaemia in most patients.
- Start at 50–100 units/kg SC × 3/week. Give IV Fe at same time. Response apparent <10 weeks; reduced doses required as maintenance. Renal Association guidelines have been produced for application and monitoring of Epo therapy. Although expensive it improves quality of life and avoids transfusion dependency and Fe overload.

Side effects of Epo

- ↑ BP.
- Pure red cell aplasia.
- Thrombotic tendency.

www.nephronline.org/standards3/

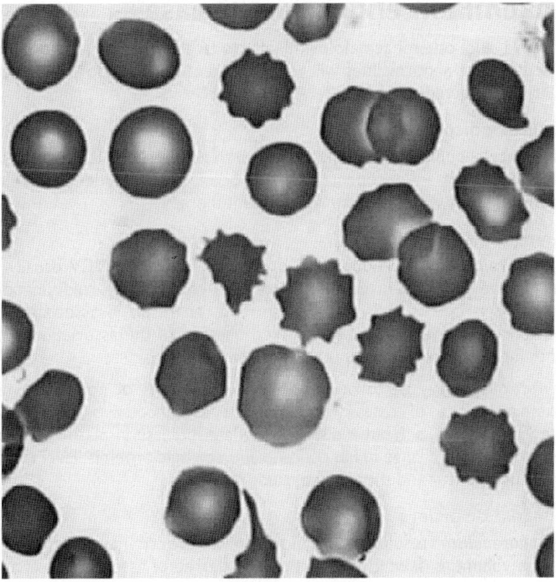

Fig. 2.1 Blood film: chronic renal failure with burr (irregular shaped) cells (📖 see Plate 1).

1. Eschbach, J.W. *et al.* (1987). Correction of the anemia of end-stage renal disease with recombinant human erythropoietin. Results of a combined phase I and II clinical trial. *N Engl J Med*, **316**, 73–8.
2. Levin, N., *et al.* (1997). National Kidney Foundation: Dialysis Outcome Quality Initiative–development of methodology for clinical practice guidelines. *Nephrol Dial Transplant*, **12**, 2060–3.

Anaemia in endocrine disease

Anaemia and other haematological effects occur in various endocrine disorders. The abnormalities will usually correct as the endocrine abnormality is corrected.

Pituitary disorders

Deficiency/hypopituitarism is associated with normochromic, normocytic anaemia; associated leucopenia may also occur. Abnormalities correct as normal function is restored, by replacement therapy.

Thyroid disorders

Hypothyroidism may produce a mild degree of anaemia; MCV usually ↑ but may be normal. Corrects on restoration of normal thyroid function. Menorrhagia occurs in hypothyroidism and can result in associated Fe deficiency. B_{12} levels should be checked because of the association with other autoimmune disorders (e.g. pernicious anaemia).

Thyrotoxicosis may be associated with mild degrees of normochromic anaemia in 20% of cases which corrects as function is normalized. Erythroid activity is ↑ but a disproportionate increase in plasma volume means either no change in Hb concentration or mild anaemia. Haematinic deficiencies occur and should be excluded.

Adrenal disorders

Hypoadrenalism results in normochromic, normocytic anaemia; the plasma volume is ↓ which masks the true degree of associated anaemia. The abnormalities are corrected by replacement mineralocorticoids.

Hyperadrenalism (Cushing's) results in erythrocytosis with a typical net increase in Hb (by 1–2g/dL). Occurs whether Cushing's is 1° or iatrogenic. Mechanism is unclear.

Parathyroid disorders—hyperparathyroidism may be associated with anaemia from impairment of Epo production, or in some cases from 2° marrow sclerosis.

Sex hormones—androgens stimulate erythropoiesis and are occasionally used to stimulate red cell production in aplastic anaemia. The influence of androgens explains the higher Hb in adult ♂ *cf.* ♀.

Diabetes mellitus when poorly controlled may be associated with anaemia; however, the majority of haematological abnormalities in diabetes mellitus result from 2° disease related complications e.g. renal failure.

1. Spivak, J.L. (2000). The blood in systemic disorders. *Lancet*, **355**, 1707–12.

Anaemia in joint disease

Rheumatoid arthritis, psoriatic arthropathy, and osteoarthritis may be complicated by anaemia. Various factors contribute to anaemia; commonly more than one is present, especially in rheumatoid arthritis. Some of the mechanisms that give rise to anaemia in rheumatoid also apply in other connective tissue disease, e.g. SLE, polyarteritis nodosa, etc.

Anaemia of chronic disorders (ACD)

ACD is a cytokine-driven suppression of red cell production. The clinical problem is to being able to recognize the presence of other contributory factors in pathogenesis of the anaemia. BM macrophages fail to pass their stored Fe to developing RBCs and a lower than expected rise in Epo suggesting some inhibition in its pathway. Marrow also appears less responsive to Epo. ↑ IL-1 has been identified. Detailed studies suggest a synergistic effect of IL-1 with T-cells to produce IFN-γ which can suppress erythroid activity. May also be ↑ levels of TNF-α which inhibits erythropoiesis through release of IFN-β from marrow stromal cells.

Typical features of ACD

- Hb range 7.0–11.0g/dL.
- MCV is usually ↔ but when longstanding the MCV is moderately ↓ (may look like Fe deficiency).
- Ferritin usually ↔ but may be ↑
- Serum Fe ↔ or ↓, TIBC ↔ or ↓. (*Note*: Fe and TIBC tests now obsolete).
- Serum transferrin receptor levels normal.
- ↑ zinc protoporphyrin level.
- BM Fe stores plentiful.

Table 2.2 Additional mechanisms of anaemia in rheumatoid disease

Autoimmune phenomena	Warm antibody AIHA in association with rheumatoid and other collagen disorders; film will show reticulocytosis and +ve DAT
	Red cell aplasia
Drug-related problems	Chronic blood loss (caused by medication)
	Drug side effects e.g. macrocytosis from antimetabolite immunosuppressives, e.g. azathioprine and methotrexate, oxidative haemolysis 2° to dapsone or sulfasalazine (occurs in normal individuals as well as those with G6PD deficiency)
	Anaemia 2° to gold therapy for rheumatoid arthritis
	Idiosyncratic reactions, unexplained or unforeseeable reactions such as marrow aplasia
	Rare autoimmune haemolysis due to mefenamic acid, diclofenac, or ibuprofen
2° to other organ prolems	Hypersplenism, Felty's syndrome in rheumatoid, renal failure in SLE or polyarteritis

Management

Supportive transfusion in symptomatic patients; coexistent Fe deficiency should be excluded and treated. Minority may be suitable for/responsive to Epo therapy.

Bleeding and Fe deficiency

Usually 2° to use of NSAIDs—consider and exclude other causes of blood loss which may occur in this patient group.

1. Bron, D., Meuleman, N., and Mascaux, C. (2001). Biological basis of anemia. *Semin Oncol*, **28**, 1–6.
2. Spivak, J.L. (2000) The blood in systemic disorders. *Lancet*, **355**, 1707–12.

Anaemia in gastrointestinal disease

Anaemia occurs in GIT disorders through mechanisms of blood loss, ACD-specific disease-related complications, or drug side effects/idiosyncrasy occurring singly or in various combinations.

Table 2.3 Blood loss in gastrointestinal disease

Acute	Immediately following acute haemorrhage—RBC indices usually ↔
	Normochromic anaemia
Acute on chronic	RBC indices show low normal or marginally ↓, especially MCV Film shows mixture of normochromic and hypochromic RBCs ('dimorphic')
Chronic	RBC indices show established chronic Fe deficiency features ↓ MCV, MCH, platelets often ↑

Anaemia in GIT disorders can be simply considered against some of the commoner problems arising through the GIT:

Oesophageal—bleeding from peptic oesophagitis, association of oesophageal web and chronic Fe deficiency.

Gastric—pernicious anaemia and B_{12} deficiency, late effects of partial or total gastrectomy producing B_{12} and/or Fe deficiency. Microangiopathic haemolytic anaemia from metastatic adenocarcinoma.

Small bowel—malabsorption states e.g. Fe and/or folate deficiency 2° to coeliac disease, malabsorption from other problems including inflammatory bowel disease; hyposplenism 2° to coeliac with or without ↓ platelets.

Large bowel—blood loss anaemia from inflammatory bowel disorders. Note: these may also be associated with ACD. Rare occurrence of autoimmune haemolysis associated with ulcerative colitis.

Pancreas—ACD associated with carcinoma or chronic pancreatitis, DIC associated with acute pancreatitis.

Liver—📖 see Anaemia in liver disease, p.41.

Drug-related anaemia arises through:
- Upper GIT irritation causing blood loss—aspirin, NSAIDs, corticosteroids.
- Bleeding due to specific drugs e.g. warfarin and heparin.
- Drug-induced haemolysis e.g. oxidative (Heinz body) haemolysis due to sulphasalazine or dapsone.
- Production impairment e.g. aplasia 2° to mesalazine.

Anaemia in liver disease

Anaemia is common in chronic liver disorders. There are several possible causes including:

- ACD—part of marrow response to chronic inflammatory processes.
- Macrocytosis ± anaemia: specific effects on membrane lipids cause ↑MCV.
- Alcohol—direct suppressive effect on erythropoiesis with ↑MCV.
- Folate deficiency: seen in alcoholic liver disease → nutritional deficiency and/or direct effect of alcohol on folate metabolism.
- Blood loss from oesophageal varices → acute or chronic anaemia.
- Hypersplenism—portal hypertension can produce marked splenic enlargement leading to hypersplenism.
- Haemolytic anaemias e.g.:
    - Autoimmune haemolytic anaemia in association with chronic active hepatitis.
    - Zieve's syndrome (hypertriglyceridaemia + self-limiting haemolysis due to acute alcohol excess).
    - Viral hepatitis may provoke oxidative haemolysis in those with G6PD deficiency.
    - Acute liver failure—DIC and MAHA may occur.
    - Acanthocytosis: acute haemolytic anaemia with acanthocytosis (spur cell anaemia). Rare. Usually late stage liver disease, with poor prognosis.

Alcohol

Even if no liver disease, chronic alcohol consumption may lead to ↑MCV (100–110fL). Anaemia may be associated with poor diet, folate deficiency, gastrointestinal bleeding and Fe deficiency. Alcohol has direct toxic effects on the marrow with reversible suppression of haemopoiesis; ↓Hb and ↓ platelets are most common.

1. Savage, D., *et al.* (1986). Anemia in alcoholics. *Medicine* (Baltimore), **65**, 322–38.
2. Wu, A., *et al.* (1974). Macrocytosis of chronic alcoholism. *Lancet*, **1**, 829–31.

Iron (Fe) deficiency anaemia

Microcytic anaemia is common and the commonest cause is chronic Fe deficiency.

Fe physiology and metabolism

Normal (Western) diet provides ~15mg of Fe/d, of which 5–10% is absorbed in duodenum and upper jejunum. Ferrous (Fe^{2+}) Fe is better absorbed than ferric (Fe^{3+}) Fe. Total body Fe store ~4g. Around 1mg of Fe/d lost in urine, faeces, sweat, and cells shed from the skin and GIT. Fe deficiency is commoner in ♀ of reproductive age since menstrual losses account for ~20mg Fe/month and in pregnancy an additional 500–1000mg Fe may be lost (transferred from mother → fetus).

Table 2.4 Causes of Fe deficiency

Reproductive system	Menorrhagia
GI tract	Oesophagitis, oesophageal varices, hiatus hernia (ulcerated; simple hiatus hernia would not cause Fe deficiency), peptic ulcer, inflammatory bowel disease, haemorrhoids, carcinoma: stomach, colorectal, (rarely angiodysplasia, hereditary haemorrhagic telangiectasia)
Malabsorption	Coeliac disease, atrophic gastritis (*Note*: may also result from Fe deficiency), gastrectomy
Physiological	Growth spurts, pregnancy
Dietary	Vegans, elderly
Genitourinary system	Haematuria (uncommon cause)
Others	PNH, frequent venesection e.g. blood donation
Worldwide	Commonest cause is hookworm infestation

Assessment

Clinical history—review potential sources of blood loss, esp. GIT loss.

Menstrual loss—quantitation may be difficult; ask about number of tampons used per day, how often these require changing, and duration.

Other sources of blood loss e.g. haematuria and haemoptysis (these are *not* common causes of Fe deficiency). Ask patient if he/she has been a blood donor—regular blood donation over many years may cause chronic Fe store depletion.

Drug therapy e.g. NSAIDs and corticosteroids may cause GI irritation and blood loss.

Past medical history e.g. previous gastric surgery (→ malabsorption). Ask about previous episodes of anaemia and treatments with Fe.

In patients with Fe deficiency assume underlying cause is blood loss until proved otherwise. In developed countries pure dietary Fe lack causing Fe deficiency is almost unknown.

Examination

- General examination including assessment of mucous membranes (e.g. hereditary haemorrhagic telangiectasia).
- Seek possible sources of blood loss.
- Abdominal examination, rectal examination, and sigmoidoscopy mandatory.
- Gynaecological examination also required.

Laboratory tests

- ↓ Hb.
- ↓ MCV (<76fL) and ↓ MCHC (*Note*: ↓ MCV in thalassaemia and ACD).
- Red cell distribution width (RDW): ↑ in Fe deficiency states with a greater frequency than in ACD or thalassaemia trait.
- Serum ferritin (measurement of Fe/TIBC generally unhelpful). *Ferritin assay preferred—low serum ferritin identifies the presence of Fe deficiency but as an acute phase protein it can be ↑, masking Fe deficiency. ↓ Fe and ↑ TIBC indicates Fe deficiency (though tests are obsolete).*
- The soluble transferrin assay (sTfR) is useful in cases where ↑ ESR. sTfR is ↑ in Fe deficiency but ↔ in anaemia in presence of ↑ ESR (e.g. rheumatoid, other inflammatory states). This assay is not universally available at present.
- % hypochromic RBCs—some modern analysers provide this parameter. ↑ % hypo RBCs are seen in Fe deficiency but also thalassaemia, CRF on Epo where insufficient Fe given.
- Zinc protoporphyrin (ZPP)—in the absence of Fe, zinc is incorporated into protoporphyrin. ↑ ZPP in Fe deficiency is a non-specific marker since ↑ ZPP is seen in any disorder that restricts Fe availability to developing RBCs e.g. infection, inflammation, cancer, etc.
- Reticulocyte Hb concentration (CHr) appears to be a sensitive method for detecting early Fe deficiency.
- Examination of BM aspirate (Fe stain) is occasionally useful.
- Theoretically FOB testing may be of value in Fe deficiency but results can be misleading. False +ve results seen in high dietary meat intake.

Treatment of Fe deficiency

Simplest, safest and cheapest treatment is oral ferrous salts, e.g. $FeSO_4$ (Fe gluconate and fumarate equally acceptable). Provide an oral dose of elemental Fe of 150–200mg/d. Side effects in 10–20% patients (e.g. abdominal distension, constipation and/or diarrhoea)—try ↓ the daily dose to bd or od. Liquid Fe occasionally necessary, e.g. children or adults with swallowing difficulties. Increasing dietary Fe intake has no routine place in the management of Fe deficiency except where intake is grossly deficient.

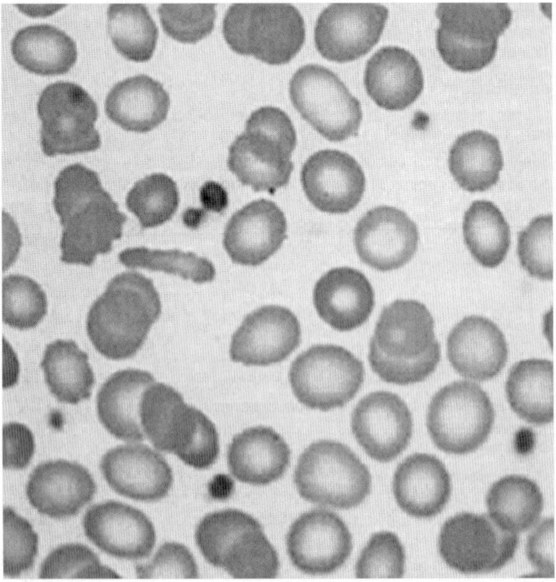

Fig. 2.2 Blood film in Fe deficiency anaemia: note pale red cells with pencil cell (top left).

Response to replacement

A rise of Hb of 2.0g/dL over 3 weeks is expected. MCV will ↑ concomitantly with Hb. Reticulocytes may ↑ in response to Fe therapy but is not a reliable indicator of response.

Duration of treatment

Generally ~6 months. After Hb and MCV are normal continue Fe for at least 3 months to replenish Fe stores.

Failure of response

- Is the diagnosis of Fe deficiency correct?
    - Consider ACD or thalassaemia trait.
- Is there an additional complicating illness?
    - Chronic infection, collagen disorder, or neoplasm.
- Is the patient complying with prescribed medication?
- Is the preparation of Fe adequate in dosage and/or formulation?
- Is the patient continuing to bleed excessively?
- Is there malabsorption?
- Are there other haematinic deficiencies (e.g. B_{12} or folate) present?
- Reassess patient: ?evidence of continued blood loss or malabsorption.

Parenteral Fe

Occasionally of value in genuine Fe intolerance, if compliance is a problem, or if need to replace stores rapidly e.g. in pregnancy or prior to major surgery. *Note*: Hb will rise no faster than with oral Fe.

Intravenous Fe

Fe may be administered IV as Fe hydroxide sucrose (ferric hydroxide with sucrose) or Fe dextran (ferric hydroxide with dextran). Facilities for cardiopulmonary resuscitation should be available though serious adverse events are uncommon.

References

1. Andrews, N.C. (1999). Disorders of iron metabolism. *N Engl J Med*, **341**, 1986–95.
2. Brugnara, C. (2000) Reticulocyte cellular indices: a new approach in the diagnosis of anemias and monitoring of erythropoietic function. *Crit Rev Clin Lab Sci*, **37**, 93–130.
3. Kuhn, L.C. and Hentze, M.W. (1992). Coordination of cellular iron metabolism by post-transcriptional gene regulation. *J Inorg Biochem*, **47**, 183–95.
4. Labbe, R.F., *et al.* (1999) Zinc protoporphyrin: A metabolite with a mission. *Clin Chem*, **45**, 2060–72.
5. Rettmer, R.L., *et al.* (1999) Zinc protoporphyrin/heme ratio for diagnosis of preanemic iron deficiency. *Pediatrics*, **104**, e37.
6. Tapiero, H., Gate, L., and Tew, K.D. (2001). Iron: deficiencies and requirements. *Biomed Pharmacother*, **55**, 324–32.

Vitamin B_{12} deficiency

B_{12} deficiency presents with macrocytic, megaloblastic anaemia ranging from mild to severe (Hb <6.0g/dL). Symptoms are those of chronic anaemia, i.e. fatigue, dyspnoea on effort, etc. Neurological symptoms may also be present—classically peripheral paraesthesiae and disturbances of position and vibration sense. Occasionally neurological symptoms occur with no/minimal haematological upset. If uncorrected, the patient may develop subacute combined degeneration of the spinal cord → permanently ataxic.

Pathophysiology

B_{12} (along with folic acid) is required for DNA synthesis; B_{12} is also required for neurological functioning. B_{12} is absorbed in terminal ileum after binding to intrinsic factor produced by gastric parietal cells. Body stores of B_{12} are 2–3mg (sufficient for 3 years). B_{12} is found in meats, fish, eggs, and dairy produce. Strictly vegetarian (vegan) diets are low in B_{12} although not all vegans develop clinical evidence of deficiency.

Presenting haematological abnormalities

- Macrocytic anaemia (MCV usually >110fL). In extreme cases RBC anisopoikilocytosis can result in MCV values just within normal range.
- RBC changes include oval macrocytosis, poikilocytosis, basophilic stippling, Howell–Jolly bodies, circulating megaloblasts.
- Hypersegmented neutrophils.
- Leucopenia and thrombocytopenia common.
- BM shows megaloblastic change; marked erythroid hyperplasia with predominance of early erythroid precursors, open atypical nuclear chromatin patterns, mitotic figures and 'giant' metamyelocytes
- Fe stores usually ↑.
- Serum B_{12} ↓.
- Homocysteine levels are ↑ in both B_{12} and folate deficiency.
- Serum/red cell folate usually ↔ or ↑.
- LDH levels markedly ↑ reflecting ineffective erythropoiesis (RBC destruction within the BM and ↓ RBC lifespan.
- Autoantibody screen in pernicious anaemia: 80–90% show circulating gastric parietal cell antibodies, 55% have circulating intrinsic factor antibodies. *Note*: parietal cell antibodies are not diagnostic since found in normals; IFA is only found in 50% of patients with PA but is diagnostic.

Management of B_{12} deficiency

- Identify and correct cause if possible.
- Investigations are undertaken and a test of B_{12} absorption is carried out (e.g. Schilling test). Urinary excretion of a test dose of B_{12} labelled with trace amounts of radioactive cobalt is compared with excretion of B_{12} bound to intrinsic factor; the test is done in two parts. B_{12} malabsorption corrected by intrinsic factor is diagnostic of pernicious anaemia (in absence of previous gastric surgery).
- Management—hydroxocobalamin 1mg IM and folic acid PO should be given immediately.

Table 2.5 Causes of B_{12} deficiency

Pernicious anaemia	Commonest, due to autoimmune gastric atrophy resulting in loss of intrinsic factor production required for absorption of B_{12}. Incidence ↑ >40 years and often associated with other autoimmune problems, e.g. hypothyroidism.
Following total gastrectomy	May develop after major partial gastrectomy.
Ileal disease	Resection of ileum, Crohn's disease.
Blind loop syndromes	E.g. diverticulae or localized inflammatory bowel changes allowing bacterial overgrowth which then competes for available B_{12}.
Fish tapeworm	*Diphyllobothrium latum.*
Malabsorptive disorders	Tropical sprue, coeliac disease.
Dietary deficiency	E.g. vegans.

- Supportive measures—bed rest, O_2, and diuretics may be needed while awaiting response. Transfusion is best avoided but 2 units of concentrated RBCs may be used for patients severely compromised by anaemia (risk of precipitating cardiac failure); hypokalaemia is occasionally observed during the immediate response to B_{12} and serum $[K^+]$ should be monitored.
- Response apparent in 3–5d with reticulocyte response of >10%; normoblastic conversion of marrow erythropoiesis in 12–24h. Patients frequently describe a subjective improvement within 24h.
- B_{12} replacement therapy—initially hydroxocobalamin 5 × 1mg IM should be given during the first 2 weeks, thereafter maintenance injections are needed 3-monthly.
- If dietary deficiency seems likely and B_{12} deficiency mild, worth trying oral B_{12} (cyanocobalamin 50–150mcg or more, daily between meals).
- Long term follow-up depends on the 1° cause. Pernicious anaemia patients require lifelong treatment and should be checked annually with a FBC and thyroid function; the incidence of gastric cancer is twice as high in these patients compared to the normal population.
- Broad spectrum antibiotics should be given to suppress bacterial overgrowth in blind loop syndrome ± local surgery if appropriate. Long term IM B_{12} may be the pragmatic solution if blind loop cannot be corrected.

1. Guidelines on the investigation and diagnosis of cobalamin and folate deficiencies. A publication of the British Committee for Standards in Haematology. BCSH General Haematology Test Force (1994). *Clin Lab Haematol*, **16**, 101–15.
2. Toh, B.H., van Driel, I.R., and Gleeson, P.A. (1997). Pernicious anemia. *N Engl J Med*, **337**, 1441–8.

Folate deficiency

Folate deficiency represents the other main deficiency cause of megaloblastic anaemia; haematological features indistinguishable from those of B_{12} deficiency. Distinction is on basis of demonstration of reduced red cell and serum folate.

►► Megaloblastic anaemia patients should never receive empirical treatment with folic acid alone. *If they lack B_{12}, folic acid is potentially capable of precipitating subacute combined degeneration of the cord.*

Pathophysiology

Adult body folate stores comprise 10–15mg; normal daily requirements are 0.1–0.2mg, i.e. sufficient for 3–4 months in absence of exogenous folate intake. Folate absorption from dietary sources is rapid; proximal jejunum is main site of absorption. Main dietary sources of folate are liver, green vegetables, nuts, and yeast. Western diets contain ~0.5–0.7mg folate/d but availability may be lessened as folate is readily destroyed by cooking, especially in large volumes of water. Folate coenzymes are an essential part of DNA synthesis, hence the occurrence of megaloblastic change in deficiency.

Diagnosis

Haematological findings are identical to those seen in B_{12} deficiency— macrocytic, megaloblastic anaemia. Other findings also similar to B_{12} except parietal cell and intrinsic factor autoantibodies usually –ve. Reduced folate levels—serum folate levels reflect recent intake, red cell folate levels give a more reliable indication of folate status.

Table 2.6 Causes of folate deficiency

↓ intake	Poor nutrition, e.g. poverty, old age, 'skid row' alcoholics
↑ requirements/losses	Pregnancy, ↑ cell turnover, e.g. haemolysis, exfoliative dermatitis, renal dialysis
Malabsorption	Coeliac disease, tropical sprue, Crohn's and other malabsorptive states
Drugs	Phenytoin, barbiturates, valproate, oral contraceptives, nitrofurantoin may induce folate malabsorption
Antifolate drugs	Methotrexate, trimethoprim, pentamidine antagonize folate *cf.* induce deficiency
Alcohol	Poor nutrition plus a direct depressant effect on folate levels which can precipitate clinical folate deficiency

Management

- Treatment and support of severe anaemia as for B_{12} deficiency.
- Folic acid 5mg/d PO (never on its own—📖 see Table 2.6), unless patient known to have normal B_{12} level.

- Treatment of underlying cause e.g. in coeliac disease folate levels and absorption normalize once patient established on gluten-free diet. Long term supplementation advised in chronic haemolysis e.g. HbSS or HS.
- Prophylactic folate supplements recommended in pregnancy and other states of ↑ demand e.g. prematurity.

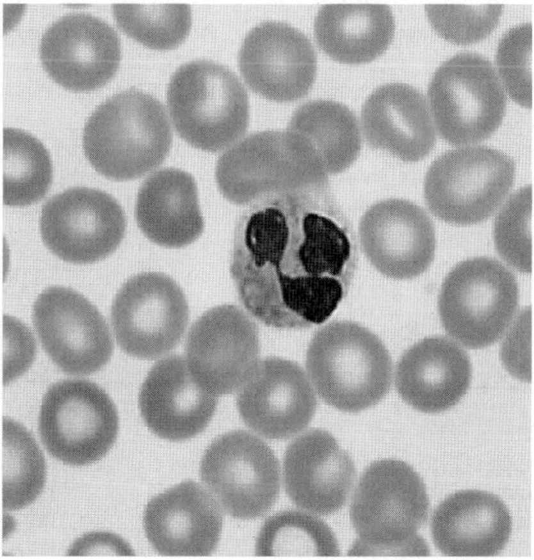

Fig. 2.3 Blood film: normal neutrophil: usually has <5 lobes. This one has 3 lobes (📖 see Plate 2).

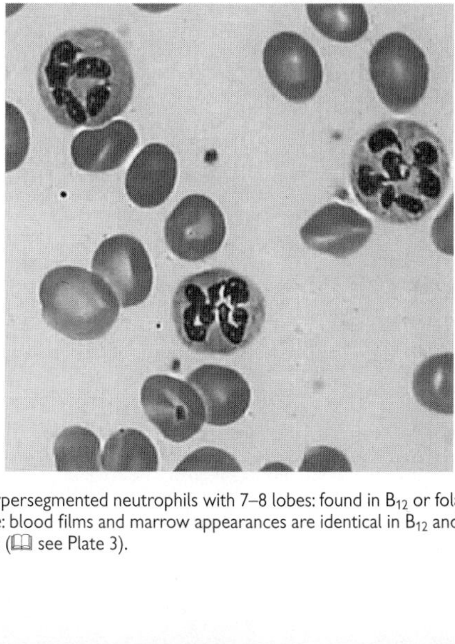

Fig. 2.4 Hypersegmented neutrophils with 7–8 lobes: found in B_{12} or folate deficiency. *Note*: blood films and marrow appearances are identical in B_{12} and folate deficiencies (📖 see Plate 3).

Other causes of megaloblastic anaemia

Megaloblastic anaemia not due to actual deficiency of either B_{12} or folate is uncommon, but may occur in the following situations.

Congenital

- Transcobalamin II deficiency—absence of the key B_{12} transport protein results in severe megaloblastic anaemia (corrects with parenteral B_{12}).
- Congenital intrinsic factor deficiency—autosomal recessive, results in failure to produce intrinsic factor. Presents as megaloblastic anaemia up to age of 2 years and responds to parenteral B_{12}.
- Inborn errors of metabolism—errors in folate pathways, also occurs in orotic aciduria and Lesch–Nyhan syndrome.
- Megaloblastosis commonly present in the congenital dyserythropoietic anaemias (📖 see Congenital dyserythropoietic anaemias, p.584).

Acquired

- MDS—often present in sideroblastic anaemia (RARS).
- Acute leukaemia—megaloblastic-like erythroid dysplasia in AML M6.
- Drug induced—2° to antimetabolite drugs including 6-mercaptopurine, cytosine arabinoside, zidovudine, and hydroxyurea.
- Anaesthetic agents—transient megaloblastic change after nitrous oxide.
- Alcohol excess—may result in megaloblastic change in absence of measurable folate deficiency.
- Vitamin C deficiency—occasionally results in megaloblastic change.

Anaemia in other deficiency states

Fe, folate, or vitamin B_{12} deficiencies account for the majority of clinically significant deficiency syndromes resulting in anaemia. Anaemia is recognized as a complication in other vitamin deficiencies and in malnutrition.

Vitamin A deficiency

Produces a chronic disorder like Fe deficiency anaemia with ↓ MCV and MCH.

Vitamin B_6 (pyridoxine) deficiency

Can produce hypochromic microcytic anaemia; sideroblastic change may occur. Pyridoxine is given to patients on antituberculous therapy with isoniazid which is known to interfere with vitamin B_6 metabolism and cause sideroblastic anaemia.

Vitamin C deficiency

Occasionally associated with macrocytic anaemia (± megaloblastic change in 10%); since the main cause of vitamin C deficiency is inadequate diet or nutrition there may be evidence of other deficiencies.

Vitamin E deficiency

Occasionally seen in the neonatal period in low birth weight infants—results in haemolytic anaemia with abnormal RBC morphology.

Starvation

Normochromic anaemia ± leucopenia occurs in anorexia nervosa; features are not associated with any specific deficiency; BM is typically hypocellular.

Haemolytic syndromes

Definition

Any situation in which there is a reduction in RBC life-span due to ↑RBC destruction. Failure of compensatory marrow response results in anaemia. Predominant site of RBC destruction is red pulp of the spleen.

Classification—3 major types

1. Hereditary *vs.* acquired
2. Immune *vs.* non-immune
3. Extravascular *vs.* intravascular

Hereditary cause suggested if history of anaemia refractory to treatment in infancy ± FH e.g. other affected members, anaemia, gallstones, jaundice, splenectomy. ***Acquired*** haemolytic anaemia is suggested by sudden onset of symptoms/signs in adulthood. ***Intravascular*** haemolysis—takes place in peripheral circulation *cf.* ***extravascular*** haemolysis which occurs in RES.

Hereditary

- Red cell membrane disorders e.g. HS and hereditary elliptocytosis.
- Red cell enzymopathies e.g. G6PD and PK deficiencies.
- Abnormal Hb e.g. thalassaemias and sickle cell disease, unstable Hbs.

Acquired—immune

Table 2.7 Acquired–immune

Alloimmune	Autoimmune
• HDN • RBC transfusion incompatibility	• Warm AIHA–1° or 2° to SLE, CLL, drugs • Cold–*Mycoplasma* or EBV infection • Cold haemagglutinin disease (CHAD) • Lymphoproliferative disorders • Paroxysmal cold haemoglobinuria (PCH)

Acquired—non-immune

- MAHA.
- TTP/HUS.
- Hypersplenism.
- Prosthetic heart valves.
- March haemoglobinuria.
- Sepsis.
- Malaria.
- Paroxysmal nocturnal haemoglobinuria.

Clinical features

Symptoms of anaemia e.g. breathlessness, fatigue. Urinary changes e.g. red or dark brown of haemoglobinuria. Symptoms of underlying disorder.

Confirm haemolysis is occurring

- Check FBC.
- Peripheral blood film—polychromasia, spherocytosis, fragmentation (schistocytes), helmet cells, echinocytes.
- ↑ reticulocytes.
- ↑ serum bilirubin (unconjugated).
- ↑ LDH.
- Low/absent serum haptoglobin (bind free Hb).
- Schumm's test (for intravascular haemolysis).
- Urinary haemosiderin (implies chronic intravascular haemolysis e.g. PNH).

Discriminant diagnostic features

Establish whether immune or non-immune—check DAT

?Immune if DAT +ve check IgG and C3 specific reagents—suggest warm and cold antibody respectively. Screen serum for red cell alloantibodies.

?Cold antibody present—examine blood film for agglutination, check MCV on initial FBC sample and again after incubation at 37°C for 2h. High MCV at room temperature due to agglutinates falls to normal at 37°C. Check anti-I and anti-i titres for confirmation. Check *Mycoplasma* IgM and EBV serology, and for presence of Donath–Landsteiner antibody (cold reacting IgG antibody with anti-P specificity).

?Warm antibody present—IgG +ve DAT only suggestive—examine film for spherocytes (usually prominent), lymphocytosis or abnormal lymphs to suggest LPD. Examine patient for nodes.

?Intravascular haemolysis—check for urinary haemosiderin, Schumm's test.

?Sepsis—check blood cultures.

?Malaria—examine thick and thin blood films for parasites.

?Renal/liver abnormality—examine for hepatomegaly, splenomegaly, LFTs and U&E.

?Low platelets—consider TTP/HUS.

?Haemoglobinopathy—check Hb electrophoresis.

?Red cell membrane abnormality—check family history and perform red cell fragility test.

?Red cell enzyme disorder—check family history and do G6PD and PK assay. *Note*: enzymes may be falsely normal if reticulocytosis since increased levels are present in young RBCs.

?PNH—check immunophenotyping for CD55 + CD59 (Ham's acid lysis test now largely obsolete).

Treatment

Treat underlying disorder. Give folic acid and Fe supplements if low.

1. Gehrs, B.C. and Friedberg, R.C. (2002). Autoimmune hemolytic anemia. *Am J Hematol*, **69**, 258–71.

Genetic control of haemoglobin production

Hb comprises 4 protein subunits (e.g. adult Hb = $2 \times \alpha + 2 \times \beta$ chains, $\alpha_2\beta_2$) each linked to a haem group. Production of different globin chains varies from embryo → adult to meet the particular environment at each stage. Globin genes are located on chromosomes 11 and 16. All globins related to α globin are located on chromosome 16; all those related to β globin are on chromosome 11. The sequence in which they are produced during development reflects their physical order on chromosomes such that ζ is the first α-like globin to be produced in life. After ζ expression stops, α production occurs ($\zeta \rightarrow \alpha$ switch). On chromosome 11 the arrangement of β-like globin genes follows the order (from left → right) $\varepsilon \rightarrow \gamma \rightarrow \delta \rightarrow \beta$ mirroring the β-like globin chains produced during development. As embryo develops into fetus, ζ production stops and α is produced. The α globin combines with γ chains and produces $\alpha_2\gamma_2$ (fetal Hb, HbF). After birth γ production ↓ and δ and β chains are produced. Adults have predominantly HbA ($\alpha_2\beta_2$) although small amounts of HbA_2 ($\alpha_2\beta_2$) and HbF are produced.

Hb switching is physiological but the mechanism is unclear. HbF ($\alpha_2\gamma_2$) binds O_2 more tightly than adult haemoglobin, ensuring adequate O_2 delivery to the fetus which must extract its O_2 from mother's circulation. After birth the lungs expand and the O_2 is derived from the air, with β production replacing that of γ, leading to an increase in adult haemoglobin ($\alpha_2\beta_2$).

Table 2.8 Structure and quantity of normal haemoglobins

Haemoglobin	Globin chains	Amount
Embryo		
Hb Gower 1	$\zeta_2\varepsilon_2$	42%*
Hb Gower 2	$\alpha_2\varepsilon_2$	24%*
Hb Portland	$\zeta_2\gamma_2$	
*by 5th week		
Fetus		
HbF	$\alpha_2\gamma_2$	85%
HbA	$\alpha_2\beta_2$	5–10%
Adult		
HbA	$\alpha_2\beta_2$	97%
HbA_2	$\alpha_2\delta_2$	2.5%
HbF	$\alpha_2\gamma_2$	0.5%

Haemoglobin abnormalities

Fall into 2 major groups: *structural abnormalities* of Hb due to alterations in DNA coding for the globin protein leading to an abnormal amino acid in the globin molecule, e.g. sickle haemoglobin (β^S). Second group of Hb disorders results from *imbalanced globin chain production*—globins produced are structurally normal but their relative amounts are incorrect and lead to the thalassaemias.

Haemoglobinopathies result in significant morbidity and mortality on a world-wide scale. Patients with these disorders are also seen in Northern Europe and the UK, especially in areas with significant Greek, Italian, Afro-Caribbean and Asian populations.

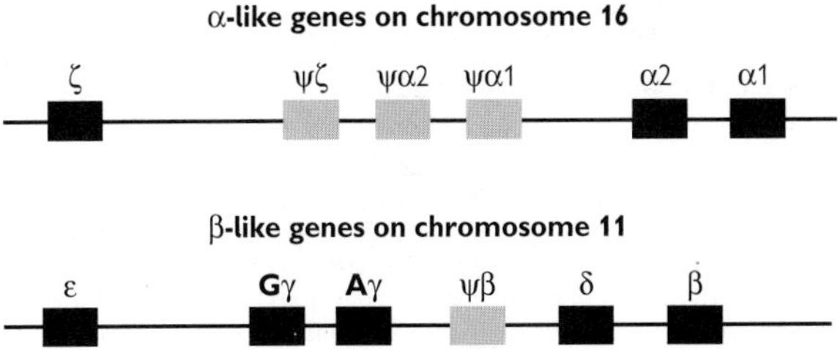

Fig. 2.5 Arrangement of α-like and β-like globin genes (ψ indicates pseudogene).

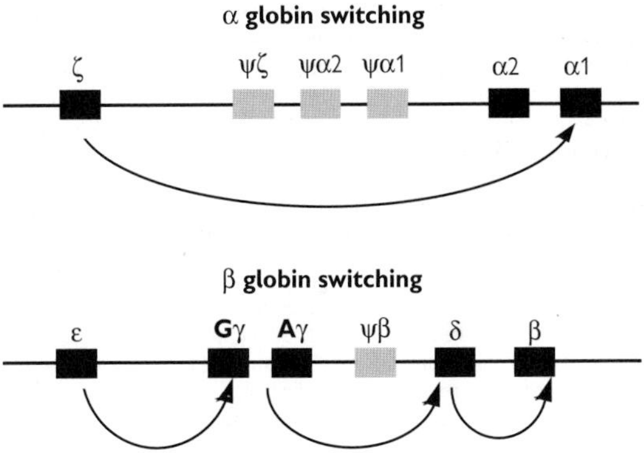

Fig. 2.6 Globin gene switching during development

1. Rund, D., *et al.* (2001). Pathophysiology of alpha- and beta-thalassemia: therapeutic implications. *Semin Hematol*, **38**, 343–9.

Sickling disorders

Sickle cell anaemia (homozygous SS, $\beta^S\beta^S$), HbSC ($\beta^S\beta^C$), HbS/β^+ or β^o thalassaemia, and HbSD ($\beta^S\beta^D$) all produce significant symptoms but homozygous sickle cell anaemia is generally the most severe. The gene has remained at high frequency due to conferred resistance to malaria in heterozygotes. Inheritance is autosomal recessive.

Sickle cell anaemia (SCA, HbSS)

Pathogenesis

Widespread throughout Africa, Middle East, parts of India and Mediterranean. Single base change in β globin gene, amino acid 6 (glu → val). Heterozygosity rates: West Africa 10–30%, African Americans and UK AfroCaribbeans 10%). Patients with SCA are the offspring of parents both of whom are carriers of the β^S gene, i.e. they both have sickle cell trait, and homozygotes for the abnormal β^S gene demonstrate features of chronic red cell haemolysis and tissue infarction. RBCs containing HbS deform (elongate) under conditions of reduced oxygenation, and form characteristic sickle cells—do not flow well through small vessels, and are more adherent than normal to vascular endothelium, leading to vascular occlusion and sickle cell crises. The vaso-occlusive process is complex and, in addition to the polymerization of globin, there is interaction of sickle cells with other types of cell and proteins. Sickle cells are more adherent to vascular endothelium than normal red cells. During vascular crises there is endothelial damage with exposure of molecules such as thrombospondin, laminin, and fibronectin. There is activation of blood coagulation with enhanced thrombin generation and hyperreactivity of platelets. Nitric oxide also plays a role, promoting the conversion of oxyhaemoglobin to methaemoglobin. NO may also play a role in vasoregulation and participates in the compensatory response to chronic vascular injury seen in sickle cell disease. Reiter 10,99

Clinical features

- Highly variable. Many have few symptoms whilst others have severe and frequent crises, marked haemolytic anaemia, and chronic organ damage. HbF level plays role in ameliorating symptoms (↑HbF→ fewer and milder crises). History may reveal a +ve family history or past history of crises.
- *Infancy*—newborns have higher HbF level than normal adult, protected during first 8–20 weeks of life. Symptoms start when HbF level falls. ↑ malaria risk. SCA often diagnosed <1 year.
- *Infection*—high morbidity and mortality due to bacterial and viral infection. Pneumococcal septicaemia (*Streptococcus pneumoniae*) well recognized. Other infecting organisms: meningococcus (*Neisseria meningitidis*), *Escherichia coli,* and *Haemophilus influenzae* (hyposplenic).
- *Anaemia*—children and adults often severely anaemic (Hb ~6.0–9.0 g/dL). Anaemia is chronic and patients generally well-adapted until episode of decompensation (e.g. severe infection) occurs.

Sickle crises

- *Vaso-occlusive*—dactylitis, chest syndrome, and girdle syndrome. Patients complain of severe bone, joint, and abdominal pain. Bone pain affects long bones and spine, and is due to occlusion of small vessels. Triggers: infection, dehydration, alcohol, menstruation, cold, and temperature changes—often no cause found.

- *Dactylitis*—mainly children. Metacarpals, metatarsals, backs of hands and feet swollen and tender (small vessel occlusion and infarction). Recurrent, can result in permanent radiological abnormalities in bones of the hands and feet (rare).
- *Acute chest syndrome*—common cause of death, seen in 40% of patients, children > adults (more severe in adults). Chest wall pain, sometimes with pleurisy, fever, and SOB. Resembles infection, infarction, or embolism. Requires prompt and vigorous treatment. Transfer to ITU if pO_2 cannot be kept >70 mmHg on air. Consider CPAP. 10% mortality. Treat infection vigorously, often due to *S. pneumoniae, H. influenzae, Mycoplasma, Legionella.*
- *Aplastic crises*—sudden ↓ in marrow production (esp. red cells). Parvovirus B19 infection is cause (invades developing RBCs). Mostly self-limiting and after 1–2 weeks the marrow begins to function normally. Top-up transfusion may be needed.
- *Haemolytic crises*—uncommon; markedly reduced red cell lifespan. May be drug-induced, 2° to infection (e.g. malaria) or associated G6PD deficiency.
- *Sequestration crises*—mainly children (30%). Pooling of large volumes of blood in spleen and/or liver. Severe hypotension and profound anaemia may result in death. Splenic sequestration is seen predominantly in children <6 years of age; often occurs following a viral infection.
- *Other problems*:
  - Growth retardation: common in children, but adult may have normal height (weight tends to be lower than normal). Sexual maturation delayed.
  - Locomotor: avascular necrosis of the head of the femur or humerus, arthritis, and osteomyelitis (*Salmonella* infection). Chronic leg ulceration is a complication of many haemoglobinopathies including sickle cell anaemia. Ischaemia is main cause. Rare in SC disease.
  - Genitourinary: renal papillary necrosis → haematuria and renal tubular defects. Inability to concentrate urine. Priapism in 10–40% males. Less common if HbF↑. Frequent UTIs in women, CRF in adults.
  - Spleen: severe pain (infarction of splenic vessels). Spleen may enlarge in early life but after repeated infarcts diminishes in size (→ hyposplenism by 9–12 months of age). Splenic function is impaired.
  - Gastrointestinal: gallstones common (2° to chronic haemolysis). Derangement of LFTs (multifactorial e.g. Fe overload, hepatitis B and C).
  - CVS: murmurs (anaemia), tachycardia.
  - Eye: proliferative retinopathy (in 30%; more common in SC disease, affecting ~50% adults), blindness (esp. HbSC), retinal artery occlusion, retinal detachment.
  - CNS: convulsions, TIAs or strokes, sensory hearing loss (usually temporary). Start transfusion programme to maintain HbS <30%. Consider chelation therapy after transfusion for 1 year.
  - Psychosocial: depression, socially withdrawn.

Laboratory features

Anaemia usual (Hb ~6.0–9.0g/dL in HbSS although may be much lower; HbSC have higher Hb). Reticulocytes may be ↑ (to ~10–20%) reflecting intense BM production of RBCs. Anaemic symptoms usually mild since HbS has reduced O_2 affinity with O_2 dissociation curve shifted to the right. MCV and MCH are normal, unless also thalassaemia trait (25% cases). Blood film shows marked variation in red cell size with prominent sickle cells and target cells; basophilic stippling, Howell–Jolly bodies, and Pappenheimer bodies (hyposplenic features after infancy). Sickle cell test (e.g. sodium dithionate) will be positive. Does *not* discriminate between sickle cell trait and homozygous disease. Serum bilirubin often ↑ (due to excess red cell breakdown).

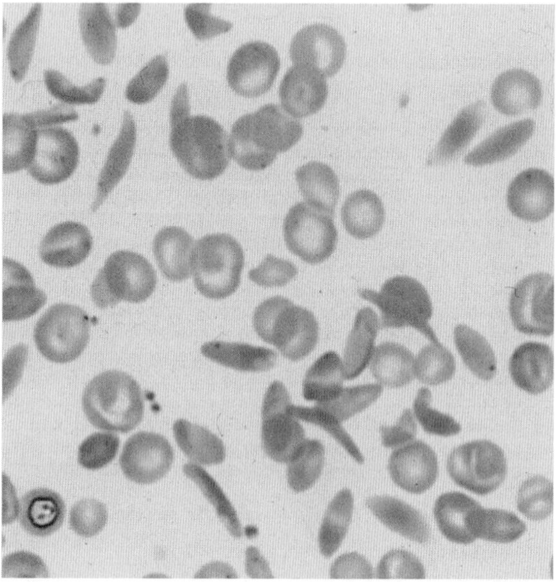

Fig. 2.7 Blood film in homozygous sickle cell disease. Note the elongated (sickled) red cells.

Confirmatory tests

Hb electrophoresis or HPLC shows 80–99% HbS with no normal HbA. HbF may be elevated to about 15%. Parents will have features of sickle cell trait.

Screening

In at-risk groups pregnant woman should be screened early in pregnancy. If both parents of fetus are carriers offer prenatal/neonatal diagnosis. Affected babies should be given penicillin daily and be immunised against *S. pneumoniae*, *H. influenzae* type b, and *Neisseria meningitidis*.

Prenatal diagnosis

May be carried out from first trimester (chorionic villus sampling from 10 weeks' gestation) or second trimester (fetal blood sampling from umbilical cord or trophoblast DNA from amniotic fluid). DNA may be analysed using restriction enzyme digestion with *Mst* II and Southern blotting, RFLP analysis assessing both parental and fetal DNA haplotypes, oligonucleotide probes specific for sickle globin point mutation, or PCR amplification followed by restriction enzyme digestion of amplified DNA. ARMS (amplification refractory mutation system) PCR is useful in ambiguous cases. In late pregnancy fetal blood sampling may be used to confirm diagnosis.

Neonatal screening programme

Aims to reduce routine childhood morbidity and mortality from sickle cell disorders where early intervention may be beneficial. Dry blood spots used with HPLC or IEF.

Management

- *General*—lifelong prophylactic penicillin 250mg bd PO with folate replacement. Pneumovax II vaccination advisable.
- *Management* during pregnancy and anaesthesia—anaesthesia should be carried out by experienced anaesthetist who is aware of complications of SCA. If the patient is unwell consider transfusion to Hb of 10g/dL, but generally transfusion not necessary.
- *Management of crises* ►► 📖 see Haematological emergencies: sickle crisis p. 658.

Management of painful crises

- 60% of patients with sickle cell disease suffer painful crises.
- May be triggered by infection, temperature changes (hot *or* cold), or stress.
- Regular parenteral opiates are useful initially but should be tapered and replaced with oral analgesia.
- Red cell transfusion is generally not required although is indicated in sudden anaemia in children (e.g. splenic sequestration), parvovirus B19 infection (with associated transient red cell aplasia), or acute chest syndrome (hypoxia).

References

1. 🖫 www.bcshguidelines.com/pdf/SICKLE.V4_0802.
2. Bonaventura, C., *et al.* (2002). Heme redox properties of S-nitrosated hemoglobin A0 and hemoglobin S: implications for interactions of nitric oxide with normal and sickle red blood cells. *J Biol Chem*, **277**, 14557–63.
3. Lottenberg, R., *et al.* (2005). An evidence-based approach to the treatment of adults with sickle cell disease. *Hematology Am Soc Hematol Educ Program*, 58–65.
4. Rees, D.C., *et al.* (2003). Guidelines for the management of the acute painful crisis in sickle cell disease. *Br J Haematol*, **120**, 744–52.
5. Steinberg, M.H. (1999). Management of sickle cell disease. *N Engl J Med*, **340**, 1021–30.

HbS—new therapies

Agents that elevate HbF levels

It has been recognized for some time that ↑ HbF levels ameliorate β thalassaemia and sickle cell disease. HbF reduces HbS polymerization and hence sickling. HbF level of >10% reduces episodes of aseptic necrosis; levels >20% HbF are associated with fewer painful crises.

Hydroxycarbamide—several studies have shown that baboons treated with cytosine arabinoside showed ↑ HbF. Similar results obtained with hydroxycarbamide which has advantages over other cytotoxics e.g. low risk of 2° malignancy with prolonged use. Hydroxycarbamide has been evaluated in a large number of clinical trials. Effects are dose-dependent and the highest elevation of HbF is seen at myelosuppressive doses. Mechanism of action: initially believed to ameliorate crises through elevation of HbF levels but it reduces the number of neutrophils, monocytes, and reticulocytes and this may be contributory. Need to monitor FBCs regularly (cytopenias).

Erythropoietin—leads to ↑ HbF but not widely used in the management of haemoglobinopathies. Evidence suggests that rHuEPO provides an additive effect when alternated with hydroxcarbamide. Dose required is high (1000–3000iu/kg × 3d/week) with co-administration of Fe supplements.

5-azacytidine—inhibitor of methyltransferase, enzyme responsible for methylation of newly incorporated cytosines in DNA. Preventing methylation of the γ globin gene leads to ↑ HbF. ►►Risk of developing 2° malignancy.

Short chain fatty acids—butyrate analogues are potent inducers of haematopoietic differentiation. Elevated concentrations of butyrate and other fatty acids in diabetic mothers is responsible for the persistently elevated HbF in the neonates born to such mothers. Initial studies involving the use of butyrate to increase HbF levels in patients with SCA appeared promising but subsequent studies have been disappointing. Mechanism of action: modulate gene expression by interacting with transcriptionally active elements of genes.

Membrane-active drugs—these help reverse cellular dehydration (sickle Hb polymerization is concentration-dependent). Some drugs block cation transport channels. Includes clotrimazole and magnesium salts.

BM transplantation—sibling donor transplants for sickle cell disease have been carried out in a number of centres. Since the mortality from sickle cell disease has dropped over recent years from 15%→1%, and with the advent of hydroxyurea therapy, there is a less compelling argument for BMT in sickle cell disease. Consider if recurrent complications or requirement for transfusion programme e.g. cerebrovascular disease.

Gene therapy—potentially curative but experimental. Globin gene transfer has been attempted with variable results. Expression of exogenous gene has been at levels too low to be of benefit.

1. Brugnara, C., *et al.* (1993). Inhibition of Ca(2+)-dependent K+ transport and cell dehydration in sickle erythrocytes by clotrimazole and other imidazole derivatives. *J Clin Invest*, **92**, 520–6.
2. Charache, S. et al (1995). Effect of hydroxyurea on the frequency of painful crises in sickle cell anemia. Investigators of the Multicenter Study of Hydroxyurea in Sickle Cell Anemia. *N Engl J Med*, **332**, 1317–22.
3. Charache, S., *et al.* (1996). Hydroxyurea and sickle cell anemia. Clinical utility of a myelosuppressive "switching" agent. The Multicenter Study of Hydroxyurea in Sickle Cell Anemia. Medicine (Baltimore), **75**, 300–26.
4. Platt, O.S. *et al.* (1994). Mortality in sickle cell disease. Life expectancy and risk factors for early death. *N Engl J Med*, **330**, 1639–44.

Sickle cell trait (HbAS)

Asymptomatic carriers have one abnormal β^S gene and one normal β gene (with 30 million carriers worldwide).

Clinical features

- Carriers are not anaemic and have no abnormal clinical features.
- Sickling rare unless O_2 saturation falls <40%. Crises have been reported with severe hypoxia (anaesthesia, unpressurized aircraft).
- Occasional renal papillary necrosis, haematuria, and inability to concentrate the urine in adults.

Laboratory features

- Hb, MCV, MCH, and MCHC normal (unless also α thalassaemia trait).
- HbS level 40–55% (if <40% then also α thalassaemia trait).
- Film may be normal or show microcytes and target cells.
- Sickle cell test will be +ve (HbSS and HbAS).

Carrier detection

Neither FBC nor film can be used for diagnostic purposes. Detection of the carrier state relies on Hb electrophoresis or HPLC (HbA ~50%; HbS ~50%).

►► Care needed during anaesthesia (*avoid hypoxia*).

Other sickling disorders

HbSC

Milder than SCA but resembles it. Patients have fewer and milder crises. Retinal damage (microvascular, proliferative retinopathy) and blindness are major complications (30–35%). Arrange regular ophthalmological review by specialist. Aseptic necrosis of femoral head and recurrent haematuria are common. ↑ risk of splenic infarcts and abscesses.

►► Beware thrombosis and PE especially in pregnancy.

Clinical

Mild anaemia (Hb 8–14g/dL) and splenomegaly common. Less haemolysis, fewer painful crises, fewer infections, and less vaso-occlusive disease than SCA. Growth and development normal. Lifespan normal. Pregnancy may be hazardous.

Film

Prominent target cells with fewer NRBC than seen in SCA. Howell–Jolly and Pappenheimer bodies (hyposplenism). Occasional C crystals may be seen.

Diagnosis

Hb electrophoresis and family studies. MCV and MCH are much lower than in HbSS.

HbSD, $HbSO_{Arab}$

Milder than HbSS. Both rare. Interactions of these globins with HbS results in reduced polymerisation. $HbD_{Punjab}^{(\beta 121\ glu \rightarrow gln)}$ and $HbO_{Arab}^{(\beta 121\ glu \rightarrow lys)}$ cause little disease on their own although there may be mild haemolysis in the homozygote. These haemoglobins cause sickle cell disease when present with HbS.

HbS/α thalassaemia

Common in Black individuals. Lessens severity of SCA by reducing the concentration of Hb in red cells.

HbS/β thalassaemia

Caused by inheritance of β^S from one parent and β thalassaemia from the other. Sickle/β° thalassaemia is severe since no normal β globin chains are produced. Sickle/β^+ thalassaemia is much milder having β globin in 5–15% of their Hb. Microcytosis and splenomegaly are characteristic. Family screening will confirm microcytosis and ↑ HbA_2 in one of the parents.

Management

Essentially as for HbSS with prompt treatment of crises (📖 p.658).

Other haemoglobinopathies

HbC disease (β6 glu→lys)

West Africa. Patients have benign compensated haemolysis. Development is normal, splenomegaly is common. Gallstones are recognized complication. The Hb may be mildly ↓. MCV and MCH ↓ and reticulocytes ↑. Blood film shows prominent target cells and occasional HbC crystals. Hb electrophoresis shows mainly HbC with some HbF. HbA is absent. Red cells said to be 'stiff'. Care with anaesthesia.

HbC trait (β6 glu→lys)

Asymptomatic. Hb is ↔. Film may be normal or show presence of target cells. HbC 30–40%.

HbD disease (e.g. D_{Punjab} β121 glu→lys)

Found in North West India, Pakistan, and Iran. Film shows target cells.

HbD trait (e.g. D_{Punjab} β121 glu→gln)

Of little consequence other than interaction with HbS. Hb and MCV ↔. Film normal or shows target cells.

HbE disease (β26 glu→lys)

South East Asia (commonest Hb variant), India, Burma, and Thailand. This Hb is moderately unstable when exposed to oxidants. May produce thalassaemic syndrome when mRNA splice mutants. There is mild anaemia, MCV and MCH ↓, reticulocytes ↔. Film shows target cells, hypochromic and microcytic red cells. There are few symptoms; underlying compensated haemolysis, mild jaundice. Liver and spleen size are normal. Treatment is not usually required.

HbE trait (β26 glu→lys)

Asymptomatic. Indices similar to β thalassaemia trait. Hb usually ↔.

HbE/β thalassaemia

Compound heterozygote. Clinical picture variable from thalassaemia minor to thalassaemia major. Most patients have moderate disease. Hb is lower than HbE; MCV and MCH are lower than Hb E trait. Reticulocytes are raised slightly at 4–6%.

Unstable haemoglobins

Congenital Heinz body haemolytic anaemia caused by point mutations in globin genes. Hb precipitates in red blood cells when there is oxidative stress → Heinz bodies. In normal Hb there are non-covalent bonds maintaining the Hb structure; loss of bonds leads to Hb denaturation and precipitation. Production of Heinz bodies leads to less deformable red cells with reduced lifespan. The degree of haemolysis varies depending on the mutation, but may be more severe if there is fever or if the patient ingests oxidant drugs.

Predominantly autosomal dominant; most patients are heterozygotes. Mainly affects β globin chain e.g. HbHammersmith (mutation involves amino acid in contact with haem pocket); HbBristol (replacement of non-polar by polar amino acid with distortion of protein).

Table 2.9 Examples of unstable haemoglobins

Haemoglobin	Mutation
Hb Koln	β_{98} val → met
Hb Zurich	β_{63} his → arg
Hb Tacoma	β_{30} arg → ser
Hb Bibba	β_{136} leu → pro
Hb Hammersmith	β_{42} phe → ser
Hb Bristol	β_{67} val → asp
Hb Poole	β_{130} trp → gly

Clinical features

- Well compensated haemolysis.
- Hb may be ↔ if unstable Hb has high O_2 affinity.
- Haemolysis exacerbated by infection and oxidant drugs.
- Jaundice and splenomegaly are common.
- Some Hbs are unstable *in vitro* but show little haemolysis *in vivo*.

Investigation

- Hb ↔ or ↓.
- MCV often ↓.
- Film shows hypochromic RBCs, polychromatic RBCs, basophilic stippling.
- Heinz bodies seen post-splenectomy.
- Reticulocytes are ↑.
- Demonstrate unstable Hb using e.g. heat or isopropanol stability tests.
- Electrophoresis may be normal.
- Brilliant cresyl blue will stain Heinz bodies—falsely +ve in neonate due to high HbF levels.
- Estimation of P_{50} may be helpful.
- DNA analysis of value in some cases.

Thalassaemias

Arise as a result of diminished or absent production of one or more globin chains. Net result is imbalanced globin chain production. Globin chains in excess form tetramers and precipitate within RBCs leading to chronic haemolysis in BM and peripheral blood. Occur at high frequency in parts of Africa, the Mediterranean, Middle East, India, and Asia. Found in high frequency in areas where malaria is endemic and thalassaemia trait probably offers some protection.

Named after affected gene e.g. in α thalassaemia the α globin gene is altered in such a way that either α globin synthesis is reduced (α^+) or abolished (α°) from RBCs. Severity varies depending on type of mutation or deletion of the α or β globin gene.

α thalassaemia

Two α globin genes on each chromosome 16, with total of 4 α globin genes per cell (normal person is designated αα/αα) making α thalassaemia more heterogeneous than β thalassaemia. Like sickle cell anaemia, patients can either have mild α thalassaemia (*α thalassaemia trait)* where 1 or 2 α globin genes are affected or they may have severe α thalassaemia if 3 or 4 of the genes are affected. α thalassaemia is generally the result of large deletions within α globin complex. High prevalence of α thalassaemia in Africa, Mediterranean regions, Middle East and South East Asia. α thalassaemia occurs from loss of linked α globin genes on one chromosome (i.e. – –/αα). Deletions in α gene of deletions in HS40 (upstream regulatory region) account for most α^{o} thalassaemia mutations. α^{+} results from deletion of one of the linked α genes (–α/αα) or inactivation due to point mutation ($\alpha^{T}\alpha$/αα). – –/αα is more common in Asian individuals while –α/–α is more common in Mediterranean and African individuals.

Silent α thalassaemia (– α/αα)

One gene deleted. Asymptomatic. ↓ MCV and MCH in minority.

α thalassaemia trait (αα/– – or –α/– α)

Asymptomatic carrier—recognized once other causes of microcytic anaemia are excluded (e.g. Fe deficiency). Hb may be ↔ or minimally ↓. MCV and MCH are ↓. Absence of splenomegaly or other clinical findings. Requires no therapy.

Haemoglobin H disease (– –/– α)

Three α genes deleted; only one functioning copy of the α globin gene/cell. Clinical features variable. May be moderate anaemia with Hb 8.0–9.0g/dL. MCV and MCH are ↓. Hepatosplenomegaly, chronic leg ulceration, and jaundice (reflecting underlying haemolysis). Infection, drug treatment, and pregnancy may worsen anaemia.

Blood film shows hypochromia, target cells, NRBC and ↑ reticulocytes. Brilliant cresyl blue stain will show HbH inclusions (tetramers of β globin, β_4, that have polymerized due to lack of α chains). Hb pattern consists of 2–40% HbH (β_4) with some HbA, A_2 and F.

Treatment

Not usually required but prompt treatment of infection advisable. Give regular folic acid especially when pregnant. Splenectomy of value in some patients with HbH disease. Needs monitoring and may require blood transfusion.

Haemoglobin Bart's hydrops fetalis (– – /– –)

Common cause of stillbirth in South East Asia. All 4 α globin genes affected. γ chains form tetramers (HbBart's, γ_4) which bind oxygen very tightly, with resultant poor tissue oxygenation. Fetus is either stillborn (at 34–40 weeks' gestation) or dies soon after birth. They are pale, distended, jaundiced, and have marked hepatosplenomegaly and ascites. Haemoglobin is ~6.0g/dL and the film shows hypochromic red cells, target cells, ↑ reticulocytes and nucleated red cells. Haemoglobin analysis shows mainly HbBart's (γ_4) with a small amount of HbH (β_4); HbA, A_2 and F are absent.

β thalassaemia

There are only 2 copies of β globin gene per cell. Abnormality in one β globin gene results in *β thalassaemia trait*; if both β globin genes are affected the patient has *β thalassaemia major* or *β thalassaemia intermedia*. Prevalent in the Mediterranean region, Middle East, India, Pakistan, and SE Asia; less common in Africa (apart from Liberia and some regions of N. Africa). Unlike α thalassaemia, most β thalassaemias are due to single point mutations (>200 identified to date; rarely due to deletions). Results in reduced β globin synthesis (β^+) or absent β globin production (β°). In β thalassaemia major, patients have severe anaemia requiring lifelong support with blood transfusion (with resultant Fe overload). There is ineffective erythropoiesis. The β thalassaemia phenotype is heterogeneous since several factors influence the disease. Recently identified α globin stabilizing protein binds free α chains, blocking production of reactive oxygen species thereby modulating the clinical picture of β thalassaemia in mice. Not yet confirmed in humans. Not obvious at birth due to presence of HbF ($\alpha_2\gamma_2$) but as γ chain production diminishes and β globin production increases effects of the mutation become obvious. Children fail to thrive, and development is affected. Hepatosplenomegaly (due to production and destruction of red cells by these organs) is typical. Children also develop facial abnormalities as the flat bones of the skull and other bones attempt to produce red cells to overcome the genetic defect. Skull radiographs show 'hair on end' appearances reflecting the intense marrow activity in the skull bones.

Investigation and management

β thalassaemia trait

- Carrier state.
- Hb may be ↓ but is not usually <10.0g/dL.
- MCV ↓ to ~63–77fL.
- Blood film: microcytic, hypochromic RBCs; target cells often present. Basophilic stippling especially in Mediterraneans.
- RCC ↑.
- HbA_2 ($\alpha_2\delta_2$) ↑—provides useful diagnostic test for β thalassaemia trait.
- Occasionally confused with Fe deficiency anaemia, however, in thalassaemia trait the serum Fe and ferritin are normal (or ↑) whereas in IDA they are ↓.
- BM shows 6 × the number of erythroid precursors as normal though this is not required to make the diagnosis of thalassaemia major.

Treatment

Not usually required. Usually detected antenatally or on routine FBC preop.

β thalassaemia intermedia

- Denotes thalassaemia major not requiring regular blood transfusion; more severe than β thalassaemia trait but milder than β thalassaemia major.
- May arise through several mechanisms e.g.
  - *Inheritance of mild β thalassaemia mutations* (e.g. homozygous β^+ thalassaemia alleles, compound heterozygote for 2 mild β^+ thalassaemia alleles, compound heterozygotes for mild plus severe β^+ thalassaemia alleles).

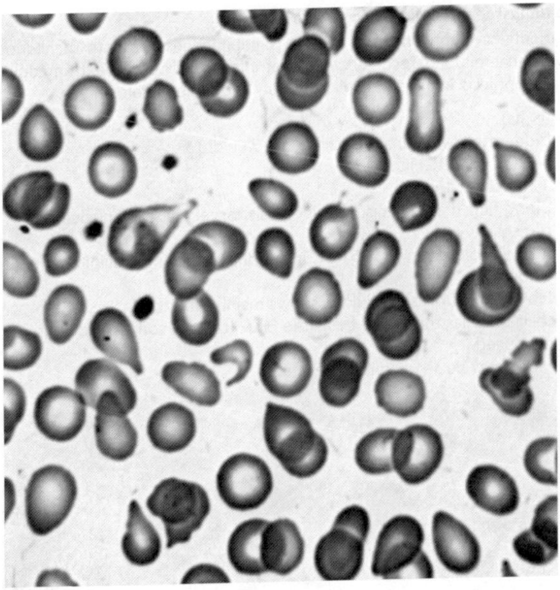

Fig. 2.8 Blood film in thalassaemia trait

- *Elevation of HbF.*
- *Coinheritance of α thalassaemia.*
- *Coinheritance of β thalassaemia trait with e.g. HbLepore.*
- *Severe β thalassaemia trait.*

Clinical

- Present with symptoms similar to β thalassaemia major but with only moderate degree of anaemia.
- Hepatosplenomegaly.
- Fe overload is a feature.
- Some patients are severely anaemic (Hb ~6g/dL) although not requiring regular blood transfusion, have impaired growth and development, skeletal deformities and chronic leg ulceration.
- Others have higher Hb (e.g. 10–12g/dL) with few symptoms.

Management

Depends on severity. May require intermittent blood transfusion, Fe chelation, folic acid supplementation, prompt treatment of infection, as for β thalassaemia major.

β thalassaemia major (Cooley's anaemia)

Patients have abnormalities of both β globin genes. Presents in childhood with anaemia and recurrent bacterial infection. There is extramedullary haemopoiesis with hepatosplenomegaly and skeletal deformities.

Clinical

- Moderate/severe anaemia (Hb ~3.0–9.0g/dL).
- ↓ MCV and MCHC.
- ↑ Reticulocytes.
- Blood film: marked anisopoikilocytosis, target cells, and nucleated red cells.
- Methyl violet stain shows RBC inclusions containing precipitated α globin.
- Hb electrophoresis or HPLC shows mainly HbF ($\alpha_2\gamma_2$). In some β thalassaemias there may be a little HbA ($\alpha_2\beta_2$) if some β globin is produced.
- HbA_2 may be ↔ or mildly elevated.

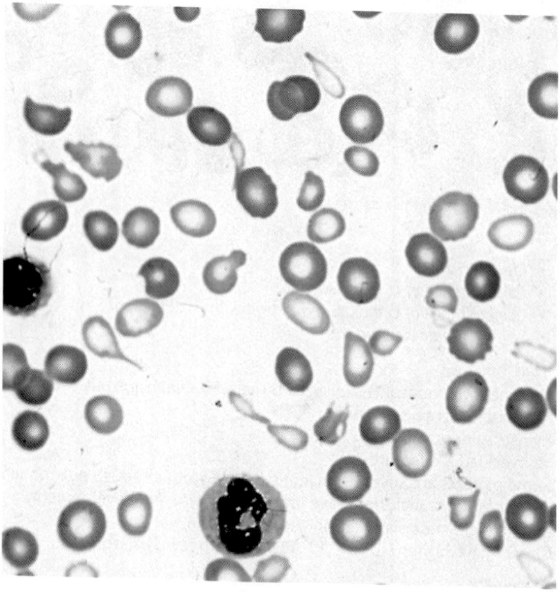

Fig. 2.9 β thalassaemia major. Note: bizarre red cells with marked anisopoikilocytosis

Management

- Regular lifelong blood transfusion (every 2–4 weeks) to maintain Hb at least 9–10g/dL and suppress ineffective erythropoiesis allowing normal growth and development in childhood.

- Fe overload (transfusion haemosiderosis) is major problem—damages heart, endocrine glands, pancreas, and liver. Desferrioxamine reduces Fe overload (by promoting Fe excretion in the urine and stool), and is given for 8–12h per day SC for 5 days/week. Compliance may be difficult, especially in younger patients. Complications of desferrioxamine include retinal damage, cataract and infection with *Yersinia* spp.
- Splenectomy may be of value (e.g. if massive splenomegaly or increasing transfusion requirements) but best avoided until after the age of 5 years due to ↑ risk of infection. Infective episodes should be treated promptly with IV antibiotics.
- BM transplantation has been carried out using sibling donor HLA-matched transplants with good results in young patients with β thalassaemia major. The procedure carries a significant procedure-related morbidity and mortality, along with GvHD (📖 BMT section pp.424–428).
- ↑ HbF levels using 5-azacytidine or hydroxycarbamide should ameliorate β thalassaemia.

Fe chelation therapies

- Desferrioxamine: parenteral, painful, compliance problems.
- Deferiprone: oral, given in 3 divided doses. Side effects include: arthralgia, nausea, other GI symptoms, LFT disturbance, leucopenia (weekly FBC recommended), Zn^{2+} deficiency.
- Deferasirox: new oral chelator, once daily, similar efficacy to desferrioxamine. Side effects include GI upset, ↑ creatinine, cytopenias.

Screening

Screen mothers at first antenatal visit. If mother is thalassaemic carrier, screen father. If both carriers for severe thalassaemia offer prenatal diagnostic testing. Fetal blood sampling can be carried out at 18 weeks' gestation and globin chain synthesis analyzed. Chorionic villus sampling at 10+ weeks' gestation provides a source of fetal DNA that can be analysed in a variety of methods: Southern blotting, oligonucleotide probes, or RFLP analysis may determine genotype of fetus. Moving towards PCR-based techniques; likely to improve carrier detection. Preimplantation diagnosis is performed using embryonic biopsies.

References

1. Dzik, W.H. (2002). Leukoreduction of blood components. *Curr Opin Hematol*, **9**, 521–6.
2. Hoffbrand, A.V., *et al.* (2003). Role of deferiprone in chelation therapy for transfusional iron overload. *Blood*, **102**, 17–24.
3. Olivieri, N.F. (1999). The beta-thalassemias. *N Engl J Med*, **341**, 99–109.
4. Rund, D., *et al.* (2005). Beta-thalassemia. *N Engl J Med*, **353**, 1135–46.
5. Shalev, O., *et al.* (1995). Deferiprone (L1) chelates pathologic iron deposits from membranes of intact thalassemic and sickle red blood cells both in vitro and in vivo. *Blood*, **86**, 2008–13.
6. Weatherall, D.J. and Provan, A.B. (2000). Red cells I: inherited anaemias. *Lancet*, **355**, 1169–75.

Other thalassaemias

Heterozygous δβ thalassaemia

Produces a picture similar to β thalassaemia trait with ↑ HbF (5–20%) and microcytic RBCs; HbA_2 is ↔ or ↓.

Homozygous δβ thalassaemia

Homozygous condition is uncommon. There is failure of production of both δ and β globins. Milder than β thalassaemia major, i.e. β thalassaemia intermedia. Represents a form of thalassaemia intermedia. Hb 8–11g/dL. Absence of HbA and HbA_2; only HbF is present (100%).

Heterozygous β thalassaemia/δβ thalassaemia

Similar to β thalassaemia major (but less severe). Hb produced is mainly HbF with small amount of HbA_2.

γδβ thalassaemia

Homozygote is not viable. Heterozygous condition is associated with haemolysis in neonatal period and thalassaemia trait in adults with ↔ HbF and HbA_2.

HbLepore

This abnormal Hb is the result of unequal crossing over of chromosomes. Affects β and δ globin genes with generation of a chimeric globin with δ sequences at NH_2 terminal and β globin at COOH terminal. Production of δβ globin is inefficient; there is absence of normal δ and β globins. The phenotype of the heterozygote is thalassaemia trait; the homozygote picture is thalassaemia intermedia.

1. BCSH haemoglobinopathy diagnosis guidelines: www.bcshguidelines.com/pdf/bjh809.pdf

Hereditary persistence of fetal haemoglobin

Heterogeneous groups of rare disorders caused by deletions or crossovers involving β and γ chain production, or non-deletional forms due to point mutations upstream of the γ globin gene, with high levels of HbF production in adult life. There is ↓ δ and β chain production with enhanced γ chain production. Globin chain imbalance is much less marked than in β thalassaemia, resulting in milder disorder. There are few clinical effects even when 100% Hb is HbF.

May be pancellular (very high levels of HbF haemoglobin synthesis with uniform distribution in RBCs) or heterocellular (↑ numbers of F cells).

Ethnic differences

- Black individuals with heterozygous pancellular HPFH have HbF levels of 15–30%.
- Greek individuals with pancellular HPFH have HbF ~10–20% (most HbF is $^{A}\gamma$).

Mechanism

Like δβ thalassaemia, HPFH frequently arises from deletions of DNA, which remove or inactivate the β globin gene (*note*: heterocellular HPFH may be result of mutations outside the β globin gene).

Heterozygous HPFH

Anaemia may be mild or absent. Haematological indices are normal. There is balanced α/non-α globin chain synthesis. HbF level ~25%.

Hb patterns in haemoglobin disorders

Table 2.10 Hb patterns in haemoglobin disorders

% Haemoglobin	A	F	A_2	S	Other
Normal	**97**	**<1**	**2–3**		
β thalassaemia trait	80–95	1–5	3–7		
β thalassaemia intermedia	30–50	50–70	0–5		
β thalassaemia major	0–20	80–100	0–13		
HPFH (Black heterozygote)	60–85	15–35	1–3		
HPFH (Black homozygote)		100			
α thalassaemia trait	85–95				Bart's 0–10% at birth
					H 5–30%
HbH disease	60–95				Bart's 20–30% at birth
HbBart's hydrops					Bart's 80–90%
HbE trait	60–65	1–2	2–3		E 30–35
HbE disease	0	5–10	5		E 95
HbE/β thalassaemia	0	30–40	–		E 60–70
HbE/α thalassaemia	13				E 80
HbD trait	50–65	1–5	1–3		D 45–50
HbD disease	1–5	1–3			D 90–95
HbD/β thalassaemia	0–7	1–7			D 80–90
HbC trait	60–70				C 30–40
HbC disease		slight ↑			C 95
Sickle trait	55–70	1	3	30–45	
Sickle cell anaemia	0	7	3	90	
Sickle/$β^+$ thalassaemia	5–30	5–15	–	60–85	
Sickle/$β^o$ thalassaemia	0	5–30	4–8	70–90	
Sickle/D	0	1–5		50	D 50%
Sickle/C	0	1	*	50–65	C 50%
HbLepore trait	80–90	1–3	2.0–2.5		Lepore 9–11%
HbLepore disease	0	70–90	0		Lepore 8–30%
HbLepore/β thalassaemia		70–90	2.5		Lepore 5–15%

Non-immune haemolysis

4 major groups
- Infections.
- Vascular (mechanical damage).
- Chemical damage.
- Physical damage.

Infection
- ***Malaria***—especially falciparum. Causes anaemia through marrow suppression, hypersplenism, and RBC sequestration. In addition there is haemolysis due to destruction of parasitized RBCs by RES and intravascular haemolysis when sporozoites released from infected RBCs. Blackwater fever refers to severe acute intravascular haemolysis with haemoglobinaemia, ↓Hb, haemoglobinuria, and ARF.
- ***Babesiosis***—Babesia (RBC protozoan). Rapid onset of vomiting, diarrhoea, rigors, jaundice, ↑T°. Haemoglobinaemia, haemoglobinuria, ARF and death.
- ***Clostridium perfringens***—septicaemia and acute intravascular haemolysis.
- ***Viral***—especially viral haemorrhagic fevers e.g. dengue, yellow fever.

Mechanical
- ***Cardiac***—turbulence and shear stress following mechanical valve replacement. General features of haemolysis: ↑ reticulocytes, ↑ LDH, ↑ plasma Hb, with ↓ haptoglobins ± ↓ platelets. Urinary haemosiderin +ve.
- ***MAHA***—📖 see Microangiopathic haemolytic anaemia, p.92.
- ***HUS/TTP***—📖 see Thrombotic thrombocytopenic purpura, p.534–536.
- ***March haemoglobinuria*** —with severe strenuous exercise e.g. running. Destruction of RBCs in soles of feet. Worse with hard soles and uneven hard ground. Mild anaemia. No specific features on film. May be associated GIT bleeding and ↓ ferritin (lost in sweat).

Chemical and physical
- ***Oxidative haemolysis***—chronic Heinz body intravascular haemolysis with dapsone or sulafasalazine in G6PD deficient people or unstable Hb (and normals if dose high enough). Film: bite cells (RBC). Heinz bodies not prominent if intact spleen. Haemolysis well compensated.
- ***MetHb***—📖 see Methaemoglobinaemia, p.91.
- ***Lead poisoning***—moderate ↓RBC lifespan. Anaemia mainly due to block in haem synthesis although lead also inhibits 5' nucleotidase (NT). Basophilic stippling on film. Ring sideroblasts in BM.
- ***O_2***—haemolysis in patients treated with hyperbaric O_2.
- ***Insect bites***—e.g. spider, bee-sting (not common with snake bites).
- ***Heat***—e.g. burns → severe haemolysis due to direct RBC damage.
- ***Liver disease***—reduced RBC lifespan in acute hepatitis, cirrhosis, Zieve's syndrome is an uncommon form of haemolysis—intravascular associated with acute abdominal pain (📖 see Anaemia in liver disease, p.41).

- ***Wilson's disease***—autosomally inherited disorder of copper metabolism, with hepatolenticular, hepatocerebral degeneration.
- ***PNH***—📖 see Paroxysmal nocturnal haemoglobinuria, p.100.
- ***Hereditary acanthocytosis***—a-β-lipoproteinaemia. Rare, inherited. Associated with retinitis pigmentosa, steatorrhoea, ataxia, and mental retardation.

Hereditary spherocytosis

Most common inherited RBC membrane defect characterized by variable degrees of haemolysis, spherocytic RBCs with ↑ osmotic fragility.

Pathophysiology

Abnormal RBC cytoskeleton: partial deficiency of spectrin, ankyrin, band 3 or protein 4.2 (leads to ↓ binding to band 4.1 protein and ankyrin). Loss of lipid from RBC membrane → spherical (*cf.* biconcave) RBCs with reduced surface area → get trapped in splenic cords and have reduced lifespan. RBCs use more energy than normal in attempt to maintain cell shape. RBC membrane has ↑ Na^+ permeability (loses intracellular Na^+) and energy required to restore Na^+ balance. Red cells are less deformable than normal.

Epidemiology

In Northern Europeans 1:5000 people are affected. In most cases inheritance is autosomal dominant although autosomal recessive inheritance has been reported.

Clinical features

Presents at any age. Highly variable clinical expression from asymptomatic to severely anaemic, but usually there are few symptoms. *Note*: phenotype is fairly uniform *within* a family. Well-compensated haemolysis; other features of haemolytic anaemia may be present e.g. splenomegaly, gallstones, mild jaundice. Occasional aplastic crises occur, e.g. with parvovirus B19 infection.

Diagnosis

- +ve family history of HS in many cases.
- Blood film shows ↑↑ spherocytic RBCs.
- Anaemia, ↑reticulocytes, ↑LDH, unconjugated bilirubin, urinary urobilinogen with ↓ haptoglobins.
- DAT–ve.

Osmotic fragility test—RBCs incubated in saline at various concentrations. Results in cell expansion and eventually rupture. Normal RBCs can withstand greater volume increases than spherocytic RBCs. +ve result (i.e. confirms HS) when RBCs lyse in saline at near to isotonic concentration, i.e. 0.6–0.8g/dL (whereas normal RBCs will simply show swelling with little lysis). Osmotic fragility more marked in patients who have not undergone splenectomy, and if the RBCs are incubated at 37°C for 24h before performing the test. *Note*: a normal result does not exclude HS and may occur in 10–20% cases.

Autohaemolysis test—since spherocytic RBCs use more glucose than normal RBCs (to maintain normal shape) red cells incubated in buffer or serum for 48h show lysis and release of Hb into solution, which can be measured. In HS RBCs release greater amounts of Hb *cf.* normal RBCs (3% *vs.* 1% in normal).

Cryohaemolysis test, osmotic gradient, ektacytometry and EMA (eosin-5-maleimide) tests have higher predictive value but tests are not specific for HS (e.g. +ve result seen in SE Asian ovalocytosis).

SDS-PAGE can be used to detect deficiency in RBC membrane protein.

Genetic analyses—e.g. DNA-based assays to detect mutations within genes for RBC membrane proteins—not routinely available.

Complications

- Aplastic crisis (e.g. parvovirus B19 infection, but may be any virus); see temporary ↓↓ reticulocytes, Hb and Hct.
- Megaloblastic changes in folate deficiency.
- ↑ haemolysis during intercurrent illness e.g. infections.
- Gallstones (in 50% patients; occur even in mild disease).
- Leg ulceration.
- Extramedullary haemopoiesis.
- Fe overload if multiply transfused.

Exclude

Other causes of haemolytic anaemia e.g. immune-mediated, unstable Hbs and MAHA, which can give rise to spherocytic RBCs.

Treatment

Supportive treatment is usually all that is required, e.g. folic acid (5mg/d). In parvovirus crisis Hb drops significantly and blood transfusion may be required. Splenectomy is 'curative' but is reserved for patients who are severely anaemic or who have symptomatic moderate anaemia. Best avoided in patients <10 years old due to risk of ↑ fatal infection post-splenectomy.

► Remember pre-splenectomy vaccines and post-splenectomy antibiotics (📖 see Splenectomy, p.704).

1. Bolton-Maggs, P.H., *et al.* (2004) Guidelines for the diagnosis and management of hereditary spherocytosis. *Br J Haematol*, **126**, 455–74.

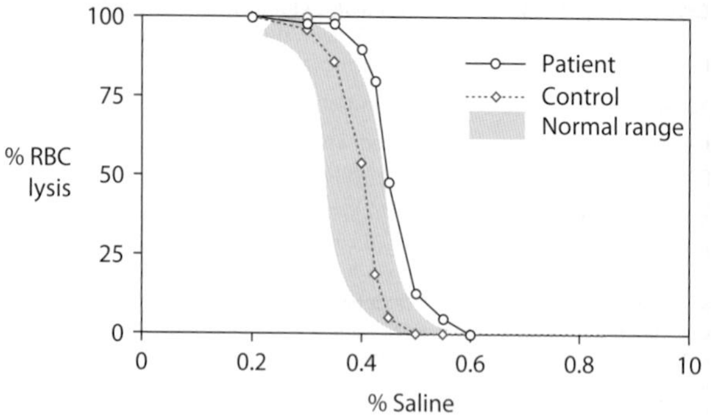

Fig. 2.10 Osmotic fragility assay: note control red cells (red) lyse at lower % saline since they are able to take up more water than spherocytic red cells before lysis occurs.

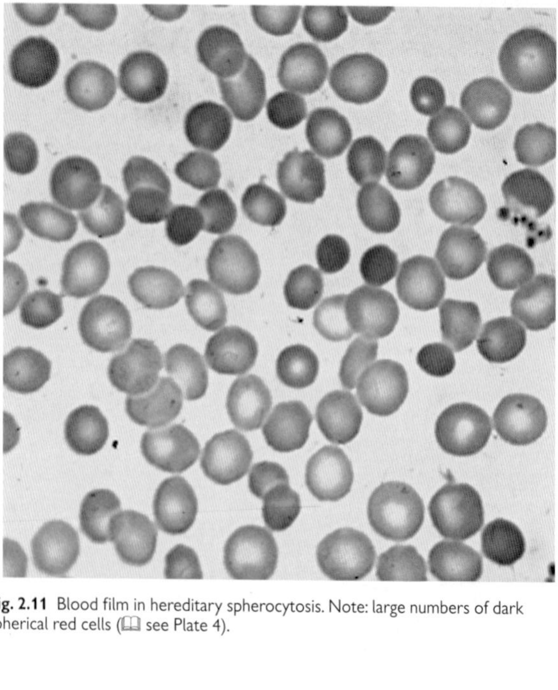

Fig. 2.11 Blood film in hereditary spherocytosis. Note: large numbers of dark spherical red cells (📖 see Plate 4).

Hereditary elliptocytosis

Heterogeneous group of disorders with elliptical RBCs.

3 major groups

- Hereditary elliptocytosis.
- Spherocytic HE.
- South East Asian ovalocytosis.

Pathophysiology

Mutations in α or β spectrin. There may be partial, complete deficiency, or structural abnormality of protein 4.1, or absence of glycophorin C.

Epidemiology

In Northern Europeans 1:2500 are affected. Inheritance is autosomal dominant. More common in areas where malaria is endemic.

Clinical features

Most are asymptomatic. Well-compensated haemolysis. A few patients have chronic symptomatic anaemia. Homozygote more severely affected.

Diagnosis

- May have +ve family history.
- Blood film shows ↑↑ elliptical or oval RBCs.
- Anaemia, ↑ reticulocytes, ↑ LDH, unconjugated bilirubin, urinary urobilinogen with ↓ haptoglobins.
- DAT is –ve.
- Osmotic fragility usually normal (unless spherocytic HE).
- Transient increase in haemolysis if intercurrent infection.

Complications

Usual complications of haemolytic anaemia e.g. gallstones, folate deficiency, etc.

Treatment

Supportive care: folic acid (5mg/d). Most patients require no treatment. In more severe cases consider splenectomy. Remember pre-splenectomy vaccines and post-splenectomy antibiotics (📖 see Splenectomy, p.704).

Spherocytic HE

Elliptical and spherical 'sphero-ovalocytes' in peripheral blood. Haemolysis and ↑ osmotic fragility distinguish it from common hereditary elliptocytosis. Molecular basis is unknown.

Southeast Asian ovalocytosis

Caused by abnormal band 3 protein. RBCs are oval with 1–2 transverse ridges. Cells have ↑ rigidity and ↓ osmotic fragility. RBCs are more resistant to malaria than normal RBCs.

Glucose-6-phosphate dehydrogenase (G6PD) deficiency

G6PD is involved in pentose phosphate shunt→generates NADP, NADPH, and glutathione (for maintenance of Hb and RBC membrane integrity, and reverse oxidant damage to RBC membrane and RBC components). G6PD deficiency is X-linked and clinically important cause of oxidant haemolysis. Affects ♂ predominantly; ♀ carriers have 50% normal G6PD activity. Occurs in West Africa, Southern Europe, Middle East, and South East Asia. >300 variants identified.

Features

- Haemolysis after exposure to oxidants or infection.
- Chronic non-spherocytic haemolytic anaemia.
- Acute episodes of haemolysis with fava beans (termed favism).
- Methaemoglobinaemia.
- Neonatal jaundice.

3 main forms of the disease, those associated with:

1. Acute intermittent haemolytic anaemia.
2. Chronic haemolytic anaemia.
3. No risk of haemolytic anaemia.

Mechanism

- Oxidants→denatured Hb→methaemoglobin→Heinz bodies →RBC less deformable→destroyed by spleen.

2 main forms of the enzyme:

- Normal enzyme is G6PD-B, most prevalent form worldwide.
- 20% of Africans are type A.
- A and B differ by one amino acid.
- Mutant enzyme with normal activity = G6PD A(+), find only in Black individuals.
- G6PD A(−) is main defect in African origin; ↓ stability of enzyme *in vivo*; 5–15% normal activity.
- 400+ variants but only 2 are relevant clinically:
    - Type A(−) = Africans (10% enzyme activity).
    - Mediterranean (with 1–3% activity).

Drug-induced haemolysis in G6PD deficiency

- Begins 1–3d after ingestion of drug.
- Anaemia most severe 7–10d after ingestion.
- Associated with low back and abdominal pain.
- Urine becomes dark (black sometimes).
- Red cells develop Heinz body inclusions (cleared later by spleen).
- Haemolysis is typically self-limiting.
- Implicated drugs shown in Table 2.11.
- But heterogeneous; variable sensitivity to drugs.
- Risk and severity are dose related.

Haemolysis due to infection and fever
- 1–2d after onset of fever
- Mild anaemia develops.
- Commonly seen in pneumonic illnesses.

Favism
- Hours/days after ingestion of fava beans (broad beans).
- Beans contain oxidants vicine and convicine→free radicals→oxidise glutathione.
- Urine becomes red or very dark.
- Shock may develop—***may be fatal***.

Table 2.11 Risk of haemolysis in G6PD-deficient individuals

Definite risk	Possible risk
Antmalarial drugs	Aspirin (1g/d acceptable in most cases)
Primaquine	Chloroquine
Pamaquine (not available in UK)	Probenecid
	Quinine and quinidine (acceptable in acute malaria)
Analgesic drugs	
Aspirin	
Phenacetin	
Others	
Dapsone	
Methylthioninium chloride (methylene blue)	
Nitrofurantoin	
4-quinolones (e.g.ciprofloxacin, nalidixic acid)	
Sulphonamides (e.g. co-trimoxazole)	

Neonatal jaundice
- May develop kernicterus (possible permanent brain damage).
- Rare in A(–) variants.
- More common in Mediterranean and Chinese variants.

Laboratory investigation
- In steady state (i.e. no haemolysis) the RBCs appear normal.
- Heinz bodies in drug-induced haemolysis (methyl violet stain).
- Spherocytes and RBC fragments on blood film if severe haemolysis.
- ↑ reticulocytes.
- ↑ unconjugated bilirubin, LDH, and urinary urobilinogen.
- ↓ haptoglobins.
- DAT –ve.

Diagnosis

Demonstrate enzyme deficiency. In suspected RBC enzymopathy, assay G6PD and PK first, then look for unstable Hb. Diagnosis is difficult during haemolytic episode since reticulocytes have ↑↑levels of enzyme and may get erroneously normal result; wait until steady state (~6 weeks after episode of haemolysis). Family studies are helpful.

Management

- Avoid oxidant drugs—see *BNF*[2].
- Transfuse in severe haemolysis or symptomatic anaemia.
- IV fluids to maintain good urine output.
- ± exchange transfusion in infants.
- Splenectomy may be of value in severe recurrent haemolysis.
- Folic acid supplements (?proven value).
- Avoid Fe unless definite Fe deficiency.

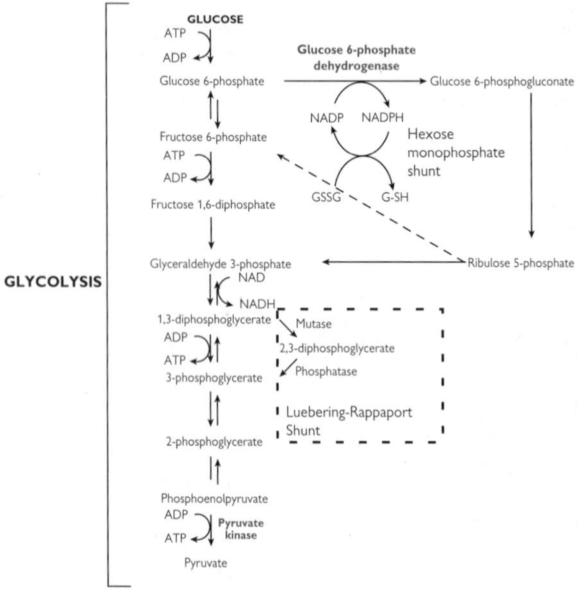

Fig. 2.12 Glycolytic pathway showing key enzymes in red.

1. Mason, P.J. *et al.* (2007). G6PD deficiency: the genotype-*phenotype* association. *Blood Rev* **21**, 267–83.
2. *British National Formulary*

Pyruvate kinase (PK) deficiency

Congenital non-spherocytic haemolytic anaemia, caused by deficiency of PK enzyme (involved in glycolytic pathway), leading to unstable enzyme with reduction in ATP generation in RBCs. O_2 curve is shifted to the right due to ↑ 2,3-DPG production.

Epidemiology

Autosomal recessive. Affected persons are homozygous or double heterozygotes.

Clinical features

Highly variable, with chronic haemolytic syndrome. May be apparent in neonate (if severe) or may present in later life.

Diagnosis

- Variable anaemia.
- Reticulocytes ↑↑.
- DAT –ve.
- LDH ↑.
- Serum haptoglobin ↓.
- Definitive diagnosis requires assay of PK level.

Complications

Aplastic crisis may be seen in viral infection (e.g. parvovirus B19).

Treatment

Dependent on severity. General supportive measures include daily folic acid (5mg/d). Transfusion may be required. Splenectomy may be of value if high transfusion requirements. In aplastic crisis (e.g. viral infection) support measures should be used.

1. Prchal, J.T., *et al.* (2005). Red cell enzymes. *Hematology Am Soc Hematol Educ Program*, 19–23.
2. Zanella, A. and Bianchi, P. (2000). Red cell pyruvate kinase deficiency: from genetics to clinical manifestations. *Baillieres Best Pract Res Clin Haematol*, **13**, 57–81.

Other red cell enzymopathies

Glycolytic pathway

- Hexokinase deficiency.
- Glucose phosphate isomerase deficiency.
- Phosphofructokinase (PFK) deficiency.
- Aldolase deficiency.
- Triosephosphate isomerase (TPI) deficiency.
- Phosphoglycerate kinase (PGK) deficiency.

Epidemiology

Incidence <1 in 10^6. Inheritance is autosomal recessive (most double heterozygote) except for phosphoglycerate kinase deficiency (X-linked recessive).

Clinical features

Similar to PK deficiency although most are more severely affected for the degree of anaemia (glycolytic block results in ↓ 2,3-DPG and left shift of O_2 dissociation curve). PFK deficiency is associated with myopathy. TPI and PGK deficiencies are associated with progressive neurological deterioration.

Diagnosis

- 📖 See Pyruvate kinase deficiency, p.87.
- Non-specific morphology with anisocytosis, macrocytosis, and polychromasia.
- Definitive diagnosis requires assay of deficient enzyme (→reference lab).

Complications

- 📖 see Pyruvate kinase deficiency, p.87.

Treatment

Folic acid (5mg/d). Transfusion may be required (beware Fe overload if high transfusion requirement). Role of splenectomy controversial.

Natural history

Similar to PK except TPI and PGK–TPI present in childhood and cause progressive paraparesis, most die <5 years old due to cardiac arrhythmias. PGK can cause exertional rhabdomyolysis and consequential renal failure. Those affected show progressive neurological deterioration.

Nucleotide metabolism—pyrimidine 5' nucleotidase deficiency

Epidemiology

Autosomal recessive. *Note*: lead poisoning causes acquired pyrimidine 5' nucleotidase deficiency.

Clinical features
- Moderate anaemia (Hb ~10g/dL).
- ↑ reticulocytes.
- ↑ bilirubin.
- Splenomegaly.

Diagnosis
- RBCs show prominent basophilic stippling.
- Pyrimidine 5' nucleotidase assay.

Treatment
Symptomatic, splenectomy is of limited value.

Drug-induced haemolytic anaemia

Large number of drugs shown to cause haemolysis of RBCs. Mechanisms variable. May be immune or non-immune.

- Some drugs interfere with lipid component of RBC membrane.
- Oxidation and denaturation of Hb: seen with e.g. sulphonamides, especially in G6PD-deficient subjects, but may occur in normal subjects if drugs given in large doses e.g.
  - Dapsone.
  - Sulfasalazine.
- *Hapten mechanism* describes the interaction between certain drugs and the RBC membrane components generating antigens that stimulate antibody production. DAT +ve.
  - Penicillins.
  - Cephalosporins.
  - Tetracyclines.
  - Tolbutamide.
- *Autoantibody mediated haemolysis* is associated with warm antibody mediated AIHA. DAT +ve.
  - Cephalosporins.
  - Mefenamic acid.
  - Methyldopa.
  - Procainamide.
  - Ibuprofen.
  - Diclofenac.
  - IFN-α.
- *Innocent bystander mechanism* occurs when drugs form immune complexes with antibody (IgM commonest) which then attach to RBC membrane. Complement fixation and RBC destruction occurs.
  - Quinine.
  - Quinidine.
  - Rifampicin.
  - Antihistamines.
  - Chlorpromazine.
  - Melphalan.
  - Tetracycline.
  - Probenecid.
  - Cefotaxime.

Laboratory features

As for autoimmune haemolytic anaemia, ↓ Hb, ↑ reticulocytes, etc.

Differential diagnosis

- Warm/cold autoimmune haemolytic anaemia.
- Congenital haemolytic disorders, e.g. HS, G6PD deficiency, etc.

Treatment

- Discontinue offending drug.
- Choose alternative if necessary.
- If DAT +ve with methyldopa no need to stop unless haemolysis.
- Corticosteroids generally unnecessary and of doubtful value.
- Transfuse in severe or symptomatic cases only.
- Outlook good with complete recovery usual.

Methaemoglobinaemia

The normal O_2 dissociation curve requires Fe to be in the ferrous form (i.e. reduced, Fe^{2+}). Hb containing the ferric (oxidized, Fe^{3+}) form is termed methaemoglobin (MetHb). MetHb is unable to bind O_2 leading to poor tissue oxygenation. In health metHb should be ≤3% total Hb. May be congenital or acquired.

Table 2.12 Methaemoglobinaemia

Methaemoglobinaemia	
Congenital	
HbM	α or β globin mutation in vicinity of Fe. Fe becomes stabilized in Fe^{3+} form. Heterozygote has 25% HbM
MetHb reductase def.	Due to deficiency of NADH-cytochrome b_5 reductase. Autosomal recessive inheritance; symptoms mainly in homozygote
Clinical features	Cyanosis from infancy. PaO_2 is normal. General health is good
Acquired	Occurs when RBCs are exposed to oxidizing agents, producing HbM. Implicated agents include: phenacetin, local anaesthetics (e.g. lignocaine), inorganic nitrates (NO_2). Patients may experience severe tissue hypoxia. HbM binds O_2 tightly and fails to release to tissues ►► HbM =50% requires urgent medical attention.

Diagnosis

May be history of exposure to oxidant drugs or chemicals. Spectrophotometry or haemoglobin electrophoresis will demonstrate HbM. Assays for MetHb reductase are available.

Treatment

In patients with congenital symptomatic HbM give ascorbate or methylthioninium chloride (methylene blue). In acquired disorder remove oxidant, if present, and administer methylthioninium chloride (methylene blue).

► If severely affected consider exchange blood transfusion.

1. Prchal, J.T., *et al.* (2005) Red cell enzymes. *Hematology Am Soc Hematol Educ Program*, 19–23.

Microangiopathic haemolytic anaemia (MAHA)

Definition

↑ RBC destruction caused when mechanical forces disrupt the physical RBC membrane integrity. Caused by trauma or vascular endothelial abnormalities.

Causes

- TTP/HUS—📖 see Haemolytic uraemic syndrome, p.536; Thrombotic thrombocytopenic purpura, p.534.
- PET/HELLP (haemolysis, elevated liver enzyme,s and low platelets).
- Malignant tumour circulations.
- Renal abnormalities e.g. acute glomerulonephritis, transplant rejection, malignant hypertension.
- Vasculitides e.g. Wegener's, PAN, SLE.
- DIC.
- Anti-cancer and other drugs e.g. mitomycin C, tacrolimus, cyclosporin, ticlopidine, cocaine
- Cardiac—prosthetic heart valves, grafts or patches, aortic stenosis and regurgitant jets.
- March haemoglobinuria.
- A–V malformations e.g. Kasabach-Merritt syndrome, A-V shunts.
- Burns.

Clinical

- Varying degree of anaemia—most severe in DIC, TTP/HUS, and HELLP.
- Often associated with ↓ platelets.
- Blood film shows marked RBC fragmentation, stomatocytes, and spherocytes.
- Reticulocytosis often very marked.
- Signs of underlying disease should be sought.

Treatment

- Diagnose and treat underlying disease.
- Give folic acid and Fe supplements if deficient.
- TTP/HUS may require plasma exchange using FFP.

1. Antman, K.H. *et al.* (1979). Microangiopathic hemolytic anemia and cancer: a review. *Medicine* (Baltimore), **58**, 377–84.
2. George, J.N. (2000). How I treat patients with thrombotic thrombocytopenic purpura-hemolytic uremic syndrome. *Blood*, **96**, 1223–9.
3. Moake, J.L. (2002) Thrombotic microangiopathies. *N Engl J Med*, **347**, 589–600.

Acanthocytosis

Abnormal RBC shape (thorn-like surface protrusions) seen in a number of conditions, inherited or acquired, affecting RBC membrane lipid structure. RBCs develop normally in marrow but once in plasma adopt characteristic shape. RBCs lose membrane and become progressively less elastic.

Inherited conditions resulting in significant acanthocytosis

- A-β-lipoproteinaemia.
- McLeod phenotype (lacking Kell antigen).
- In(Lu) phenotype.
- In association with abnormalities of band 3 protein.
- Hereditary hypo-β-lipoproteinaemia.

Acquired conditions resulting in significant acanthocytosis

- Severe liver disease.
- Myelodysplastic syndromes.
- Neonatal vitamin E deficiency.

Inherited conditions resulting in mild acanthocytosis

- McLeod phenotype heterozygote.
- PK deficiency.

Acquired conditions resulting in mild acanthocytosis

- Post-splenectomy and hyposplenic states.
- Starvation including anorexia nervosa.
- Hypothyroidism.
- Panhypopituitarism.

A-β-lipoproteinaemia

Autosomal recessive. Congenital absence of β apolipoprotein. ↑ cholesterol:phospholipid ratio. RBC precursors normal. Usually obvious in early life with associated malabsorption of fat (including vitamins A, D, E, and K). Sphingomyelin accumulates.

Haematological abnormalities

- Mild haemolytic anaemia.
- 50–90% circulating RBCs are acanthocytic.
- Reticulocytes mildly ↑.

McLeod phenotype

- ↓ expression of Kell antigen on RBC.
- Mild (compensated) haemolytic anaemia.
- 10–85% acanthocytic RBCs in peripheral blood.

1. Cooper, R.A. (1980). Hemolytic syndromes and red cell membrane abnormalities in liver disease. *Semin Hematol*, **17**, 103–12.

2. McBride, J.A., *et al.* (1970). Abnormal kinetics of red cell membrane cholesterol in acanthocytes: studies in genetic and experimental abetalipoproteinaemia and in spur cell anaemia. *Br J Haematol*, **18**, 383–97.

Autoimmune haemolytic anaemia

RBCs react with autoantibody ± complement→premature destruction of RBCs by reticuloendothelial system.

Mechanism

RBCs opsonized by IgG, recognized by Fc receptors on RES macrophages→phagocytosis. If phagocytosis incomplete remaining portion of RBC continues to circulate as *spherocyte* (*note*: phagocytosis usually complete if complement involved).

Seen in:

- Haemolytic blood transfusion reactions.
- Autoimmune haemolytic anaemia.
- Drug-induced haemolysis (some).

Table 2.13 Types of autoimmune haemolyte anaemia.

Warm antibody induced	Idiopathic
	2° to lymphoproliferative disease e.g. CLL, NHL
	2° to other autoimmune diseases e.g. SLE
Cold antibody induced	Idiopathic
	Cold haemagglutinin disease (CHAD)
	2° to *Mycoplasma* infection
	Infectious mononucleosis
	Lymphoma
Paroxysmal cold haemoglobinuria	Idiopathic
	2° to viral infection
	Congenital or tertiary syphilis

Warm antibody induced haemolysis

Extravascular RBC destruction by RES mediated by warm-reacting antibody. Most cases are idiopathic with no underlying pathology, but may be 2° to lymphoid malignancies e.g. CLL, or autoimmune disease such as SLE.

Epidemiology

Affects predominantly individuals >50 years of age.

Clinical features

- Highly variable symptoms, asymptomatic or severely anaemic.
- Chronic compensated haemolysis.
- Mild jaundice common.
- Splenomegaly usual.

Diagnosis

- Anaemia.
- Spherocytes on peripheral blood film.
- ↑↑ reticulocytes.
- Neutrophilia common.
- RBC coated with IgG, complement, or both (detect using DAT).
- Autoantibody —often pan-reacting but specificity in 10–15% (Rh, mainly anti-e, anti-D, or anti-c).
- ↑ LDH.
- ↓ serum haptoglobin.
- Consider underlying lymphoma (BM, blood, and marrow cell markers).
- Autoimmune profile—to exclude SLE or other connective tissue disorder.

Treatment

Prednisolone 1mg/kg/d PO tailing off after response noted (usually 1–2 weeks). If no response consider immunosuppression e.g. azathioprine or cyclophosphamide. Splenectomy should be considered in selected cases. IVIg (0.4g/kg/d for 5d) useful in refractory cases, or where rapid response required. Rituximab (anti-CD20) is emerging as a useful agent for a range of refractory autoimmune disorders, including AIHA. Regular folic acid (5mg/d) is advised.

1. Gehrs, B.C. and Friedberg, R.C. (2002). Autoimmune hemolytic anemia. *Am J Hematol*, **69**, 258–71.

2. Zecca, M., *et al.* (2003). Rituximab for the treatment of refractory autoimmune hemolytic anemia in children. *Blood*, **101**, 3857–61.

Cold haemagglutinin disease (CHAD)

Describes syndrome associated with acrocyanosis in cold weather due to RBC agglutinates in blood vessels of skin. Caused by RBC antibody that reacts most strongly at temperatures <32°C. Complement is activated →RBC lysis→haemoglobinaemia and haemoglobinuria. May be idiopathic (1°) or 2° to infection with *Mycoplasma* or EBV (infectious mononucleosis).

Clinical features

- Elderly.
- Acrocyanosis (blue discoloration of extremities e.g. fingers, toes) in cold conditions.
- Chronic compensated haemolysis.
- Splenomegaly usual.

Diagnosis

- Anaemia.
- ↑↑ reticulocytes.
- Neutrophilia common.
- +ve DAT—C3 only.
- ± Autoantibodies—IgG or IgM
  - Monoclonal in NHL.
  - Polyclonal in infection-related CHAD.
- IgM antibodies react best at 4°C (thermal amplitude 4–32°C).
- Specificity
  - Anti-I (*Mycoplasma*).
  - Anti-i (infectious mononucleosis)—causes little haemolysis in adults since RBCs have little anti-i (cf. newborn i >> I).
- ↑ LDH.
- ↓ serum haptoglobin.
- Exclude underlying lymphoma (BM, blood, and marrow cell markers).
- Autoimmune profile to exclude SLE or other connective tissue disorder.

Treatment

- Keep warm.
- Corticosteroids generally of little value.
- Chlorambucil or cyclophosphamide (greatest value when there is underlying B-cell lymphoma, occasionally helpful in 1° CHAD).
- Plasma exchange may help in some cases.
- If blood transfusion required use in-line blood warmer.
- Splenectomy occasionally useful (*note*: liver is main site of RBC sequestration of C3b-coated RBCs)
- Infectious CHAD generally self-limiting.

Natural history

Prolonged survival, spontaneous remissions not unusual, with periodic relapses.

Leucoerythroblastic anaemia

Definition

A form of anaemia characterized by the presence of immature white and RBCs in the peripheral blood. Mature white cells and platelets are also often reduced.

Causes

Marrow infiltration by:

- 2° malignancy: commonly breast, lung, prostate, thyroid, kidney, colon.
- Myelofibrosis (a primary myeloproliferative disorder, 📖 see Idiopathic myelofibrosis, p.286).
- Other haematological malignancy e.g. myeloma and Hodgkin's disease.
- Rarely, severe haemolytic or megaloblastic anaemia.

Marrow stimulation by:

- Infection, inflammation, hypoxia, trauma (common in ITU patients).
- Massive blood loss.

When due to marrow infiltration, there is often associated neutropenia ± thrombocytopenia. In cases with marrow stimulation there is often neutrophilia and thrombocytosis.

Investigations

- FBC and blood film. Typical film appearances are of ↑ poly-chromasia due to reticulocytosis, nucleated RBCs, poikilocytosis (tear drop forms common in infiltrative causes), myelocytes and band forms, occasionally even promyelocytes and blast cells.
- Clotting screen—where cause is 2° malignancy or infective, DIC may occur.

BM is usually diagnostic

- Hypercellular BM with normal cell maturation, typical of marrow stimulation causes.
- Infiltration with neoplastic cells of a 2° malignancy may be identified as abnormal clumps with characteristic morphology—immunohistochemistry may identify the 1° source e.g. PSA for prostate.
- Increase in reticulin fibres running in parallel bundles identifies fibrotic infiltrative cause—usually myelofibrosis, but may occur with other haematological malignancy.

Treatment

- Diagnose and treat underlying cause if possible.
- Supportive transfusions as required, management of BM failure (📖 see Management of chronic bone marrow failure, p.686)

1. Oster, W. *et al.* (1990). Erythropoietin for the treatment of anemia of malignancy associated with neoplastic bone marrow infiltration. *J Clin Oncol*, **8**, 956–62.

Aplastic anaemia

Definition

A gross reduction or absence of haemopoietic precursors in all 3 cell lineages in BM resulting in pancytopenia in peripheral blood. Although this encompasses all situations in which there is myelosuppression, the term is generally used to describe those in which spontaneous marrow recovery is unusual.

Incidence

Rare ~5 cases per million population annually. Wide age range, slight increase around age 25 years and >65 years. 10 × more common in Orientals.

Causes

Divided into categories where aplasia is regarded as:

- *Inevitable:*
  - TBI dose of >1.5Gy (note: >8Gy always fatal in absence of graft rescue).
  - Chemotherapy e.g. high dose busulfan.
- *Hereditary:*
  - Fanconi syndrome—stem cell repair defect resulting in abnormalities of skin, facies, musculo-skeletal system, and urogenital systems.
  - BM failure often delayed until adulthood.
- *Idiosyncratic:*
  - Chronic benzene exposure.
  - Drug-induced, but not dose related—mainly gold, chloramphenicol, phenylbutazone, NSAIDs, carbamazepine, phenytoin, mesalazine.
  - Genetic predisposition demonstrated for chloramphenicol.
- *Post-viral:*
  - Parvoviral infections—classically red cell aplasia but may be all elements. Devastating in conjunction with chronic haemolytic anaemia e.g. aplastic sickle crisis.
  - Hepatitis viruses A, B, and C, CMV and EBV.
- *Idiopathic:*
  - Constitute the majority of cases.

Classification (Table 2.14)

- According to severity most clinically useful.
- Defines highest risk groups.

Table 2.14 Classification of severity in aplastic anaemia

Severe	2 of the following:	
	Neutrophils	$<0.5 \times 10^9$/L
	Platelets	$<20 \times 10^9$/L
	Reticulocytes	<1%
Very severe	Neutrophils	$<0.2 \times 10^9$/L and infection present

Clinical features

Reflects the pancytopenia. Bleeding from mucosal sites common, with purpura, ecchymoses. Infections, particularly upper and lower respiratory tracts, skin, mouth, peri-anal. Bacterial and fungal infections common. Anaemic symptoms usually less severe due to chronic onset.

Diagnosis and investigation

- FBC and blood film show pancytopenia, MCV may be ↑, film morphology unremarkable.
- Reticulocytes usually absent.
- BM aspirate and trephine show gross reduction in all haemopoietic tissue replaced by fat spaces—important to exclude hypocellular MDS or leukaemia—the main differential diagnoses.
- Flow cytometry using anti-CD55 and anti-CD59 will show lack of both membrane proteins. Ham's acid lysis test is now largely obsolete.
- Specialized cytogenetics on blood to exclude Fanconi syndrome (📖 see Fanconi's anaemia, p.590).

Complications

- Progression to more severe disease.
- Evolution to PNH—occurs in 7%.
- Transformation to acute leukaemia occurs in 5–10%.

Treatment

- Mild cases need careful observation only. More severe will need supportive treatment with red cell and platelet transfusions and antibiotics as needed. Blood products should be CMV –ve, and preferably leucodepleted to reduce risk of sensitization.
- Specific treatment options are between allogeneic transplant and immunosuppression.
- Sibling allogeneic transplant treatment of choice for those <50 years with sibling donor. Should go straight to transplant avoiding immunosuppression and blood products if possible.
- Matched unrelated donor transplant should be considered in <25 years age group.
- Immunosuppressive options include anti-lymphocyte globulin (ALG) ± ciclosporin. Response to ALG may take 3 months. Refractory or relapsing patients may respond to a second course of ALG from another animal.
- Ciclosporin post-ALG looks promising.
- Androgens or danazol may be useful in some cases.

1. Abkowitz, J.L. (2001). Aplastic anemia: which treatment? *Ann Intern Med*, **135**, 524–6.
2. Young, N.S. and Barrett, A.J. (1995). The treatment of severe acquired aplastic anemia. *Blood*, **85**, 3367–77.
3. Young, N.S., *et al.* (1997). The pathophysiology of acquired aplastic anemia. *N Engl J Med*, **336**, 1365–72.

Paroxysmal nocturnal haemoglobinuria

Definition

Rare acquired clonal abnormality of the haemopoietic stem cell leading to chronic haemolysis, ↑ risk of VTE and BM suppression rendering them more sensitive to complement-mediated lysis, most noticeable in RBCs. Cells lack phosphatidylinositol glycoproteins (PIG) transmembrane anchors. Caused by mutation in X-linked *PIG-A* gene.

Incidence

Rare. Aplastic anaemia is closely related.

Clinical features

- Chronic intravascular haemolytic anaemia particularly overnight (?due to lower blood pH). Infections trigger acceleration of haemolysis.
- WBC and platelet production also often ↓.
- Chronic haemolysis may induce nephropathy.
- Haemoglobinuria usually results in Fe deficiency.
- ↑↑ tendency to venous thrombosis particularly at atypical sites e.g. hepatic vein (Budd–Chiari syndrome), sagittal sinus thrombosis.
- Fatigue, dysphagia, and impotence occasionally seen.
- BM failure often accompanies PNH.

Diagnosis and treatment

- FBC, blood film—polychromasia and reticulocytosis (*cf.* AA).
- BM aspirate and trephine biopsy—usually hypoplastic with ↑ fat space but with erythropoietic nests or islands distinct from AA.
- Ham's test (acidified serum lysis) is invariably +ve though non-specific and seldom used now.
- Cellular immunophenotype shows altered PIG proteins, CD55, and CD59.
- Urinary haemosiderin +ve.

Complications

- May progress to more severe aplasia.
- Transforms to acute leukaemia in 5%.
- Serious thromboses in up to 20%.

Treatment

- Chronic disease—supportive care may be satisfactory in mild cases.
- Fe replacement usually required.
- Trial of steroid/androgens/danazol may ↓ symptoms and transfusion need.
- ALG/ciclosporin may be indicated for more severe cases as for aplastic anaemia.
- Acute major thromboses should be treated aggressively with urgent thrombolysis and 10 days of heparin. Long-term warfarin mandatory. Consider warfarin prophylaxis after any one clotting episode.
- Severe cases <50 years should be considered for sibling allogeneic transplant if they have a donor—consider MUD in <25 years age group if no sibling donor.

- Eculizumab—humanized monoclonal antibody against complement C5. Inhibits terminal complement activation. Recent TRIUMPH study showed that eculizumab able to stabilize Hb and ↓ transfusion requirements in classical PNH. ↑ risk of neisserial infection and patients require vaccination against *Neisseria meningitidis* 2 weeks before receiving study drug.

Prognosis

Median survival from diagnosis is 9 years. Major cause of mortality is thrombosis and marrow failure. Molecular genetic basis now established—could be a candidate disease for gene transplantation.

1. Hillmen, P., *et al.* (2004). Effect of eculizumab on hemolysis and transfusion requirements in patients with paroxysmal nocturnal hemoglobinuria. *N Engl J Med*, **350**, 552–9.
2. Hillmen, P. *et al.* (1995). Natural history of paroxysmal nocturnal hemoglobinuria. *N Engl J Med*, **333**, 1253–8.
3. Moyo, V.M., *et al.* (2004). Natural history of paroxysmal nocturnal haemoglobinuria using modern diagnostic assays. *Br J Haematol*, **126**, 133–8.
4. Rosse, W.F. (1997). Paroxysmal nocturnal hemoglobinuria as a molecular disease. *Medicine* (Baltimore), **76**, 63–93.

Pure red cell aplasia

Definition

A group of disorders characterized by reticulocytes <1% in PB, <0.5% mature erythroblasts in BM but with normal WBC and platelets. Incidence rare. May be caused by abnormal stem cells or 2° to autoimmune disease, viral infection, or chemicals. Congenital and acquired forms exist.

Table 2.15 Classification of red cell aplasia

Congenital	Diamond–Blackfan anaemia (DBA), see Congenital red cell aplasia, p.570	
Acquired	Childhood:	Transient erythroblastopenia of childhood (TEC)
	Adults:	1° autoimmune or idiopathic
		2° chronic: thymoma, haematological malignancies especially CLL, pernicious anaemia, some solid tumours, SLE, RA, malnutrition with riboflavin deficiency
		2° transient: infections especially Parvovirus B19, CMV, HIV, many drugs e.g. chloramphenicol, gold, dapsone, rifampin, sulfasalazine
		Recent interest following red cell aplasia in renal patients treated with SC Epo

Clinical features

- Lethargy usually only symptom of the anaemia since slow onset.
- No abnormal physical signs except of any underlying disease.

Diagnosis and investigations

- FBC shows severe normochromic, normocytic anaemia with reticulocytes <1%. WBC and platelets normal.
- BM shows absence of erythroblasts but is normocellular (distinguishes from aplastic anaemia).

Treatment

- Treat underlying cause first if identified.
- Remove thymoma.
- If due to parvovirus B19, try IVIg.
- Assume immune origin if no other cause found and give prednisolone 60mg od PO as starter dose ~40% response. Failure of response, try ciclosporin or ALG or azathioprine.

Prognosis

- 15% spontaneous remission. 65% will respond to immunosuppression.
- 50% will relapse but 80% of relapsers will respond again.
- A few progress to AA or AML.

1. Raghavachar, A. (1990) Pure red cell aplasia: review of treatment and proposal for a treatment strategy. *Blut*, **61**, 47–51.

Iron (Fe) overload

Fe is an essential metal but overload occurs when intake of Fe exceeds requirements and occurs due to the absence in humans of a physiological mechanism to excrete excess Fe. Sustained ↑ Fe intake (dietary or parenteral) may result in Fe accumulation, overload, and potentially fatal tissue damage. Fe absorption is regulated at the enterocyte level by HFE and other proteins.

Timing and pattern of tissue damage is determined by rate of accumulation, the quantity of total body Fe and distribution of Fe between reticuloendothelial (RE) storage sites and vulnerable parenchymal tissue. Fe accumulation in parenchymal cells of the liver, heart, pancreas, and other organs is the major determinant of clinical sequelae.

Haemochromatosis

- Inherited (autosomal recessive) occurring in up to 0.5% population (N. Europe).
- 10–13% N. European Caucasians are heterozygotes.
- Haemochromatosis locus is tightly linked to the HLA locus on chromosome 6p and up to 10% of the population are heterozygous.
- Single missense mutation found in the homozygous state in 80% of patients.
- The gene designated *HFE* is an MHC class Ib gene.
- 2 mutations in *HFE* cause most cases of HH. C282Y is the most important. Most HH patients have this mutation (individuals homozygous for C282Y account for ~90% cases of HH). Heterozygotes do not develop Fe overload providing there are no additional risk factors (e.g. alcohol, hepatitis). The second is H63D; this is less penetrant. A small proportion develop Fe overload. Compound heterozygotes (C282Y/H63D) may develop mild Fe overload. A third (uncommon) mutation is S65C.
- Homozygotes develop symptomatic Fe overload.

Caused by failure to regulate Fe absorption from bowel causing progressive increase in total body Fe. Parenchymal accumulation occurs initially in liver then pancreas, heart, skin, and other organs rather than RE sites. Symptoms do not usually develop until middle age when body Fe stores of ≥15–20g have accumulated. Environmental factors (e.g. alcohol use in males and menstruation in females) affect rate of accumulation and age at presentation. Clinical expression of haemochromatosis is seen 10 × more commonly in ♂. Only 25% of heterozygotes show evidence of minor increases in Fe stores and clinical problems do not occur.

Clinical manifestations of Fe overload only occur in homozygotes and presentation as 'bronze diabetes' is characteristic (📖 see Table 2.16).

Evaluation of Fe status

- Most useful indirect measure of Fe stores is serum ferritin estimation (useful surrogate marker of total body Fe stores). Rises to maximum concentration of 4000mcg/L and may underestimate extent of Fe overload in some patients. *Note*: may be spuriously ↑ by infection, inflammation, or neoplasia.

Table 2.16 Clinical features of Fe overload (homozygous haemochromatosis)

• Skin pigmentation	• Slate grey or bronze discolouration
• Hepatic dysfunction	• Hepatomegaly, chronic hepatitis, fibrosis, • cirrhosis, hepatocellular carcinoma (20–30%)
• Diabetes mellitus	• Retinopathy, nephropathy, neuropathy, vascular complications
• Gonadal dysfunction	• Hypogonadism, impotence
• Other endocrine dysfunction	• Hypothyroidism, hypoparathyroidism, adrenal insufficiency
• Abdominal pain	• Unknown aetiology (25%)
• Cardiac dysfunction	• Cardiomyopathy, heart failure, dysrhythmias (10–15%)
• Chondrocalcinosis	• Arthropathy

- The % transferrin saturation provides confirmatory evidence but no measure of the extent of Fe overload. Useful screening test. If >60% in ♂ or 45–50% in ♀ repeat and investigate further.
- Liver biopsy provides a direct albeit invasive measure of Fe stores (% Fe concentration by weight) and visual assessment of Fe distribution, and the extent of tissue damage. Indicated if LFTs abnormal or serum ferritin >1000mcg/L.
- MRI T2* useful tool for assessment of Fe overload in heart, liver and other sites.
- SQUID (Superconducting Quantum Interference Device) uses high-power magnetic field and detectors that measure the interference of Fe within the field. Linear correlations have been demonstrated between SQUID measurements and liver biopsy Fe levels.

Diagnosis

May be difficult to differentiate haemochromatosis from Fe overload 2° to other causes, particularly that associated with chronic liver disease. Recent identification of *HFE* gene will provide a tool for more definitive diagnosis and screening of relatives (previously performed by serum ferritin estimation).

Management

- Aim to reduce ferritin to <50mcg/L and prevent complications of overload.
- Achieved by regular venesection (500mL blood = 200–250mg Fe) on weekly basis until Fe deficiency develops (may take many months).
- Hb should be measured prior to each venesection and response to therapy can be monitored by intermittent measurement of the serum ferritin.
- Once Fe deficiency develops a maintenance regimen can be commenced with venesection every 3–4 months.
- Avoid alcohol, exogenous Fe.
- Liver cirrhosis and hepatoma risk are not reversible.

Natural history

Cirrhosis and hepatocellular carcinoma are the most common causes of death in patients with haemochromatosis and are due to hepatic Fe accumulation. Cirrhosis does not usually develop until the hepatic Fe concentration reaches 4000–5000mcg/g of liver (normal 50–500mcg/g). Hepatocellular carcinoma is the cause of death in 20–30% but does not occur in the absence of cirrhosis which increases the risk over 200 ×. If venesection can be commenced prior to the development of cirrhosis and other complications of haemosiderosis the life expectancy is that of a normal individual. Reduction of Fe overload by venesection has only a small effect on symptomatology which has already developed: skin pigmentation diminishes, liver function may improve, cardiac abnormalities may resolve, diabetes and other endocrine abnormalities may improve slightly, arthropathy is unaffected.

1. Beutler, E., *et al.* (2002). Penetrance of 845G-->A (C282Y) HFE hereditary haemochromatosis mutation in the USA. *Lancet*, **359**, 211–18.

2. Bulaj, Z.J., *et al.* (2000). Disease-related conditions in relatives of patients with hemochromatosis. *N Engl J Med*, **343**, 1529–35.

3. Olynyk, J.K. *et al.* (1999). A population-based study of the clinical expression of the hemochromatosis gene. *N Engl J Med*, **341**, 718–24.

4. Sanchez, A.M. *et al.* (2001). Prevalence, donation practices, and risk assessment of blood donors with hemochromatosis. *JAMA*, **286**, 1475–81.

Transfusion haemosiderosis

Fe overload occurs in patients with transfusion dependent anaemia, notably thalassaemia major, Diamond–Blackfan syndrome, aplastic anaemia, and acquired refractory anaemia. In many of these conditions Fe overload is aggravated by physiological mechanisms which promote increased dietary absorption of Fe in response to ineffective erythropoiesis. Each unit of blood contains 200–250mg Fe and average transfusion dependent adult receives 6–10g of Fe/year. Distribution of Fe is similar to haemochromatosis with primarily liver parenchymal cell accumulation followed by pancreas, heart, and other organs. Cardiac deposition occurs in patients who have received 100 units of blood (20g Fe) without chelation, and is followed by damage to the liver, pancreas, and endocrine glands.

Clinical features of Fe overload in children who require transfusion support for hereditary anaemia are listed. Similar problems excluding those related to growth and sexual maturation develop in patients who commence a transfusion programme for acquired refractory anaemia in later life.

Features of transfusion haemosiderosis in hereditary anaemia

- Growth retardation in second decade.
- Hypogonadism—delayed or absent sexual maturation.
- Skin pigmentation—slate grey or bronze discolouration.
- Hepatic dysfunction—hepatomegaly, chronic hepatitis, fibrosis, cirrhosis, hepatocellular carcinoma.
- Diabetes mellitus.
- Other endocrine dysfunction—rarely hypothyroidism, hypoparathyroidism, adrenal insufficiency.
- Cardiac dysfunction—cardiomyopathy, heart failure, dysrhythmias (main cause of death).
- Death from heart disease in adolescence.

Management

- Fe chelation therapy by parenteral desferrioxamine is the mainstay of treatment for patients with transfusion haemosiderosis, who remain anaemic. Haemosiderosis due to previous transfusions in conditions where Hb now normal e.g. treated AML, may be venesected to remove Fe.
- Regular treatment is required in transfusion dependent children if they are to avoid the consequences of Fe overload in the second decade of life.
- SC administration of desferrioxamine by portable syringe pump over 9–12h on 5–7 nights/week is a common regimen.
- Ascorbic acid supplementation may help mobilize Fe and increase excretion with desferrioxamine but can cause hazardous redistribution of storage Fe.
- Early and regular desferrioxamine infusion ↓ hepatic Fe and improves hepatic function, promotes growth and sexual development, and protects against heart disease and early death.
- Deferiprone and deferasirox are both oral agents which are being increasingly used instead of desferrioxamine.

Natural history

The prognosis of the underlying haematological condition in transfusion dependent elderly patients may eliminate the need for Fe chelation. In others with a longer life expectancy, IV infusion of desferrioxamine with each blood transfusion may adequately delay the rate of Fe accumulation.

Other causes of haemosiderosis

Dietary Fe overload may also occur as a result of chronic over-ingestion of Fe-containing traditional home-brewed fermented maize beverages peculiar to sub-Saharan Africa, which overwhelms physiological controls on Fe absorption. Fe stores may >50g and Fe is initially deposited in both hepatocytes and Kupffer cells but when cirrhosis develops, accumulates in the pancreas, heart, and other organs. Over-ingestion of medicinal Fe may possibly have a similar though less dramatic effect but is certainly harmful to patients with Fe-loading disorders. The excessive Fe absorption seen in patients with chronic liver disease is associated with accumulationin Kupffer cells rather than hepatic parenchyma. Rare congenital defects associated with Fe overload have been reported.

White blood cell abnormalities

Neutrophilia

Neutrophils are derived from same precursor as monocytes. Cytoplasm contains granules; the nucleus has 3–4 segments. Functions include chemotaxis—neutrophils migrate to sites of inflammation by chemotactic factors e.g. complement components (C5a and C3), and cytokines. Cytotoxic activity is via phagocytosis and destruction of particles/invading microorganisms (latter often antibody coated = *opsonized*). Granules contain cationic proteins→lyse Gram –ve bacteria, 'defensins', myeloperoxidase—interacts with H_2O_2 and HCl→hypochlorous acid (HOCl); lysozyme (hydrolyses bacterial cell walls); superoxide (O_2^-) and hydroxyl (OH^-) radicals. Neutrophil lifespan is ~1–2d in tissues.

Normal neutrophil count 2.0–7.5 × 10^9/L (neonate differs from adult; 📖 Normal ranges, p.800).

Neutrophilia is defined as an absolute neutrophil count >7.5 × 10^9/L.

Mechanisms

- ↑ production.
- Accelerated/early release from marrow→blood.
- Demargination (marginal pool→circulating pool).

Causes

- Infection (bacterial, viral, fungal, spirochaetal, rickettsial).
- Inflammation (trauma, infarction, vasculitis, rheumatoid disease, burns).
- Chemicals e.g. drugs, hormones, toxins, haemopoietic growth factors e.g. G-CSF, GM-CSF, adrenaline, corticosteroids, venoms.
- Physical agents e.g. cold, heat, burns, labour, surgery, anaesthesia.
- Haematological e.g. myeloproliferative disease, CML, PPP (1° proliferative polycythaemia), myelofibrosis, chronic neutrophilic leukaemia.
- Other malignancies.
- Cigarette smoking.
- Post-splenectomy.
- Chronic bleeding.
- Idiopathic.

Investigation

History and examination. Ask about cigarette smoking, symptoms suggesting occult malignancy.

Other investigations

- ESR.
- CRP.

Treatment

Usually treatment of underlying disorder is all that is required.

Leukaemoid reaction

May resemble leukaemia (hence name); see ↑ WBC (myeloblasts and promyelocytes prominent). Occurs in severe and/or chronic infection, metastatic malignancy.

Neutropenia

Defined as absolute peripheral blood neutrophil count of $<2.0 \times 10^9$/L. Racial variation: Black and Middle Eastern people may have neutrophil count of $<1.5 \times 10^9$/L normally.

Congenital neutropenia syndromes

- *Kostmann's syndrome*— 📖 Paediatric haematology, p.593.
- *Chediak–Higashi*— 📖 Paediatric haematology, p.599.
- *Shwachman–Diamond syndrome*— 📖 Paediatric haematology, p.593.
- *Cyclical neutropenia*—3–4-week periodicity; often 21d cycle, lasts 3–6d.
- *Miscellaneous*—transcobalamin II deficiency, reticular dysgenesis, dyskeratosis congenita.

Acquired neutropenia

Table 3.1 Acquired neutropenia: commenest causes

Infection	Viral, e.g. influenza, HIV, hepatitis, overwhelming bacterial sepsis
Drugs	Anticonvulsants (e.g. phenytoin)
	Antithyroid (e.g. carbimazole)
	Phenothiazines (e.g. chlorpromazine)
	Antiinflammatory agents (e.g. phenylbutazone)
	Antibacterial agents (e.g. cotrimoxazole)
	Others (gold, penicillamine, tolbutamide, mianserin, imipramine, cytotoxics)
Immune mediated	Autoimmune (antineutrophil antibodies)
	SLE
	Felty's syndrome (rheumatoid arthritis + neutropenia + splenomegaly; no correlation between spleen size and degree of neutropenia)
As part of pancytopenia	
Bone marrow failure	Leukaemia, lymphoma, LGLL, haematinic deficiency, anorexia
Splenomegaly	Any cause

Clinical features

When severe neutropenia: throat/mouth infection, oral ulceration, septicaemia.

Diagnosis

Examine peripheral blood film, check haematinics, autoimmune profile, anti-neutrophil antibodies, haematinics, bone marrow aspirate and trephine biopsy if indicated (e.g. severe or prolonged neutropenia, or features suggestive of infiltration of marrow failure syndrome).

Treatment

Consists of prompt antibiotic therapy if infection, IVIg and corticosteroids may be helpful but effects unpredictable. In seriously ill patients consider use of G-CSF (need to exclude underlying leukaemia before starting therapy with growth factors). Consider prophylaxis with low dose antibiotics (e.g. ciprofloxacin 250mg bd) and antifungal (e.g. fluconazole 100mg od) agents. Drug-induced neutropenia usually recovers on stopping suspected agent (may take 1–2 weeks).

1. Bux, J. *et al.* (1998). Diagnosis and clinical course of autoimmune neutropenia in infancy: analysis of 240 cases. *Blood*, **91**, 181–6.

2. Dale, D.C., *et al.* (2002). Cyclic neutropenia. *Semin Hematol*, **39**, 89–94.

Lymphocytosis and lymphopenia

Lymphocytes are small cells with a high N:C ratio; some (e.g. natural killer cells) have prominent cytoplasmic granules. Two principal types: B and T lymphocyte. B-cells express monoclonal surface (not cytoplasmic) IgM and often IgD. B-cell stimulation through cross linkage of surface Ig molecules or via effector T cells causes their differentiation into plasma cells. Predominant role is humoral immunity via Ig secretion.

T cells are derived from stem cells that undergo maturation in thymus and express T-cell receptor molecule (CD3) on cell surface. Responsible for cell-mediated immunity e.g. delayed hypersensitivity, graft rejection, contact allergy, and cytotoxic reactions against other cells.

Lymphocytosis (peripheral blood lymphocytes >4.5 $\times$ 10^9/L)

- Leukaemias and lymphomas including: CLL, NHL, Hodgkin's disease, acute lymphoblastic leukaemia, hairy cell leukaemia, Waldenström's macroglobulinaemia, heavy chain disease, mycosis fungoides, Sézary syndrome, large granular lymphocyte leukaemia, ATLL.
- Infections e.g. EBV, CMV, *Toxoplasma gondii*, rickettsial infection, *Bordetella pertussis*, mumps, varicella, coxsackievirus, rubella, hepatitis virus, adenovirus.
- 'Stress' e.g. myocardial infarction, sickle crisis.
- Trauma.
- Rheumatoid disease (occasionally).
- Adrenaline.
- Vigorous exercise.
- Post-splenectomy.
- β thalassaemia intermedia.

Lymphopenia (peripheral blood lymphocytes <1.5 $\times$ 10^9/L)

- Malignant disease e.g. Hodgkin's disease, some NHL, non-haematopoietic cancers, angioimmunoblastic lymphadenopathy.
- MDS.
- Collagen vascular disease e.g. rheumatoid, SLE, GvHD.
- Infections e.g. HIV.
- Chemotherapy.
- Surgery.
- Burns.
- Liver failure.
- Renal failure (acute and chronic).
- Anorexia nervosa.
- Fe deficiency (uncommon).
- Aplastic anaemia.
- Cushing's disease.
- Sarcoidosis.
- Congenital disorders (rare) such as SCID, reticular dysgenesis, agammaglobulinaemia (Swiss type), thymic aplasia (DiGeorge's syndrome), ataxia telangiectasia.

Eosinophilia

Differential diagnosis

Common

- Drugs (huge list e.g. gold, sulphonamides, penicillin); erythema multiforme (Stevens–Johnson syndrome).
- Parasitic infections: hookworm, *Ascaris*, tapeworms, filariasis, amoebiasis, schistosomiasis.
- Allergic syndromes—asthma, eczema, urticaria.

Less common

- Pemphigus.
- Dermatitis herpetiformis (DH).
- Polyarteritis nodosa (PAN).
- Sarcoid.
- Tumours esp. Hodgkin's.
- Irradiation.

Rare

- Hypereosinophilic (Loeffler's) syndrome.
- Eosinophilic leukaemia.
- AML with eosinophilia esp. M4Eo (📖 see Table 4.1, p.122).

Discriminating clinical features

- Drugs—history of exposure, time course of eosinophilia with resolution on cessation of drug.
- Allergic conditions—history of eczema, urticaria, or typical rashes. Symptoms and signs of asthma.
- Parasites—history of exposure from foreign travel, symptoms and signs of Fe deficiency anaemia (hookworm is commonest cause world-wide). Blood film may show filariasis. Stool microscopy and culture for ova, cysts, and parasites for amoebiasis, *Ascaris*, *Taenia*, schistosomiasis.
- Skin diseases—typical appearances confirmed by biopsy e.g. dermatitis herpetiformis and pemphigus.
- PAN—renal failure, neuropathy, angiography and ANCA positivity.
- Sarcoid—multi-system features with non-caseating granulomata in biopsy of affected tissue or on BM biopsy; high serum ACE.
- Hodgkin's—lymphadenopathy, hepatosplenomegaly—BM or node biopsy.
- Hypereosinophilic syndrome—history of allergy, cough, fever, and pulmonary infiltrates on CXR, may be cardiac involvement. Eosinophils on blood film have normal morphology and granulation. Diagnosis on exclusion of similar causes.
- Eosinophilic leukaemia—eosinophils on blood film have abnormal morphology with hyperlobular and hypergranular forms. BM heavily infiltrated with same abnormal cells. Other signs of myeloproliferative disease may be present.
- AML M4Eo—blasts with myelomonoblastic features on BM and blood film (📖 see Table 4.1, p.122).

Basophilia and basopenia

Basophils are found in peripheral blood and marrow (≡ mast cells in tissues). Short lifespan (1–2d), cannot replicate. Degranulation results in hypersensitivity reactions (IgE Fc receptors trigger), flushing, etc.

Basophilia (peripheral blood basophils >0.1 × 10^9/L)

- Myeloproliferative disorders:
  - CGL.
  - Other chronic myeloid leukaemias.
  - PRV.
  - Myelofibrosis.
  - Essential thrombocythaemia.
  - Basophilic leukaemia.
- AML (rare).
- Hypothyroidism.
- IgE-mediated hypersensitivity reactions.
- Inflammatory disorders e.g. rheumatoid disease, ulcerative colitis.
- Drugs e.g. oestrogens.
- Infection e.g. viral.
- Irradiation.
- Hyperlipidaemia.

Basopenia (peripheral blood basophils <0.1 × 10^9/L)

- As part of generalized leucocytosis e.g. infection, inflammation.
- Thyrotoxicosis.
- Haemorrhage.
- Cushing's syndrome.
- Allergic reaction.
- Drugs e.g. progesterone.

Monocytosis and monocytopenia

Bone marrow monocytes give rise to blood monocytes and tissue macrophages. Part of RES. Other components of RES: lung alveolar macrophages; pleural and peritoneal macrophages; Kupffer cells in liver; histiocytes; renal mesangial cells; macrophages in lymph node, spleen and marrow.

Contain 2 sets of granules: (1) lysosomal (acid phosphatase, arylsulphatase and peroxidase), and (2) function of second set unknown.

Monocytosis (peripheral blood monocytes >0.8 × 10^9/L)

Common

- Malaria, trypanosomiasis, typhoid (commonest world-wide causes).
- Post-chemotherapy or stem cell transplant esp. if GM-CSF used.
- Tuberculosis.
- Myelodysplasia (MDS).

Less common

- Infective endocarditis.
- Brucellosis.
- Hodgkin's lymphoma.
- AML (M4 or M5).

Discriminating clinical features

- Malaria—identification of parasites on thick and thin blood films.
- Trypanosomiasis—parasites seen on blood film, lymph node biopsy, or blood cultures.
- Typhoid—blood culture, faecal and urine culture, and BM culture.
- Infective endocarditis—cardiac signs and blood cultures.
- Tuberculosis—AFB seen and cultured in sputum, EMU, blood, or BM, tuberculin positivity on intradermal challenge, caseating granulomata on biopsy of affected tissue or BM.
- Brucellosis—blood cultures and serology.
- Hodgkin's—lymphadenopathy, hepatosplenomegaly, eosinophilia, biopsy of node or BM.
- MDS—typical dysplastic features on blood film or BM (📖 see Myelodysplastic syndromes, p.222).
- AML (M4 or M5) —monoblasts on blood film and BM biopsy. Skin and gum infiltration common, (📖 see Acute myeloblastic leukaemia, p.120).

Monocytopenia (peripheral blood monocytes <0.2 × 10^9/L)

- Autoimmune disorders e.g. SLE.
- Hairy cell leukaemia.
- Drugs e.g. glucocorticoids, chemotherapy.

Mononucleosis syndromes

Definition

Constitutional illness associated with atypical lymphocytes in the blood.

Clinical features

Peak incidence in adolescence: may be subclinical or acute presentation consisting of fever, lethargy, sweats, anorexia, pharyngitis, lymphadenopathy (cervical>axillary>inguinal), tender splenomegaly ± hepatomegaly, palatal petechiae, maculopapular rash especially if given ampicillin. Rarely also pericarditis, myocarditis, encephalitis. Usually self-limiting illness but complications include lethargy persisting for months or years (chronic fatigue syndrome), depression, autoimmune haemolytic anaemia, thrombocytopenia, 2° infection, and splenic rupture.

Causes

EBV, CMV, *Toxoplasma*, *Brucella*, Coxsackie and adenoviruses, HIV seroconversion illness.

Pathophysiology

In EBV related illness, EBV infection of B lymphocytes results in immortalisation and generates a T cell response (the *atypical lymphocytes*) which controls EBV proliferation. In severe immunodeficiency following prolonged use of cyclosporin, oligoclonal EBV-related lymphoma may develop which usually regresses with reduction of immunosuppressive therapy but may evolve to a monoclonal and aggressive lymphoma e.g. after MUD stem cell transplant. In malarial Africa, EBV infection is associated with an aggressive lymphoma—Burkitt's lymphoma (📖 Burkitt's lymphoma, p.198).

Diagnosis—haematological features

- Atypical lymphocytes on blood film (recognized by the dark blue cytoplasmic edge to cells and invagination (scalloping) around RBCs).
- Usually lymphocytosis with mild neutropenia.
- Occasionally anaemia due to cold antibody mediated haemolysis (anti-i)—identify with cold haemagglutinin titre.
- Paul–Bunnell/monospot test for presence of heterophile antibody +ve when cause is EBV but only in the first few weeks. False +ves can occur in lymphoma.
- ↑ bilirubin and abnormal LFTs.
- Serological testing should include EBV capsid Ag, CMV IgM, Toxoplasma titre, Brucella titre, HIV 1 and 2 Ag and Ab.
- Immunophenotype of peripheral blood B lymphocytes shows polyclonality (distinguishes from lymphoma and other lymphoproliferative disorders).

Treatment

Rest and symptom relief are mandatory. No other specific treatment has been shown to influence outcome.

Chapter 4
Leukaemia

Acute myeloblastic leukaemia (AML)

Malignant tumour of haemopoietic precursor cells of non-lymphoid lineage, almost certainly arising in the BM.

Incidence

Commonest acute leukaemia in adults; 3 per 100,000 annually. ↑ frequency with age (median 64 years; incidence 35/100,000 at age 90). Infrequent in children <15 years. 66% are >60 years of age.

Aetiology

Unclear—association with pre-existing myelodysplasia, prior cytotoxic chemotherapy (particularly alkylating agents and epipodophyllotoxins), ionizing radiation, benzene exposure, constitutional chromosomal abnormalities (e.g. Down (older patients) and Fanconi syndromes) and smoking.

Diagnosis

- FBC—usually shows leucocytosis, anaemia, and thrombocytopenia.
- Blood film—usually contains blasts.
- BM aspirate—≥20% blasts.
- Trephine biopsy—to exclude fibrosis and multilineage dysplasia.
- Immunophenotyping to differentiate AML from ALL: CD3, CD7, CD13, CD14, CD33, CD34, CD64, CD117, cytoplasmic myeloperoxidase (MPO).
- Cytochemistry—MPO or SB, combined esterase.
- Cytogenetic analysis—to identify prognostic group.
- Molecular analysis—RT-PCR for *AML1-ETO, CBFB-MYH11*, or *PML-RARA*; FISH in selected cases.

Morphological classification

The French–American–British (FAB) system is based on predominant differentiation pathway and degree of differentiation (Table 4.1). Although superceded by the WHO classification (Table 4.2) the FAB classification remains useful for preliminary classification of a newly diagnosed patient before the cytogenetics result is known.

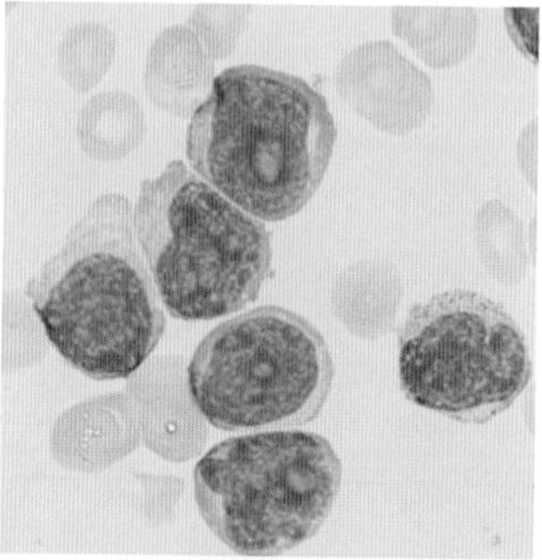

Fig. 4.1 BM showing myeloblasts in AML (📖 see Plate 5).

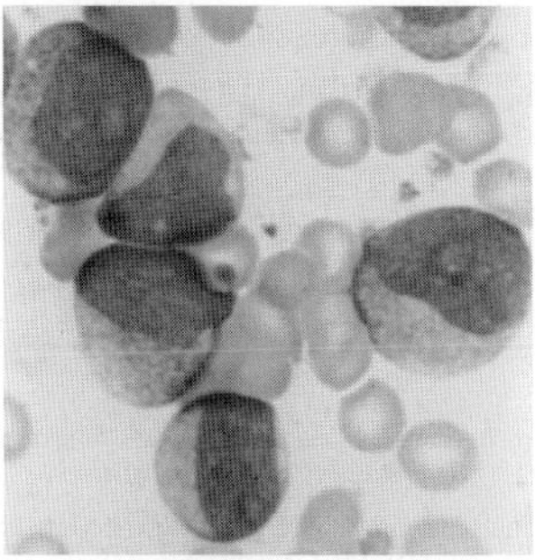

ig. 4.2 BM showing myeloblasts in AML (see Plate 6).

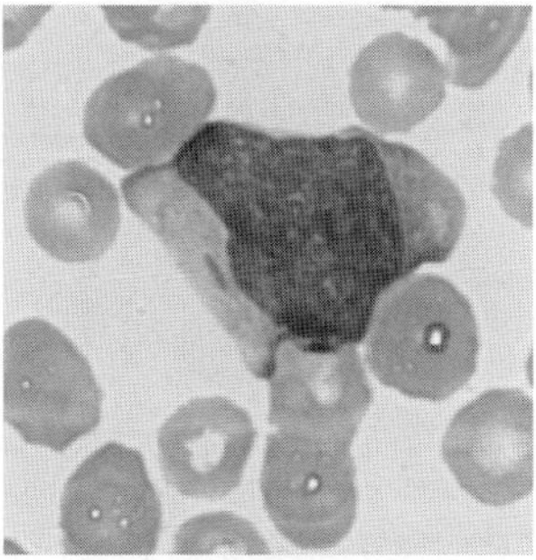

ig. 4.3 AML: myeloblast with large Auer rod (left) (see Plate 7).

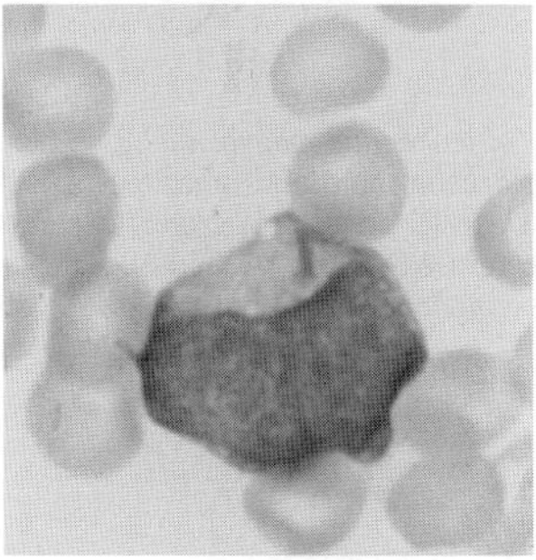

ig. 4.4 AML: myeloblast with large Auer rod (top of cell) (see Plate 8).

Table 4.1 FAB morphological classification of AML [1,2,3]

M0	AML with minimal differentiation (SB and MPO cytochemistry negative but myeloid immunophenotyping; may also express CD4 and CD7); 3% of cases.
M1	AML without maturation (<10% promyelocytes/myelocytes or monocytes; may have Auer rods) 20% of cases.
M2	AML with maturation (≥10% promyelocytes/myelocytes; < 20% monocytes; may have Auer rods; t(8;21)) commonest subtype: 30% of cases.
M3	Acute promyelocytic leukaemia (APL; >30% promyelocytes; multiple Auer rods (faggot cells); t(15;17)) 10% of cases.
M3v	Microgranular variant of APL (high WBC count; minimal granulation; Auer rods rare; t(15;17)).
M4	Acute myelomonocytic leukaemia (mixed myeloid (>20% blasts and promyelocytes) and monocytic (≥20%) maturation; monocytic cells are non-specific esterase +ve; may have Auer rods) 20% of cases.
M4Eo	M4 variant with 5–30% eosinophils; associated with inv(16) chromosome abnormality. 5% of cases
M5a	Acute monoblastic leukaemia (poorly differentiated subtype with ≥80% monocytoid cells of which ≥80% are monoblasts; Auer rods unusual) 10–15% cases are M5a or M5b.
M5b	Acute monocytic leukaemia (differentiated subtype with ≥80% monocytoid cells including NSE-+ve cells with typical monocytic appearance; Auer rods rare)
M6	Acute erythroleukaemia (myeloblasts sometimes with Auer rods plus ≥50% bizarre often multinucleated erythroblasts; erythroblasts often PAS-positive) 3–5% of cases but 10–20% of 2° leukaemias.
M7	Acute megakaryoblastic leukaemia (difficult to diagnose morphologically; often dry tap due to fibrosis; requires immunophenotyping with anti-platelet antibodies or electron microscope analysis of platelet peroxidase) rare.

Cytochemistry

Formerly mainstay of leukaemia diagnosis—SB, myeloperoxidase (MPO) and esterase (chloroacetate and non-specific esterase) stains are +ve in AML and –ve in ALL (<3% blasts +ve). *Note*: M0 and M7 AML are MPO –ve. Non-specific esterase (NSE) is +ve in monocytic cells. Cytochemistry is not essential if 4-colour flow cytometry and estimation of cytoplasmic MPO is available.

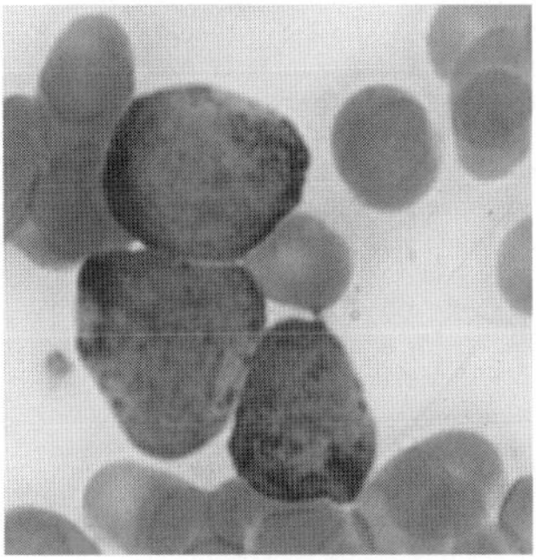

Fig. 4.5 AML: Sudan Blac k stain (dark granules clearly seen in myeloblasts) (📖 see Plate 9).

WHO classification of acute myeloid leukaemia[4]

Although the FAB classification provides a morphological classification of AML the correlation between morphology and both genetic and clinical features is imperfect. The WHO classification correlates morphological, genetic, and clinical features to categorize cases of AML into unique clinical and biological subgroups. The WHO system should be used for the definitive diagnosis and classification of AML.

In the WHO classification the blast threshold for the diagnosis of AML is reduced from 30% to 20% BM blasts (i.e. most patients previously diagnosed as RAEB-t are classified as AML with multilineage dysplasia) and patients with clonal recurring abnormalities t(8;21)(q22;q22), inv(16)(q13q22), t(16;16)(p13;q22), or t(15;17)(q22;q12) should be considered to have AML regardless of the blast percentage.

Table 4.2 WHO classification of acute myeloid leukaemia[4]

Acute myeloid leukaemia with recurrent genetic abnormalities
- Acute myeloid leukaemia with t(8;21)(q22;q22), (AML1/ETO)
- Acute myeloid leukaemia with abnormal BM eosinophils and inv(16)(q13;q22) or t(16;16)(p13;q22), (CBβ/MYH11)(=FAB M4Eo)
- Acute promyelocytic leukaemia with t(15;17)(q22;q12), (PML/RARα), and varients (= FAB M3)
- Acute myeloid leukaemia with 11q23 (MLL) abnormalities

Acute myeloid leukaemia with multilineage dysplasia
- Following MDS or MDS/MPD
- Without antecedent MDS or MDS/MPD, but with dysplasia in at least 50% of cells in 2 or more myeloid lineages

Acute myeloid leukaemia and myelodysplastic syndromes, therapy-related
- Alkylating agent/radiation-related type
- Topoisomerase II inhibitor-related type (some may be lymphoid)
- Others

(continued)

Table 4.2 WHO classification of acute myeloid leukaemia (*continued*)

Acute myeloid leukaemia, not otherwise categorized
Categorize as:
- Acute myeloid leukaemia, minimally differentiated (=FAB M0)
- Acute myeloid leukaemia, without maturation (=FAB M1)
- Acute myeloid leukaemia, with maturation (FAB M2)
- Acute myelomonocytic leukaemia (=FAB M4)
- Acute monoblastic/acute monocytic leukaemia (=FAB M5a/5b)
- Acute erythroid leukaemia: erythroid/myeloid (≥50% erythroid precursors plus ≥20% blasts;= FAB M6) and pure erythroleukaemia (≥80% immature erythroid precursors)
- Acute megakaryoblastic leukaemia (=FAB M7)
- Acute basophilic leukaemia
- Acute panmyelosis with myelofibrosis (=acute myelofibrosis)
- Myeloid sarcoma

Immunophenotyping

Monoclonal antibodies to cell surface antigens reliably differentiate AML from ALL and confirm the diagnosis of M0, M6, and M7 (see Table 4.3).

Table 4.3 Immunophenotypic diagnosis of acute leukaemia

Panel of monoclonal antibodies to differentiate AML and ALL	
Myeloid	Anti-MPO; CD13; CD33; CD45; CDw65; CD117
B lymphoid	CD19; cytoplasmic CD22; cytoplasmic CD79a; CD10
T lymphoid	Cytoplasmic CD3; CD2; CD7
Immunophenotypic patterns in AML subtypes	
Undifferentiated (M0)	Anti-MPO; CD13; CD33; CD34; CDw65; CD117; negative cytochemistry; lymphoid markers
Myelomonocytic (M1–M5)	anti MPO; CD13; CD33; CDw65; CD117
Monocytic (M4 & M5)	Stronger expression of CD11b & CD14
Erythroid (M6)	Anti-glycophorin A
Megakaryocytic (M7)	CD41; CD61

Bain, B.J. *et al.* (2002) Revised guideline on immunophenotyping in acute leukaemias and chronic lymphoproliferative disorders. *Clin Lab Haematol*, **24**, 1–13.
http://www.bcshguidelines.com/pdf/CLH135.PDF

Lineage infidelity

It is sometimes impossible to define a single lineage for leukaemic blasts on the basis of phenotypic marker expression. The expression of markers of more than one cell lineage by a leukaemic cell is termed lineage infidelity and may reflect abnormal gene expression in the clone or abnormal maturation of an early uncommitted precursor. Blasts can display cytochemical and immunophenotypic markers of both myeloid and lymphoid precursors. Up to 50% of myeloid leukaemias may be positive for lymphoid antigens, most commonly CD2 (34%) and CD7 (42%) and this does not appear to have prognostic significance.

Biphenotypic leukaemias

A minority of acute leukaemias (~7%) have 2 distinct leukaemic cell populations on phenotyping and are characterized as biphenotypic leukaemias. Most commonly these cell populations express B-lymphoid and myeloid markers and are associated with a high frequency of t(9;22)(q34;q11), the Ph chromosome. These patients have variable response rates. Some may display 'lymphoid' features such as marked lymphadenopathy and high blast counts.

Cytogenetic analysis

Should be performed in all cases of acute leukaemia. It detects translocations and deletions that provide independent prognostic information in AML.

'Favourable risk' cytogenetics (irrespective of other genetic abnormalities)

- t(8;21)(q22;q22): FAB M2; 5–8% adults <55 years, rare older; fusion gene *AML1/ETO*.
- inv(16)(p13;q22) or t(16;16)(p13;q22): FAB M4Eo; 10% adults <45 years, rare older; fusion gene *CBFβ/MYH11*.
- t(15;17)(q21;q11): FAB M3; 15% adults <45 years, rare older; fusion gene *PML-RARα*. Variants: t(11;17)(q23;q11) fusion gene *PLZF-RARα*; t(5;17)(q32;q11) fusion gene *NPM-RARα*; t(11;17)(q13;q11) fusion gene *NuMA-RARα*.

'Intermediate risk' cytogenetics

- Normal karyotype: any FAB type; 15–20% adults.
- + 8: any FAB type; 10% adults.
- Abnormal 11q23*: >50% infant AML cases; 5–7% adults; fusion gene *MLL*.
- Others: del(9q)*; del(7q)*; +6; +21; +22; –Y and 3–5 complex. abnormalities* plus other structural or numerical defects not included in the good risk or poor risk groups.

'Poor risk' cytogenetics

- –5/del(5q): any FAB type; >10% adults >45 years.
- –7/del(7q): any FAB type; >10% adults >45 years.
- Complex karyotypes (>5 abnormalities*).
- Others: t(6;9)(p23;q34); t(3;3)(q21;q96); 20q; 21q; t(9;22); abn 17p.

Note: This classification is based on the MRC-UK scheme[5]. Abnormalities marked * are classed as 'unfavourable' i.e. 'poor risk' in the scheme used by US Cooperative Groups[6].

Molecular analysis

FISH and RT-PCR methods add sensitivity and precision to the detection of translocations, deletions, and aneuploidy in cases where conventional cytogenetics fails or gives normal results.

RT-PCR detects minimal residual disease overlooked by conventional methods and monitoring by quantification of PML-RARA transcript numbers in APL can identify patients at higher risk of relapse. This may also be useful in patients with t(8;21) or inv(16) as well.

Presence of an activating mutation of the *FLT3* gene with internal tandem repeats (25–30% of all AML patients) is predictive for poor outcome in all cytogenetic subgroups.

Mutations of the nucleophosphmin (*NPM*) gene which normally produces a protein with diverse functions including regulation of the p53 pathway, are found in many cases with a 'normal' karyotype and are associated with a favourable response to induction therapy. Abnormal localization of NPM in the cytoplasm can be detected by immunohistochemistry (NPMc+).[7]

Clinical features

- Acute presentation usual; often critically ill due to effects of BM failure.
- Symptoms of anaemia: weakness, lethargy, breathlessness, lightheaded-ness, and palpitations.
- Infection: particularly chest, mouth, perianal, skin (*Staphylococcus*, *Pseudomonas*, HSV, *Candida*).
- Fever, malaise, sweats.
- Haemorrhage (especially M3 due to DIC): purpura, menorrhagia and epistaxis, bleeding gums, rectal, retina.
- Gum hypertrophy and skin infiltration (M4, M5).
- Signs of leucostasis e.g. hypoxia, retinal haemorrhage, confusion, or diffuse pulmonary shadowing.
- Hepatomegaly occurs in 20%, splenomegaly in 24%; the latter should raise the question of transformed CML; lymphadenopathy is infrequent (17%).
- CNS involvement at presentation is rare in adults with AML.

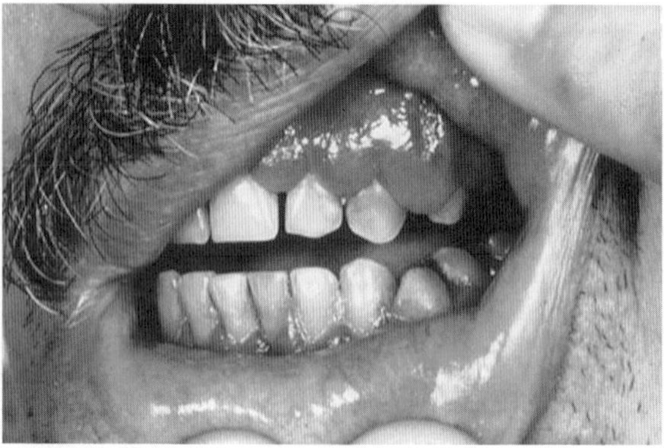

Fig. 4.6 Gum hypertrophy in AML (see Plate 10).

Investigations and diagnosis

- FBC and blood film.
- Infectious mononucleosis serology in a young person; consider CMV and toxoplasma serology.
- BM aspirate ± biopsy (omit if peripheral blast count high and patient considered for palliative treatment).
- BM cytogenetics and molecular analysis.
- Immunophenotyping of blood or marrow blasts.
- WBC usually ↑ with blasts on film—but WBC may be low.
- Hb, neutrophils, and platelets usually ↓.

- BM infiltrated with blasts (≥20%)
- Further recommended investigations—📖 see Acute leukaemia—investigation, 📖 p.668.

Differential diagnosis

- ALL, blast crisis of CML, infectious mononucleosis (in younger patients).

Emergency treatment

- Seek expert help immediately.
- Intensive cardiovascular and respiratory resuscitation may be needed for septic shock or massive haemorrhage.
- Immediate empirical broad spectrum antibiotic treatment for neutropenic sepsis.
- Leucapheresis if peripheral blast count high (hyperleucocytosis; >100 × 10^9/L: 3 × risk of early death) or signs of leucostasis (retinal haemorrhage, reduced conscious level, diffuse pulmonary shadowing on CXR, or hypoxia) —📖 p655. *Note*: **NOT** in APL —📖 p.131.
- Intensive hydration (± alkalinization of the urine) to prevent acute tumour lysis syndrome in patients with a high peripheral blast cell count (>100 × 10^9/L)—📖 see Tumour lysis syndrome, p.684.
- Urgent chemotherapy is almost never necessary (*cf.* APL); can usually be delayed until necessary clinical and laboratory assessments available.

Supportive treatment

- Explain diagnosis and offer counselling—the word *'leukaemia'* and prospect of prolonged chemotherapy are often distressing.
- RBC and platelet transfusion support will continue through treatment:
  - CMV –ve products for potential SCT recipients until status known.
  - Irradiated products for patients treated with purine analogues.
  - Platelet transfusion to maintain count >10 × 10^9/L, unless septic, on antibiotics, haemorrhagic or other haemostatic abnormality (>20 × 10^9/L); in bleeding APL >50 × 10^9/L.
- Start neutropenic infection prophylaxis regimen (📖 Prophylaxis regimen for neutropenic patients, 📖 p.674); prophylactic antibiotics not currently recommended in BCSH guidelines.
- Start hydration aiming for urine output >100mL/h throughout induction therapy.
- Start allopurinol or rasburicase (recommended in patients with WBC >100 × 10^9/L) to prevent hyperuricaemia.
- Insert tunnelled central venous catheter (📖 see Technique, p.690).
- Routine use of growth factors is not recommended.

Chemotherapy[8,9]

Initial aim of chemotherapy is to eliminate leukaemic cells and achieve complete haematological remission (CR), defined as normal BM cellularity (blast cells <5% and normal representation of trilineage haematopoiesis), normalization of peripheral blood count with no blast cells, neutrophils ≥1.5 × 10^9/L, platelets ≥100 × 10^9/L and Hb>10g/dL. Leukaemia is undetectable by conventional morphology but may be demonstrated by more sensitive molecular techniques (when available) and CR is not synonymous with cure. CR may result from a three-log kill from 10^{12} leukaemic cells at diagnosis to 10^9 at CR.

AML treatment consists of two phases:

1. *Remission induction* to achieve CR: usually 1–2 courses of anthracycline-containing combination chemotherapy; assess BM response after 3–4 weeks.
   - Typically daunorubicin 45–60mg/m^2 IV × 3 days plus cytarabine 200mg/m^2/day as 12h IV infusion or divided dose bd bolus × 7–10d.
2. *Consolidation therapy*—essential to reduce leukaemia burden further and reduce risk of relapse; optimum number unknown, usually 2–4; if CR after 1 induction course, 2nd induction course is 1st consolidation; may include 'intensification' phase or autologous or allogeneic transplant if poor risk:
   - Typically each cycle introduces new non-cross resistant agents, e.g. m-amsacrine and etoposide or mitoxantrone in combination with cytarabine at standard or intermediate (9g/m^2/cycle) dose or single-agent high dose cytarabine (18g/m^2/cycle).

- *Enter patient into national or international multicentre clinical trial if possibl***e.** Randomized studies are based on large patient numbers and compare incremental experimental therapy with best treatment arm from previous trials. Allows access to novel therapies, e.g. gemtuzamab ozogamicin (anti-CD33 immunoconjugate).
- Treatment protocols are generally age related; patients >60 years will only tolerate less intensive treatments and rarely transplantation.
- Outline treatment for patients <60 years is 4–5 courses of intensive combination chemotherapy; each followed by 2–3 week period of profound myelosuppression where good supportive therapy is essential.
- Risk stratification using prognostic factors may determine consolidation therapy in some clinical trials or for patients off-study.
- Patients who have resistant disease with >15% BM blasts after course 1 or adverse risk cytogenetic or molecular features should be considered for alternative treatment for high-risk AML preferably within study.
- Major complications are infective episodes which may be bacterial (Gram +ve and Gram –ve) or fungal (*Candida* and *Aspergillus*); less commonly viral (esp. HSV, HZV) and haemorrhage.
- Maintenance therapy has been abandoned in AML as there is no evidence of benefit; in some cases it may be useful in some elderly patients unfit for intensive therapy.
- Effectiveness of therapy assessed by CR rate, relapse free or disease-free survival, and overall survival.

Stem cell transplantation (SCT)[8,9]

- Allogeneic SCT from a HLA-compatible sibling donor should be offered to younger patients (<45 years) with poor-risk AML in 1st CR. Relapse risk falls to 20% from 50% with conventional chemotherapy but transplant-related mortality (7–25%) erodes this advantage.
- Sibling donor SCT is an option for those with intermediate (standard) risk AML. Intensive consolidation is the preferred option for patients with favourable cytogenetics for whom SCT should be reserved as salvage treatment in the event of relapse.
- Some older patients with poor risk AML or beyond 1st CR may benefit from allogeneic SCT with a reduced intensity conditioning regimen.

- Unrelated donor grafts have higher toxicity but may be indicated in patients with poor-risk disease and in 2nd CR.
- Autologous SCT is an option for intensive consolidation of patients (<65 years) with intermediate or poor-risk AML in 1st CR. It has lower procedure-related mortality and morbidity than an allograft but lacks a GvL effect and has a relapse rate of 40–50%.
- Haplo-identical SCT may be undertaken in younger patients with poor-risk AML or beyond 1st CR in the context of a clinical trial.

Prognosis

- 70–80% of patients aged <60 years will achieve a CR with a modern regimen and good supportive care; more intensive induction and consolidation regimens reduce the risk of relapse.
- Relapse risk at 5 years in patients <60 years with favourable risk cytogenetics is 29–42%; intermediate risk 39–60%; poor risk 68–90%.
- 50–60% of patients aged ≥60 years achieve CR with induction treatment (rate drops with each decade) but relapse occurs in 80–90%; a higher proportion have poor risk karyotype, previous myelodysplasia and co-morbidity; treatment-related morbidity and mortality is high.

Prognostic factors

The most important prognostic factors predicting for achievement of remission and for subsequent relapse are:

- Advancing patient age: <50 years favourable; >60 years unfavourable.
- Presence of specific cytogenetic abnormalities (📖 p.125) classifies 'favourable', 'intermediate', and 'poor risk' groups.
- Failure to achieve CR with 1st cycle of induction therapy predicts for relapse.
- Mutation of *FLT3* gene predicts for poor outcome in all cytogenetic subgroups.
- History of antecedent MDS or leukaemogenic therapy: unfavourable.
- Presenting blast count: $<25 \times 10^9$/L favourable; $>100 \times 10^9$/L unfavourable.
- FAB subtype: M3, M4Eo favourable; M0, M5a, M5b, M6, M7 unfavourable.

Management of relapse[8,9]

- 50% of patients in CR after conventional chemotherapy will relapse.
- Most relapses occur in the first 2–3 years; <50% achieve 2nd CR.
- Younger age and longer duration of first CR (> 6 months) are good prognostic factors for achieving 2nd CR.
- ~50% of patients achieve 2nd CR with further therapy containing intermediate to high dose cytarabine (e.g FLAG: fludarabine, cytarabine, G-CSF); <10% survive > 3 years without a transplant.
- Allogeneic stem cell transplantation from HLA-matched sibling may be the treatment of choice for a younger patient (<45) who achieves 2nd CR after relapse. Patients who achieve 2nd CR with chemotherapy should proceed to allograft as soon as possible thereafter. Long term DFS rates of 40–50% have been achieved.
- Matched unrelated donor SCT may be used in younger patients without a compatible sib and can achieve DFS >30%.

- Older patients beyond 1st CR may be benefit from a transplant with reduced intensity conditioning.
- Autologous SCT is restricted to older patients and younger patients without a sibling or matched unrelated donor.
- In younger patients with relapsed AML refractory to 2 cycles of conventional chemotherapy, allogeneic SCT can achieve prolonged DFS in 20–30%.
- Donor lymphocyte infusion (DLI) may be used to treat recurrence after an allogeneic transplant.

AML in the elderly

- Older patients (>60 years) have poorer prognosis, less frequent favourable cytogenetics, more frequent unfavourable cytogenetics, more frequent 2° leukaemia, more frequent MDR overexpression, ↑ resistance to chemotherapy and ↑ treatment-related toxicity.
- Standard chemotherapy regimens may be appropriate in patients <70 years with good performance status (WHO 0–2), WBC $<100 \times 10^9$/L, no adverse cytogenetics or MDR expression. Aggressive salvage for relapse is rarely appropriate.
- Non-intensive chemotherapy in combination with good supportive care may control the WBC, minimize hospitalization and provide optimum quality of life. Low dose SC cytarabine or oral hydroxycarbamide, etoposide, or melphalan may be used in this way.
- In some patients supportive care alone, including transfusion support, may be appropriate.

AML in pregnancy

- Chemotherapy should be avoided in the 1st trimester if possible due to the high risk of fetal malformation. The option of termination should be discussed with the mother.
- Chemotherapy in the 2nd and 3rd trimesters is associated with ↑ risk of abortion, premature delivery, fetal growth retardation, and neonatal pancytopenia. Early induction of labour between cycles should be discussed.
- Single agent ATRA is the safest approach for APL in 2nd or 3rd trimesters; AVOID in first trimester as teratogenic.

Extramedullary disease

- Ranges from gum and skin infiltration in M4/M5 AML to tumour-like masses (chloroma, granulocytic sarcoma) at any site.
- Chloroma associated with t(8;21) CD56+, high presenting WBC but may occur without evidence of marrow or blood involvement by AML.
- Chloroma may be misdiagnosed as DLBC NHL if no blasts in blood; immunohistochemistry will differentiate.
- Treat with systemic anti-leukaemic chemotherapy.

CNS disease

- Occurs in 0.5% at diagnosis; 5% of AML patients in CR relapse in CNS.
- Often followed by BM relapse if not already evident.
- IT prophylaxis shows no benefit in AML.
- Treat with IT cytarabine and systemic re-induction chemotherapy.

Acute promyelocytic leukaemia (APL)

APL (FAB M3) requires a different therapeutic approach that relates to its biology. Risk of DIC prior to and during initial therapy due to release of thromboplastins from leukaemic cells is an indication for urgent treatment. Rapid confirmation of presence of PML-RARA fusion protein (due to t(15,17)) by PML immunofluorescence test or FISH analysis predicts favourable response to all-*trans*-retinoic acid (ATRA) or arsenic trioxide (ATO). The variant PLZF-RARA fusion (t(11;17) 1%) confers resistance.

ATRA should be started as soon as APL is suspected. ATRA induces differentiation of abnormal clone by overcoming molecular block resulting from t(15;17) translocation and reduces the risk of DIC. ATRA alone cannot achieve sustained remission; in combination with anthracycline chemotherapy, 70% of patients may be cured. Current 1st line therapy is ATRA + anthracycline induction followed by anthracycline consolidation.

ATRA syndrome is a complication that may follow ATRA therapy: marked neutrophilia, fever, pulmonary infiltrates, hypoxia and fluid overload. Treat with dexamethasone 10mg bd IV. Discontinue ATRA in severe cases.

Molecular monitoring is useful as persistence of the abnormal *PML-RARA* fusion product after therapy detected by RT-PCR predicts relapse. ATO is a useful agent to achieve 2nd CR in patients with *PML-RARA*-positive APL who relapse but most are consolidated by transplantation.

References

1. Bennett, J.M., *et al.* (1985). Proposed revised criteria for the classification of acute myeloid leukaemia. *Annals of Internal Medicine*, **103**, 626–9.
2. Bennett, J.M., *et al* (1985). Criteria for the diagnosis of acute leukaemia of megakaryocytic lineage (M7). A report of the French-American-British Cooperative Group. *Annals of Internal Medicine*, **103**, 460–2.
3. Bennett, J.M., *et al.* (1991). Proposals for the recognition of minimally differentiated acute myeloid leukaemia (AML-M0). *British Journal of Haematology*, **78**, 325–9.
4. Jaffe, E.S., *et al.* (2001). *Tumours of Haematopoietic and Lymphoid Tissues. World Health Organization Classification of Tumours*. IARC Press, Lyon.
5. Grimwade, D. *et al.* (2001). The predictive value of hierarchical cytogenetic classification in older adults with acute myeloid leukemia (AML): analysis of 1065 patients entered into the United Kingdom Medical Research Council AML11 trial. *Blood*, **98**, 1312–20
6. Smith, M.A. *et al.* (1996). The secondary leukemias: challenges and research directions. *J Natl Cancer Inst*, **88**, 407–18.
7. Dohner, K. *et al.* (2005). Mutant nucleophosmin (NPM1) predicts favorable prognosis in younger adults with acute myeloid leukemia and normal cytogenetics: interaction with other gene mutations. *Blood*, **106**, 3740–6.
8. Milligan, D.W., *et al.* (2006). Guidelines on the management of acute myeloid leukaemia in adults. *British Journal of Haematology*, **135**, 450–74.
9. http://www.bcshguidelines.com/fulltext/guideline.asp?id=5584

Acute lymphoblastic leukaemia (ALL)

Malignant tumour of haemopoietic precursor cells of lymphoid lineage.

Incidence

Commonest malignancy in childhood with the majority of cases in the 2–10 age group (median 3.5 years). Five times more frequent in childhood than AML. Rare leukaemia in adults, 0.7 to 1.8/100,000 annually. In adults, peaks at 15–24 years with further peak in old age (2.3/100,000 >80 years).

Aetiology

Unknown. Predisposing factors are ionizing radiation (AML is more common) and congenital predisposition in Down (20-fold in childhood), Bloom's, Klinefelter's, and Fanconi syndromes. Chemicals, pollution, viruses, urban/rural population movements, father's radiation exposure, radon levels, and proximity to power lines have all been postulated.

Table 4.4 Morphological classification (French–American–British, FAB)

L1	Small monomorphic type—small homogeneous blasts, single inconspicuous nucleolus, regular nuclear outline; commonest subtype in children; <50% of adults.
L2	Large heterogeneous type—larger blasts, more pleomorphic and multinucleolate, irregular frequently clefted nuclei with conspicuous nucleoli; commonest in adults.
L3	Burkitt cell type—large homogeneous blasts, prominent nucleoli, abundant strongly basophilic cytoplasm with vacuoles; associated with B-cell phenotype.

Immunophenotyping

A panel of monoclonal antibodies differentiates ALL from AML (📖 Table 4.3, p.124). A further panel of B-and T-lineage markers and lymphocyte maturation markers subclassify ALL.

Immunological classification of ALL

B lineage ~85%

- *Pro B-ALL*: HLA-DR+, TdT+, CD19+ (5% children; 11% adults).
- *Common ALL*: HLA-DR+, TdT+, CD19+, CD10+ (65% children; 51% adults).
- *Pre B-ALL*: HLA-DR+, TdT+, CD19+, CD10±, cytoplasmic IgM+ (15% children; 10% adults).
- *B-cell ALL*: HLA-DR+, TdT-, CD19+, CD10±, surface IgM+ (3% children; 4% adults)

T lineage ~15%

- *Pre-T ALL*: TdT+, cytoplasmic CD3+, CD7+ (1% children; 7% adults).
- *T-cell ALL*: TdT+, cytoplasmic CD3+, CD1a/2/3+, CD5+ (11% children; 17% adults).

Cytogenetic analysis

- Provides important prognostic information in both children and adults.
- Abnormalities detected in up to 85%. Major abnormalities are clonal translocations: t(9;22), t(4;11), t(8;14), t(1;19), or t(10;14) and other structural abnormalities (9p, 6q, or 12p). With the exception of t(9;22) each has an incidence in the order of 5–10% or less in adults.
- If no structural abnormalities present, abnormalities are classified by the modal chromosome number: <46 (hypodiploid); 46 with other structural abnormalities (pseudodiploid); 47–50 (hyperdiploid); >50 (hyper-hyperdiploid).
- t(9;22)(q34;q11), the Philadelphia (Ph) chromosome, found in 5% of children and 25% of adults with ALL; very strong adverse prognostic factor in both; resultant BCR-ABL hybrid product is same 210 kDa protein detected in CML in 33% but ia smaller 180 kDa protein in 66%; can be used for MRD detection. Ph+ ALL rarely cured by chemotherapy.
- t(1;19) associated with precursor B-cell ALL.
- t(4;11) occurs in 80% of infants with ALL and 6% of adults; fuses the *MLL* gene from 11q23 to the *AF4* gene from 4q21 which can be detected by PCR; all these abnormalities associated with refractory disease and early relapse.
- t(8;14) is associated with B-cell ALL (L3 morphology) and occurs in 5% of cases (dysregulates the *c-myc* proto-oncogene); variant *c-myc* translocations occur in t(2;8) & t(8;22). NB WHO reclassification.
- t(12;21)(p13;q22) is most common specific abnormality in childhood ALL (~25%); associated with *TEL-AML1* translocation and good prognosis; much less common in adults (~2%).
- Hyper-hyperdiploidy (>50 chromosomes) confers favourable prognosis (~25% children; ~5% adults); combined +4, +10 confers a favourable outcome in B-cell precursor ALL; patients with hypoploidy (<46 chromosomes) and pseudodiploidy have a poor prognosis.
- t(11;19) with *MLL-ENL* fusion and overexpression of *HOX11* confers good prognosis in T-cell ALL.

Molecular analysis

FISH and RT-PCR methods add sensitivity and precision to the detection of prognostically significant translocations, deletions, and aneuploidy in cases where cytogenetics fails or gives normal results. Analysis of specific translocations, Ig or T-cell receptor rearrangements allows detection of MRD permitting risk-stratified consolidation therapy.

Clinical features

- Acute presentation usual; often critically ill due to BM failure:
  - Anaemia: weakness, lethargy, breathlessness, lightheadedness, and palpitations.
  - Infection: particularly chest, mouth, perianal, skin (*Staphylococcus*, *Pseudomonas*, HSV, *Candida*).
  - Fever, malaise, sweats.
  - Haemorrhage: purpura, menorrhagia, and epistaxis, bleeding gums, rectal, retina.

- Signs of leucostasis e.g. hypoxia, retinal haemorrhage, confusion, or diffuse pulmonary shadowing.
- Bone or joint pain is more common in children.
- Mediastinal involvement in 15%; may cause SVC obstruction especially T-ALL.
- CNS involvement in 6% at presentation; may cause cranial nerve palsies especially facial nerve, sensory disturbances, and meningism.
- Signs include widespread lymphadenopathy in 55%, mild-to-moderate splenomegaly (49%), hepatomegaly (45%), and orchidomegaly.

Differential diagnosis

- In adults: AML, aplastic anaemia, infectious mononucleosis, lymphoma with blood spill, transformed CML.
- In childhood: AML, aplastic anaemia, infectious mononucleosis, pertussis, neuroblastoma, rhabdomyosarcoma, Ewing's sarcoma,

Investigations and diagnosis

- FBC and blood film.
- BM aspirate ± biopsy.
- BM cytogenetics and molecular analysis.
- Immunophenotyping of blood or marrow blasts.
- Total WBC usually high with blast cells on film but may be low (aleukaemic leukaemia).
- Hb, neutrophils, and platelets often low; clotting may be deranged.
- BM heavily infiltrated with blasts (≥20%).
- CXR and CT scan needed if ALL has B-cell or T-cell phenotype for abdominal or mediastinal lymphadenopathy respectively.
- Lumbar puncture mandatory to detect occult CNS involvement but may be postponed until treatment reduces high peripheral blast count to prevent seeding (*Note*—fundoscopy, CT scan of head and platelet transfusion usually required).

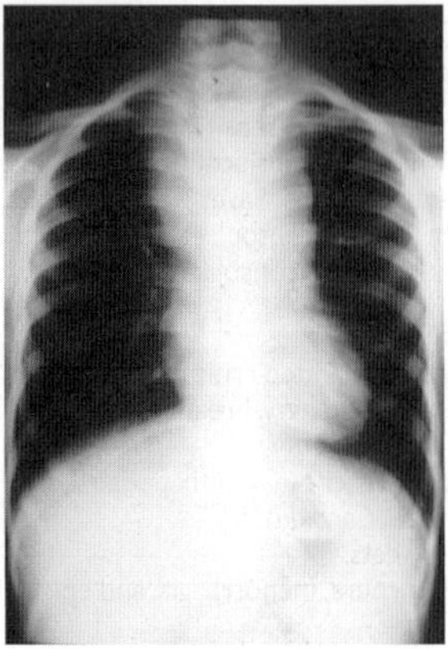

Fig. 4.7 Mediastinal mass in T-ALL.

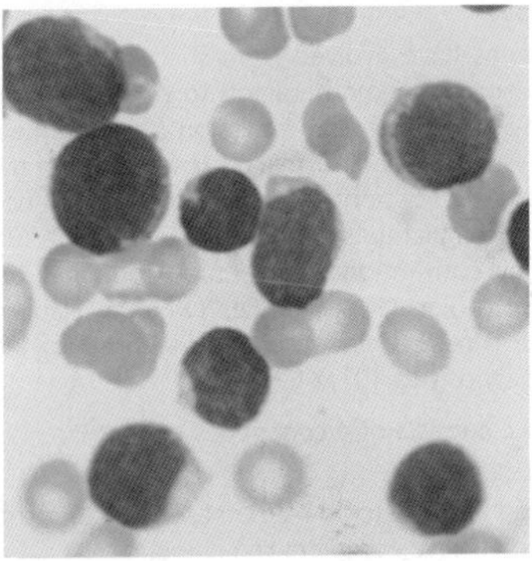

Fig. 4.8 BM: lymphoblasts in ALL L1 (📖 see Plate 11).

Emergency treatment

►► Seek expert help immediately.

- Cardiovascular and respiratory resuscitation may be needed if septic shock or massive haemorrhage.
- Immediate empirical broad spectrum antibiotic treatment for neutropenic sepsis.
- Leucapheresis may be needed if peripheral blast count high or signs of leucostasis (retinal haemorrhage, reduced conscious level, diffuse pul-monary shadowing on CXR or hypoxia).
- LP if meningism (note precautions already discussed).

Supportive treatment

- Provide explanation and offer counselling—the word *'leukaemia'* and prospect of prolonged chemotherapy are often distressing.
- RBC and platelet transfusion support will continue through treatment:
  - CMV –ve products for potential SCT recipients until status known.
  - Irradiated products for patients treated with purine analogues.
  - Platelet transfusion to maintain count $>10 \times 10^9$/L, unless septic, on antibiotics, haemorrhagic or other haemostatic abnormality ($>20 \times 10^9$/L).
- Start neutropenic regimen (📖 Prophylactic regimen for neutropenic patients, p.674) as prophylaxis against infections.
- Start hydration aiming for urine output >100mL/h throughout induction therapy (📖 Tumour lysis syndrome, p.684—a special problem in B-cell or T-cell ALL).
- Start allopurinol to prevent hyperuricaemia (*Note*: interaction with 6-mercaptopurine: discontinue allopurinol or reduce dose of 6-MP) or rasburicase (especially with high counts).
- Insert tunnelled central venous catheter (📖 see Technique, p.690).

Chemotherapy

Adult ALL regimens have evolved from successful treatments for childhood ALL. Initial aim of chemotherapy is to eliminate leukaemic cells and achieve complete haematological remission (CR), defined as normal BM cellularity (blast cells <5% and normal representation of trilineage haematopoiesis), normalization of peripheral blood count with no blast cells, neutrophils $\geq 1.5 \times 10^9$/L, platelets $\geq 100 \times 10^9$/L and Hb>10g/dL. Leukaemia is undetectable by conventional morphology but may be demonstrated by more sensitive molecular techniques (when available) and CR is not synonymous with cure. CR may result from a three-log kill from 10^{12} leukaemic cells at diagnosis to 10^9 at CR.

Treatment for ALL consists of 4 contiguous phases*[1–3]*:

1. *Remission induction*

- Vincristine, prednisolone (or dexamethasone), daunorubicin, and asparaginase to achieve complete remission.
- More intensive induction using more anthracycline improves leukaemia-free survival.

2. *Consolidation therapy*

- To further reduce or eliminate tumour burden and risk of relapse and development of drug-resistant cells; consists of alternating cycles of induction agents and other cytotoxics.
- Usually includes several *'intensification'* phases; combinations of methotrexate at high dose, cytarabine, etoposide, *m*-amsacrine, mitoxantrone (mitozantrone), and idarubicin.

3. *CNS prophylaxis*

- Cranial irradiation (18–24 Gy in 12 fractions over 2 weeks) plus IT chemotherapy (methotrexate ± cytarabine or prednisolone) early in the consolidation phase.
- Irradiation avoided in childhood ALL due to side-effects and replaced by high dose systemic methotrexate plus IT therapy.
- IT therapy continued in consolidation and maintenance phases.
- CNS prophylaxis reduces CNS relapse from 30% to 5%.

►► Simultaneous administration of IV vincristine and IT methotrexate MUST be avoided as errors can be fatal.

4. *Maintenance therapy*

- Necessary for all patients who do not proceed to SCT.
- Daily 6-MP PO and weekly methotrexate PO with doses to limits of tolerance plus cyclical IV vincristine, oral prednisolone and IT methotrexate for 2–3 years.

or allogeneic stem cell transplantation

- Option for adults <50 years with a compatible sib; leukaemia-free survival superior after 1st remission allograft in patients with high risk disease (40% vs. <10% for Ph/BCR-ABL+ ALL); treatment-related mortality up to 30%.
- In low risk patients SCT should be reserved for second CR.
- Matched unrelated donor transplant: option in younger patients (<40 years) with very high risk disease (Ph/BCR-ABL+ ALL) but up to 48% treatment-related mortality.

or autologous stem cell transplantation

- Alternative for adults up to 60 years without compatible donor: lower treatment related mortality (up to 8%); no clear survival advantage over maintenance therapy in 1st remission for most patients but may improve survival in very high risk disease without allograft option.

Enrol in high quality multi-centre trial if possible:

- Major complications are infective episodes which may be bacterial (Gram +ve and Gram –ve), viral (esp. HSV, HZV) and fungal (*Candida* and *Aspergillus*).
- In the longer term, relapse is the main complication.

BCR-ABL+ ALL[4]

- *Imatinib mesylate* is included in regimen of patients with BCR-ABL + ALL as several small studies suggest improved CR, LFS, and OS.
- Eligible patients should receive SCT early in 1st CR.

Mature B-cell ALL/Burkitt's cell leukaemia[5]

- FAB L3—Burkitt cell type: distinct treatment approach.
- No longer ALL in WHO classification: Burkitt's lymphoma/Burkitt's cell leukaemia.
- Higher incidence of CNS disease at diagnosis and relapse.
- Treated with shorter more intensive cycles including high dose methotrexate, high dose cytarabine and fractionated cyclophosphamide: e.g. CODOX-M/IVAC 📖 p.724
- Improved prognosis; 75% CR; >65% LFS at 1 year: 40% DFS

T-cell ALL[6]

- Higher incidence of CNS disease at diagnosis and relapse.
- High cure rates when treated with cyclophosphamide containing regimens yielding DFS of 50–70%.

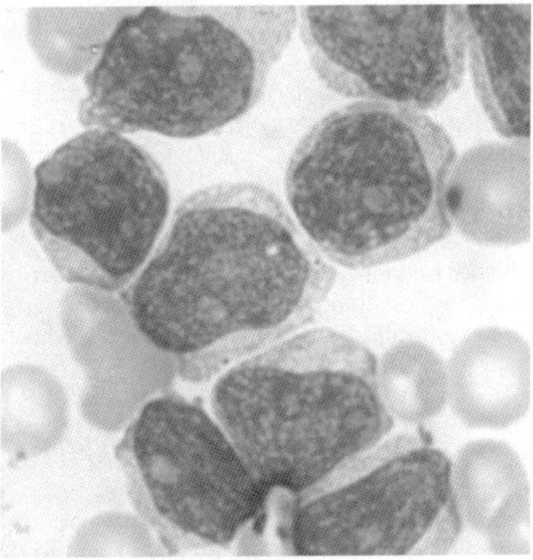

Fig. 4.9 BM: T-cell ALL showing numerous lymphoblasts (📖 see Plate 12).

CNS leukaemia

- ↑ risk with high-risk genetics, T-cell ALL and high blast count.
- Presents with headache, vomiting, lethargy, nuchal rigidity or cranial or peripheral nerve dysfunction.
- Clinical examination may reveal papilloedema, meningism, neurological deficit, and LP shows blasts in CSF.
- Treat with intensified IT triple therapy plus 18 Gy cranial irradiation; IT methotrexate, cytarabine and hydrocortisone 2–3 × times weekly over 3–4 weeks until 2 consecutive CSF samples are –ve; insertion of an Ommaya reservoir facilitates such frequent IT therapy.
- If relapse, will require systemic re-induction as BM relapse often present or follows.
- Poor prognosis.

Minimal residual disease detection

Flow cytometry for clonal immunophenotypes or FISH or RT-PCR for fusion proteins or clonal Ig/TCR gene rearrangements identified at diagnosis can detect minimal residual disease (MRD) at a sensitivity of 10^{-3}–10^{-6}. Morphological and molecular CR can be distinguished and detection of MRD after initial therapy in childhood ALL has strong –ve prognostic implications. Residual disease level of <0.01% on completion of induction therapy identifies patients with a very good outcome. Patients with ≥1% at the end of induction or ≥0.1% later, have very high risk of relapse and are candidates for intensified therapy.

Prognosis

- Overall ~75% of adults with ALL achieve a CR with a modern regimen and good supportive care; more intensive induction and consolidation reduces relapse risk but adds toxicity; results in patients >50 years are less good.
- Median remission duration of CR is around 15 months. 35–40% of adults with ALL treated with intensive chemotherapy survive 2 years.
- In contrast to high cure rate in childhood ALL, leukaemia free survival (LFS) in adult ALL in general is <30% at 5 years (patients >50 years 10–20%). LFS after chemotherapy in patients without adverse risk factors is >50% but <10% for very high risk Ph/BCR-ABL+ ALL; hence latter should have an allograft in 1st CR if possible.

Prognostic factors

Prognosis in adult ALL is much poorer than childhood ALL (cure rate ~80%) due to higher frequency of poor prognostic features and treatment-related toxicity. The most important prognostic factors are listed. These are useful for risk stratification to identify patients who require more intensive therapy e.g. SCT, in first CR.

- Patient age (<50 years CR >80%, LFS>30%; ≥50 years CR <60%, LFS <20%).
- High leucocyte count (>30 × 10^9/L in B precursor-ALL; >100 × 10^9/L in T-ALL) poor risk.
- Immunophenotype: pro-B-ALL and pro-T-ALL have poorer outcomes; common pre-B-ALL still poor; mature B-cell ALL and T-cell ALL have better outcomes due to the use of more intensive regimens.

- Cytogenetics: Ph/BCR-ABL+ very poor prognosis: <10% LFS after chemotherapy; for others (see Cytogenic analysis, p.133).
- Long time to CR (>4 weeks): poor risk.
- High MRD level after induction ($>10^{-3}$); persistent/increasing MRD during consolidation: poor risk.

Management of relapse

- Relapse rate highest within first 2 years but may occur after 7 years.
- 20% occur outside BM, generally CNS; testis and other sites occur in 5%.
- Isolated extramedullary relapse often followed by haematological relapse; these patients require local treatment followed by systemic re-induction therapy.
- Best predictive factor for response is duration of first CR (better >18 months).
- 50–60% of patients achieve a short 2nd CR (generally <6 months);
- prompt SCT offers only prospect of LFS and cure.
- Patients with BCR-ABL+ALL on maintenance imatinib at relapse have prospect (70%) of up to 6 months haematological response to dasatinib.

References

1. Finiewicz, K.J. and Larson, R.A. (1999). Dose-intensive therapy for adult acute lymphoblastic leukemia. *Semin Oncol*, **26**, 6–20.
2. Thomas, X. *et al.* (2004). Outcome of treatment of adults with acute lymphoblastic leukaemia: analysis of the LALA-94 trial. *J Clin Oncol*, **22**, 4075–86.
3. Pui, C.-H. and Evans, W.E. (2006). Treatment of acute lymphoblastic leukaemia. *N Engl J Med*, **354**, 166–78.
4. Wassmann, B. *et al.* (2006). Alternating versus concurrent schedules of imatinib and chemotherapy as front-line therapy for Philadelphia-positive acute lymphoblastic leukemia (Ph+ ALL). *Blood*, **108**, 1469–77.
5. Lee, E.J. *et al.* (2001). Brief-duration high-intensity chemotherapy for patients with small noncleaved-cell lymphoma or FAB L3 acute lymphocytic leukemia: results of cancer and leukemia group B study 9251. *J Clin Oncol*, **19**, 4014–22.
6. Larson, R.A. *et al.* (1995). A five-drug remission induction regimen with intensive consolidation for adults with acute lymphoblastic leukemia: cancer and leukemia group B study 8811. *Blood*, **85**, 2025–37.

Chronic myeloid leukaemia (CML)

Malignant tumour of pluripotent haemopoietic stem cell. The clonal marker is found in all three myeloid lineages and in some B and T lymphocytes demonstrating a primitive origin. Characterized by ↑↑ granulocytes with left shift and the presence of the Ph chromosome.

Incidence

Rare disease. Frequency 1.25 per 100,000. Accounts for 15% adult leukaemias. Rare in children. Median age of onset 50 years. Slight ♂ excess.

Aetiology

Unknown. Irradiation is only known epidemiological factor. BCR-ABL fusion proteins appear to play a role in the pathogenesis of CML and have been shown to transform haemopoietic progenitor cells *in vivo* and *in vitro*. ↑ proliferation, affect differentiation, and block apoptosis.

Classification

Classified as a myeloproliferative disorder (📖 WHO classification of chronic myeloproliferative diseases, p.254) with which it shares a number of clinical features but it also has unique biological features.

Natural history

- Biphasic or triphasic disease—chronic phase (CP), accelerated phase (AP), and blast crisis (BC); 50% transform directly from CP to BC.
- >85% patients present in CP: defined by absence of features of AP or BC.
- Duration of CP varies (typically 3–6 years; median 4.2 years).
- Transformation least likely in 2 years immediately after diagnosis but occurs at an annual rate of 20–25% thereafter.
- AP characterized by blood counts and organomegaly becoming increasingly refractory to therapy; some have constitutional symptoms; generally brief (Table 4.5).
- BC resembles acute leukaemia with >20% blasts and promyelocytes in blood or marrow; rapidly fatal (Table 4.6).

Table 4.5 WHO criteria for accelerated phase

Blasts 10–19% of WBCs in peripheral blood and/or nucleated BM cells
Peripheral blood basophils ≥20%
Persistent thrombocytopenia (<100 × 10^9/L) unrelated to therapy or persistent thrombocytosis (>1000 × 10^9/L) unresponsive to therapy
↑ spleen size and ↑ WBC count unresponsive to therapy
Cytogenetic evidence of clonal evolution

Table 4.6 WHO criteria for blast crisis

Blasts ≥20% of peripheral blood WBCs in or of nucleated BM cells
Extramedullary blast proliferation
Large foci or clusters of blasts in the BM biopsy

The widely used MD Anderson definition of AP is similar; other criteria differ: cytogenetic evolution in the absence of other criteria for AP remains CP in a Leukaemia-Net review[2].

Clinical symptoms and signs

- 30% asymptomatic at diagnosis; present after routine FBC.
- Fatigue, lethargy, weight loss, sweats.
- Splenomegaly in >75%; may cause (L) hypochondrial pain, satiety, and sensation of abdominal fullness.
- Gout, bruising/bleeding, splenic infarction, and occasionally priapism.
- Signs include: moderate-to-large splenomegaly (40% >10cm), hepatomegaly (2%), lymphadenopathy unusual.
- Occasional signs of leucostasis at presentation.

Diagnosis and investigations

- FBC and blood film show ↑ WBC (generally $>25 \times 10^9$/L, often $100–300 \times 10^9$/L): predominantly neutrophils and myelocytes; basophilia; sometimes eosinophilia.
- Anaemia common; platelets typically ↔ or ↑.
- Neutrophil alkaline phosphatase (NAP) score ↓ (no longer routine) and ESR ↓ in absence of infection.
- LDH and urate levels ↑.
- BM shows marked hypercellularity due to myeloid hyperplasia (blasts <10% in chronic phase; >10% in AP; >20% blasts in BC); trephine biopsy useful to assess marrow fibrosis.
- Cytogenetic analysis of blood or marrow for t(9;22).
- Molecular analysis by real-time quantitative reverse transcription polymerase chain reaction (RQ-PCR) for *BCR-ABL* transcripts to obtain baseline for subsequent monitoring. FISH analysis of blood or marrow will confirm presence of *BCR-ABL*.

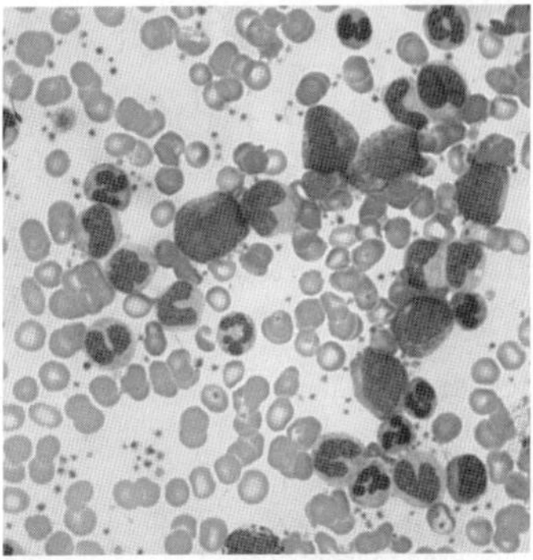

Fig. 4.10 Peripheral blood film in CML: note large numbers of granulocytic cells at all stages of differentiation (low power) (📖 see Plate 13).

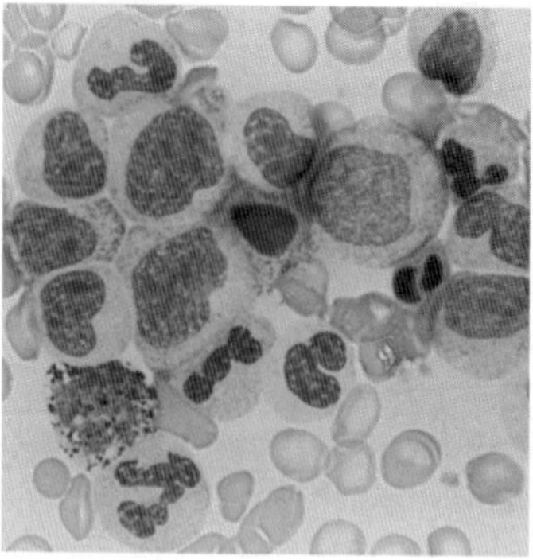

Fig. 4.11 Peripheral blood film in CML (high power) (see Plate 14).

Cytogenetic and molecular analysis

- Characterized in >80% patients by the presence of the Ph chromosome. Reciprocal translocation between chromosomes 9 and 22, (t9;22)(q34;q11), involving two genes, *BCR* and *ABL* that form a fusion gene *BCR-ABL* on chromosome 22. This produces an aberrant 210 kDa protein ($p210^{BCR\text{-}ABL}$) that is constitutively active and has greater tyrosine kinase activity than the normal ABL protein.
- 10% of patients have variant translocations involving chromosome 22 ± 9 and other chromosomes.
- A further 8% with typical clinical features lack the Ph chromosome, i.e. have Ph-–ve CML; half of these have the hybrid *BCR-ABL* gene: Ph-–ve, BCR-ABL-+ve CML.
- Accelerated phase is marked by the acquisition of new cytogenetic abnormalities in 50–80% of patients.
- Myeloid blast crisis associated with additional copies of Ph chromosome, +8 and i (17q).
- Lymphoid blast crisis associated with chromosome 7 anomalies.

Differential diagnosis

Differentiate CP from leukaemoid reaction due to infection, inflammation or carcinoma (NAP ↑ or normal; absent Ph chromosome) and CMML (absolute monocytosis; trilineage myelodysplasia; absent Ph chromosome); 5% present with predominant thrombocytosis and must be differentiated from ET (NAP ↑ /normal; absent Ph chromosome).

Prognostic factors

- Sokal score based on age, spleen size, platelet count, and % blasts in blood at diagnosis used to identify good, moderate, and poor prognosis groups; based on patients treated with chemotherapy; (Table 20.4, p 806).
- Hasford calculation adds effect of basophilia and eosinophilia at diagnosis; based on patients treated with interferon-α.

- Either can be used to predict the cytogenetic response to imatinib 400mg od of a newly diagnosed patient in CP and Sokal predicts molecular response in IRIS study[3].
- Molecular analysis e.g. gene profiling may prove more informative.
- Early cytogenetic response to imatinib is another important prognostic factor: PCyR at 6 months, 80% probability of CCyR at 2 years; minor or minimal CyR at 6 months, 50% probability; no CyR at 6 months, 15% probability.

Treatment of chronic phase

- ***Imatinib*** 400mg PO od first-line treatment of choice in newly diagnosed patients in CP (NICE approved[4]); continue to intolerance, failure or sub-optimal response. Long term outcome not yet assessed.
- Imatinib is a small molecule signal transduction inhibitor that specifically targets BCR-ABL and some other tyrosine kinases.
  - Achieves 96% complete haematological response (CHR), 87% major cytogenetic response (MCyR), and 76% complete cytogenetic response (CCyR)[5]; 50% major molecular response (3 log ↓)[3].
  - 5-year follow-up of IRIS trial shows 69% CCyR at 12 months ↑ to 87% at 60 months; 7% progressed to AP or BC; 89% overall survival at 5 years[6].
  - Most patients achieve MCyR within first 6 months of therapy; patients with MCyR have lower risk of relapse; CCyR predicts for EFS.
  - Commonest side effects: myelosuppression, oedema, nausea, rash, cramps, fatigue, diarrhoea, headache, arthralgia, and abnormal LFTs.
  - Add G-CSF to maintain neutrophils $>1.0 \times 10^9$/L or interrupt therapy and reduce dose if necessary (not < 300mg/d); if platelets $<50 \times 10^9$/L interrupt therapy and reduce dose if necessary; add erythropoietin for grade 3–4 anaemia; interrupt therapy and reduce dose for ≥grade 2 hepatotoxicity; topical or systemic steroid for rash; supportive management of other grade 3 toxicity; interrupt and consider 300mg/d for other grade 4 toxicity.
  - Consider change to dasatinib, nilotinib or clinical trial if not tolerated.
  - Imatinib 800mg/d *vs.* 400mg/d being compared in clinical studies.
- Commence allopurinol.
- Consider leukapheresis in patients with leucostasis or priapism.
- Symptomatic leukocytosis may respond to hydroxycarbamide, apheresis or imatinib; symptomatic thrombocytosis may respond to hydroxycarbamide, anti-platelet agents, anagrelide, or apheresis.
- HLA-type patients aged <50 years and sibs; 30% have a compatible sibling donor; if no compatible sib and aged <40, perform preliminary search to determine prospective unrelated donor availability.
- Allogeneic SCT is the only curative treatment but carries significant morbidity and mortality; important that each patient is aware of treatment options, risks, and benefits.
- Only exceptions to imatinib as first-line therapy of choice are children with HLA-matched sib and patients with syngeneic twin.
- Indication for and outcome of SCT are age, donor, and transplant centre dependent; discuss in high risk CML patients with low transplant risk.

Definitions of response to treatment

Table 4.7 Haematological response

Complete (CHR):
Platelets <450 × 10^9/L
WBC <10 × 10^9/L
Differential: no immature granulocytes and <5% basophils
Non-palpable spleen
Monitoring: check 2 weekly until CHR achieved and confirmed × 2; then every 3 months.

Table 4.8 Cytogenetic response (examination of ≥ 20 marrow metaphases)

Complete (CCyR):	Ph+ metaphases 0%
Partial (PCyR):	Ph+ 1–35%
Major (MCyR):	CCyR + PCyR
Minor:	Ph+ 36–65%
Minimal:	Ph+ 66–95%
Monitoring: check at least every 6 months until CCyR achieved and confirmed × 2; then at least every 12 months.	

Table 4.9 Molecular response (assessed on peripheral blood cells)

Complete:	Transcripts not detectable
Major (MMolR):	≤0.1% (≡ 3 log reduction against International Scale)
Monitoring: check every 3 months; confirm × 2; mutational analysis in case of failure, sub-optimal response or transcript level increase	

Disease monitoring

- Disease monitoring is critical to modern management of CML and selection of appropriate risk-adjusted therapy.
- Goals of therapy in order are CHR, CCyR, MMolR and 'complete' molecular response.
- BM cytogenetics of value until CCyR; RQ-PCR for *BCR-ABL* transcripts more sensitive for patients in CCyR with imatinib (>75%).

3-month evaluation

- CHR: continue same dose of imatinib.
- Not in CHR: dasatinib/SCT/clinical trial/(interferon-α if unable to tolerate imatinib or dasatinib).

6-month evaluation (including BM cytogenetics)
- CCyR: continue same dose of imatinib.
- PCyR or Minor CyR: continue same dose of imatinib or increase as tolerated (max 600–800mg).
- No CyR or cytogenetic relapse: dasatinib/ increase imatinib as tolerated (max 600–800mg)/clinical trial/SCT.

12-month evaluation (including BM cytogenetics)
- CCyR: continue same dose of imatinib.
- PCyR: continue same dose of imatinib or increase as tolerated (max. 600–800mg).
- Minor CyR or no CyR or cytogenetic relapse: increase imatinib as tolerated (max. 600–800mg)/ dasatinib/clinical trial/SCT.

18-month evaluation (including BM cytogenetics if not CCyR at 12 months)
- CCyR: continue same dose of imatinib.
- PCyR or Minor CyR, no CyR or cytogenetic relapse: increase imatinib as tolerated (max 600–800mg)/ dasatinib/SCT/clinical trial.

Patients in CCyR
- RQ-PCR for BCR-ABL transcript levels every 3 months (consider BM cytogenetics every 12–18 months for clonal cytogenetic abnormalities).
- MMolR after 12 months associated with a better EFS and PFS[1]; rise in level associated with mutations or loss of response.
- Repeat RQ-PCR in one month if rising transcript level (1 log ↑).
- If confirmed, monitor monthly; perform ABL kinase domain mutation analysis.
- Significance of mutations unclear; not consistently associated with relapse; several associated with resistance to imatinib; T315I associated with resistance to imatinib, dasatinib, and nilotinib.

Table 4.10 Definitions of failure and sub-optimal response

Time	Failure	Sub-optimal response	Warnings
Diagnosis	Not applicable	Not applicable	High risk score; Del(9q+); Additional chromosome abnormalities (ACA) in Ph+ cells
3 months	No HR (stable disease or progression)	Less than CHR	
6 months	Less than CHR; No CyR (Ph+ >95%)	Less than PCyR (Ph+ >35%)	
12 months	Less than PCyR (Ph+ >35%)	Less than CCyR	Less than MMolR
18 months	Less than CCyR	Less than MMolR	
Any time	Loss of CHR*; Loss of CCyR**; Mutation (high level insensitivity e.g. T315I)	ACA in Ph+ cells***; Loss of MMolR***; Mutation (low level insensitivity)	Any rise in transcript level; Other chromosome abnormalities in Ph–ve cells

*Confirm on 2 occasions unless associated with progression to AP/BC; **Confirm on 2 occasions unless associated with CHR loss or progression to AP/BC; ***Confirm on 2 occasions unless associated with CHR or CCyR loss.

Actions

- *Intolerance*: SCT or interferon-α ± cytarabine or novel agent.
- *Failure*: dose-escalate imatinib (provided tolerated at 400mg/d and no highly insensitive mutation) or discontinue imatinib and consider SCT or second-line TK-inhibitor: dasatinib or nilotinib.
- *Sub-optimal response*: re-assess and consider imatinib dose-escalation or treatment change now or in near future; offer SCT to those with high risk score or other warning features.
- *Warnings*: features suggesting possible incipient resistance to imatinib and/or progression to advanced phase; needs closer monitoring and consideration of dose escalation, SCT, or investigational agents.

Other agents

- ***Dasatinib***[9–11]: FDA-approved for use in patients with CML no longer responding to or intolerant of imatinib. Orally active ABL kinase inhibitor that binds to both active and inactive conformations of ABL kinase domain. START-C trial of 70mg bd in 186 imatinib-resistant or intolerant CP patients: 90% CHR, 52% MCyR; 2% progressed or died after MCyR; 92% PFS after 8 months. Good results also in imatinib-resistant or intolerant patients in AP (Major HR 64%; MCyR 33%) and BC (Major HR ~33%; MCyR 31% in myeloid BC, 50% in lymphoid BC). The most frequently reported adverse effects are fluid retention, pleural effusion, diarrhoea, skin rash, headache, haemorrhage, fatigue, nausea, dyspnoea, and myelosuppression. 100mg od recommended for CP patients due to reduced toxicity and improved tolerability. 70mg bd in AP and BC.

- ***Nilotinib:*** orally active (400mg bd), highly selective inhibitor of BCR-ABL tyrosine kinase; 20–50 × more potent than imatinib in imatinib-resistant cell lines. Early studies show high response rates in imatinib-resistant or intolerant CP (74% CHR; 40% CCyR) and in AP (24% CHR; 16% CCyR). Low toxicity. Not yet FDA/NICE approved.
- ***Hydroxycarbamide*** may be used to control leucocytosis or thrombocytosis and may 'normalize' FBC and reduce spleen size in CP in elderly imatinib intolerant. Maintenance 1–1.5g PO od. No effect on cytogenetics or natural history. Side effects: rash, mouth ulcers and diarrhoea.
- ***Interferon-α*** (IFN-α) at a dose of 3 million IU SC 3 times weekly corrects haematological abnormalities in 75% and produces 10–15% CCyR and 15–30%. MCyR. Role in SCT-ineligible, TK-inhibitor intolerant.
  - Treatment with IFN-α is associated with longer time to progression and longer survival (27–53% at 10 years) than hydroxycarbamide treatment, most significantly in patients with CCyR and MCyR. Adding cytarabine increases CCyRs to 25–35% but does not improve survival.
  - IFN-α side effects (malaise, febrile reactions, anorexia and weight loss, depression) reduce quality of life and are not tolerable for many patients.
  - Polyethylene glycol-IFN administered once weekly and has a more favourable side effect profile.

Allogeneic SCT

- Matched sibling SCT is treatment of choice for patients <50 years who fail to achieve MCyR but only 30% have matched sibling.
- Transplant related mortality ~ 20%.
- Best outcomes in patients aged <30 years in CP <1 year from diagnosis.
- Overall survival (OS) at 18 years: first CP SCT 50%; later SCT 20%; cumulative incidence of relapse at 18 years: first CP SCT 25%; later SCT 37%.
- Monitor peripheral blood with RQ-PCR for *BCR-ABL* every 3 months for 2 years then 6 months for 3 years once Ph –ve engraftment achieved.
- If available, use unrelated allogeneic SCT for <25 years age group and consider <40 years but transplant related mortality rises to 45%.
- Reduced intensity conditioning lowers treatment related toxicity in older patients; long-term impact not yet assessed; clinical trial only.

Complications

- Modest ↑ infection risk—sometimes atypical organisms.
- Progression to BC (75% myeloid, 25% lymphoid).
- Lymphoid BC: treat with TK inhibitor or modified ALL protocol (may survive >12 months). Follow with SCT where possible.
- Myeloid BC usually refractory to conventional chemotherapy, survival 2–5 months; may get brief response with TK inhibitor. SCT where possible.

Prognosis

- Median OS with hydroxycarbamide was 5.5 years (range 3 months–22 years).
- IFN-α achieved 27–53% OS at 9–10 years.
- Imatinib improves OS (89% at 5 years), freedom from progression (84% at 54months), CHR (95%), CCyR (76%), MMolR (55% at 2 years), compliance, toxicity and quality of life. 'Complete' molecular remission (–ve RQ-PCR for BCR-ABL at 10^{-5}–10^{-6}) variable (4–34%); probably not cured. Progression to AP/BC 0.9–2.8%/year in first 4 years of treatment.
- Sibling matched SCT: all ages, leukaemia-free survival 50% at 5 years; OS 60% and EFS 50% at 10 years; MUD SCT: all ages, 5-year OS 40%.
- BC median OS 6 months.

Treatment of advanced phase CML[8, 12]

- Patients presenting in AP or BC not previously treated with imatinib should receive imatinib 600–800mg od.
- Previously untreated patients in AP have 37% CHR rate and 19% CCyR rate, prolongation of time to progression (40% at 3 years) and improved survival. Eligible patients should receive SCT.
- A proportion of patients in BC respond to imatinib 600–800mg od (25% CHR) but response duration is short (median ≤10 months). Follow with chemotherapy and/or SCT for responders where possible.
- Patients who progress on imatinib may respond to dasatinib or other TK inhibitors. SCT should be offered where possible.
- SCT offers eligible patients with advanced phase CML the only prospect of prolonged survival and possible cure. Results are significantly less good than for SCT in CP (0–10% 5-year survival in BC) though achievement of second CP pre-SCT improves results after BC.
- Relapse after SCT has been successfully treated with imatinib, dasatinib and with donor lymphocyte infusions (DLI) (60–80% response in molecular or cytogenetic relapse); GvHD is a side effect of DLI but is less frequent with incremental doses.

References

1. Jaffe, E.S., *et al.* (2001). *Tumours of Haematopoietic and Lymphoid Tissues. World Health Organization Classification of Tumours*. IARC Press, Lyon.
2. Baccarani, M., *et al.* (2006). Evolving concepts in the management of chronic myeloid leukaemia: recommendations from an expert panel on behalf of European LeukaemiaNet. *Blood*, **108**, 1809–20.
3. Hughes, T.P., *et al.* (2003). Frequency of major molecular responses to imatinib or interferon alfa plus cytarabine in newly diagnosed chronic myeloid leukemia. *N Engl J Med*, **349**, 1421–32.
4. www.nice.org.uk
5. O'Brien, S.G., *et al.* (2003). Imatinib compared with interferon and low dose cytarabine for newly diagnosed chronic phase chronic myeloid leukaemia. *N Engl J Med*, **348**, 994–1004;

6. Druker, B.J., *et al.* (2006). Five-year follow-up of patients receiving Imatinib for chronic myeloid leukaemia. *N Engl J Med*, **355**, 2408–17.
7. Hughes, T.P., *et a.l* (2006). Monitoring CML patients responding to treatment with tyrosine kinase inhibitors–recommendations for 'harmonizing' current methodology for detecting BCR-ABL transcripts and kinase domain mutations and for expressing results. *Blood*, **108**, 28–37.
8. Goldman, J. (2007). Recommendations for the management of BCR-ABL-positive chronic myeloid leukaemia.
   🖫 www.bcshguidelines.com/pdf/CML_guidelines_270707.pdf
9. Hochhaus, A., *et al.* (2007). Dasatinib induces notable hemaologic and cytogenetic responses in chronic phase chronic myeloid leukaemia after failure of imatinib therapy. *Blood*, **109**, 2303–9.
10. Guilhot, F., *et al.* (2007). Dasatinib induces significant hemaologic and cytogenetic responses in patients with imatinib-resistant or intolerant chronic myeloid leukaemia in accelerated phase. *Blood*, **109**, 4143–50.
11. Cortes, J., *et al.* (2007). Dasatinib induces complete hemaologic and cytogenetic responses in patients with imatinib-resistant or intolerant chronic myeloid leukaemia in blast crisis. *Blood*, **109**, 3207–13.
12. NCCN Practice Guidelines (2007).
    🖫 www.nccn.org/professionals/physician_gls/PDF/cml.pdf

Chronic lymphocytic leukaemia (B-CLL)

Progressive accumulation of mature-appearing, functionally incompetent, long-lived B lymphocytes in peripheral blood, BM, lymph nodes, spleen, liver, and sometimes other organs.

Incidence

Commonest leukaemia in Western adults (25–30% of all leukaemias). 2.5/100,000 per annum. 20–30 × more common in Western Caucasian and black populations than in India, China, and Japan. Predominantly disease of elderly (in over 70s, >20/100,000). Median age at diagnosis 65 years. ♂ : ♀ ratio ~2:1.

Aetiology

Unknown. No causal relationship with radiation, chemicals, or viruses. Small proportion familial. ↑ lymphoid malignancies in 1st and 2nd degree relatives of patients with CLL. Genetic factors suggested by low incidence in Japanese even after emigration. Lymphocyte accumulation appears to result from defects in intracellular apoptotic pathways: 90% of CLL cases have high levels of BCL-2 which blocks apoptosis.

Clinical features and presentation

- 70–80% asymptomatic; lymphocytosis (>5.0 x 10^9/L) on routine FBC.
- With more advanced disease: lymphadenopathy: painless, often symmetrical, splenomegaly (66%), hepatomegaly and ultimately BM failure due to infiltration causing anaemia, neutropenia, and thrombocytopenia.
- Recurrent infection due to acquired hypogammaglobulinaemia: esp. herpes zoster.
- Patients with advanced disease: weight loss, night sweats, general malaise.
- Autoimmune phenomena occur; DAT +ve in 10–20% cases, warm antibody AIHA in <50% these cases. Autoimmune thrombocytopenia in 1–2%.

Diagnosis

FBC: lymphocytosis >5.0 × 10^9/L; usually >20 × 10^9/L, occasionally >400 × 10^9/L; anaemia, thrombocytopenia, and neutropenia absent in early stage CLL; autoimmune haemolysis ± thrombocytopenia may occur at any stage.
Blood film: lymphocytosis with 'mature' appearance; characteristic artefactual damage to cells in film preparation produces numerous 'smear cells' (note: absence of smear cells should prompt review of diagnosis); spherocytes, polychromasia and ↑ retics if AIHA; ↓ platelets if BM failure or ITP. In 15% of patients morphology is 'atypical' with >10% prolymphocytes (CLL/PLL) or >15% lymphoplasmacytoid cells/cleaved nuclei.
Immunophenotyping: differentiates CLL from other lymphocytoses (📖 Table 4.15, p.158). First line panel: CD2; CD5; CD19; CD23; FMC7; SmIg (κ/λ); CD22 or CD79b. CLL characteristically:

- CD2 and FMC7 –ve.
- CD5, CD19, and CD23 +ve.
- SmIg, CD22, CD79b weak; κ or λ light chain restricted.

Immunoglobulins: immuneparesis (hypogammaglobulinaemia) common; monoclonal paraprotein (usually IgM) <5%.

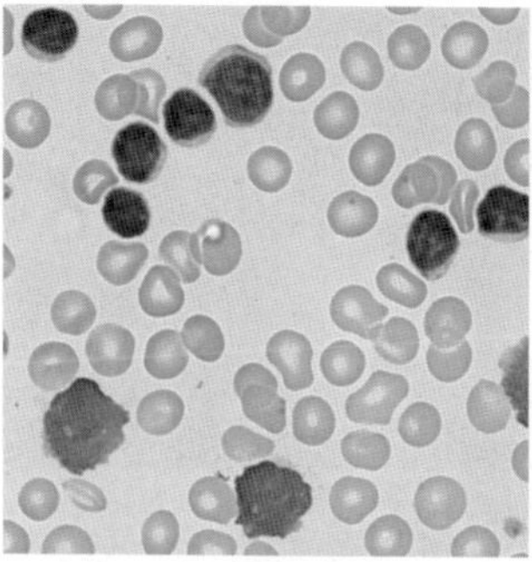

Fig. 4.12 Blood film in CLL showing smear cells (bottom of field) (see Plate 15).

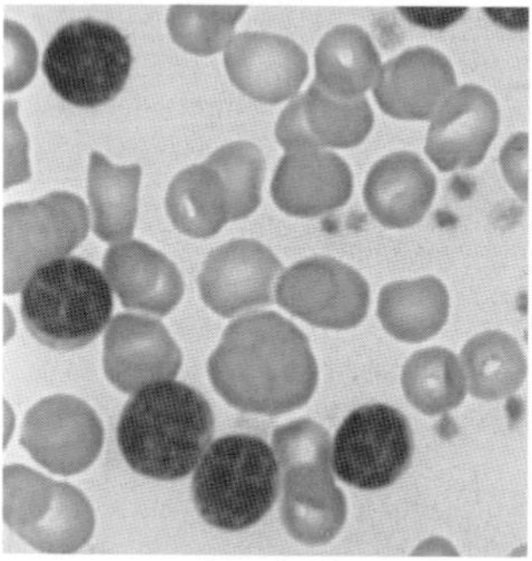

Fig. 4.13 Blood film in CLL.

BM: >30% 'mature' lymphocytes.
Trephine biopsy: provides prognostic information: infiltration may be nodular (favourable); interstitial; mixed; diffuse (unfavourable).
Lymph node biopsy: rarely required; appearances of lymphocytic lymphoma; may be useful if diagnosis uncertain or to exclude transformation to lymphoma in patients with bulky lymphadenopathy.
Cytogenetics: prognostic value; abnormalities in >80% using FISH. Clonal evolution over time. 11q– and 17q– associated with advanced disease. 11q–, 17q– very unfavourable; isolated 13q– favourable; isolated 6q– intermediate.

- 13q– (55%) if isolated (14–40%), favourable, median OS 133 months.
- 11q– (18%; *ATM* gene), median OS 79 months; fludarabine refractory.
- 12q+ (16%) if isolated, neutral prognostically.
- 17p– (7%; *p53* mutation), median OS 32 months; fludarabine refractory.
- 6q– (7%) associated with plasmacytoid lymphoid cells.
- +12 associated with atypical morphology and disease progression.

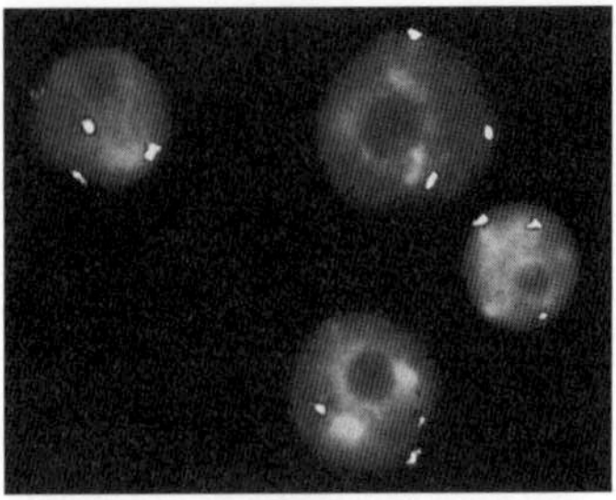

Fig. 4.14 FISH showing trisomy 12 (3 bright spots in each nucleus, each of which represents chromosome 12). Reproduced with permission from Souhami, R.L. *et al* (2001). *Oxford Textbook of Oncology*, 2e. Oxford University Press, Oxford.

Other tests: direct antiglobulin test; reticulocyte count; U&E; urate; LFTs; LDH; β2-microglobulin; imaging e.g. CXR, CT, or ultrasound as necessary for symptoms; newer prognostic indicators CD38 and/or Zap 70 expression by flow cytometry or immunochemistry.

Differential diagnosis

Morphology and immunophenotyping (📖 Table 4.15, p.158) will usually differentiate CLL from other chronic lymphoproliferative disorders.

Scoring system in B-cell lymphoproliferative disorders

Devised to facilitate diagnosis based on the antigen profile of CLL using a panel of 5 monoclonal antibodies.[1]

Table 4.11 Scoring system for CLL diagnosis

Marker		(Score)		(Score)
Smlg	weak	(1)	moderate/strong	(0)
CD5	positive	(1)	negative	(0)
CD23	positive	(1)	negative	(0)
FMC7	negative	(1)	positive	(0)
CD22/79b	weak	(1)	Strong	(0)

Total scores for CLL range from 3–5 and for non-CLL cases from 0–2.

Poor prognostic factors[2,3]

- ♂ sex.
- Advanced clinical stage (📖 see Clinical staging, p.153).
- Initial lymphocytosis >50 × 10^9/L.
- >5% prolymphocytes in blood film.
- Diffuse pattern of infiltrate on trephine.
- Blood lymphocyte doubling time <12 months.

- Cytogenetic abnormalities 11q–, 17p–, or complex.
- p53 mutations (occurs in 10–15%)—correlates with refractory CLL.
- Unmutated IgVH genes (≤2%)—predicts advanced/progressive disease.
- Cytoplasmic ZAP 70 expression (>20%)—correlates with IgVH status.
- CD38 expression (>30%)—independent of IgVH status.
- ↑ serum β_2-microglobulin—correlates with stage and poor response.
- ↑ serum LDH.
- ↑ serum thymidine kinase—predicts disease progression.
- ↑ soluble CD23—predicts disease progression.
- Poor response to therapy.

'Atypical CLL' includes those with >10% prolymphocytes 'CLL/PLL' which may show an aberrant phenotype (SmIg strong +ve, FMC7/CD79b +ve) is associated with trisomy 12 and p53 abnormalities and a more aggressive course.

Clinical staging

2 systems are used to classify patients as low, intermediate, or high risk—Rai modified staging (Table 4.12) and Binet clinical staging (Table 4.13).

Table 4.12 Rai modified staging

Level of risk	Stage		Median survival (% of patients)
Low	0	Lymphocytosis alone	>13 years (30%)
Intermediate	I	Lymphocytosis and lymphadenopathy	8 years (25%)
	II	Lymphocytosis, spleno-, or hepatomegaly	5 years (25%)
High	III	Lymphocytosis, anaemia (Hb <11.0g/dL)*	2 years (10%)
	IV	Lymphocytosis, thrombocytopenia (<100 × 10^9/L)*	1 year (10%)

*Not due to autoimmune anaemia or thrombocytopenia.

Table 4.13 Binet clinical staging

Stage	Clinical features	Median survival (% of patients)
A	No anaemia or thrombocytopenia <3 lymphoid regions enlarged	12 years (60%)
B	No anaemia or thrombocytopenia ≥3 lymphoid regions enlarged	5 years (30%)
C	Anaemia (Hb ≤10g/dL) and/or thrombocytopenia (≤100 × 10^9/L)	2 years (10%)

Initial clinical management

- Choice between observation, traditional alkylator-based palliation, or in fit patients, aiming for CR as those who achieve CR live longer.
- Management of a patient with CLL is based on:
  - Age, performance status, and co-morbidities.
  - Clinical stage, presence of symptoms, disease activity, and prognostic factors.

Early stage CLL

- Patients with asymptomatic lymphocytosis should be observed.
- Evidence that treatment improves outcome only in Rai stage III and IV or Binet stage B and C, ∴ monitor Rai stage 0–II or Binet stage A patients until treatment indicated for progressive or symptomatic disease.
  - *Note*: some patients have very indolent, '*smouldering CLL*': Binet stage A, non-diffuse BM involvement; lymphocytes $<30 \times 10^9$/L, Hb >12g/dL, lymphocyte doubling time >12 months; Binet stage A with somatic mutation of IgVH gene, median survival 25 years.

NCI-WG indications for treatment[4]

- Constitutional symptoms due to CLL: ≥10% weight loss in 6 months; extreme fatigue; fevers >38°C for ≥2 weeks without infection; night sweats without infection.
- Progressive marrow failure: development of or worsening anaemia and/or thrombocytopenia.
- Autoimmune haemolytic anaemia and/or thrombocytopenia unresponsive to steroids.
- Massive (>6cm below LCM) or progressive splenomegaly.
- Massive (>10cm nodes or clusters) or progressive lymphadenopathy.
- Progressive lymphocytosis with ↑ >50% over 2 months or anticipated doubling time of <6 months.

Advanced or progressive disease

- Initial decision to adopt a 'palliative' approach treating symptomatic disease with minimum toxicity or to aim for prolonged disease-free survival with hope of improved overall survival.
- ***Chlorambucil:*** alkylating agent; traditional 'palliative' first-line therapy; dose 6–10mg/d (0.1–0.2mg/kg/d) PO for 7–14d in 28d cycles until disease stabilized (usually 6–12 cycles). Improves FBC and shrinks lymph nodes and spleen in 45–86%; CR 3–7%. Median response ~1 year. No effect on survival (~50% at 5 years). Further responses achieved in most good responders on progression. Side effect myelosuppression. Prolonged use ↑ risk of myelodysplasia or 2° leukaemia. Cyclophosphamide an alternative but offers no advantage.
  - Higher doses of chlorambucil (15mg/d to maximum response or toxicity) followed by twice weekly maintenance for 3 years improves response rate (89%) and survival (median 68 months).
  - CVP (📖 p.741) gives a more rapid response rate but no difference in progression-free or overall survival.
- Avoid ***prednisolone*** except for autoimmune complications or initial 1–2 weeks in very cytopenic patients with extensive BM infiltration.
- ***Fludarabine:*** purine analogue; dose 40mg/m²/d PO **or** 25mg/m²/d IV × 5d q28 (6–8 cycles). Achieves 70–80% overall responses (OR), ~2 year

duration, 27% CRs and 73 months median survival. In UK fludarabine therapy is **not recommended** by NICE for first-line therapy of CLL (February 2007[5]), only for patients who have failed other treatment. Widely used elsewhere. Side effects include immune suppression, infection, myelosuppression, and autoimmune haemolytic anaemia or thrombocytopenia.

- ***Fludarabine plus cyclophosphamide (FC)*** (📖 p.732) achieved better OR (94%), CR (38%), and progression-free survival (PFS) at 5 years (36%) than fludarabine monotherapy (80%, 15%, and 10%) and chlorambucil (72%, 7%, and10%) in large randomized study[6] suggesting this is the best option for all age groups. No significant difference in overall survival.
- *Note*: purine analogues cause profound lymphodepletion with risk of opportunistic infection due to *P. jiroveci*, *M. tuberculosis*, herpes zoster, and other organisms. Patients should receive co-trimoxazole prophylaxis (480mg bd tiw) throughout therapy and for 3 months post therapy and irradiated cellular blood products indefinitely to prevent GvHD.
- ***Cladribine:*** another purine analogue; achieves up to 75% OR, 38% CR, and ~2 year response. Less widely used.
- ***Alemtuzumab:*** humanized anti-CD52 monoclonal antibody (30mg IV or SC tiw up to 18 weeks); preferentially eliminates CLL cells from blood, marrow, and spleen; 81% OR and 19% CR as initial therapy. Approved in USA for initial therapy and fludarabine-refractory CLL. Appears effective in 17p- CLL refractory to alkylators and fludarabine. Side effects: immunosuppression and virus reactivation (HZV and CMV – monitor weekly during and after treatment by CMV-PCR). Irradiate cellular blood products indefinitely to prevent GvHD. Septrin prophylaxis of *P. jiroveci* for 6 months after treatment.
- ***Rituximab:*** anti-CD20 chimeric monoclonal antibody (375mg/m^2/wk × 4 weeks); less effective monotherapy than alemtuzumab; day 1 dose added to fludarabine initial therapy improves CRs to 47%; added to fludarabine + cyclophosphamide (FCR) improves CRs to 66% and 57% MRD–ve by RT-PCR.

Assessment of response

Table 4.14 NCI-WG response criteria for CLL[4]

Criteria	Complete response	Partial response	Progressive disease
Symptoms	None		Richter's syndrome *or*
Lymph nodes	None	≥50% decrease	≥50% increase or new nodes *or*
Liver/spleen	Not palpable	≥50% decrease	≥50% increase or new *or*
Lymphocytes	≤4.0 × 10^9/L	≥50% decrease	≥50% increase
Haemoglobin	>110g/L (untransfused)	>110g/L (untransfused) or 50% improvement*	

(continued)

Table 4.14 NCI-WG response criteria for CLL[4] (*continued*)

Criteria	Complete response	Partial response	Progressive disease
Neutrophils	≥1.5 × 10^9/L	≥1.5 × 10^9/L *	
Platelets	>100 × 10^9/L	>100 × 10^9/L *	
BM aspirate	<30% lymphocytes		
BM trephine	No interstitial or nodular infiltrate	May be residual lymphoid nodules	

*≥ 1 of these features required for PR; features should be present for ≥2 months for CR or PR. Stable disease is defined as all other patients.

MRD assessment

- MRD assessment more relevant now CR achievable.
- Assessed by allele-specific PCR for Ig heavy chain variable gene or 4-colour cytofluorimetry.
- MRD –ve status after alemtuzumab predicts longer remission duration and survival; detection of MRD after FCR predicts for relapse.

Second line and subsequent treatment

Treatment is indicated for symptomatic or progressive disease. Treatment and response are determined by stage, adverse prognostic factors, and number, quality, and duration of responses to prior treatments.

- Prior responders to ***chlorambucil*** often respond on one or more further occasions. Further responses usually poorer and shorter. Resistance inevitably develops. Only 7% respond when fludarabine resistant.
- ***Fludarabine*** achieves a 35–46% OR rate in patients resistant to chlorambucil. NICE guidance recommends fludarabine as second line therapy in patients who have failed or are intolerant of an alkylating agent. 66% of patients with an initial response to fludarabine >1 year will respond again to fludarabine. Not recommended if previous AIHA.
- ***Fludarabine + cyclophosphamide*** (📖 p.732) achieves a response rate of 38% in patients previously refractory to fludarabine alone.
- ***CHOP*** (📖/p.720) achieves 13–27% OR in patients refractory to chlorambucil and 38% OR in patients refractory to fludarabine. Remains useful in patients unsuitable for fludarabine due to haemolytic anaemia.
- ***High dose methylprednisolone*** (1g/m^2/day × 5 days q28) achieves up to 77% OR rate; median duration 9 months. May be of particular use in patients refractory to fludarabine with bulky disease and/or p53 mutations. Infection frequent. Contraindicated in patients with active peptic ulceration. Caution with diabetes and CCF.
- ***Alemtuzumab*** achieves 39% OR rate in fludarabine resistant patients and appears effective in some refractory patients with p53 mutations. Not so effective in bulky nodal disease (>5cm). Combination with

fludarabine may be effective in CLL resistant to either agent alone. Trials underway to evaluate role in clearing MRD after fludarabine.
- ***Rituximab*** achieves only limited responses as a single agent in previously treated CLL. In combination with fludarabine + cyclophosphamide (*FCR*) a high response rate achieved in previously treated patients including 20% CR in chlorambucil resistant CLL.

Stem cell transplantation
- ***Autologous SCT*** has been carried out after high dose chemotherapy ± TBI for younger (<55 years) patients with advanced or poor risk CLL who achieve CR or good PR with fludarabine. Prolonged responses (~50% 5 year DFS). Not curative. ↑ risk of second malignancy and MDS (19% and 9% at median ~3 years). Optimal timing uncertain. Remains investigational.
- ***Allogeneic SCT*** has been successful in small numbers of younger, symptomatic patients with high risk CLL and HLA-matched siblings or unrelated donors. Clear GvL effect. Some patients may be cured (40–60% DFS at 3–6 years) but high treatment-related morbidity and mortality (24–46%). May salvage some refractory patients <50 years. Reduced-intensity conditioning lowers toxicity and is under investigation.

Treatment of complications
- Advise patients to report infection promptly as immunocompromised. Highest risk in elderly, advanced stage, and fludarabine treatment. Prophylactic antibiotics or monthly ***IVIg*** may reduce recurrent infections in patients with hypogammaglobulinaemia but has no effect on survival.
- ***Autoimmune cytopenias:*** manage symptomatic AIHA or ITP with corticosteroids in the first instance; IVIg, chemotherapy, rituximab, or splenectomy may be required; test patients with pure red cell aplasia for parvovirus infection; treat with prednisolone, ciclosporin, or ATG.
- ***Radiotherapy*** helpful for persistent or bulky lymphadenopathy; splenic irradiation is sometimes helpful palliation in frail patients with symptomatic splenomegaly who are unfit for splenectomy.
- ***Splenectomy*** may sometimes be useful for massive splenomegaly, hypersplenism or refractory cytopenia (RR 50–88%).
- ***Lymphomatous transformation*** (Richter's syndrome) occurs in <10%; occurs in all stages; median interval from diagnosis 24 months; abrupt onset; progressive LN ↑; fever; weight loss; high LDH; usually diffuse large B-cell NHL but ~10% Hodgkins-like histology; chemoresistant; median survival 4 months with CHOP, better with ABVD for Hodgkins-like.

Prognosis
CLL remains an incurable disease with current therapy apart from a few allografted patients. Most patients with early stage, asymptomatic CLL die of other unrelated causes. Infection is a major cause of morbidity and mortality in symptomatic patients. Advanced stage patients eventually develop refractory disease and BM failure. Terminally some refractory patients develop prolymphocytic transformation. A second malignancy (skin, colon) occurs in up to 20%.

Cell markers in chronic lymphoproliferative disorders

Table 4.15 Mature B-cell lymphoproliferative disorders

Marker	CLL	PLL	HCL	SMZL	FL	MCL
Surface Ig	weak	++	++	++	++	+
CD5	++	–/+	–	–	–	++
CD10	–	–/+	–	–	+	–
CD11c	–/+	–	+	+/–	–	–
CD19	++	++	++	++	++	++
CD20	–/+	++	+	++	++	++
CD22	–/weak	++	++	++	+/–	+/–
CD23	++	+/–	–	–/+	–/+	–
CD25	+/–	–	++	–/+	–	–
CD79b	weak/–	++	+	++	++	++
FMC7	–/+	+	+	++	++	++
CD103	–	–	+	–/+	–	–
HC2	–	–	+	–/+	–	–
Cyclin D1	–	+	–/weak	–	–	++

CLL, chronic lymphocytic leukaemia; PLL, prolymphocytic leukaemia; HCL, hairy cell leukaemia; SMZL, splenic marginal zone lymphoma; FL, follicular lymphoma; MCL, mantle cell lymphoma.

Table 4.16 Mature T-cell lymphoproliferative disorders

Marker	T-LGLL	NK-LGLL	T-PLL	ATL	SS
TdT*	–	–	–	–	–
CD2	+	+	+	+	+
CD3	++	–	++	++	++
CD4	–	–	+/–	++	++
CD5	+	+	+	+	+
CD7	–/+	–	+++	–	–/+
CD8	++	–	–/+	–	–
CD16	+	+	–	–	–
CD25	–	–	–/+	++	–
CD56	–/+	+	–	–	–
Other		CD11b+		HTLV1+	
		CD57+			
Genotype	TCRR+	TCRR–	TCRR+	TCRR+	TCRR+

T-LGLL, T-cell large granular lymphocyte leukaemia; NK-LGLL, NK-cell large granular lymphocyte leukaemia; T-PLL, T cell prolymphocytic leukaemia; ATL, adult T cell leukaemia/lymphoma; SS, Sézary syndrome. *TdT: terminal deoxynucleotidyl transferase dif-ferentiates these cells from lymphoblasts of ALL. TCRR, clonally re-arranged T-cell receptor.

References

1. Moreau, E.J. *et al.* (1997). Improvement of the chronic lymphocytic leukemia scoring system with the monoclonal antibody SN8 (CD79b). *Am J Clin Pathol*, **108**, 378–82.
2. Montserrat, E. (2006). New prognostic markers in CLL. *Hematology 2006*, 279–84.
3. Seiler, T. et al (2006). Risk stratification in chronic lymphocytic leukaemia. *Semin Oncol*, **33**, 186–94.
4. Cheson, B.D. *et al* (1996). National Cancer Institute-Sponsored Working Group guidelines for chronic lymphocytic leukemia: revised guidelines for diagnosis and treatment. *Blood*, **12**, 4990–7.
5. www. NICE.org.uk/TA119february2007.
6. Catovsky, D. *et al* (2007). Assessment of fludarabine plus cyclophosphamide for patients with chronic lymphocytic leukaemia (the CLL4 Trial): a randomized controlled trial. *Lancet*, **370**, 230–9.
7. Oscier, D. *et al* (2004). Diagnosis and management of chronic lymphocytic leukaemia: A guideline. *Brit J Haematol*, **125**, 294–315.
8. http://www.bcshguidelines.com/pdf/chronicLL_050504.pdf
9. Gribben, J.G. (2005). Salvage therapy for CLL and the role of stem cell transplantation. *Hematology 2005*, 292–8.
10. Montserrat, E. *et al* (2006). How I treat refractory CLL *Blood*, **107**, 1276–83.
11. Wierda, W. (2006). Current and investigational therapies for patients with CLL. *Hematology 2006*, 285–94.

Prolymphocytic leukaemia (PLL)

Uncommon aggressive clinicopathological variant of CLL with characteristic morphology and clinical features. B-cell and rare T-cell forms recognized.

Epidemiology

Median age at presentation is 67 years; ♂:♀ ratio 2:1. Accounts for <2% cases of 'CLL'. B-PLL 75%; T-PLL 25%.

Clinical features

- Symptoms of BM failure and constitutional symptoms—lethargy, weight loss, fatigue, etc.
- Massive splenomegaly, typically >10cm below costal margin may cause abdominal pain. Hepatomegaly common.
- Minimal lymphadenopathy in B-PLL, generalized lymphadenopathy more common in T-PLL.
- Skin lesions occur in 25% T-PLL as do serous effusions.

Investigation and diagnosis

- FBC: high WBC (typically $>100 \times 10^9$/L; commonly $>200 \times 10^9$/L in T-PLL); anaemia and thrombocytopenia usually present.
- Differential shows >55% (often >90%) prolymphocytes.
- Morphology: large lymphoid cells, abundant cytoplasm (B-PLL mainly), prominent single central nucleolus.
- BM diffusely infiltrated.
- Immunophenotype: 📖 see Table 4.15, p.158
- Cytogenetics—B-PLL: 14q+ in 60%; t(11;14)(q13;q32)in 20%; *p53* gene abnormalities in 75%; 6q– and chromosome 1 abnormalities also described; T-PLL 14q11 abnormalities in >70%; loss of heterozygosity in 11q22–23 region affecting *ATM* gene expression in 67%; +8 in 50%.

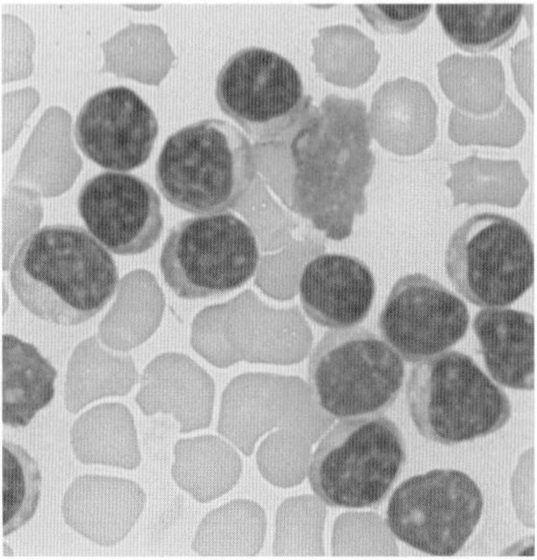

Fig. 4.15 Blood film in PLL: cells are larger than those seen in CLL have large prominent nucleoli and moderate chromatin condensation (📖 see Plate 16).

Differential diagnosis

B-PLL and CLL are not always easily distinguished and mixed 'CLL/PLL' is recognized (>10%, <55% prolymphocytes). Clinical features, morphology, and notably markers (📖 Table 4.15, p.158) used to distinguish PLL from other lymphoproliferative disorders.

Management

- PLL is typically resistant to chlorambucil.
- ***Splenectomy*** may be symptomatically helpful, 'debulking', but must be followed with other therapy.
- ***Splenic irradiation*** offers symptomatic relief if unfit for splenectomy.
- ***Combination chemotherapy:*** CHOP may achieve responses in about 33% and prolongs survival in younger patients.
- ***Purine analogue therapy:*** fludarabine, cladribine, or deoxycoformycin may produce responses in some patients with B-PLL; the combination of fludarabine and rituximab is under investigation in B-PLL.
- ***Alemtuzumab:*** anti-CD52 monoclonal antibody produces responses in both B-PLL and T-PLL. In T-PLL CR rates of 40–60% have been achieved; may last several months and permit high dose therapy with autologous or allogeneic SCT in eligible patients; some prolonged survival.
- ***Rituximab:*** anti-CD20 monoclonal antibody produces complete responses in B-PLL that may last several months and permit subsequent SCT in eligible patients.
- ***SCT:*** in view of the poor prognosis of both B- and T-PLL, younger patients who achieve a CR should be considered for allogeneic SCT where possible or autologous SCT.

Natural history

PLL is a relentlessly progressive disease and treatment is unsatisfactory. T-PLL carries poor prognosis with median survival 6–7 months. Median survival in B-PLL is 3 years.

Hairy cell leukaemia and variant

Uncommon low grade B-cell lymphoproliferative disorder associated with splenomegaly, pancytopenia, and typical 'hairy cells' in blood and BM.

Epidemiology

Accounts for 2% of leukaemias in adults, 8% of chronic lymphoproliferative disorders in West. Rare in Japan. No known aetiological factors. Presents in middle age (>45 years) with ♂:♀ ratio of 4:1

Clinical features

- Typically non-specific symptoms: lethargy, malaise, fatigue, weight loss, and dyspnoea.
- 15% present with infections, often atypical organisms due to monocytopenia.
- ~30% have recurrent infection; 30% bleeding or easy bruising.
- Splenomegaly in 80% (massive in 20–30%), hepatomegaly in 20%.
- Lymphadenopathy rare (<5%).
- Pancytopenia may be an incidental finding on a routine FBC.
- Vasculitic polyarthritis and visceral involvement similar to polyarteritis nodosa occurs in some patients with HCL.

Investigation and diagnosis

- FBC: moderate-to-severe pancytopenia; Hb <8.5g/dL 35%.
- Blood film: low numbers of 'hairy cells' in 95%; florid leukaemic features unusual.
- Hairy cells: kidney shaped nuclei, clear cytoplasm and irregular cytoplasmic projections (more notable on EM).
- WBC differential: neutropenia, $<1.0 \times 10^9/L$ in 75%; monocytopenia is a consistent feature.
- Cytochemistry: +ve for tartrate-resistant acid phosphatase (TRAP) in 95%; now identified by flow cytometry using antibody to TRAP.
- Immunophenotyping: typically CD11c, CD25, CD103, HC2+; differentiates HCL from other chronic lymphoproliferative disorders (📖 Table 4.15, p.158).
- BM: aspiration often unsuccessful—'dry tap' due to ↑ BM fibrosis; trephine shows diagnostic features with focal or diffuse infiltration of HCL where cells have characteristic 'halo' of cytoplasm confirmed by immunocytochemistry with anti-CD20/DBA-44 and anti-TRAP.
- Abdominal CT for intra-abdominal lymphadenopathy (15–20%).

Differential diagnosis

Confirmation of diagnosis may be difficult because of low numbers of circulating leukaemic cells and dry tap on marrow aspiration; trephine biopsy usually diagnostic; differential diagnosis includes myelofibrosis and other low grade lymphomas notably splenic marginal zone lymphoma.

Prognostic factors

No established staging system. Response to therapy is probably the best prognostic indicator. Bulky abdominal lymphadenopathy at diagnosis correlates with poor response to first-line therapy.

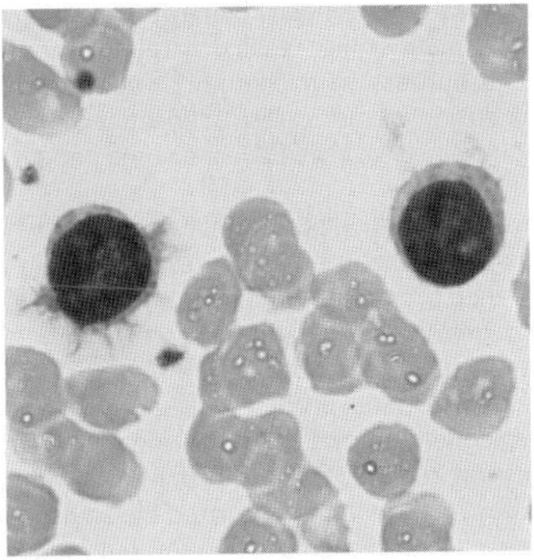

Fig. 4.16 Peripheral blood film in HCL showing typical 'hairy' lymphocytes (medium power) (see Plate 17).

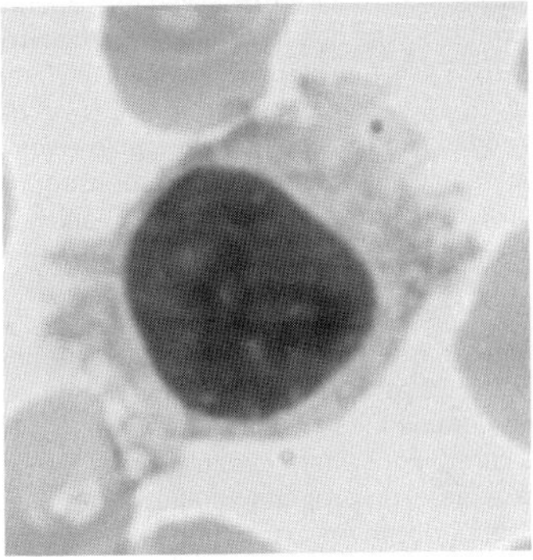

Fig. 4.17 Peripheral blood film in HCL showing typical 'hairy' lymphocytes (high power) (see Plate 18).

Management

- In <10% patients, often elderly with minimal or no splenomegaly and cytopenia, the disease remains relatively stable and may be observed.
- Therapy is required in patients with Hb <10g/dL, neutropenia <1.0 × 10^9/L, thrombocytopenia <100 × 10^9/L, symptomatic splenomegaly, recurrent infection, extralymphatic involvement, autoimmune complications, florid leukaemia, or progressive disease.
- Supportive management is important particularly in the early stages of therapy where cytopenias can worsen: treat infections promptly. *Note*: ↑ incidence of atypical mycobacterial infections in HCL.
- Cladribine: purine analogue; widely used as first-line therapy; continuous infusion of 0.1mg/kg/d × 7 days through PICC line

produces 80% CR rate, remainder PR; may be given as 2 hour infusion (0.14mg/kg/d × 5d) with similar results; platelet response in 2–4 weeks; temporary myelosuppression, maximum 1 week after infusion; avoid co-trimoxazole during infusions (rash); repeat at 6 months if no CR; 54% progression-free survival at 12 years; some patients probably cured.

- Deoxycoformycin alternative purine analogue; 4mg/m^2 IV bolus every 2 weeks to maximum response plus 2 cycles (generally 6–10); check creatinine clearance pre-therapy (must be >60mL/min for full dose; half dose >40mL/min) improvement begins after 2 cycles; maximum response generally 4–7 months; up to 90% OR; 75% CR; 15% continued CR at 8 years; some patients probably cured.
- After purine analogue therapy CD4 lymphodepletion causes immunosuppression: requires *P. jiroveci* prophylaxis with cotrimoxazole for 6 months after treatment and irradiated blood products indefinitely.
- IFN- α may be useful initial therapy (tiw) for 2–4 months before a purine analogue in patients with profound cytopenias.
- G-CSF may be useful in patients with severe neutropenia.
- Allopurinol should be given with initial therapy to prevent gout.
- Splenectomy: now rarely required; reserved for patients unresponsive to therapy or with bleeding due to severe thrombocytopenia. Non-curative but 40–70% will improve FBC for median 20 months without further therapy. OS 70% at 5 years. Histology shows characteristic infiltration of red pulp and atrophy of white pulp. Avoid drug therapy for 6 months after splenectomy to assess response.
- Monitor response to therapy at 3 months by trephine biopsy stained for CD20/DBA-44 and TRAP.

Natural history

Hairy cell leukaemia treated with a purine analogue is associated with prolonged survival (95% at 5 years, 80–87% at 10–12 years), with many patients achieving durable CRs (PFS 60% at 12 years with 2CdA); some patients may be cured. For others careful application of available treatments at disease relapse or progression allows prolonged, good quality survival. Late relapses occur. An association with second malignancy has been reported.

Second line and subsequent therapy

Immediate retreatment is not always necessary when relapse is identified. If a remission of >5 years has been achieved then a further remission with the same agent is likely. 2CdA treatment for relapse achieves 52% CR and 83% OR. The second remission is likely to be shorter (35 months v 42 months with 2CdA). Early relapse or resistance may benefit from an alternative purine analogue, IFN-α, or rituximab.

- ***IFN-α:*** 3 million units SC 3 × weekly continued for 12–18 months may be useful for HCL refractory to purine analogues; initial therapy achieves PR in up to 80% but CR in <5%; lower responses later in disease; generally normalization of blood counts occurs within 6 months and responses persist 12–15 months after discontinuation. Side effects notably flu-like symptoms and fatigue cause intolerance in some patients.

- ***Rituximab:*** 375mg/m^2 /wk iv x 4–12; offers an alternative to patients resistant to purine analogues. 26–80% ORs and 10–55% CRs have been reported with median responses of 14–73 months.

Hairy cell variant

Describes a very rare variant of HCL where the presenting WBC count is high due to circulating leukaemic cells (40–60 × 10^9/L) and monocytopenia is absent. Cells are villous but have a central round nucleus and a distinct nucleolus-like PLL. Marrow is aspirated easily due to low reticulin but the trephine appearance is similar to HCL and associated neutropenia. Immunophenotype differs from typical HCL: CD11c+, CD25, and HC2 –ve, CD103 usually –ve. Response to deoxycoformycin or IFN-α is poor but chlorambucil appears active in this form, and the variant generally follows an indolent course.

1. Chadha, P. *et al* (2005.) Treatment of hairy cell leukaemia with 2-chlorodeoxyadenosine (2-CdA): long term follow-up of the Northwestern University experience. *Blood*, **106**, 241–6.

Splenic marginal zone lymphoma (SMZL)

Formerly 'splenic lymphoma with villous lymphocytes' (SLVL). Rare B-cell lymphoproliferative disorder (<1% NHL) usually associated with marked splenomegaly and moderate lymphocytosis with irregular cytoplasmic borders. Probably arises in marginal zone of the spleen. Some cases may be antigen driven, notably those associated with hepatitis C infection.

Clinical features

- Non-specific symptoms, e.g. fatigue, abdominal discomfort.
- Affects older patients, median age at diagnosis ~65 years; rare <50.
- Moderate-to-massive splenomegaly.
- Hepatomegaly in 50%.
- Peripheral lymphadenopathy rare (splenic hilar LN frequently ↑).
- Auto-immune phenomena in 10%: AIHA, cold agglutinins, ITP, lupus anticoagulant, acquired von Willebrand's syndrome.
- Symptoms of cryoglobulinaemia in rare patients with concomitant hepatitis C infection.

Laboratory features

- Anaemia and thrombocytopenia in 25–30% usually due to hypersplenism. Neutropenia not marked.
- Total WBC ↑ due to lymphocytosis 95%; not grossly elevated (usually $<40 \times 10^9$/L; *cf.* PLL).
- Morphology: intermediate size lymphocytes, larger than typical CLL cells, round/oval nuclei; clumped chromatin, indistinct nucleoli, usually with villous cytoplasmic projections at one/both poles; not in all cases.
- Monocytopenia not a feature (*cf.* HCL).
- Immunophenotype: CD19+, CD20+, CD79b+, FMC7+, moderate-to-strong SmIg+; CD10–; most CD23–; usually CD5– CD25–; 20% CD25+ but CD11c– & CD103– differentiating from HCL; NB some DBA44+; 20% CD5+ but CD23– CD79b+ differentiating from CLL; cyclin D1– differentiates CD5+ SMZL from MCL; 📖 Table 4.15, p.158.
- Monoclonal serum paraprotein in up to 30%; usually IgM; sometimes IgG, rarely IgA; free urinary light chains in 66%.
- LDH usually normal; ↑ serum β_2-microglobulin.
- BM aspirate may show lymphocytosis (some plasmacytoid) with typical immunophenotype; biopsy may be normal (10%) but usually shows moderate patchy/nodular lymphoid infiltration; some interstitial or diffuse; intrasinusoidal CD20+ lymphoma cells characteristic of SMZL.
- Cytogenetic/molecular abnormalities in 80% but none specific; 7q– most frequent (26–79%); +3, Ig gene translocations, 17p– also recur.
- Genes involved in B-cell receptor signalling, AKT1 signalling, TNF signalling and NF-κB activation consistently deregulated.
- Spleen histology: characteristic with nodular infiltration involving the white pulp (*cf.* HCL).
- Rare patients with hepatitis C infection respond to treatment of this.

Differential diagnosis

Main differentials are MCL (especially 20% CD5+ SMZL) CLL, PLL, HCL, and hairy cell variant. Diagnosis requires careful morphological and immunophenotypic assessment (📖 Table 4.15, p.158).

Prognosis

Generally follows an indolent course with >50% survival at 5 years. Over 10% may require no treatment. Hgb <12g/dL, elevated LDH and albumin <35g/L have been used to identify 3 prognostic groups: low risk (no adverse factors; 41% of patients; 5-year cause specific survival (CSS) 88%); intermediate risk (1 factor; 34%; CSS 73%) and high risk (≥2 factors; 25%; CSS 50%). Loss, mutation, or overexpression of *p53* gene, CD38 expression, and unmutated IgV_H genes associated with poor outcome. Median survival >10 years from diagnosis. Transformation to diffuse large B-cell NHL occurs in ~10% in a median of 2–4 years: suggested by 'B-symptoms', lymphadenopathy, CNS involvement, and circulating 'blasts'.

Treatment

- Asymptomatic patients with modest splenomegaly and no significant cytopenias may be observed.
- Optimal therapy not yet defined.
- Splenectomy is recommended for bulky enlargement or hypersplenism (and/or to confirm diagnosis in some cases) and can correct cytopenias and associated symptoms for >5 years.
- Splenic irradiation is a safe and effective alternative to splenectomy in some cases and may be repeated.
- Progression after splenectomy may respond to chlorambucil (44% response rate; no CRs), fludarabine (very high response rates in small studies), and/or rituximab (very high response rates in small studies). Toxic effects with purine analogues may be marked in elderly patients; all patients should receive prophylactic co-trimoxazole and irradiated blood products.
- Rare patients with hepatitis C infection have high response rate to interferon-α or ribavirin.
- Treatment of transformation should follow that of diffuse large B-cell NHL.

1. Oscier, D. *et al* (2005). Splenic marginal zone lymphoma *Blood Rev*, **19**, 39–51.

2. Arcaini, L. *et al* (2006). Splenic marginal zone lymphoma. *Blood*, **107**, 4643–9.

Mantle cell lymphoma (MCL)

Pre-germinal centre B-cell derived lymphoid neoplasm defined in the WHO/REAL classification (📖 Table 5.1, p.181) by clinical, morphological, immunophenotypic, cytogenetic, and molecular criteria.

Incidence and aetiology

4–8% of adult NHL cases. Aetiology unknown. t(11;14)(q13;q32) involves *IgH* gene on chromosome 14, juxtaposes and dysregulates *BCL-1* with overexpression of cyclin D1, a protein involved in cell cycle regulation.

Clinical features and presentation

- Commonly ♂ >50 years; median age 63, range 35–85; ♂:♀ ratio 4:1.
- B symptoms (fever, night sweats, weight loss) 40%. Fatigue, abdominal distension, and symptoms related to extranodal disease.
- Lymphocytosis in peripheral blood may prompt referral as '?CLL'.
- Commonly advanced disease at presentation (87%) with generalized lymphadenopathy (57%); splenomegaly (47%); hepatomegaly (18%).
- Extranodal involvement, particularly in GI tract is common (18%), also lungs and CNS.
- Stage IV disease at diagnosis in 70%.

Diagnosis and investigation

- FBC: 36% have lymphocytosis; anaemia and mild thrombocytopenia only in very advanced disease.
- Blood film: intermediate size lymphocytes; nucleus often has clefts and indentations; smear cells unusual (*cf.* CLL).
- Immunophenotype: critical to diagnosis (📖 Table 4.15, p.158); SmIg strongly+ CD5+, CD10–, CD19+, CD20+, CD23–, CD43+, CD79b+, cyclin D1+ Bcl6–; rarely CD5–.
- Cytogenetics: t(11;14) in 50–90% by FISH techniques.
- BM trephine biopsy demonstrates involvement in >70% with nodular, paratrabecular, interstitial, or diffuse patterns similar to CLL.
- Lymph node biopsy: mantle zone expansion or diffuse effacement of nodal architecture by uniform 'centrocytes'; characteristic immunochemistry pattern: CD5+, CD10–, CD79b+, cyclin-D1+. Blastoid variant has larger cells with higher proliferative activity (Ki67+ cells) and more aggressive clinical course.
- Most patients have elevated LDH and serum β2-microglobulin
- Up to 30% have detectable paraprotein band, usually IgM.
- CT of chest, abdomen, and pelvis may confirm widespread disease.
- Colonoscopy helpful in some cases; colon involvement common.
- LP indicated in patients with blastoid variant to exclude CNS disease.

Differential diagnosis

In patients with lymphocytosis differentiation from CLL by immunophenotype: strong SmIg+, CD23–, and cyclin-D1+; from PLL when CD5+ by morphology; from follicular lymphoma by CD5+, CD10–, and cyclin D1+.

Prognostic factors

Stage using Ann Arbor system (📖 Table 5.8, p.210). International Prognostic Index (📖 Table 5.3, p.184) not generally as useful as in diffuse large B-NHL. Age >70 years, HB <12g/dL, and poor performance status are unfavourable. Blastoid variant, high proliferation index (Ki67), cytogenetic abnormalities, *p53* mutations, leukaemic phase, and ↑ β_2-microglobulin associated with worse prognosis.

Prognosis

MCL generally aggressive disease with poor prognosis. Median survival 3 years; 5–10% survive 10 years. Most develop progressive refractory disease. A small number follow a more indolent course. No evidence that MCL is cured by either conventional chemotherapy or autologous SCT.

Initial management

- Optimal therapy not defined. Enrol patients in clinical trial if available.
- ***COP or CHOP:*** overall response rates of 50–90% including 30–50% CR. Median freedom from progression <1 year. No clear survival advantage for anthracycline containing regimens.
- ***Fludarabine–cyclophosphamide(FC)*** (📖 p.732) has a high response rate (63%) and is under investigation as initial therapy ± rituximab. Cladribine and clofarabine also have activity in MCL and are in trials.
- ***Rituximab***, anti-CD20 monoclonal antibody, produces responses as a single agent (OR 35%; CR 10–15%; median duration 1 year); addition to CHOP ***(R-CHOP)*** improves CR rate (34% *vs.* 7%) but not time to progression (16–18 months); adding R to FC (***FCR***) or to FCM (FC + mitoxantrone) improves OR, CR, and PFS; maintenance role under evaluation.
- ***Chlorambucil*** as a single agent may be appropriate for elderly patients and those with co-morbidities.
- ***Hyper-CVAD ± rituximab*** (📖 p.734) used in USA as first-line therapy for younger patients (<65 years); achieves up to 87% CR and 97% overall responses with 64% freedom from progression at 36 months. High treatment-related toxicity. ***R-EPOCH*** (📖 p.729) is an alternative intensive regimen. Relapse in median 15–18 months without adjuvant SCT.
- Some evidence that consolidation of initial good response with high dose therapy (optimal regimen not defined) and ***allogeneic or autologous SCT*** in eligible patients prolongs remission; autograft not curative; reduced-intensity conditioning allografts under clinical trial.

Refractory or relapsed MCL

- Optimal therapy not defined. Enrol in clinical trial when possible.
- Consider FC, FCR, FCMR (FCR + mitoxantrone), or FMD (fludarabine, mitoxantrone + dexamethasone) in fludarabine-naïve patients. Consider Hyper-CVAD ± R in others if fit enough.
- Consolidation of response to salvage therapy with autologous SCT may benefit a subset of patients but continuous pattern of relapse.
- ***Bortezomib:*** proteasome inhibitor; single agent (1.3mg/m^2 IV d1, 4, 8, and 11 in 21d cycle × 8 cycles) achieves 31% OR in relapsed or refractory MCL; median duration 9 months; in trials in combination

with chemotherapy; FDA approved December 2006 for MCL patients who have received at least 1 prior therapy.

- ***Thalidomide***, ^{131}I-tositumomab, ^{90}Y- ibritumomab and lenalidomide show single-agent activity; in trials in combination with chemotherapy and rituximab. Thalidomide (200–400mg od until progression) + rituximab (375mg/m^2 IV x 4) achieved 81% OR and 31% CR with median PFS 20mo in a small study; may be suitable for older patients.

1. Ganti, A.K. *et al* (2005). Hematopoietic stem cell transplantation in mantle cell lymphoma. *Ann Oncol*, **16**, 618–24.

2. Romaguera, J.E. *et al.* (2005). High rate of durable remissions after treatment of newly diagnosed aggressive mantle-cell lymphoma with rituximab plus hyper-CVAD alternating with rituximab plus high-dose methotrexate and cytarabine. *J Clin Oncol*, **23**, 7013–23.

3. Fisher, R.I. *et al.* (2006). Multicenter phase II study of bortezomib in patients with relapsed or refractory mantle cell lymphoma. *J Clin Oncol*, **24**, 4867–74.

4. Schulz, H. *et al* (2007). Immunochemotherapy with rituximab and overall survival in patients with indolent or mantle cell lymphoma: a systematic review and meta-analysis. *J Natl Cancer Inst*, **99**, 706 –14.

Large granular lymphocyte leukaemia (LGLL)

Uncommon clonal lymphoproliferative disorders, characterized by an increase in LGLs in blood. Heterogeneous—may be either T-cell or NK-cell phenotype; each may follow an indolent or aggressive course.

T-cell LGLL

- Most frequent form of LGLL, 85% of LGL patients.
- Aetiology unclear—?chronic antigen stimulation by exogenous agents e.g. HTLV or by autoantigens.

Clinical features

- Median age at diagnosis 60 years; ♂=♀.
- Usually asymptomatic; modest lymphocytosis on routine FBC with large granular lymphocytes $>2 \times 10^9$/L (NR $0.2–0.4 \times 10^9$/L).
- 80% develop neutropenia; ~45% $<0.5 \times 10^9$/L.
- Occasional presentation with chronic fatigue or recurrent bacterial infections—usually mucocutaneous.
- Arthralgia, itching, rash (25%), mouth ulcers; association with seropositive rheumatoid arthritis in 25–35% and Felty's syndrome (neutropenia + splenomegaly + rheumatoid arthritis).
- Splenomegaly 20–50% of cases. Lymphadenopathy rare.

Laboratory findings

- Hb and platelets usually normal; chronic neutropenia (80%) and mild anaemia (48%) may be present. Thrombocytopenia 20%.
- Mild/moderate lymphocytosis (usually $<10 \times 10^9$/L); medium-large cells; eccentric nucleus; abundant cytoplasm and distinct azurophiliic granules.
- Phenotyping: most type as 'cytotoxic' T cells (CD3+ CD8+ CD16+ CD56– CD57+); variants co-express CD4 and CD8, CD4 alone or neither; weak expression of CD5 and CD7 distinguishes from reactive LGLs
- Clonal rearrangement of T-cell receptor genes (TCRβ & γ) confirms diagnosis by RFLP and Southern blotting (TCRβ) and PCR (TCRγ).
- Polyclonal hypergammaglobulinaemia, rheumatoid factor and antinuclear antibodies occur in 50% even without joint disease.
- BM involvement often subtle; may be diffuse or nodular usually non-paratrabecular; anti-CD3 immunohistochemistry helps.
- No characteristic cytogenetic pattern; <10% abnormal.

Differential diagnosis

Reactive lymphocytosis (screen for infection especially EBV); other T-cell lymphoproliferative disorders (immunophenotype; 📖 Table 4.16, p.159).

Prognosis and management

- Incurable but generally stable benign disease. Asymptomatic patients require observation only.
- Care is essentially supportive with prompt treatment of infection with appropriate broad spectrum antibiotics.
- Treatment indicated by development of recurrent infections, severe neutropenia, symptomatic anaemia or thrombocytopenia or symptomatic splenomegaly or systemic symptoms.

- Immunosuppression with low dose methotrexate (10mg/m^2 PO weekly), ciclosporin (2mg/kg PO bd) or cyclophosphamide (50–100mg PO od) effective in ~50% of patients with persistent severe neutropenia; treat for at least 4 months to assess response; indefinite treatment may be necessary to sustain response; more side effects with ciclosporin.
- Symptoms may improve without improved neutrophil count; failure to eradicate clone does not prevent improvement in cytopenias.
- Corticosteroids in modest dosage may improve neutropenia but predispose to infection, including fungal infections; responses less durable; may improve response rate if added to methotrexate or cyclophosphamide during 1st month of therapy; do not exceed 1 month; prophylactic antibiotics can be helpful in severe neutropenia on steroid therapy.
- G-CSF may be of value in symptomatic chronic neutropenia.
- Alemtuzumab and purine analogue drugs are reported to be effective as single agents in refractory T-LGLL.

Aggressive T-cell LGLL

- Rare; affects younger age-group: median age 41 years, range 9–64.
- Present with rapidly progressive B symptoms, hepatosplenomegaly, lymphadenopathy, lymphocytosis, anaemia, and/or thrombocytopenia.
- Poor prognosis; survival 2 months–2 years.
- Diagnosis by aggressive course plus FBC: LGLs >0.5 × 10^9/L, many >10 × 10^9/L; Immunophenotype: CD3+, CD8+, CD56+, TCR$\alpha\beta$, or variants; clonally rearranged TCR β and γ genes.
- Differentiate from:
  - Indolent T-cell LGLL: indolent clinical course, neutropenia, autoimmune disease, and CD56–.
  - Aggressive NK-LGLL: sCD3–, germline TCR genes, intracellular clonal episomal EBV; usually Asian patient.
- Optimal therapy undefined; treat with ALL-type regimen including CNS prophylaxis followed by SCT in first CR.

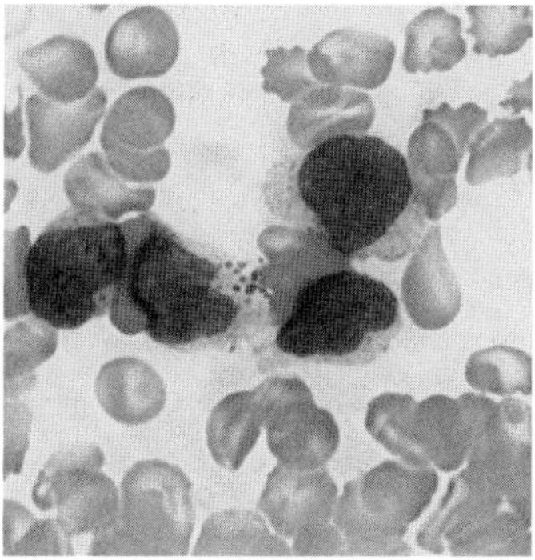

Fig. 4.18 Blood film showing large granular lymphocytes in LGL leukaemia.

Chronic NK-cell LGLL

- ~5% of LGL patients; median age 58; ♂:♀ ratio ~3:1.
- Aetiology unclear, ?role of viral infection.

Clinical and laboratory features

- Indolent disorder with favourable prognosis.
- Persistently elevated LGLs (~2×10^9/L).
- No fever, hepatosplenomegaly, or lymphadenopathy.
- Mild neutropenia and/or anaemia may occur; less severe and less frequent than in indolent T-cell LGLL.
- Immunophenotype: typically CD2+, CD3–, CD8–, CD16+, CD56+, CD57 variable.
- Demonstration of clonality and differential diagnosis from reactive NK-cell lymphocytosis can be difficult; panels vs. NK-associated antigens can be helpful; reactive lymphocytosis associated with viral infection and connective tissue disorders and rarely last >6 months; differentiate from indolent T-cell LGLL by immunophenotype and TCR clonal studies.

Treatment

As for indolent T-cell LGLL

Aggressive NK-cell LGLL

- ~10% of LGL patients; most prevalent in younger Asian patients.
- Median age 39 years; ♂=♀.
- Association with EBV infection—?aetiological role.

Clinical and laboratory features

- Acute presentation with B symptoms, hepatosplenomegaly, and cytopenia. DIC and multi-organ failure may occur.
- BM: diffuse infiltration by NK cells.
- Diagnosis by immunophenotype CD2+, CD3–, CD56+, usually CD57–; germline TCR genes; clonal episomal EBV.
- Cytogenetics: del(6q21-q25) and –17p13 most common.

Treatment

CHOP-type therapy ineffective. Consider ALL-type regimen with CNS prophylaxis as initial therapy; consolidate responders with SCT.

1. Alekshun, T.J. and Sokol, L. (2007). Diseases of large granular lymphocytes. *Cancer Control*, **14**, 141–50. http://www.medscape.com/viewarticle/556140

Adult T-cell leukaemia-lymphoma (ATL)

Aggressive neoplasm of CD4-+ve T-lymphocytes caused by HTLV-I with a distinct geographical distribution.

Incidence

Highest incidence among populations where HTLV-I infection endemic: Kyushi district of SW Japan, Caribbean, parts of Central and South America, Central and West Africa. Incidence 2/1000 ♂ and 0.5–1/1000 ♀ seropositive for HTLV-I (37% ♂ >40) in SW Japan. Risk 2.5% at 70 years. Non-endemic cases generally originate from these areas.

Aetiology

HTLV-I involved in multi-step pathogenesis. HTLV-I provirus in ATL cells; all patients with ATL are seropositive for prior HTLV-I infection. Transfer of live infected cells required for infection; 3 major routes: mother to infant (mainly by breast milk); parenteral transmission; sexual transmission. Not all infected patients develop ATL: during long latent period (40–60 years) viral products notably Tax and *HBZ*, host epigenetic changes, genetic factors, and immunity influence neoplastic transformation

Clinical subtypes

4 subtypes described: acute, chronic, smouldering, and lymphomatous forms. Acute subtype most common (66%), median survival 6 months despite therapy. Other forms have longer survival but often progress to the acute form after several months. Median survival of lymphomatous subtype ~1 year and chronic subtype ~2 years. The smouldering subtype is most indolent and is associated survival >24 months.

Clinical features and presentation

- Median age at diagnosis 58 years (range 20–90); ♂:♀ ratio 1:4.
- History of residence or origin in HTLV-I endemic area usual.
- Usually short history of rapidly increasing ill health.
- Opportunistic infection common.
- Acute subtype: abdominal pain, diarrhoea, pleural effusion, ascites, and respiratory symptoms (often due to leukaemic infiltration of lungs).
- Lymphadenopathy 60%; hepatomegaly 26%, splenomegaly 22%; skin lesions 39% in acute subtype.
- Lymphomatous subtype: prominent lymphadenopathy; few circulating cells. Chronic subtype: mild ↑ WBC; some skin lesions, ↑ LN, organomegaly. Smouldering subtype: few ATL cells, skin lesions, and occasional pulmonary involvement.

Diagnosis and investigation

- FBC: WBC usually markedly ↑ (up to 500×10^9/L) in acute form but may be normal; anaemia and thrombocytopenia common.
- Blood film: large numbers of lymphoid cells with marked nuclear irregularity occasionally multilobulated with 'floral' or 'clover leaf' appearance (Fig. 4.19).
- Immunophenotyping: generally CD2+, CD3+, CD4+, CD5+, CD7–, CD8–, CD25+, HLA-DR+ T cells; rarely CD4–, CD8+ or CD4+, CD8+ (📖 Table 4.16, p.159).

- Serology: +ve for HTLV-I.
- Cytogenetics: multiple abnormalities described; no consistent pattern.
- Serum chemistry: hypercalcaemia in 33–50% of patients at diagnosis; 70% during disease course due to ↑ osteoclasts.
- BM: diffuse infiltration by ATL cells.
- Monoclonal integration of HTLV-I provirus in lymphoid cells can be demonstrated by Southern blotting.

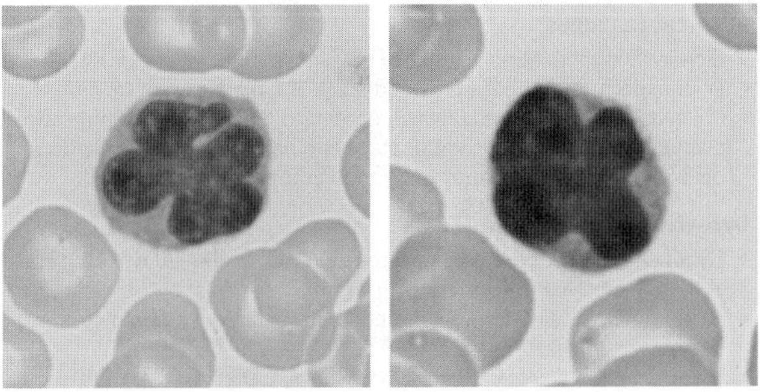

(a) (b)

Fig. 4.19 Peripheral blood films showing typical ATL cell with lobulated 'clover leaf' nucleus' (📖 see Plate 19 and Plate 20).

Prognostic factors

Poor prognostic features

- ↑ LDH.
- Hypercalcaemia.
- Hyperbilirubinaemia.
- ↑ WBC.

Management and prognosis

- Treatment unsatisfactory; poor prognosis in acute and lymphomatous ATL: median survivals 6 and 10 months respectively. Death is usually due to opportunistic infection.
- Patients with acute and lymphomatous ATL require immediate treatment; patients with chronic or smouldering ATL may be observed.
- Biweekly CHOP (with G-CSF) achieves 66% OR with 25% CR; median survival <1 year; OS at 3 years ~13%.
- More intensive treatment (VCAP-AMP-VECP) improves responses (OR 72%; CR 40%); median survival ~1 year; OS at 3 years ~24%.
- Infectious complications are frequent with chemotherapy.
- Allogeneic SCT can achieve median DFS up to 18 months. GvL effect appears important. Reduced-intensity conditioning safer in older patients (most >50 years). Donors should be HTLV-I seronegative as donor cell transformation to ATL reported.

1. Yasunaga, J. and Matsuoka, M. (2007). Human T-cell leukaemia virus type 1 induces adult T-cell leukaemia: from clinical aspects to molecular mechanisms. *Cancer Control*, **14**, 133–40. 🖫 http://www.medscape.com/viewarticle/556137.

Sézary syndrome (SS)

Leukaemic phase of a low grade 1° cutaneous mature T-cell lymphoma (mycosis fungoides; MF).

Incidence

Occurs in up to 20% of cases of 1° cutaneous T-cell lymphoma; median age 52 years; ♂:♀ ratio 2:1.

Clinical features

- Generally diagnosed as a result of FBC in a patient with exfoliative erythroderma; not necessarily end-stage and may present *de novo*.
- MF classically progresses through eczematoid plaque stage, infiltrative plaque stage, and overt tumour stage and has characteristic histology on skin biopsy (epidermotropism and Pautrier microabscesses).

Investigations and diagnosis

- FBC: generally moderate leucocytosis (WBC rarely $>20 \times 10^9$/L); Hb and platelets usually normal.
- Blood film: typically reveals large numbers of large lymphoid cells with characteristic 'cerebriform' folded nucleus.
- Immunophenotyping: CD2+, CD3+, CD4+, CD5+, CD7–, CD8–, CD25– T cells.
- Cytogenetics: no typical pattern.

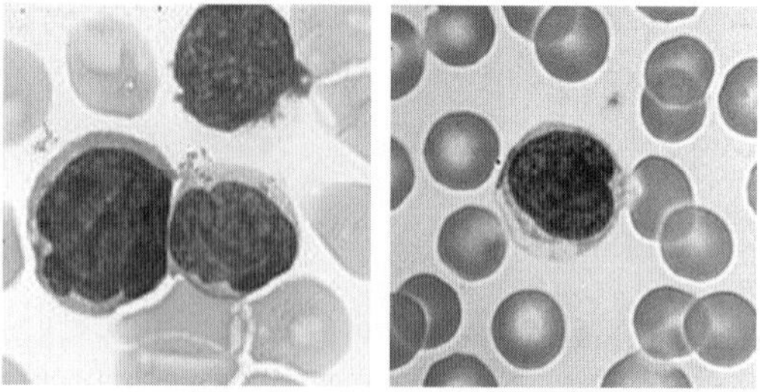

(a) (b)

Fig. 4.20 Blood film in SS showing typical cerebriform nuclei. Image (b) is reproduced with permission from Souhami, R. L. *et al* (2002). *Oxford Textbook of Oncology*, 2e. Oxford University Press, Oxford (📖 see Plate 21).

Management and prognosis

Patients with SS have a poor prognosis. High Sézary cell count, loss of CD5 and CD7, and chromosomal abnormalities associated with poor outcome. There is no evidence that single agent or combination chemotherapy (CVP or CHOP) improves survival. High response rates achieved but short durations. May palliate symptoms. Median survival 6–8 months. Allogeneic SCT should be considered in younger patients as it may be curative.

1. Rosen, S.T. and Querfield, C. (2006). Primary cutaneous T-cell lymphomas. *Hematology 2006*, 323–30.

Chapter 5

Lymphoma

Non-Hodgkin lymphoma (NHL)

NHL is a diagnosis applied to a group of histologically and biologically heterogeneous clonal malignant diseases arising from the lymphoid system.

Epidemiology

The annual incidence in Western countries is 14–19 cases per 100,000 (i.e. 4% of all cancers) and has ↑ at a rate of 3–4% per annum since the 1970s. Incidence ↑ with age. ♂:♀ ratio 3:2. The ↑ incidence is only in part due to ↑ mean age of the population, improvements in diagnosis, the HIV pandemic, and immunosuppressive therapy.

Aetiology

The rearrangement and mutation of immunoglobulin genes that occur in B-cell differentiation and the response to antigen offers an opportunity for genetic accidents such as translocations or mutations involving immunoglobulin gene loci that have been characterized in many lymphomas. Most translocations involve genes associated with either proliferation (e.g. *c-MYC*) or apoptosis (e.g. *BCL-2*). Factors associated with NHL are:

- Congenital immunodeficiency: ataxia telangiectasia, Wiskott–Aldrich syndrome, X-linked combined immunodeficiency (?EBV infection important).
- Acquired immunodeficiency: immunosuppressive drugs, transplantation, HIV infection (typically high grade and often occur in extranodal sites e.g. brain).
- Infection: HTLV-I (ATL); EBV (Burkitt lymphoma, Hodgkin lymphoma and immunodeficiency related high grade lymphomas); *Helicobacter pylori* (gastric mucosa-associated lymphoid tissue (MALT) lymphomas).
- Environmental toxins: association with exposure to agricultural pesticides, herbicides and fertilisers, solvents and hair dyes.
- Familial: risk ↑ 2–3-fold in close relatives (?genetic or environmental).

Classification

The World Health Organization (WHO) classification of lymphoid neoplasms (📖 Table 5.1) refined the Revised European American Lymphoma (REAL) classification (📖 Table 5.2) producing a list of clinico-pathologically well characterized lymphomas using morphology, immunophenotype, genotype, ↔ cell counterpart, and clinical behaviour. Inter- and intraobserver reproducibility is 85–95%. In Europe and USA 85% of lymphomas are B-cell type.

The clinical behaviour of lymphomas informs management strategies in clinical practice and current treatment protocols are still based on classification systems that group histological diagnoses into indolent (low grade) and aggressive (intermediate and high grade or simply high grade) NHL. More biologically relevant classification of lymphoma diagnosis using the WHO system and emerging therapeutic options based on immunological and molecular characteristics may increase the diagnosis-specific nature of therapy in the future.

Table 5.1 WHO classification of lymphoid neoplasms[1,2]

B-cell neoplasms

Precursor B-cell neoplasms

- Precursor B-lymphoblastic leukaemia/lymphoma (precursor B-cell acute lymphoblastic leukaemia)

Mature (peripheral B-cell) neoplasms

- B-cell chronic lymphocytic leukaemia/ small lymphocytic lymphoma
- B-cell prolymphocytic leukaemia
- Lymphoplasmacytic lymphoma
- Splenic marginal zone B-cell lymphoma (± villous lymphocytes)
- HCL
- Plasma cell myeloma/plasmacytoma
- Extranodal marginal zone B-cell lymphoma of MALT type
- Nodal marginal zone B-cell lymphoma (± monocytoid B-cells)
- Follicular lymphoma
- Mantle cell lymphoma
- Diffuse large B-cell lymphoma
    - Mediastinal large B-cell lymphoma
    - 1° effusion lymphoma
- Burkitt lymphoma/leukaemia

T-cell neoplasms

Precursor T-cell neoplasms

- Precursor T-lymphoblastic leukaemia/lymphoma (precursor T-cell acute lymphoblastic leukaemia)
- Blastoid NK-cell lymphoma

Mature (peripheral) T-cell and NK-cell neoplasms

- T-cell prolymphocytic leukaemia
- T-cell large granular lymphocytic leukaemia
- Aggressive NK-cell leukaemia
- Adult T-cell leukaemia/lymphoma (HTLV-I+)
- Extranodal NK/T-cell lymphoma, nasal type
- Enteropathy type T-cell lymphoma
- Hepatosplenic T-cell lymphoma
- Subcutaneous panniculitis-like T-cell lymphoma
- Mycosis fungoides/Sézary syndrome
- Primary cutaneous anaplastic large cell lymphoma, T/null cell
- Peripheral T-cell lymphoma (not otherwise specified)
- Angioimmunoblastic T-cell lymphoma
- Primary systemic anaplastic large cell lymphoma, T/null-cell

Hodgkin lymphoma

Nodular lymphocyte predominant Hodgkin lymphoma

Classical Hodgkin lymphoma

- Nodular sclerosis Hodgkin lymphoma (grades 1 and 2)
- Lymphocyte-rich classical Hodgkin lymphoma
- Mixed cellularity Hodgkin lymphoma
- Lymphocyte depleted Hodgkin lymphoma

Table 5.2 'Clinical grade' and frequency of lymphomas in the REAL classification[3]

Diagnosis	% of all cases
Indolent lymphomas (low risk)	
Follicular lymphoma (*Note*: grade I and II; grade III intermediate risk)	22%
Marginal zone B-cell, MALT lymphoma	8%
Chronic lymphocytic leukaemia/small lymphocytic lymphoma	7%
Marginal zone B-cell, nodal	2%
Lymphoplasmacytic lymphoma	1%
Aggressive lymphomas (intermediate risk)	
Diffuse large B-cell lymphoma	31%
Mature (peripheral) T-cell lymphomas	8%
Mantle cell lymphoma	7%
Mediastinal large B-cell lymphoma	2%
Anaplastic large cell lymphoma	2%
Very aggressive lymphomas (high risk)	
Burkitt lymphoma	2%
Precursor T-lymphoblastic	2%
Other lymphomas	7%

Presentation

The features at presentation reflect a spectrum from 'low grade' lymphoma (typically, widely disseminated at diagnosis but with indolent course; non-destructive growth patterns) to 'high grade' lymphoma (short history of localized rapidly enlarging lymphadenopathy ± constitutional upset: drenching night sweats, >10% weight loss and/or fever; destructive growth patterns).

In Europe and the USA almost 75% of adults present with nodal disease, usually superficial painless lymphadenopathy. 25% are extranodal (~50% in the Far East) and may present with oropharyngeal involvement (5–10%), GI involvement (15%), CNS involvement (5–10%, esp. high grade NHL), skin involvement (esp. T-cell lymphomas), or autoimmune cytopenias. Patients with GI involvement have a higher frequency of oropharyngeal involvement (Waldeyer's ring) and vice versa. Hepatosplenomegaly is common in advanced disease.

Diagnostic and staging investigations

- Histological diagnosis by expert haematopathologist: biopsy of lymph node or extranodal mass with immunohistochemistry ± molecular analysis. *Note.* FNA is inadequate for reliable diagnosis and grading.
- Detailed history including 'B symptoms'.
- Physical examination including Waldeyer's ring.
- FBC, plasma viscosity/ESR, and blood film.
- Performance status.
- LDH.

- Serum β2-microglobulin.
- U&E, uric acid, LFTs.
- Serum protein electrophoresis.
- BM trephine biopsy.
- CXR.
- CT chest, abdomen, and pelvis to define nodal and extranodal disease.
- Useful in some patients:
  - PET scan or Gallium scan.
  - Neck CT.
  - LP and CT or MRI head/spine for patients with CNS symptoms.
  - LP also for high grade disease with BM, testicular, paranasal sinus, parameningeal, peri-orbital or paravertebral involvement, HIV+ or lymphoblastic or Burkitt histology.
  - MRI spine.
  - Bone scan.
  - HIV test (especially in Burkitt lymphoma and CNS lymphoma).
  - *H. pylori* testing in gastric MALT lymphoma.

Staging helps to define prognosis and select therapy. Also helps assess response to therapy. The Ann Arbor staging system developed for Hodgkin lymphoma also used in NHL (📖 Hodgkin lymphoma, p.210).

Laboratory features

- Normochromic normocytic anaemia common.
- Leucoerythroblastic film if extensive BM infiltration ± pancytopenia.
- Hypersplenism (occasionally).
- PB may show lymphoma cells in some patients: moderate lymphocytosis in MCL; cleaved 'buttock' cells in FL and blasts in high grade disease.
- LFTs abnormal in hepatic infiltration.
- Serum LDH and β2-microglobulin are useful prognostic factors.
- Lymph node biopsy provides the best material for classification and precise diagnosis using morphology, immunohistochemistry and genetic features e.g. translocations or immunoglobulin and T-cell receptor gene rearrangement. FNA is not adequate for diagnosis or grading.
- WHO classification recommends FL is graded histologically based on the average number of centroblasts or 'large transformed cells' (LTCs) in 10 neoplastic follicles at +40 high power field (HPF) examination:
  - Grade 1, 0–5 LTCs/HPF.
  - Grade 2, 6–15 LTCs/HPF.
  - Grade 3a >15 LTCs/HPF with many residual small cells.
  - Grade 3b >15 LTCs/HPF in monotonous sheets.
  - This grading does not appear to be clinically predictive but a diffuse component >50% confers inferior survival similar to DLBCL and recommended treatment for Grade 3b is R-CHOP.
- ~20% of patients with SLL or FL have a serum paraprotein, usually IgM and usually low level.

Prognostic factors

- Histologic grade.
- Performance status.
- Constitutional ('B'-) symptoms unfavourable.

- Age (unfavourable >60 years).
- Disseminated disease (stage III–IV) unfavourable.
- Extranodal disease (unfavourable ≥2 extranodal sites).
- Bulky disease (unfavourable if >10 cm).
- Raised serum LDH (unfavourable if ↑).
- Raised serum β_2-microglobulin unfavourable.
- High proliferation rate by Ki-67 immunochemistry unfavourable.
- BCL-2 expression poor risk in DLBCL (not with R-CHOP treatment)
- BCL-6 expression favourable in DLBCL (not with R-CHOP treatment)
- *P53* mutations unfavourable.
- T-cell phenotype unfavourable.
- High grade transformation from low grade NHL unfavourable.
- Gene expression profile in DLBCL (GCB favourable; ABC poor)

The International Prognostic Index (IPI)[4] was developed for aggressive NHL and validated in all clinical grades of NHL as a predictor of response to therapy (in the pre-rituximab era), relapse and survival (Table 5.3). One point is awarded for each of the following characteristics to identify 4 risk groups:

- Age > 60 years.
- Stage III or IV.
- ≥ 2 extranodal sites of disease.
- Performance status ≥2.
- Serum LDH raised.

Table 5.3 IPI[4]

Score	IPI risk group	%CR	5-year CR-DFS	5-year OS
0 or 1	Low	87%	70%	73%
2	Low/intermediate	67%	50%	51%
3	Intermediate/high	55%	49%	43%
4 or 5	High	44%	40%	26%

The age-adjusted IPI[4] is designed for patients aged ≤60 years who may be eligible for more intensive therapy (Table 5.4). One point is awarded for each of the following characteristics:

- Stage III or IV.
- Raised serum LDH.
- Performance status ≥ 2.

Table 5.4 Age-adjusted IPI[4]

Score	IPI risk group (patients ≤60)	%CR	5-year CR-DFS	5-year OS
0	Low	92%	86%	83%
1	Low/intermediate	78%	66%	69%
2	Intermediate/high	57%	53%	46%
3	High	46%	58%	32%

A revised International Prognostic Index (R-IPI)[5] has been developed for patients with DLBCL treated with R-CHOP as addition of monoclonal antibody therapy has altered the survival of IPI prognostic groups. R-IPI uses the same risk factors as IPI to identify 3 distinct groups (Table 5.5).

Table 5.5 R-IPI[5]

Score	R-IPI risk group	% patients	4-year PFS	4-year OS
0	Very good	10%	94%	94%
1 or 2	Good	45%	80%	79%
3, 4 or 5	Poor	45%	53%	55%

The Follicular Lymphoma Prognostic Index (FLIPI)[6] provides better prognostic information in patients with follicular lymphoma as only ~11% are high risk on IPI. FLIPI may be used to assess the need for early treatment and its likely outcome. One point is awarded for each of the following risk factors to identify 3 risk groups:

- Age >60 years.
- Ann Arbor stage III or IV.
- Haemoglobin <12g/dL.
- Raised serum LDH.
- Number of nodal sites ≥5.

Table 5.6 FLIPI[6]

Score	FLIPI risk group	% patients	5yr OS	10yr OS
0 or 1	Low	36	91%	71%
2	Intermediate	37	78%	51%
≥ 3	High	27	52%	36%

References

1. Harris, N.L. *et al.* (1994). A revised European-American classification of lymphoid neoplasms: a proposal from the International Lymphoma Study Group. *Blood*, **84**, 1361–92
2. Jaffe, E.S. *et al.* (2001). In Kleihues, P. Sobin, L. (eds.) *WHO Classification of Tumours*. ARC Press, Lyon.
3. A clinical evaluation of the International Lymphoma Study Group classification of non-Hodgkin's lymphoma. The Non-Hodgkin's Lymphoma Classification Project. (1997) *Blood*, **89**, 3909–18.
4. A predictive model for aggressive non-Hodgkin's lymphoma. The international Non-Hodgkin's Lymphoma Prognostic Factors. (1993) *N Engl J Med*, **329**, 987–94.
5. Sehn, L.H. *et al.* (2007). The revised International Prognostic Index (R-IPI) is a better predictor of outcome than the standard IPI for patients with diffuse large B-cell lymphoma treated with R-CHOP *Blood*, **109**, 1857–61.
6. Solal-Celigny P. *et al.* (2004). Follicular lymphoma international prognostic index. *Blood*, **104**: 1258–65.

Indolent lymphoma

Clinical features

Up to 40% of cases; typically slowly progressive disorders.

Follicular lymphoma

Most common in middle and old age (median age 55 years); presents with painless lymphadenopathy at ≥1 sites, effects of BM infiltration, constitutional symptoms (15–20%) or pressure effects of bulky nodes (ureter, spinal cord, or orbit); LN may fluctuate in size; at diagnosis, 66% stage III or IV, 70% BM involvement, 15–20% localized stage I or II disease; median survival ~8–10 years; ~30% may transform to high grade DLBCL (often resistant to treatment; median survival 12 months). *Note*: cases of FL with high proportion of centroblasts (>50%) on histology follow a more aggressive clinical course and are treated as aggressive lymphomas.

Marginal zone lymphoma

Takes 3 forms:

- MALT lymphomas—associated with local invasion at site of origin, e.g. stomach, small bowel, salivary gland, or lung; gastric MALT lymphomas present with long history of dyspepsia, abdominal pain ± GI bleeding; diagnosis by endoscopy and biopsy; localized in 80–90% and respond to antibiotic treatment for *H. pylori*; good prognosis (>80% 5-year survival).
- Nodal marginal zone lymphoma (MZL)/monocytoid B-cell lymphoma; rare; associated with Sjögren's syndrome and Hashimoto's thyroiditis; usually localized to ocular adnexa, thyroid, parotid, lung, or breast.
- Splenic MZL related to SLVL (📖 p.166); elderly patients with marked splenomegaly ± hypersplenism, BM involvement ± villous lymphocytosis, lymphadenopathy absent.

Small lymphocytic lymphoma

Nodal form of CLL (📖 p.150); generally age >60 years; disseminated peripheral lymphadenopathy and splenomegaly; lymphocyte count <4.5 $\times 10^9$/L; BM involvement in 80%; constitutional symptoms <20%; serum paraprotein, usually IgM in 30%; median survival 8–10 years; some patients evolve into CLL, others to DLBCL.

Lymphoplasmacytic lymphoma

Occurs in older patients; usually isolated lymphadenopathy ± serum paraprotein; usually IgM, symptoms of hyperviscosity if markedly ↑ (📖 Waldenström's macroglobulinaemia, p.366).

Immunohistochemical and cytogenetic features

Follicular lymphomas

- Pan-B markers; CD5–, CD10+, BCL–2+. t(14;18)(q32;q21) in 90% (*cf.* reactive lymphoid hyperplasia with normal follicles BCL-2–).
- A survival predictor score has been developed from gene expression profiles representing immune response genes of infiltrating non-malignant cells.

Treatment of indolent lymphoma

FL and SLL comprise the majority of patients. Both diseases are usually responsive to chemotherapy and radiotherapy but unless truly localized, inevitably recur. There is no firm evidence of a curative therapy for advanced disease. Many patients have few or no symptoms and a decision to initiate treatment and the treatment chosen must take account of individual quality of life issues. At each stage, pros and cons of treatment options should be shared with the patient to reach an agreed treatment decision. Median OS with traditional treatment 8–10 years.

Initial treatment of localized FL and SLL (stage I/II)

Involved field radiotherapy (35–40Gy) may be curative in the 15–30% of patients with localized disease. 5-year DFS >50% may be expected. Recurrence generally occurs outside radiation field. Late relapses occur. OS ~80% at 5 years, ~60% at 10 years. Addition of chemotherapy e.g. CVP improves DFS but not OS.

Initial management of advanced (stage III/IV) FL (histological grade 1 and 2) and SLL

Histological grade 3b FL is usually treated like DLBCL. Traditionally management of newly diagnosed patients with other types of FL/SLL involved a decision between (i) 'watchful waiting' or (ii) conventional chemotherapy and/or radiotherapy. Symptomatic patients require treatment at diagnosis. 'Watchful waiting' in others was based on studies showing similar overall survival but better 'quality of life' in asymptomatic patients in whom therapy was deferred until indicated, compared to those in whom therapy was initiated at diagnosis. Newer more effective therapeutic options are prompting a re-evaluation of this approach.

'Watchful waiting'

Therapy may be deferred for many months/years after diagnosis in asymptomatic patients with low bulk disease until clinical symptoms or complications develop. Patients may have better QoL and avoid exposure to cytotoxic agents but must be monitored closely (every 3 months for 1 year then every 3–6 months) to prevent or identify insidious complications promptly. OS >80% at 5 years.

Indications for treatment

- B symptoms: unexplained weight loss, fever, or night sweats.
- Cytopenia.
- Bulky disease.
- Steady progression.
- Threatened end-organ function.
- Transformation.
- Patient preference.

Therapy

Enter patient in clinical trial where possible; otherwise treatment generally involves one of the following:

- *R-CVP:* (📖 p.741.) Addition of rituximab to CVP improves responses (OR 81% *vs.* 57%; CR 41% *vs.* 10%; median time to failure (TTF) 34 *vs.*

15 months; OS 83% *vs.* 77%)[1] and in the UK, is NICE approved for 1st-line therapy of stage III/IV FL but not for SLL (TA110; 09/06).[2]

- *Chlorambucil (Clb):* superceded as 1st choice in FL but may still have a place in elderly patients; still widely used in SLL in UK; (0.1–0.2 mg/kg/d × 7–14d PO, q28 or 0.4–0.6mg/kg every 2 weeks) or cyclophosphamide (50–150mg/d PO) as single agents or with prednisolone; OR 50–80% after 12–18 months treatment; most relapse < 5 years; convenient oral regimen; well tolerated but prolonged or repeated use causes myelosuppression.
- *'Simple' combination chemotherapy* (e.g. 📖 CVP, p.741): traditional alternative to Clb; more rapid response (useful in bulky disease or symptomatic patients) but otherwise similar: OR 80–90%; median response 1.5–3 years; few durable remissions; IV and oral regimen; higher CR rate, longer PFS but no OS advantage *vs.* Clb; causes alopecia.
- *'High grade' regimens:* high 'CR' rates (~60%) with CHOP-type regimens but continuous pattern of relapse and OS not convincingly improved in indolent FL (histological grades I and II). FL histological 'grade 3b' treated as 'high grade' with R-CHOP (📖 p.740); achieves responses equivalent to DLBCL (📖 see 196) but higher relapse rate. R-CHOP is widely used in USA as first line therapy for FL.
- *Purine analogues:* fludarabine has OR rate of ~75% (~40% CRs) in untreated patients with FL. Combination with cyclophosphamide (📖 FC, 📖 p.732) increases response rates (89% CRs) and response duration. Combination with mitoxantrone (FM) achieves 91% ORs, 43% CRs and 2-year DFS of 63% (reviewed in reference 3). In CLL/SLL fludarabine achieves higher response rates and durations than Clb but no OS advantage. Prophylaxis of *P. jiroveci* by co-trimoxazole required during and for 6 months after therapy and also of HZV by aciclovir in some patients. Cellular blood products must be irradiated for 6 months after therapy. FCR is widely used for SLL in USA.
- *Monoclonal antibody therapy:* rituximab is humanized anti-CD20 monoclonal antibody, licensed by FDA and European Medicine Agency (EMA) for (i) treatment of patients with relapsed/refractory CD20+ FL; (ii) 1st-line treatment of CD20+ FL in combination with CVP chemotherapy (R-CVP is NICE approved 1st-line therapy for stage III/IV FL 📖 p.741); (iii) treatment of CD20+ low grade NHL in stable disease or PR or CR after CVP. Single agent 375mg/m^2 infusion weekly x 4 achieves 72% OR, 36% CR rates in untreated patients and median TTP 2 years.[4] Less good responses with bulky disease. May be useful for elderly or infirm patient, if available. In a randomized trial, the same dose every 6 months as maintenance therapy after response to chemotherapy achieved median PFS of 31 months *vs.* 7 months though no OS benefit.[5] A number of other maintenance schedules demonstrate prolonged DFS. NICE, FDA and EMA have approved maintenance therapy for patients responding to CVP. Rituximab has also been used for '*in vivo* purging' prior to stem cell harvest. Toxicity is mild. Risk of anaphylaxis with first course (📖 see p.742).
- *Chemoimmunotherapy:* combination of rituximab with chemotherapy regimens enhances OR rates, CR rates, DFS, and OS in newly diagnosed patients with indolent NHL. R-CVP (NICE-approved;

see p.741), R-CHOP, FCR and R-MCP achieve better responses than CVP, CHOP, FC and MCP (reviewed in reference 3).
- *Radiotherapy* may be useful for treatment of local problems due to bulky disease e.g. cord compression.

Other treatment options for indolent lymphomas

- ***IFN-α maintenance:*** several large randomized trials demonstrate a beneficial effect on survival for patients treated with ≥9 million U/week administered with and after intensive chemotherapy for >18 months or until progression; side effects reduce QoL and the attraction of this therapy.
- ***Radioimmunotherapy:*** *tositumomab,* ^{131}I-radiolabelled murine anti-CD20 monoclonal antibody; β and γ emission; a single infusion achieves very high response rates (95% OR and 75% CR) in untreated patients with median PFS >6 years;[6] up to 68% OR and 38% CR in treated patients and better and more prolonged responses than prior chemotherapy achieved; transient mild-to-moderate myelosuppression; antimurine antibodies develop especially in untreated patients. A phase II trial of a single infusion after CHOP therapy improved the CR rate 2-fold.[7] Remains investigational in early stage disease. Currently may be best used for early 'salvage' in chemo- or rituximab-resistant patients. *Ibritumomab tiuxetan* ^{90}Yt-labelled murine anti-CD20 monoclonal antibody; beta emission only; achieves good response rates (OR 74%, CR 15%) in relapsed FL refractory to rituximab.
- ***Total lymphoid (or nodal) irradiation:*** may achieve very high CR rates with 5-year DFS rates >60% but is rarely used due to toxicity.
- ***Autologous SCT:*** 3 randomized trials of auto-SCT *vs.* IFN-α maintenance after initial chemotherapy in FL (reviewed in reference 3). Auto-SCT can achieve ~80% CR rate; and up to 65% DFS at 5 years but not yet a convincing improvement in OS. Continuing risk of relapse. Risk of myelodysplasia and 2nd malignancy. First CR auto-SCT remains investigational. Improved responses with FCR make this less attractive.
- ***Allogeneic SCT:*** relatively few allografts have been undertaken. Most use TBI-containing conditioning. CR rate >80% and relapse rates lower than after autograft (12% *vs.* 55% at 5 years) and very few after 2 years. Some patients may be cured. The benefit of better disease control is offset by a higher treatment-related mortality (15–30%). Reduced-intensity conditioning reduces toxicity, preserves the GvL effect and widens the availability of this treatment. Allo-SCT should be considered in appropriate patients with poor prognosis disease e.g. 1° refractory or early relapse after R-CVP (reviewed in reference 3).

Treatment of relapsed FL/SLL

Relapsed asymptomatic disease is not necessarily an indication for further treatment. When indolent lymphoma progresses after partial or complete response to initial therapy, it is important to rule out transformation to DLBCL (esp. if LDH ↑, LN rapidly enlarging, constitutional symptoms, extranodal disease). Therapy should be chosen in the context of the patient's goals (palliative *vs.* potentially curative), performance status, previous treatment(s) and response(s).

- In recurrent indolent NHL, further responses can be achieved with previous therapy in many patients who have achieved a durable response (>12 months). Resistance ultimately develops.
- Rituximab as a single agent achieves ~50% ORs (6% CRs) in Clb/CHOP treated patients; median duration 13 months.[8] On relapse 40% will respond again. In the UK, NICE recommends its use in chemoresistant disease (TA37; 03/02) when all other options have been exhausted.
- R-CHOP offers a higher OR (85% *vs.* 72%) and CR (30% *vs.* 16%) and median PFS (33 months *vs.* 20 months) over CHOP in relapsed FL and maintenance rituximab offers further improvements in median PFS (52months *vs.* 15 months) and OS at 3 years (85% *vs.* 77%).[9]
- Fludarabine ± cyclophosphamide (FC)/± mitoxantrone and dexamethasone (FND) achieves responses in most Clb/CVP treated patients.
- Radioimmunotherapy is an option for relapsed or rituximab refractory FL especially in patients ineligible for high dose therapy and auto-SCT.
- Auto-SCT may offer younger patients with relapsed FL a survival advantage with a 4-year OS 71–77% vs. 46% for conventional chemotherapy in the CUP trial.[10] Not curative. Allo-SCT using reduced intensity conditioning has achieved 73% OS and 65% PFS at 3 years.[11]

Regimens for advanced stage indolent lymphoma

SLL	***FL***
1st line	*1st line*
Chlorambucil±prednisolone	R-CVP
CVP±R*	R-CHOP*
CHOP±R*	F±R*
F±R*	FMD±R*
FC±R*	Rituximab
	Chlorambucil
2nd line	*2nd line*
Chlorambucil±prednisolone	F±R*
CVP±R*	FC±R*
F±R*	Radioimmunotherapy*
FC±R*	Autologous SCT
CHOP±R*	Rituximab
Alemtuzumab*	Allogeneic SCT

**not approved in UK by NICE*

High grade transformation

Recognized clinically in up to 50% of patients with FL, invariably to DLBCL. Less frequent in other indolent NHL subtypes. Median time to transformation in FL 3.5 years, 15% risk at 10 years, 22% risk at 15 years. ↑ risk with grade 3 histology and high risk FLIPI score.[12] Other risk factors are low albumin, high β_2-microglobulin, and absence of CR with initial therapy. Course is progressive, response to treatment poor and survival short (median 1.2 year). Treatment dependent on prior therapy. Enter in clinical trial if available. CHOP type therapy ± high dose therapy and auto-SCT can achieve ~50% CR rate. Prognosis poor if CR is not achieved. Palliation may be appropriate.

Treatment of marginal zone lymphomas (MZL)

Gastric MALT lymphoma (extranodal MZL)

Generally stage I_E; eradication of *H. pylori* with clarithromycin, amoxicillin, and omeprazole for 2 weeks achieves CR in up to 80% of patients with 80% OS at 10 years. Regression of lesions can take 3–18 months Re-stage 3-monthly with biopsy to rule out DLBCL. Regimen should be repeated if still *H. pylori* +ve and no progression. Late relapses occur. Local radiotherapy (RT; 30–33 Gy) can achieve CR in non-responders (frequent in t(11;18) +ve), those who progress and *H. pylori* –ve patients. Single agent chlorambucil or rituximab if RT contraindicated. For more widespread disease with symptoms, non-responders, or recurrence post RT, treat as for stage III/IV indolent NHL.

Non-gastric MALT lymphomas

Simple combination regimens, chlorambucil or local radiotherapy (20–30 Gy) generally achieve good responses; otherwise manage as for FL.
Nodal MZL: therapy similar to FL.
Splenic MZL: 📖 see p166.

References

1. Marcus, R.E. *et al.* (2005). CVP chemotherapy plus rituximab compared with CVP as first-line treatment for advanced follicular lymphoma. *Blood*, **105**, 1417–23.
2. 🖫 www.nice.org.uk/guidance/index
3. Gribben, J.G. (2007). How I treat indolent lymphoma. *Blood*, **109**, 4617–26.
4. Witzig, T.E. *et al.* (2005). Rituximab therapy for patients with newly diagnosed, advanced stage, follicular grade I non-Hodgkin's lymphoma: a phase II trial in North Central Cancer Treatment Group. *J Clin Oncol*, **23**, 1103–8.
5. Hainsworth, J.D. *et al.* (2005). Maximising therapeutic benefit of rituximab: maintenance therapy versus re-treatment at progression in patients with indolent non-Hodgkin's lymphoma – a randomized phase II trial of the Minnie Pearl Cancer Research Network. *J Clin Oncol*, **23**, 1088–95.
6. Kaminski, M.S. *et al.* (2005). 131I-Tositumomab therapy as initial treatment for follicular lymphoma. *N Engl J Med*, **352**, 441–9.
7 Press, O.W. *et al.* (2003). A phase 2 trial of CHOP chemotherapy followed by tositumomab/iodine I121 tositumomab for previously untreated follicular non-Hodgkin lymphoma: Southwest Oncology Group protocol S9911. *Blood* **102,** 1606–12.
8. McLaughlin, P. *et al.* (1998). Rituximab chimeric anti-CD20 monoclonal antibody therapy for relapsed indolent lymphoma: half of patients respond to a four-dose treatment program. *J Clin Oncol*, **16**, 2825–33
9. van Oers, M.H. *et al.* (2006). Rituximab maintenance improves clinical outcome of relapsed/resistant follicular non-Hodgkin's lymphoma, both in patients with and without rituximab during induction: results of a prospective randomized phase III intergroup trial. *Blood*, **108**, 3295–3301.
10. Schouten, H.C. *et al.* (2003). High dose therapy improves progression-free survival and survival in relapsed follicular non-Hodgkin's lymphoma: results from the randomized European CUP trial. *J Clin Oncol*, **21**, 3918–27.
11. Morris, E. *et al.* (2004). Outcomes after alemtuzumab-containiing reduced-intensity allogeneic transplantation regimen for relapsed and refractory non-Hodgkin's lymphoma. *Blood*, **104**, 3865–71.
12. Gine, E. *et al.* (2006). The Follicular Lymphoma Prognostic Index (FLIPI) and the histological subtype are the most important factors to predict histological transformation in follicular lymphoma. *Ann Onc*, **17**, 1539–45.

Aggressive lymphomas

Clinical features

~50% of cases of lymphoma; rapidly progressive if untreated.

Diffuse large B-cell lymphoma: most common lymphoma worldwide; ~30% of all lymphomas; occurs at all ages, generally >40 years; presents with localized stage I or II disease in 50% of patients but disseminated extranodal disease is not uncommon; constitutional symptoms in 33%; extranodal sites in 30-40% most commonly GI. CNS involvement more frequent in patients with testicular or BM involvement. Ascites and pleural effusions are common end-stage symptoms. Histological subtypes: anaplastic, immunoblastic, intravascular, lymphomatoid granulomatous, multi-lobulated, plasmablastic, primary effusion, T-cell rich.

T-cell rich B-cell lymphoma: subtype of DLBCL; occurs in younger patients; more aggressive with early BM involvement.

Mediastinal large B-cell lymphoma: typically occurs in women <30 years; anterior mediastinal mass sometimes causes superior vena cava obstruction; tendency to disseminate to other extranodal sites including CNS; cure rate with R-CHOP therapy similar to DLBCL (📖 see p.196).

Mantle cell lymphoma: usually elderly; median 63 years; B symptoms 50%; usually disseminated at diagnosis: BM involvement 75%, GI involvement 15–20%; poor therapeutic outcome: partial responses and eventual chemoresistance; median survival 3–4 years (📖 p.168).

Mature (peripheral) T-cell lymphomas (PTCL): several conditions; most frequent PTCL-unspecified (PTCLU); most common T-cell NHL in West but more common in Far East; median age 56; ♂:♀ ratio 2:1; variable clinical behaviour; nodal form more common in West, more aggressive and less responsive to therapy than DLBCL; heterogeneous group of extranodal forms (common in Asia, particularly EBV+ nasal type with nasal obstruction, discharge, and facial swelling); 80% stage III–IV at diagnosis; constitutional symptoms, BM and skin involvement common; 30–40% 5-year OS with combination therapy; IPI has predictive value.

Angio-immunoblastic T-cell lymphoma (AITL): PTCL; occurs in elderly (median 57–68 years); constitutional symptoms, generalized lymphadenopathy, hepatosplenomegaly, pruritic skin rash, arthritis, polyclonal hypergammaglobulinaemia, DAT+ve haemolytic anaemia, cryoglobulinaemia, cold agglutinins, and eosinophilia; 33% progress to immunoblastic lymphoma; poor prognosis.

Anaplastic large cell lymphoma (ALCL): PTCL; 3 subtypes: systemic ALK+ usually younger patients and children; typically lymphadenopathy at single site; (median age <30 years and chemosensitive); systemic ALK- (median age 50–60; unfavourable); 1° cutaneous ALK– ALCL (good prognosis); may spontaneously resolve; occasional LN spread; rarely widespread.

Enteropathy type T-cell lymphoma (ETTL): PTCL subtype; occurs in gluten-sensitive enteropathy; abdominal pain, weight loss, small bowel obstruction and perforation; poor prognosis, median OS 7.5 months.

Mycosis fungoides: mature T-cell lymphoma; presents as localized or generalized plaque or erythroderma; lymphadenopathy in 50%; median survival 10 years but prognosis poor with lymphadenopathy, blood (📖 Sézary syndrome, p.178) or visceral involvement.

Immunohistochemical and cytogenetic features

Diffuse large B-cell lymphoma:[1] pan-B markers (CD20+, CD79a+), generally sIg+; Ki67 <90% favours DLBCL (*cf.* Burkitt >99%); probably multiple unrecognized entities; 2 subgroups delineated by gene expression profiling using DNA microarrays: germinal centre-B-cell profile (GCB subtype: favourable; ~60% 5-year OS) and activated B-cell profile (ABC subtype: unfavourable; ~30% 5-year OS). Der(3)(q27) involving *BCL-6* gene mutations 35%; t(14;18) 25%; t(8;14) 15%.

Mediastinal large B-cell lymphoma: pan-B markers (CD20+, CD79a+), often CD30+; sIg–; gene expression profile similar to classical Hodgkin's lymphoma.

Mantle cell lymphoma: pan-B markers; CD5+, strong sIg, CD23–, cyclin-D1+. t(11;14)(q13;q32) in 70%.

Mature (peripheral) T-cell lymphomas: pan-T markers (CD3+, CD2+); TdT– (*cf.* precursor T-lymphoblastic TdT+); Ki-67 has prognostic value.

Angioimmunoblastic T-cell lymphoma: characteristic PAS+ arborizing venules in LN; pan-T markers, CD4+, TdT–, CD10+, sometimes BCL-6+, CXCL13 overexpression; B-cells are EBV+.

Anaplastic large cell lymphoma: Pan-T markers but often CD3-; CD4+; TdT–, CD30+, ALK+, or ALK–. t(2;5)(p23;q35) in 60%. 1° cutaneous always ALK–.

1. Rosenwald, A. *et al.* (2002). The use of molecular profiling to predict survival after chemotherapy for diffuse large B-cell lymphoma. *N Engl J Med*, **346**, 1937–47.

Initial treatment of aggressive lymphomas

Many patients can be cured by combination chemotherapy or by radiotherapy.

Localized DLBCL

Stage I and non-bulky (mass <10cm) stage II disease without adverse prognostic factors have usually been treated with 3 cycles of CHOP followed by involved field radiotherapy (IF-RT; 30–36Gy); achieves 99% OR, 77% PFS, and 85% long-term survival. Superior to RT alone (15% relapse in irradiation field) and to 8 cycles of CHOP. In good risk patients 6 × R-CHOP alone may be superior[1] and R-CHOP × 3 plus IF-RT gives PFS and OS>90%.[2] Patients with bulky disease and/or local extranodal disease are better treated with 6–8 courses of R-CHOP plus IF-RT (30–40 Gy).[3] Patients with localized testicular DLBCL should receive 6–8 courses of R-CHOP with intrathecal therapy followed by scrotal RT due to risk of CNS and contralateral testicular relapse.[4] In the UK, NICE recommend that in localized disease, rituximab is used only in clinical studies.[5]

Advanced stage DLBCL

Several regimens have curative potential. CR rates from 50-80%. CHOP (📖 p.720) became standard therapy because of ease of administration and tolerability. ~30% of patients were cured using CHOP alone with more salvaged by 2nd-line therapy. A prospective randomized trial comparing CHOP, m-BACOD, ProMACE-CytaBOM, and MACOP-B revealed no significant difference in response rates, time to treatment failure or survival.[6] Addition of rituximab to CHOP improves response, failure-free survival, and OS. In a randomized study of 400 elderly patients with DLBCL, R-CHOP initial therapy improved the CR rate (76% *vs.* 63%), EFS (57% *vs.* 38%), and OS (70% *vs.* 57%) at 2 years with no added toxicity.[7] This was sustained on longer follow-up (5-year OS 58% *vs.* 45%)[8] and confirmed in younger patients with DLBCL (3-year EFS 79% *vs.* 59%).[1] A Canadian population based study shows survival in DLBCL ↑ ~20% as a result of rituximab availability.[9] R-CHOP x 6-8 has been endorsed by NICE[5] for use as 1st-line therapy in CD20+ DLBCL stage II, III, or IV. *Note*: patients with testicular, sinus, BM, or epidural involvement should receive concomitant IT MTX and/or cytarabine (4–8 doses). Consider adjuvant RT to any site of bulk disease (>10cm) at diagnosis. Data do not support maintenance rituximab. Intensification of initial therapy is under investigation with the addition of etoposide (R-EPOCH) or a 14- rather than 21d cycle (R-CHOP-14) (📖 p.720 & p.740).

Response assessment

Evaluate response to initial therapy by CT after 3–4 courses to identify non-response or progression despite therapy. Complete 6–8 courses if ≥50%PR has been achieved. Repeat all +ve studies on completion of therapy. Gallium or PET scans are useful to determine whether residual masses represent persistent active tumour. Biopsy should be considered if masses are +ve after therapy. Patients with only PR at the end of initial therapy may be considered for a clinical trial or autologous SCT if eligible.

Consolidation therapy in DLBCL

More intensive protocols may be appropriate for high-risk groups of patients (risk-adapted therapy). Consolidation of 1st CR by high dose therapy and autologous SCT has been examined. Improved DFS (and OS in 1 of 3 studies) was demonstrated for patients with ≥2 adverse factors on IPI. Further studies are in progress. Patients in IPI high-intermediate or high risk groups (but note R-IPI) may benefit from intensive consolidation and SCT should be discussed with eligible high risk patients in 1st CR. SCT is only likely to benefit patients who achieve CR after standard chemotherapy.[4]

Follow-up

Patients who achieve CR should be reviewed every 3 months for 24 months then every 6 months for 36 months.[3] Review should include history, physical examination, FBC, renal and liver biochemistry, and LDH. Apparent relapse from CR should be confirmed by biopsy before initiating therapy.[4] For 2nd-line therapy 📖 see p.201.

Mantle cell lymphoma

Incurable with conventional therapy but does not follow an indolent course. Enrol in clinical trial when possible. Otherwise decide whether patient is SCT-candidate and suitable for intensive approach. Chlorambucil, CVP, or CHOP may be appropriate for a frail elderly patient. CHOP OR rate ~80% (CR ~50%) with PFS <18 months and OS 3 years; not markedly different from CVP. Regimens such as FC or FCR (📖 p.732) achieve better responses. Rituximab alone achieves OR rate ~35% (14% CR) with median TTP <1 year. R-CHOP (📖 p.740) improves responses and widely used in USA but not approved for MCL in UK by NICE. R-HyperCVAD (📖 p.734) alternating with MTX and cytarabine very intensive with high toxicity: 89%CR; 3-year FFS 80% in patients <65 years[10] and R-EPOCH (📖 p.729)[11] improve response rates though relapse remains common in 15–18 months unless consolidated by autologous or allogeneic SCT. Rituximab pre-harvest acts as in vivo purge increasing the proportion of PCR –ve collections. Suitable patients with a sibling allogeneic SCT option should receive an allograft. Relapsed patients with MCL who have not received SCT and respond to salvage therapy achieve further remissions with HDT and autologous SCT but further relapse usual. Enter relapsed and refractory patients into clinical trials where possible. Bortezomib in combination with chemotherapy and/or rituximab, FC, FCR, rituximab + thalidomide, lenalidamide + rituximab, and radioimmunotherapy all have activity and are in clinical trials.

Mature (peripheral) T/NK cell lymphoma

No consensus on optimal therapy;[12] clinical trial enrolment recommended; ***ALK+ ALCL*** is chemosensitive (5-year OS 60–90% following CHOP-type therapy) and CHOP therapy is often effective (+IF-RT for stage I/II) with SCT reserved for relapse in eligible patients; ***ALK- ALCL*** is less sensitive (11–46% 5-year OS) and for stage III/IV consideration should be given to SCT consolidation of 1st CR or to salvage PR; ***PTCLU*** has inferior outcome with CHOP to DLCBL (5-year OS <30%) and SCT consolidation should be considered for stage III/IV in 1st CR or to salvage PR; ***AITL*** may respond to 7d trial of prednisolone (1mg/kg)[3] and CHOP-type therapy can achieve 50–70% CR but 5-year OS only 10–30% due to early relapse or infective deaths; consider SCT to consolidate 1st CR or to salvage PR for stage III/IV; ***Nasal NK/T lymphomas*** may respond to local RT plus chemotherapy and CNS prophylaxis.

Regimens for aggressive lymphoma

DLBCL	*MCL*
1st line	*1st line***
R-CHOP 21	R-CHOP*
R-EPOCH*	FCR*
R-CHOP 14	R-EPOCH*
	R-HyperCVAD* + MA
*2nd line***	*2nd line*
R-DHAP	Bortezomib†
R-ESHAP	FCR*
R-ICE	Thalidomide + R*
R-mini-BEAM	

* R *not approved in UK by* NICE; ***consolidate with SCT where possible* † *not approved in UK by NICE*

Very aggressive lymphomas

Clinical features

~10% cases of NHL; require prompt treatment.

Burkitt lymphoma

- Endemic BL: presents in childhood/adolescence in Africa with large extranodal tumours in jaw or abdominal viscera; 90% associated with EBV infection; aggressive but curable disease.
- Sporadic BL: often children, rare in adults (median age 31 years); presents with rapidly growing lymphadenopathy, often intra-abdominal mass arising from a Peyer's patch or mesenteric node; BM, CNS, and blood involvement frequent; 30% associated with EBV infection; also associated with HIV infection; aggressive but curable disease in non-HIV-associated cases.

Lymphoblastic lymphoma

Young patients (median age 15 years; >50% of childhood lymphomas); share features with ALL; T-cell LBL more frequent (85%) and usually associated with thymic mass; 33–50% present with BM involvement; CNS involvement common; commonly progresses to ALL; aggressive but potentially curable in children.

Immunohistochemical and cytogenetic features

Burkitt lymphoma

Pan-B markers, CD10+, sIg+, Ki67 >99% favours BL (cf. DLBCL <90%), TdT–. 80% t(8;14)(q24;q32), 15% t(2;8)(q11;q24), 5% t(8;22)(q24;q11) juxtapose *c-MYC* with Ig gene loci and cause MYC overexpression but not diagnostically useful as expressed in ↔ cells and other lymphomas. Endemic cases have raised antibody titres to EBV antigens and multiple copies of EBV DNA in tumour (unusual in sporadic cases). Presence of t(14;18) associated with poor response to therapy.

Precursor B-lymphoblastic: pan-B markers, sIg–, CD10+, TdT+; variable cytogenetics.

Precursor T-lymphoblastic: pan-T markers, TdT+; variable cytogenetics.

Initial treatment of very aggressive lymphomas

These lymphomas display an exponential growth rate, a tendency to involve BM and meninges. There is a high risk of tumour lysis and good pre-treatment hydration plus rasburicase are essential.

Non-endemic Burkitt lymphoma (BL)

Successful treatment of BL in children has informed adult treatment. High remission rates and long-term DFS achieved with intensive short duration (3–6 months) multi-agent chemotherapy regimens including high dose MTX, high dose cytarabine, etoposide, ifosfamide, and CNS prophylaxis. Protocols designed for lymphoblastic lymphoma or ALL are clearly inferior to specific BL protocols. 90% EFS rates in childhood BL. Treatment of adults with BL with intensive regimens including intrathecal therapy such as CODOX-M/IVAC (📖 p.724) improves response and survival rates (~50% curable) though not to childhood results. The role of high dose therapy is uncertain but it should be considered in relapsed patients. Meningeal involvement still carries poor prognosis.

Follow-up

Patients who achieve CR should be reviewed every 2 months for 12 months then every 3 months for 12 months then every 6 months. For 2nd-line therapy (📖 see p.201).

Lymphoblastic lymphoma

Management in adults follows more successful intensive regimens in childhood based on ALL treatment (including CNS prophylaxis and maintenance). High CR rates (~85%) and 5 year DFS up to 45% reported. The poor outlook for patients has led to evaluation of high-dose therapy with autologous or allogeneic SCT early in its management. Consider allograft in eligible relapsed patients.

Adult T-leukaemia/lymphoma: 📖 see p.176.

Role of FDG-PET scanning in lymphoma[13]

CT is a reliable technique for pre-treatment staging but is inadequate for assessment of patients with apparent incomplete resolution of, usually previously bulky, nodal sites after therapy. Pre-treatment PET/CT not currently standard but does facilitate interpretation of equivocal post-therapy scans especially in HL and DLBCL. At restaging a +ve PET scan is predictive of relapse in DLBCL (~85%) and HL (~65%) and the –ve predictive value is stronger (85%). PET is more accurate than CT for response assessment (~80% v 50%). Variable FDG uptake by lymphomas: DLBCL, MCL, and HL generally avid; indolent lymphomas generally much less avid, FL best, MZL less good and SLL generally poor. T-NHL variable.

False +ves occur due to inflammation, infection granulomatous disease, brown fat, thymic hyperplasia in HL, marrow and splenic hyperplasia after G-CSF, previous radiotherapy. Delay of at least 3 weeks after chemotherapy and 8–12 weeks after radiotherapy recommended. False –ves occur due to lesions below scanner resolution (5–10mm), too brief an interval between injection and scan (2h recommended), masking of tumour by physiological uptake by brain, heart or GI tract, hyperglycaemia reducing uptake by tumour.

Table 5.7 Response criteria for lymphoma (including PET)[14]

Response	Definition	Nodal masses	Spleen, liver	BM
Complete response (CR)	Disappearance of all evidence of disease	(a) FDG-avid or PET +ve prior to therapy: mass of any size permitted if PET –ve; (b) Variably FDG-avid or PET –ve: regression to ↔ size on CT	Not palpable, nodules disappeared	Infiltrate cleared on repeat biopsy; if indeterminate by morphology, immunohisto-chemistry should be –ve
Partial response (PR)	Regression of measurable disease and no new sites	≥50% decrease in SPD of up to 6 largest dominant masses; no increase in size of other nodes (a) FDG-avid or PET +ve prior to therapy: ≥1 +ve at previously involved site (b) Variably FDG-avid or PET –ve: regression on CT	≥50% decrease in SPD of nodules (for single nodule in greatest transverse diameter); no increase in size of liver or spleen	Irrelevant if +ve prior to therapy; cell type should be specified.
Stable disease (SD)	Failure to achieve CR/PR or PD	(a) FDG-avid or PET +ve prior to therapy; PET +ve at prior sites of disease and no new sites on CT or PET (b) Variably FDG-avid or PET –ve; no change in size of previous lesions on CT		
Relapsed disease or progressive disease (PD)	Any new lesion or increase ≥50% of previously involved sites from nadir	Appearance of a new lesion(s) >1.5cm in any axis, ≥50% increase in SPD of >1 node, or ≥50% increase in longest diameter of a previously identified node >1cm in short axis. Lesions PET +ve if FDG-avid lymphoma or PET +ve prior to therapy	>50% increase from nadir in the SPD of any previous lesions	New or recurrent involvement

Salvage therapy in aggressive and very aggressive lymphoma

Patients who relapse or fail to achieve remission with initial therapy have a poor prognosis. Without effective 2nd-line (salvage) therapy, almost all die of progressive lymphoma in a median period of 3–4 months. A significant proportion of patients with DLBCL who relapse from 1st CR can be salvaged but prognosis for primary refractory NHL is very poor.

Conventional chemotherapy

Although relatively high CR rates have been reported with several salvage regimens, <10% patients with relapsed or refractory NHL will achieve long-term DFS. The addition of rituximab to EPOCH and ICE salvage regimens improves response rates. Several 2nd-line regimens are available for patients relapsing from 1st CR or with refractory disease but none is clearly superior: DHAP ± R (📖 p.728), ESHAP ± R (📖 p.730), ICE ± R (📖 p.736), MINE ± R (📖 p.738), or mini-BEAM ± R (📖 p.739). Eligible patients (age <65 years) who respond to 2nd-line therapy (PR or CR) should receive high dose therapy (e.g. BEAM (📖 p.718)) and autologous SCT. ~50% of those achieving CR are long term disease-free survivors and may be cured.[12] RT may be administered to sites of bulk disease. Patients ineligible for SCT should be treated in a clinical trial.

High dose therapy and SCT

High dose therapy (generally BEAM, BEAC, or CBV) and autologous SCT is used to treat patients with relapsed or refractory aggressive or very aggressive NHL. A significant proportion of patients with DLBCL are cured (5-year EFS 46%; OS 53%) and its superiority to conventional dosage salvage therapy (5-year EFS 12%; OS 32%) was demonstrated in a randomized trial.[15] Best results are obtained when lymphoma still responsive to conventional dosage therapy and SCT performed in a state of minimal residual disease. HDT is generally preceded by 1–2 cycles of combination therapy e.g. mini-BEAM, DHAP, ESHAP with aim of testing chemo-responsiveness, inducing minimal residual disease and harvesting PBSCs. Syngeneic and allogeneic transplants have been used less frequently but are associated with cures. Patients who relapse after autologous SCT can sometimes be salvaged with an allogeneic SCT. Rituximab and IFN-α can achieve prolonged survival in some patients relapsing after SCT.[4]

Monoclonal antibody therapy

Single agent rituximab produces responses in ~30% relapsed DLBCL. More useful in combination therapy where it appears to enhance responses to ICE and DHAP. ^{90}Y-ibritumomab tiuxetan achieved ~50% OR in patients with DLBCL ineligible for SCT who failed induction or relapsed from CR, median PFS of 3.5–6 months and OS ~22 months.[16] It has also been used to consolidate the response to R-CHOP in high risk patients. ^{131}I-tositusimab has been combined with etoposide and cyclophosphamide followed by autologous SCT. Epratuzumab, against CD22, is in clinical trials in combination with R-CHOP. Bevacizumab, against vascular endothelial growth factor, is also under investigation in NHL.

New agents

Bortezomib, lenalidamide and mTOR inhibitors are in clinical trial in combination or as single agents.

AIDS-related lymphoma

Burkitt lymphoma, DLBCL, or 1° CNS lymphoma most common. The latter is generally seen in patients with very low CD4 counts. Hodgkin lymphoma and indolent lymphoma less frequent. Incidence of NHL has decreased as a result of highly active antiretroviral therapy (HAART). CODOX-M/IVAC achieves comparable results in HIV-+ve patients with BL. DLBCL should be treated with CHOP. Omit rituximab as it is associated with ↑ infection and no net benefit in outcome. Administer HAART, prophylactic intrathecal chemotherapy, and full dose regimens with G-CSF support.

Post-transplantation LPDs

Occurs in <2% of organ transplant recipients. Risk highest in heart-lung recipients. Monomorphic DLBCL most common; associated with immunosuppressive therapy (esp. ATG) and EBV (main risk EBV mismatch). Tends to involve donor organ and multiple extranodal sites. Treat with local therapy, reduction of immunosuppression and single agent rituximab (achieves OR ≤75% CR ≤69%).

References

1. Pfreundschuh, M. *et al.* (2006). CHOP-like chemotherapy plus rituximab versus CHOP-like chemotherapy alone in young patients with good-prognosis diffuse large B-cell lymphoma: a randomized controlled trial by the Mabthera International Trial (MinT) Group. *Lancet Oncol*, **7**, 379–91.
2. Miller, T.P. *et al.* (2006). Diffuse aggressive histologies of non-Hodgkin lymphoma: treatment and biology of limited disease. *Semin Hematol*, **43**, 207–12.
3. NCCN Clinical Practice Guidelines in Oncology: Non-Hodgkin's Lymphomas V.3.2007 www.nccn.org
4. Armitage, J.O. (2007). How I treat patients with diffuse large B-cell lymphoma. *Blood*, **110**, 29–36.
5. NICE Technology Appraisal 65, September 2003.
6. Fisher, R.I. *et al.* (1993). Comparison of a standard regimen (CHOP) with three intensive chemotherapy regimens for advanced non-Hodgkin's lymphoma. *N Engl J Med*, **328**, 1002–6.
7. Coiffier, B. *et al.* (2002). CHOP chemotherapy plus rituximab compared with CHOP alone in elderly patients with diffuse large-B-cell lymphoma. *N Engl J Med*, **346**, 235–242
8. Feugier, P. *et al.* (2005). Long-term results of the R-CHOP study in the treatment of elderly patients with diffuse large B-cell lymphoma: a study of the Groupe d'Etude des Lymphomes de l'Adulte. *J Clin Oncol*, **23**, 4117–26.
9. Sehn, L.H. *et al.* (2005). Introduction of combined CHOP plus rituximab therapy dramatically improved outcome of diffuse large B-cell lymphoma in British Columbia. *J Clin Oncol*, **23**, 5027–33.
10. Lenz, G. *et al* (2005). Immunochemotherapy with rituximab and cyclophosphamide, doxorubicin, vincristine and prednisolone significantly improves response and time to treatment failure but not long term outcome in patients with previously untreated mantle cell lymphoma: results of a prospective randomized trial of the German Low Grade Lymphoma Study Group (GLSG) *J Clin Oncol*, **23**, 1984–92.
11. Dreyling, M. *et al.* (2005). Early consolidation by myeloablative radiochemotherapy followed by autologous stem cell transplantation in first remission significantly prolongs progression-free survival in mantle cell lymphoma: results of a prospective randomized trial of the European MCL Network. *Blood*, **105**, 2677–84.
12. Greer, J. (2006). Therapy of peripheral T/NK neoplasms. *Hematology 2006*, 331–7.
13. Seam, P. *et al.* (2007). The role of FDG-PET scans in patients with lymphoma. *Blood*, **110**, 3507–16.

14. Cheson, B.D. *et al.* (2007). Revised response criteria for malignant lymphoma. *J Clin Oncol,* **25**, 579–86.

15. Philip, T. *et al.* (1995) Autologous bone marrow transplantation as compared with salvage chemotherapy in relapses. of chemotherapy -sensitive non-Hodgkin's lymphoma. *N Engl J Med,* **333**, 1540–5.

16. Morschhauser, F. *et al.* (2007). Efficacy and safety of Yttrium-90 ibritumomab tiuxetan in patients with relapsed and refractory diffuse large B-cell lymphoma not appropriate for autologous stem cell transplantation. *Blood,* **110**, 54–8.

CNS lymphoma

1° CNS lymphoma (PCNSL)[1–3]

- 2–3% of NHL cases; 3% of all brain tumours.
- Incidence ↑ 3 × two decades ago partly due to HIV pandemic; occurs in severe AIDS (CD4s < 50/μL) hence incidence has fallen with early intervention with HAART.
- Non-HIV related PCNSL occurs in ages 55–70 years; immunocompromised often younger.
- Usually classified as a diffuse large B-cell lymphoma; Burkitt-like occasionally in immunocompromised patients.
- Commonly involves frontal lobes, corpus callosum, or deep periventricular structures; may involve eyes, meninges, or spinal cord; systemic lymphoma uncommon.
- Multiple lesions in 20–40% at diagnosis especially in immunocompromised patients; invariable later in disease course.
- Commonly presents with focal neurological deficit, cognitive or personality change, language deficits, paresis, symptoms of raised intracranial pressure (headache and vomiting); 10% seizures; 40% evidence of leptomeningeal spread: confusion, cranial neuropathies, and cauda equina syndrome; spinal cord disease causes neck or back pain or myelopathy.
- LP (if safe) for CSF cytology gives variable results: flow cytometry and PCR analysis for Ig gene re-arrangement may help.
- Diagnosis by gadolinium-enhanced magnetic resonance and stereotactic needle biopsy.
- N.B. diagnostic accuracy is improved by avoiding routine use of steroids for cerebral oedema; use parenteral mannitol as osmotic therapy.
- Slit-lamp eye examination recommended to exclude malignant uveitis.
- Most important prognostic factors are age and performance status.
- Poor prognosis improved by addition to whole brain radiotherapy (WBRT) of systemic chemotherapy including high dose MTX (≥3.5g/m^2) plus procarbazine ± high dose cytarabine ± other agents (optimum combination unclear) ± IT MTX (esp. if LP +ve) ± IT cytarabine; MTX requires creatinine clearance ≥50mL/min.
- Combined chemoradiotherapy (including high dose MTX) improves survival with >95% responses and median survival 30–60 months (RT alone 12–18 months).
- 50% relapse risk; most relapses in CNS, others mainly leptomeningeal and ocular, <10% systemic.
- Delayed neurotoxicity common (5-year cumulative incidence 24%), esp. >60 years: progressive subcortical dementia, psychomotor slowing, memory dysfunction, behavioural changes, ataxia, urinary dysfunction, and incontinence;
- Due to risk of neurotoxicity some centres defer or avoid WBRT especially in older patients but this compromises response duration;
- Where used, fractionated WBRT (24–36Gy) recommended following CR with MTX; with <CR, additional limited field of 45Gy to tumour.
- Consolidation of a response to high dose MTX-based therapy (without WBRT) with thiotepa-busulfan-cyclophosphamide followed by SCT has

produced prolonged responses in a small number of patients with poor prognostic features; significant toxicity; should be in clinical trial.
- Patients who relapse after a response to high dose MTX may respond again or to WBRT if not previously administered.

Ocular lymphoma

- intraocular lymphoma presents as ocular floaters and blurred vision; progresses to involve both eyes; 50% develop brain involvement; 15% of PCNSL develop concurrent or later eye involvement;
- standard therapy is fractionated radiotherapy (35-40 Gy over 5 weeks) to globe and contralateral globe with systemic chemotherapy (including high dose MTX) to prevent CNS relapse

2° CNS lymphoma

- Usually meningeal involvement; occurs in up to 10% of cases of NHL.
- IT MTX, cytarabine and prednisolone twice weekly until CSF clear then weekly × 6 ± cranial irradiation as for ALL.
- Insertion of Ommaya reservoir facilitates administration.
- Simultaneous systemic therapy including high dose MTX and cytarabine (penetrate CNS) normally necessary.
- Poor prognosis; median survival <3 months.

1. DeAngelis, L.M. and Iwamoto, F.M. (2006). An update on therapy for primary central nervous system lymphoma. *Hematology 2006,* 311–16.

2. Hochberg, F.H. et *al.* (2007). Primary CNS lymphoma. *Nat Clin Pract Neurol,* **3,**: 24–35.

3. NCCN Clinical Practice Guidelines in Oncology: Central Nervous System Cancers V.I.2007 www.nccn.org

Hodgkin lymphoma (HL, Hodgkin's disease)

First described by Thomas Hodgkin in 1832. The lineage of the neoplastic cells was controversial for >160 years. Single cell PCR for Ig gene amplification demonstrated that the neoplastic cells in HL are clonal germinal centre (GC) or post-GC B-lymphocytes.

Incidence

- 1% cancer registrations per annum. Annual incidence ~3 per 100,000 in Europe and USA (less common in China and Japan).
- Bimodal age incidence—major peak between 20 and 29 years and minor peak at 60 years; median age 35; >90% of cases age 16–65.
- Overall higher incidence in ♂.
- Nodular sclerosing (NS) histology is most common subtype in young adults (>75% of NS cases are <40 years) and peak at this age is confined to NS subtype and has a ♀ preponderance.

Risk factors

- Associated with high socioeconomic status in childhood (esp. NS in young adults) and with Caucasians in the USA.
- Familial aggregations frequently reported: 99 × ↑ risk in identical twins; 7 × risk for siblings of young adults (no increase for sibs of older adults); ?genetic or environmental effect.
- Considerable evidence linking EBV to HL: 4 × ↑ risk of HL in individuals with history of infectious mononucleosis with median interval of 4,1 years;[1] EBV encoded nuclear RNAs detected in Reed–Sternberg (RS) cells; 26–50% cases +ve for EBV by molecular analysis (esp. mixed cellularity HL).
- HIV infected patients have ~8 × ↑ risk of HL; usually good CD4 counts; usually EBV+; associated with advanced stage at presentation, unusual sites, and poorer outcome.

Pathophysiology

Both forms of HL are B-cell lymphomas.

- *RS cells* in classical HL appear to be transformed post-germinal centre B-cells with re-arranged but non-expressed Ig genes (due to crippling mutations) destined for apoptosis that survive through several mechanisms including latent EBV infection, NF-κB expression and a permissive inflammatory cell infiltrate. Aneuploidy and 14q abnormalities frequent.
- *L&H cells* in nodular lymphocyte-predominant HL are neoplastic germinal centre B-cells that express BCL-6, frequently have translocations involving *bcl-6* but usually EBV –ve.

Histology and classification

Immunological analysis has resulted in reclassification of HL into 2 distinct entities in the WHO classification of lymphoid neoplasia (📖 Table 5.1, p.181): classical HL and nodular lymphocyte-predominant HL which has a different immunophenotype, natural history, and response to therapy.

'Classical' HL

Large mononuclear (Hodgkin cells) or binucleate/multinuclear RS cells make up only 1–2% of the cellularity of the lymph node. These cells are CD30+ and typically CD3–, CD15+, CD20–, CD45–, CD75–, CD79a–. The predominant cells are an infiltrate of lymphocytes, plasma cells, eosinophils, and histiocytes containing scattered neoplastic cells and a variable degree of fibrosis. Differential diagnosis: anaplastic large cell lymphoma; peripheral T-cell NHL; DLBCL; T-cell rich B-cell lymphoma; mediastinal large B-cell lymphoma.

There are four histological subtypes of classical HL:

- *Nodular sclerosing HL (NSHL):* ~80%; prominent bands of fibrosis and nodular growth pattern; lacunar Hodgkin cells; variable numbers of RS cells. Sub-divided into grade I (~80% of NS) and grade II (~20%) based on cellularity of nodules, amount of sclerosis and number and atypia of neoplastic cells. Grade II may be more aggressive.
- *Mixed cellularity HL (MCHL):* ~17%; mixed infiltrate of lymphocytes, eosinophils, and histiocytes with classical RS cells.
- *Lymphocyte depleted HL (LDHL):* rare; diffuse hypocellular infiltrate with necrosis, fibrosis, and sheets of RS cells.
- *Lymphocyte rich classical HL (LRCHL):* uncommon; diffuse predominantly lymphoid infiltrate with scanty RS cells of 'classical' phenotype.

Nodular lymphocyte-predominant HL (NLPHL)

3–8%; contains large atypical B cells and lymphocytic and histiocytic (L&H) 'popcorn' cells. These are CD30–, CD15–, CD3–, CD20+, CD45+, CD75+, CD79a+ and BCL-6 protein+, EMA–. Typical RS cells absent. L&H cells associated with CD4+/CD57+ T-cell rosettes. Nodules contain CD21+/CD35+ follicular dendritic cell meshwork. No evidence of EBV. Differential diagnosis: T-cell rich B-cell lymphoma; lymphocyte-rich classical HL.

Clinical features

- Presentation commonly with painless 'rubbery' supradiaphragmatic lymph node enlargement; frequently cervical gland(s).
- Initial mode of spread occurs predictably to contiguous nodal chains. Often involves supraclavicular and axillary glands and other sites.
- Waldeyer's ring involvement is rare and suggests a diagnosis of NHL.
- Lymphadenopathy in HL may wax and wane during observation.
- Spleen involved in ~30% but palpable splenomegaly only 10%, hepatomegaly 5%.
- Abdominal lymphadenopathy is unusual without splenic involvement.
- Supradiaphragmatic disease ± intra-abdominal involvement is usual, and regional disease limited to subdiaphragmatic sites is uncommon (except NLPHL).
- Bulky mediastinal and hilar lymphadenopathy may produce local symptoms (e.g. bronchial or SVC compression) or direct extension (e.g. to lung, pericardium, pleura, or rib). Pleural effusions in 20%.
- Extranodal spread may also occur via bloodstream (e.g. to BM (1–4%), lung, or liver). Presence of disseminated extranodal disease is generally accompanied by generalized lymphadenopathy and splenic involvement; usually a late event.

- ~33% patients have ≥1 associated constitutional 'B' symptoms at presentation: weight loss >10% body weight during the previous 6 months, unexplained fever, or drenching night sweats. 'B' symptoms correlate with disease extent, bulk, and prognosis. Further systemic symptoms associated with HL (but not 'B' symptoms) are generalized pruritus and alcohol-induced lymph node pain.
- A defect in cellular immunity has been documented in patients with HL rendering them more susceptible to TB, fungal, protozoal and viral infections including *P. jiroveci* and HZV.
- NSHL occurs typically in young adults (median age 26 years); usually localized involving cervical, supraclavicular, and mediastinal nodes; good prognosis if stage I/II.
- MCHL median age 30 years but more prevalent in paediatric and older patients; associated with advanced stage and intermediate prognosis.
- LDHL more common in older adults; often extensive disease relatively poor prognosis.
- LRCHL ♂>♀; tendency to localized disease; favourable prognosis.
- NLPHL more frequent in ♂ (2–3 ×); median age 35 years; typically localized at presentation; usually cervical or inguinal; infrequent 'B' symptoms; indolent course; late relapses occur; increased risk of DLBCL (2–5%); otherwise favourable prognosis; 10-year OS 80–90%.

Investigation, diagnosis, and staging

- Seek 'B' symptoms, alcohol intolerance, pruritus, fatigue, and performance status in history.
- Document extent of nodal involvement and organomegaly by clinical examination.
- Confirm diagnosis by lymph node excision biopsy; FNA inadequate; image guided core needle biopsy, laparotomy, mediastinoscopy, or mediastinotomy may be necessary to obtain a tissue diagnosis.
- Multiple biopsies of suspicious nodes may be necessary because reactive hyperplastic nodes may occur.
- Clinical staging now standard; routine staging laparotomy for 'pathological staging' abandoned as a result of wider use of chemotherapy and better imaging; useful only if result may substantially reduce treatment.
- Clinical staging includes the initial biopsy site and all other abnormalities detected by non-invasive methods.
- Pathological staging requires biopsy confirmation of abnormal sites.
- FBC: may show normochromic normocytic anaemia, reactive leucocytosis, eosinophilia, and/or a reactive mild thrombocytosis.
- ESR/plasma viscosity; U&E; LFTs; urate; LDH.
- CXR.
- CT chest, abdomen and pelvis to define occult nodal and extranodal involvement; PET scan if equivocal CT; CT neck sometimes helpful.
- BM trephine biopsy to exclude marrow involvement in patients with stage IB/IIB or stage III/IV disease (not essential in stage IA/IIA disease); BM may show reactive features.
- Isotope bone scan, MRI or PET scan may be necessary.
- Biopsy of other suspicious sites may be necessary e.g. liver or bone.
- Pregnancy test in premenopausal women.
- Fertility counselling.

- Semen cryopreservation in young ♂ prior to chemotherapy or pelvic radiotherapy; may be unsuccessful in those with 'B' symptoms.
- Oophoropexy in premenopausal ♀ if pelvic RT considered.
- Pneumococcal, HIB, and meningococcal immunization if splenic radiotherapy planned.
- HIV serology if risk factors present or unusual presentation.
- Cardiac ejection fraction and pulmonary function tests if ABVD or BEACOPP planned.

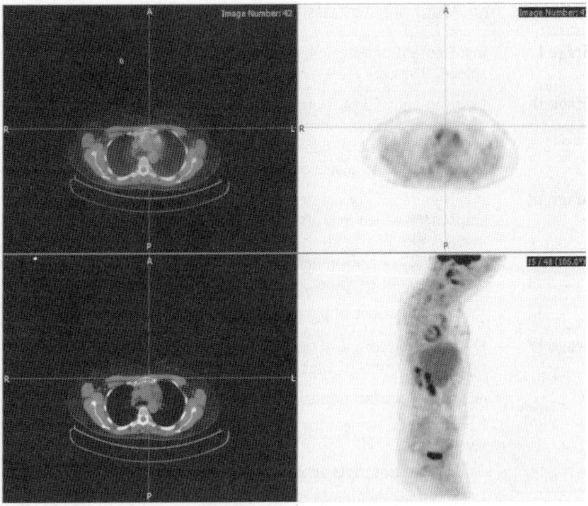

Fig. 5.1 PET and CT scans in patient with nodular sclerosing Hodgkin lymphoma demonstrating active disease (moderate FDG uptake on PET) in residual anterior mediastinal mass on CT after ABVD chemotherapy (📖 see Plate 22).

Ann Arbor staging (Cotswolds modification)

Accurate staging is critical to selection of the most appropriate therapy. The Ann Arbor staging classification has strong prognostic value and is determined by the number of lymph node regions (not sites) involved and the presence or absence of 'B' symptoms (📖 Table 5.8). The Cotswolds modification reflects the use of modern imaging techniques and recognizes and clarifies differences in disease distribution and bulk.

Table 5.8 Ann Arbor staging classification (Cotswolds modification)

Stage I	Involvement of a single lymph node (LN) region / structure (e.g. spleen, thymus, Waldeyer's ring) or single extralymphatic site (I_E)
Stage II	Involvement of 2 or more LN regions on the same side of the diaphragm; localized involvement of 1 extranodal organ/site and LN regions on same side of diaphragm (II_E); number of anatomical sites indicated by a subscript, e.g. II_3.
Stage III	Involvement of LN regions/structures on both sides of the diaphragm, which may also be accompanied by localized involvement of an extranodal organ/site (III_E), involvement of spleen (III_S) or both (III_{SE})
III_1	± involvement of spleen, splenic hilar, coeliac or portal nodes
III_2	With involvement of para-aortic, iliac, or mesenteric nodes
Stage IV	Diffuse involvement of one or more extranodal sites (e.g. BM, liver, or other extranodal sites not contiguous with LN—*cf.* 'E' below).
A	Absence of constitutional symptoms
B	Fevers >38°C, weight loss >10% in 6 months or drenching night sweats
	Additional subscripts applicable to any disease stage:
X	Bulky disease (widening of mediastinum by >33% or mass ≥10cm)
E	Involvement of a single extranodal site contiguous or proximal to known nodal site.

Clinical imaging criteria

- Lymph node involvement: >1cm on CT scan is considered abnormal.
- Spleen involvement: splenomegaly may be 'reactive'; filling defects on CT or USS confirm involvement.
- Liver involvement: hepatomegaly insufficient; filling defect on imaging and abnormal LFTs confirm involvement.
- Bulky disease: ≥10cm in largest dimension or mediastinal mass greater than one third the maximal intrathoracic diameter.

FDG-PET scanning

- Role of FDG PET scanning in lymphoma 📖 p.199. FDG-PET often useful at staging if CT equivocal PET alone has not replaced CT for pretreatment staging in HL despite higher sensitivity (>80%) and specificity (~90%); stage altered in only 15–20% and treatment altered in 5–10%.[2] Low dose PET/CT will ultimately become routine practice.

- A pre-therapy PET scan facilitates interpretation of equivocal post-therapy PET scans.
- PET has clear role in restaging after therapy completed particularly if CT shows residual mass(es) as can distinguish viable tumour from fibrosis. High –ve predictive value (NPV; ~85%). Lower +ve predictive value (PPV; ~65%) due possibly to effects of previous RT.
- PET scan after 2 cycles of chemotherapy for HL may be as accurate as later scans and superior to CT; shown to be predictive of PFS and OS with PPV 69% and NPV 95% in one study.[3] Another study of PET after 2 cycles found 2-year FFS of 95% for PET–ve patients *vs.* 12.8% for PET+.[4]

Initial therapy

- Treatment results for HL have improved dramatically over the last 4 decades and a patient aged <60 years now has a >80% prospect of cure.
- The aim of 'risk-adapted therapy' is to provide each patient with the best probability of cure while minimizing early and late treatment-related morbidity.
- Treatment is determined by stage, symptoms, disease bulk, and patient characteristics such as age and comorbidities.
- Clinical trials remain essential to evaluate therapeutic regimens in order to achieve this objective for all patients without over-treatment.
- Patients with classical HL are generally divided into 3 treatment groups: early favourable, early unfavourable (intermediate), and advanced stage. Therapy of stage I/II NLPHL reflects its indolent nature.

Early stage HL

Prognostic factors

Prognostic factors for patients with stage I/II HL that identify favourable and unfavourable groups have been identified by French and German study groups and define treatment groups and these are now widely applied in Europe to inform treatment choice. There are small differences in the risk factors identified and treatment groups defined (GHSG adds IIB with large mediastinal mass or extranodal disease to the advanced stage group[5]). In the USA, a similar approach is adopted using B symptoms and bulky disease (mediastinal mass >1/3 maximum intrathoracic diameter on CXR or >35% thoracic diameter at T5–6 or any other mass >10cm on CT) to identify patients who require more therapy: NCCN Guidelines recommend that non-bulky stage I/II B HL are treated like stage III/IV HL.[6] See Table 5.9.

Table 5.9 European study group risk factors and treatment groups in Hodgkin lymphoma

	EORTC/GELA	GHSG
Risk factors (RF)	A. Large mediastinal mass*	A. Large mediastinal mass*
	B. Age ≥50 years	B. Extranodal disease
	C. Elevated ESR**	C. Elevated ESR**
	D. ≥4 involved regions	D. ≥3 involved regions
Treatment groups		
NLPHL	Supradiaphragmatic CS I/II; no RFs	CS I/II; no RFs
Early stage favourable	Supradiaphragmatic CS I/II; no RFs	CS I/II; no RFs
Early stage unfavourable (Intermediate)	Supradiaphragmatic CS I/II; with ≥1 RF	CS I, CSIIA with ≥1 RF; CS IIB with C/D but not A/B
Advanced stage	CS III/IV	CS IIB with A/B; CS III/IV

EORTC, European Organisation for Research and Treatment of Cancer; GELA, Groupe d'Etude des Lymphomes de l'Adulte; GHSG, German Hodgkins Study Group * mediastinal mass ratio > 0.35 (mass ≥10cm widely applied); ** ESR >50mm/h or >30 in presence of 'B' symptoms.

- Other identified risk factors have been: ♂ gender, MC, or LD histology, disease distribution (HL confined to upper cervical nodes—good; infra-diaphragmatic disease—poor), anaemia, and low serum albumin.

Classical HL, favourable stage I/II: no risk factors

About 30% of patients have favourable early stage HL at presentation.

Aim: cure with minimal side effects.

- Enter patient in multicentre randomized trial when possible.
- Treatment of choice: combined modality treatment (CMT) with abbreviated chemotherapy, usually ABVD × 2–4 cycles (📖 p.716) + involved field RT (IFRT; 20–30Gy) to sites of disease (avoid high cervical regions when possible and axillae in women).
- CMT aims to eliminate local HL with reduced toxicity by limited field RT and treat occult HL with small number of cycles of chemotherapy.
- Expected outcome: >90% FFS and >95% OS at 5 years.
- Extended field RT/subtotal nodal irradiation (EFRT) was abandoned due to 25–30% relapse rate and high risk of 2° malignancy, cardiac toxicity, and pulmonary dysfunction (40% at 25–30 years).
- Better disease control achieved with CMT: 3 × doxorubicin and vinblastine + EFRT *vs.* EFRT (3-year FFS 94% *vs.* 81%).[7]
- CMT + IFRT is superior to EFRT (EORTC H7 trial 10-year EFS 88% *vs.* 78%; both 92% 10-year OS).[8] The EORTC H8F trial shows the superiority of abbreviated chemotherapy + IFRT compared to EFRT (5-year EFS 98% *vs.* 74%; 10-year OS 97% *vs.* 92%).[9,10]

- Randomized comparison of MOPP or ABVD (both +EFRT) showed ↑ RFS, similar OS and ↓ myelotoxicity and infertility in ABVD arm.[11]
- Randomized trials now evaluating further reductions in treatment intensity seeking reduced toxicity by reduction to 2 cycles of ABVD, omission of bleomycin and dacarbazine, 20Gy RT or use of ABVD alone. Role of PET scans at 2 cycles to tailor further therapy also being examined. No clear answer yet on interim analyses.

Alternative therapeutic options

- *Stanford V* x 2 cycles (📖 p.744) for 8 weeks then IFRT (30Gy within 3 weeks of last chemotherapy) is dose dense CMT with ↓ cumulative doses of doxorubicin, nitrogen mustard, and bleomycin, added etoposide and intensive RT; effective in early stage HL (~95% FFP and ~97% 3-year OS).

or

- *Subtotal lymphoid irradiation* (36–40Gy mantle ± paraaortic-spleen or inverted Y): selected patients who cannot tolerate chemotherapy may be treated with RT alone. It has been argued that relapse after RT can usually be salvaged by chemotherapy thus sparing most patients toxicity from CMT. A very favourable subgroup (stage I, age <40 years, no 'B' symptoms, ESR <50, ♀ and MT ratio <0.35) may achieve 65–75% FFS and >90% OS at 10 years following EFRT alone. However, long-term toxicity from EFRT is significant.

or

- *Chemotherapy alone* (CT) is an option for highly selected patients in whom RT is contra-indicated. In these patients, ABVD × 6 is recommended. This approach may further reduce long-term toxicity but early results of CT not convincing: EORTC/GELA H9-F trial CT-alone arm closed due to inferior 4-year EFS (69% *vs.* 85% and 88% with additional 20Gy and 36Gy IFRT) but EBVP regimen not equivalent to ABVD.[12] Subset analysis in NCI-C/ECOG study showed comparable results between ABVD × 6 and EFRT for favourable patients (CMT superior for unfavourable group).[13] A single centre study with 152 patients showed no significant difference in 5-year FFP and OS between ABVD × 6 and CMT but not powered to detect important differences.[14] Further results are awaited.

Stage IA patients with subdiaphragmatic disease should receive chemotherapy ± involved field radiotherapy avoiding extended pelvic/abdominal fields that are myeloablative and sterilizing in women.

Restaging

If CMT is planned restaging including PET/CT should be undertaken at completion of chemotherapy (4 cycles of ABVD/2 cycles of Stanford V). IFRT should then be administered. If RT is not planned, 2 further cycles of ABVD should be administered to patients in CR or Cru (uncertain) after 4 cycles. Patients who fail to achieve CR on completion of therapy or have progressive disease should proceed to salvage therapy.

Classical HL unfavourable stage I/II: ≥1 risk factor

Aim: cure with some acceptable side effects.

- Enter patient in multicentre randomized trial when possible.
- CMT is widely regarded as essential in these patients.

- Chemotherapy alone is inadequate in patients with bulky disease.
- Optimal regimen, number of cycles and dose of RT not defined.
- ABVD (📖 p.716) × 6 cycles + IFRT (bulky disease 30–36Gy; non-bulky disease 20-30Gy) is widely used.
- Expected outcome: ~85% DFS and ~90% OS at 5 years. ~15% will relapse within 5 years and ~5% have primary refractory disease.
- Alternative therapeutic option: Stanford V (📖 p.744) x 3 cycles (12 wks) + IFRT within 3 weeks (36Gy to initial sites >5cm or involved spleen, 30Gy to other involved sites).
- Clinical trials are evaluating intensified chemotherapy but IFRT appears essential in this group of patients.

Restaging

Restaging including PET/CT should be undertaken after 4 cycles of ABVD or 3 cycles of Stanford V. If –ve/CR, administer IFRT after 2 further cycles of ABVD or within 3 weeks if on Stanford V. If +ve/PR after 4 x ABVD, administer 2 further cycles and restage; if then –ve/CR administer IFRT; if then +ve, biopsy to confirm diagnosis and consider IFRT *vs.* salvage therapy. If progressive disease or no change on PET/CT after 3 × Stanford V, rebiopsy and proceed to salvage therapy.

Classical HL advanced stage (III/IV)

About 30% of patients have stage III/IV HL at presentation. Advanced stage HL has been curable with combination chemotherapy for over three decades. The first widely used regimen, MOPP achieved 80% OR and long-term DFS in ~50%.[15,16] but has been superceded by ABVD.[17]

Prognostic factors

The *International Prognostic Score (IPS)* for advanced HL has been developed to distinguish patients who may be cured by conventional therapy from those who require more intensive therapy.[18] 7 unfavourable factors were identified from a study of 1618 patients and combined into a simple prognostic score predictive of 5-year FFP and OS (📖 Table 5.10):

- Serum albumin <40g/L.
- Hb <10.5g/dL.
- ♂ gender.
- Stage IV disease.
- Age ≥45 years.
- WBC ≥15 × 10^9/L.
- Lymphopenia <0.6 x 10^9/L or <8% of differential.

Patients with no adverse factors had 84% 5-year FFP. Each additional factor reduced FFP by ~7% until patients with 4–7 factors have ~40%-5 year FFP. 3 main risk groups may be identified with wide consensus that the high risk group require more intensive therapy, e.g. escalated BEACOPP:

- IPS score 0–1 (low risk): 29% patients, 79% FFP and 90% OS at 5 years.
- IPS score 2–3 (intermediate risk): 52% pts, ~64% FFP, ~80% OS at 5 years.
- IPS score 4–7 (high risk): 19% patients, 47% FFP and 59% OS at 5 years.
- Other identified risk factors have been: serum LDH, MC or LD histology, disease distribution (BM involvement, inguinal LN involvement), serum soluble CD30, presence of CD15, activated cytotoxic T-cells, bcl-2 +, β2-microglobulin, EBV expression.

Table 5.10 International Prognostic Score (IPS) for advanced HL

Number of factors	% of patients	5-year FFP (%)	5-year OS (%)
0–1	29	79	90
2	29	67	81
3	23	60	78
4–7	19	47	59

Combination chemotherapy

- Enter patient in a multicentre randomized clinical trial when possible.
- ABVD (📖 p.716) has become the standard regimen for patients with advanced HL (stage III/IV) not enrolled in a clinical trial.
- In a landmark randomized trial of 361 patients 6–8 cycles of ABVD was equivalent to 12 cycles of MOPP-ABVD alternating regimen with lower toxicity (CR 82% *vs.* 83%; 5-year FFS 61% *vs.* 65%) and superior to 6–8 cycles of MOPP (CR 67%; 5-year FFS 50%).[19]
- ABVD has much lower risk of infertility than MOPP and is not associated with ↑ risk of leukaemia but the anthracycline component may exacerbate cardiac and pulmonary complications of mediastinal RT.
- ABVD seems to offer the best and most reliable balance between efficacy and toxicity compared to MOPP/ABV (5-year FFS 63%; OS 81%)[20] a modified Stanford V, MOPPEBVCAD (5-year FFS 78%; OS 90%),[21] ChlVPP/PABlOE and ChlVPP/EVA;[22] multidrug regimens toxic >45 years.
- ABVD often poorly tolerated by elderly patients due to cumulative doses of doxorubicin and bleomycin; G-CSF may be necessary; pulmonary toxicity reported in 30% of patients, fatal in ~2%.[20]

Alternative therapeutic options

- *Stanford V* : (📖 p.744) brief duration dose intensified regimen, 3 cycles of weekly low cumulative doses of alkylators, doxorubicin, bleomycin, and additional etoposide over 12 weeks followed by IFRT (36Gy) to sites of bulk disease (≥5cm); FFP 89%, OS 96% at 5 years in single centre study with best results in IPS 0-2 (FFP 94% *vs.* 75%)[23]; fertility preserved in high proportion; very low risk of leukaemia; less good results have been obtained elsewhere especially in poor risk patients; results awaited of US intergroup randomized trial vs. ABVD (E2496) in advanced HL and IPS 0-2; may not be adequate therapy if IPS >3.

or

- *Escalated BEACOPP*: (📖 p.717) based on a mathematical model suggesting that more rapid administration and dose escalation could increase DFS; BEACOPP combines bleomycin, etoposide, doxorubicin, cyclophosphamide, vincristine, procarbazine, and prednisolone; escalated BEACOPP adds G-CSF to intensify doses of cyclophosphamide, etoposide, and doxorubicin; randomized comparison of escalated BEACOPP *vs.* BEACOPP *vs.* COPP-ABVD (all 8 cycles) in advanced HL showed superiority over COPP-ABVD for 5 years FFS (87% *vs.* 76% *vs.* 69%) that was evident in all IPS groups, and OS (91% *vs.* 88% *vs.* 83%)[24] and has been ↑ at 10 years (FFS 82% *vs.* 70% *vs.* 64%;

OS 86% vs. 80% vs. 75%);[25] grade 3 /4 acute haematological toxicity marked, fertility impaired in both sexes and 14 cases of AML (3.2%) reported at 10 years; nonetheless this regimen widely adopted for poor risk patients (IPS >4); not for >65 years; **N.B**. even standard BEACOPP too toxic in patients ≥ 65years (21% acute mortality);[26] results awaited of intergroup randomized trial of escalated BEACOPP × 4 plus standard BEACOPP × 4 *vs*. ABVD × 8 (EORTC 20012) in patients aged <60 years with advanced HL and IPS≥3.

Adjuvant radiotherapy

IFRT is an integral part of Stanford V and is frequently given to bulky mediastinal disease after completion of other chemotherapy (CT). A meta-analysis suggested an overall 11% improvement in DFS *vs*. no therapy and greatest benefits for NSHL (least for MC and LD), for mediastinal bulk rather than other sites and no benefit in stage IV or vs. further CT (better OS with CT).[27] Late toxicity ↑ by RT. Lack of OS benefit attributed to ↑ 2nd malignancy and poorer response and OS on relapse after combined modality therapy. EORTC randomized trial demonstrated no benefit from RT for patients in CR after 8 × MOPP/ABV but benefit in PR patients.[28] Ongoing studies are evaluating the role of PET to identify a risk group who may benefit from RT.

Autologous SCT consolidation

A randomized study in poor risk patients demonstrated no advantage for autologous SCT after 4 cycles of CT *vs*. 4 further courses of CT.[29]

Evaluation of response

- Restage by physical examination and repetition of abnormal investigations at initial staging. PET/CT is extremely useful.
- The revised response criteria for lymphoma (📖 p.200) are also used in HL with the added *Cotswolds response criteria:*
  - CR: complete resolution of all radiological and laboratory evidence of active HL.
  - CRu: 'uncertain CR', identifies presence of a residual mass that remains stable or regresses on follow-up.
- Perform initial restaging after 4 courses of ABVD chemotherapy to ensure adequate response and to determine total duration of therapy:
  - If CR/CRu, administer 2 more cycles of ABVD (total 6 cycles) ± IFRT (20–36 Gy) to bulky sites then final restage to confirm stability of minor abnormalities.
  - If <CRu or PET+ CRu administer 2 more cycles of ABVD and rescan – if CR/CRu, administer 2 more cycles of ABVD (total 8 cycles) ± IFRT (20–36 Gy) to bulky sites; final restage may be necessary to confirm stability of minor abnormalities.
  - If progressive disease at any restaging or persistent <CRu or PET+ CRu on 2nd restaging, proceed to 2nd-line CT, RT, or salvage therapy dependent on disease sites and patient characteristics.
- For BEACOPP, perform initial restaging after 4 cycles then 4 further cycles if CR/CRu (total 8 cycles) then final restage to confirm stability of minor abnormalities; add IFRT (30–40Gy) to initial sites >5cm if CR/CRu achieved after 8 cycles after initial <CRu or PET+ CRu.

- For Stanford V, perform initial restaging on completion of chemotherapy then if CR or PR administer IFRT to initial sites >5cm or CT/PET+ spleen within 3 weeks; if progressive disease or no change in scan from pretreatment staging, biopsy and proceed to salvage therapy.
- Residual masses sometimes persist on CT at completion of therapy, notably in mediastinum: may be residual fibrotic tissue with no viable tumour. PET scan is best method to exclude active disease; if –ve obviates need for invasive biopsy.

Follow-up and monitoring for late complications[6]

- Review and check FBC, ESR and chemistry every 2–4 months for 1–2 years, then every 3–6 months for 3–5 years. TSH annually if RT to neck.
- CXR every 3–6 months for first 2–3 years then annually.
- Annual influenza immunization especially after chest RT or bleomycin.
- Annual mammogram/breast MRI starting 5–8 years post-therapy or age 40 years if earlier, if RT above diaphragm.
- Annual BP, serum glucose and lipid screen after 5 years.
- Pneumococcal immunization every 5–7 years if splenic RT or splenectomy.
- Consider spiral CT at 5 years if increased risk of lung cancer.
- Baseline exercise stress test/ECG at 10 years then annually.

Salvage therapy

- 5–10% 1° refractory HL; 10–30% will relapse, 90% within 2 years.
- >50% of patients relapsing from 1° RT of early stage HL are cured by ABVD; very few now treated with RT alone.
- Durable FFP and prolonged survival not generally achieved by conventional CT for patients refractory to or relapsing after initial CT.
- High-dose therapy (HDT) and autologous SCT is the best option for patients with 1° *refractory HL* but most patients will relapse; a GHSG report HDT achieved 31% 5-year FFS and 43% OS for HDT *vs.* 17% and 26% for all patients; low Karnofsky score, age >50 years and failure to achieve temporary remission to 1st line are adverse factors for OS.[30] A MSKCC study showed that response to 2nd line standard CT is predictive of response to HDT (≥25%PR 10-year EFS 60% *vs.* 17% <25%PR).[31]
- *Relapsed patients* with classical HL should undergo biopsy and restaging.[6]
- HDT and autologous SCT is standard salvage therapy for most patients relapsing after CT; randomized trials by BNLI[32] and GHSG[32] demonstrated better EFS and PFS after HDT compared to salvage CT; up to 80% CR and >50% EFS after 3 years irrespective of duration of remission.
- Precede HDT with 1–2 cycles salvage CT, e.g. DHAP (📖 p.728), ESHAP (📖 p.730), ICE (📖 p.736), mini-BEAM (📖 p.739) to establish chemosensitivity (prognostic), ↓ bulk (HDT most effective with minimal residual disease) and harvest PBSCs; no regimen clearly superior.
- HDT (generally BEAM or CBV) may be followed by IFRT to bulky sites at relapse; low morbidity and mortality (<5%) in selected patients.
- Patients ineligible for HDT (age >70 years or co-morbidity) require individualized therapy: IFRT for localized relapse, CMT or CT (ESHAP, MINE, EVA, GND); remission <12 months, B symptoms, and advanced stage are adverse factors for OS.

- Allogeneic SCT with standard conditioning associated with high early mortality; EBMT case-matched study showed 4-year OS 24% *vs.* 60% for autologous SCT[34]; reduced intensity conditioning lowers risk and DLI can be effective, showing possible GVL effect;[35] remains investigational.
- Patients who relapse after HDT have a poor prognosis and responses to further treatment are generally brief though median survival is 2 years.
- New drugs: vinorelbine and gemcitabine are under study in combinations. Each may be used as single agent palliative therapy as may vinblastine and lomustine; early trials of anti-CD30 have been disappointing.

Late complications of therapy

- 10–15 years after treatment the risk of late complications of therapy exceeds the risk of relapse.
- Treatment-induced *sterility* is frequently seen in ♂ after treatment with MOPP and MOPP-like regimens regardless of age (90% azoospermic 1 year after ≥6 courses); ABVD produces significantly less infertility. Abnormal menstruation due to MOPP more common in women over 30 years (60–70%) and less common in those <20 (20–30%).
- *Premature menopause* more common after MOPP in older ♀.
- ABVD + mantle RT causes higher incidence of post-irradiation *paramediastinal fibrosis* causing persistent effort dyspnoea.
- Patients cured of HL have ↑ risk of *second malignancy;* relative risk 6.4.
- *Solid tumours*: commonly breast, lung, melanoma, soft tissue sarcoma, stomach, and thyroid; comprise >50% of 2nd malignancies; proportion increases as follow-up lengthens; risk ~13% at 15 years and ~22% at 25 years; associated with RT, dose, and volume and young age at time of treatment; 75% occur within radiation fields; breast cancer occurs within 30 years of treatment in 30% of women treated with thoracic RT at age <30 years; lung cancer risk ↑ 20 × in heavy smokers after thoracic RT for HL and 7 × in light or non-smokers.
- *Acute myeloblastic leukemia* risk ~3% at 10 years after treatment; peak incidence between 5–9 years; risk ↓10 years after therapy; particularly associated with MOPP chemotherapy (5% risk within 5 years), age >40 years and RT dose >30Gy to mediastinum; risk 10 years after ABVD <1%.
- *NHL* risk 7%; rises after 10 years and declines after 15 years; no clear association with type of therapy.
- *Cardiac toxicity*: myocardial infarction, radiation-induced pericarditis, valvular disease, and congestive failure occur at ↑ frequency in patients previously treated for HL; higher risk in patients <40 years at treatment: risk of coronary artery disease up to 6% at 10 years and 10–20% at 20 years.
- *Pulmonary toxicity*: generally mild, usually asymptomatic changes in pulmonary function; associated with mediastinal irradiation and bleomycin containing chemotherapy (ABVD).
- *Thyroid toxicity*: 50% risk at 20 years after radiation to the neck and upper mediastinum; highest risk ages 15–25 years; usually hypothyroidism, minority hyperthyroidism, Hashimoto's thyroiditis, nodules or cancer.
- Risks may be significantly lower with advances in radiation technology and use of lower doses and IF rather than EFRT but justify studies of chemotherapy alone in early stage HL.
- Patients treated with HDT and autologous SCT have ↑ incidence of myelodysplasia and AML; azoospermia in males and pre-mature ovarian failure in females is usual.

Nodular lymphocyte predominant HL (NLPHL)

- ***Early stage non-bulky NLPHL*** with unilateral high cervical or epitrochlear lymphadenopathy may be treated with IFRT alone; localized inguinal or femoral NLPHL may be treated by regional RT only; 90% OS at 10 years; at median follow up >7 years, more die of treatment-related toxicity than recurrent HL; observation after excision biopsy and rigorous staging may be appropriate in some patients; single agent rituximab (anti-CD20) treatment may be effective: 100% OR but, median FFP 10 months; less effective in bulky disease, stage III/IV and >2 nodal regions.[36]
- ***Stage III/IV NLPHL:*** chemotherapy is indicated as good responses achieved when formerly treated as 'HD' (96% CR and 74% FFS and 89% OS at 8 years);[37] standard HL regimens widely used though some use alkylator-based or CHOP-type regimens ± rituximab; symptomatic patients not candidates for chemotherapy may benefit from RT or single agent rituximab (not NICE-approved in UK).

References

1. Hjalgrim, H. et *al* (2003). Characteristics of Hodgkin's lymphoma after infectious mononucleosis. *N Engl J Med*, **349**, 1324–32.
2. Seam, P. *et al.* (2007). The role of FDG-PET scans in patients with lymphoma. *Blood*, **110**, 3507–16.
3. Hutchings, M. *et al.* (2006). FDG-PET after two cycles of chemotherapy predicts treatment failure and progression-free survival in Hodgkin lymphoma. *Blood*, **107**, 52–9.
4. Gallamini A *et al.* (2006). The predictive value of positron emission tomography scanning performed after two courses of standard therapy on treatment outcome in advanced stage Hodgkin's disease. *Haematologica* **91**:475–481.
5. Sasse, S. *et al.* (2006). Combined modality treatment for early stage Hodgkins lymphoma: the GHSG experience. *Haematologica Reports*, **2**, 19–22.
6. NCCN Clinical Practice Guidelines in Oncology Hodgkin Disease/Lymphoma v.1.2007. www.nccn.org/professionals/physician_gls/PDF/hodgkins.pdf
7. Press, O.W. *et al.* (2001). Phase III randomized intergroup trial of subtotal lymphoid irradiation versus doxorubicin, vinblastine and subtotal lymphoid irradiation for stage IA to IIA Hodgkin's disease. *J Clin Oncol*, **19**, 4238–44.
8. Noordijk, E.M. *et al.* (2006). Combined modality therapy for clinical stage I or II Hodgkin's lymphoma: long-term results for the European Organisation for Research and Treatment of Cancer H7 randomized controlled trials. *J Clin Oncol*, **24**, 3128–35.
9. Hagenbeek, A. *et al.* (2000). Three cycles of MOPP/ABV hybrid and involved field irradiation in favourable supradiaphragmatic clinical stages I-II Hodgkin's disease: preliminary results of the EORTC-GELA H8F randomized trial in 543 patients. *Blood*, **96**, 676a (abstract)
10. Ferme, C. *et al.* (2007). Chemotherapy plus involved-field radiation in early-stage Hodgkin's disease. *N Engl J Med*, **357**, 1916–27.
11. Carde, P. *et al.* (1993). Clinical staging versus laparotomy and combined modality with MOPP versus ABVD in early stage Hodgkin's disease: the H6 twin randomized trials from the EORTC Lymphoma Co-operative Group *J Clin Oncol*, **11**, 2258–72.
12. Eghbali, H. *et al.* (2005). Comparison of three radiation dose levels after EBVP regimen in favourable supradiaphragmatic clinical, stages I-II Hodgkin's lymphoma: preliminary results of the EORTC/GELA H9-F trial. *Blood*, **106**, 240a (abstract).
13. Meyer, R.M. *et al.* (2005). Randomized comparison of ABVD chemotherapy with a strategy that includes radiation therapy in patients with limited-stage Hodgkin's lymphoma: National Cancer Institute of Canada Clinical Trials Group and the Eastern Cooperative Oncology Group. *J Clin Oncol*, **23**, 4634–42.
14. Straus, D.J. *et al.* (2004). Results of a prospective randomized clinical trial of doxorubicin, bleomycin, vinblastine and dacarbazine (ABVD) followed by radiation therapy (RT) versus ABVD alone for stages I, II and IIA nonbulky Hodgkin disease. *Blood*, **104**, 3483–9.
15. Devita, V.T. Jr *et al.* (1970). Combination chemotherapy in the treatment of advanced Hodgkin's disease. *Ann Intern Med*, **73**, 881–95.
16. Longo, D.L. *et al.* (1986). Twenty years of MOPP therapy for Hodgkin's disease. *J Clin Oncol*, **4**, 1295–1306.

17. Bonnadonna, G. and Santoro, A. (1982). ABVD chemotherapy in the treatment of Hodgkin's disease. *Cancer Treatment Reviews,* **9**, 21–35.
18. Hasenclever, D. and Diehl, V. (1998). A prognostic score for advanced Hodgkin's disease. International Prognostic Factors Project on Advanced Hodgkin's Disease. *N Engl J Med,* **339**, 1506–14
19. Canellos, G.P. *et al.* (1992). Chemotherapy of advanced Hodgkin's disease with MOPP, ABVD, or MOPP alternating with ABVD. *N Engl J Med,* **327**, 1478–84.
20. Duggan, D.B. *et al.* (2003). Randomized comparison of ABVD and MOPP/ABV hybrid for the treatment of advanced Hodgkin's disease: report of an intergroup trial. *J Clin Oncol,* **21**, 607–14.
21. Gobbi PG *et al.* (2005). ABVD versus modified Stanford V versus MOPPEBVCAD with optional and limited radiotherapy in intermediate- and advanced-stage Hodgkin's lymphoma: final results of a multicenter randomized trial by the Intergruppo Italiano linfomi. *J Clin Oncol,* **23**, 9198–207.
22. Johnson, P.W. *et al.* (2005). Comparison of ABVD and alternating or hybrid multidrug regimens for the treatment of advanced Hodgkin's lymphoma: results of the United Kingdom Lymphoma Group LY09 Trial. *J Clin Oncol,* **23**, 9208–18.
23. Horning, S.J. *et al.* (2002). Stanford V and radiotherapy for locally extensive and advanced Hodgkin's disease: mature results of a prospective clinical trial. *J Clin Oncol,* **20**, 630–7.
24. Diehl, V. *et al.* (2003). Standard and increased-dose BEACOPP chemotherapy compared with COPP-ABVD for advanced Hodgkin's disease. *N Engl J Med,* **348**, 2386–95.
25. Andreas, E. *et al.* (2007). Long-term follow up of BEACOPP escalated chemotherapy in patients with advanced Hodgkin lymphoma on behalf of the German Hodgkin Study Group. *Blood,* **110**, 70a (abstract).
26. Ballova, V. *et al.* (2005). A prospectively randomized trial carried out by the German Hodgkin Study Group (GHSG) for elderly patients with advanced Hodgkin's disease comparing BEACOPP baseline and COPP-ABVD (study HD9elderly) *Ann Oncol,* **16**, 124–31.
27. Loeffler, M. *et al.* (1998). Meta-analysis of chemotherapy versus combined modality treatment trials in Hodgkin's disease. International Database on Hodgkin's Disease Overview Study Group. *J Clin Oncol,* **16**, 818–29.
28. Aleman, B.M. *et al.* (2003). Involved field radiotherapy for advanced Hodgkin's lymphoma. *N Engl J Med,* **348**, 2396–2406.
29. Federico, M. *et al.* (2003). High-dose therapy and autologous stem cell transplantation versus conventional therapy for patients with advanced Hodgkin's lymphoma responding to front-line therapy. *J Clin Oncol,* **21**, 2320–5.
30. Josting, A. *et al.* (2000). Prognostic factors and treatment outcome in primary progressive Hodgkin's lymphoma: a report from the German Hodgkin Lymphoma Study Group. *Blood,* **96**, 1280–6.
31. Moskowitz, C.H. *et al.* (2004). Effectiveness of high dose chemoradiotherapy and autologous stem cell transplantation for patients with biopsy-proven primary refractory Hodgkin's disease. *Br J Haematol,* **124**, 645–52.
32. Linch, D.C. *et al.* (1993). Dose intensification with autologous bone-marrow transplantation in relapsed and resistant Hodgkin's disease: results of a BNLI randomized trial. *Lancet,* **341**, 1051–4.
33. Schmitz, N. *et al.* (2002). Aggressive conventional chemotherapy with autologous haemopoietic stem-cell transplantation for relapsed chemosensitive Hodgkin's disease: a randomized trial. *Lancet,* **359**, 2065-71.
34. Peniket, A.J. *et al.* (2003). An EBMT Registry matched study of allogeneic stem cell transplants for lymphoma: allogeneic transplantation is associated with a lower relapse rate but a higher procedure related mortality rate than autologous transplantation. *Bone Marrow Transplant,* **31**, 667–8.
35. Peggs, K.S. *et al.* (2005). Clinical evidence of a graft-versus-Hodgkin's lymphoma effect after reduced-intensity allogeneic transplantation. *Lance,t* **365**, 1934–41.
36. Ekstrand, B.C. *et al.* (2003). Rituximab in lymphocyte-predominant Hodgkin disease: results of a phase 2 trial. *Blood,* **101**, 4285–9.
37. Diehl, V. *et al.* (1999). Clinical presentation, course and prognostic factors in lymphocyte-predominant Hodgkin's disease and lymphocyte-rich classical Hodgkin's disease. *J Clin Oncol,* **17**, 776–83.

Chapter 6

Myelodysplasia

Myelodysplastic syndromes (MDS)

The myelodysplastic syndromes (MDS) are a group of biologically and clinically heterogeneous clonal disorders characterized by ineffective haematopoiesis and peripheral cytopenia due to ↑ apoptosis and by a variable tendency to evolve to BM failure or acute myeloblastic leukaemia.

Incidence

Predominantly affects the elderly but may occur at any age; median age 69; annual incidence 4/100,000 in general population; rising from 0.5/100,000 aged <50 years to 89/100,000 aged ≥80 years.

Risk factors

- Age.
- Prior cancer therapy: notably with radiotherapy, alkylating agents (chlorambucil, cyclophosphamide, melphalan; peak 4–10 years after therapy) or epipodophyllotoxins (etoposide, teniposide; peak within 5 years). Often seen after autologous SCT (20% of patients with NHL). *Note*: prolonged alkylator therapy also used in rheumatology and other specialties.
- Environmental toxins: notably benzene and other organic solvents; related to intensity and duration of exposure; also smoking, petroleum products, fertilizers, semi-metal, stone dusts, and cereal dusts.
- Genetic: rare familial syndromes; MDS ↑ in children with Schwachman–Diamond syndrome, Fanconi anaemia, and neurofibromatosis type 1.

Pathophysiology

- Clonal haematopoietic stem cell disorder characterized by stepwise genetic progression possibly due to a combination of genetic predisposition and environmental exposures.
- Early mutations cause differentiation arrest and dysplasia with later mutations leading to proliferation, clonal expansion, and AML.
- Recurring cytogenetic abnormalities well recognized but molecular pathogenesis and basis for progression as yet undefined.
- The *MLL* gene at 11q23 is up-regulated (with *HOXA9* activation) in significant % of MDS and AML) patients including normal karyotypes.[1]
- Abnormalities in the marrow microenvironment described: e.g. aberrant cytokine production (↑ inhibitory pro-apoptotic cytokines including TNF- α, IL-6, TGF-β, IFN- α, and Fas ligand) and altered stem cell adhesion.
- MDS marrow stem cells display lowered apoptotic threshold to TNF- α, IFN-α, and anti-Fas antibodies and less response to haemopoietic growth factors.
- Early indolent pro-apoptotic MDS transforms to aggressive proliferative MDS as genetic lesions accumulate (*ras, FLT3, FMS*, and *p53* mutations associated with disease progression).
- Symptoms relate not only to the degree of cytopenia but to impaired function of granulocytes and platelets and may occur at near-↔ or ↔ levels.

1. Poppe, B. *et al.* (2004). Expression analyses identify MLL as a prominent target of 11q23 amplification and support an etiologic role for MLL gain of function in myeloid malignancies. *Blood*, **103**, 229–35.

Classification

2 systems are currently widely used. The NCCN Guidelines endorse the use of both systems in diagnosis, risk assessment, and management.[1]

French–American–British (FAB) system

- Morphology-based classification used since 1982.[2]
- Defines 5 subtypes.
- Requires dysplastic changes in ≥2 lineages.
- Useful for predicting prognosis and risk of evolution to acute leukaemia.

FAB classification

- *Refractory anaemia (RA):* cytopenia of 1 peripheral blood (PB) lineage; normo- or hypercellular marrow with dysplasia ≥2 lineages; <1% PB blasts; <5% BM blasts. 25% of patients.
- *Refractory anaemia with ringed sideroblasts (RARS):* defined as for RA plus ringed sideroblasts constituting >15% nucleated erythroid cells; 15% of patients.
- *Refractory anaemia with excess blasts (RAEB):* cytopenia of ≥2 PB lineages; dysplasia of all 3 BM lineages; <5% PB blasts; 5–20% BM blasts; 35% of patients.
- *Refractory anaemia with excess blasts in transformation (RAEB-t):* cytopenia of ≥2 PB lineages; dysplasia of all 3 BM lineages; ≥5% PB blasts; 21–30% BM blasts or Auer rods in blasts; 15% of patients.
- *Chronic myelomonocytic leukaemia (CMML):* PB monocytosis (>1×10^9/L); <5% PB blasts; ≤20% BM blasts; 10% of patients.

World Health Organization (WHO) system[3] (Table 6.1)

- Reclassification of MDS based on morphology, karyotype, and clinical features that defines more homogeneous subgroups and provides valuable prognostic information useful for clinical decision-making.[4–6]
- Unilineage dysplasia accepted for diagnosis of RA or RARS provided it persists ≥6months and other causes of dysplasia are excluded.
- Lower threshold for diagnosis of AML from 30%→20% blasts in PB or BM; eliminates FAB category 'RAEB-t'.
- Addition of new category 'refractory cytopenia with multilineage dysplasia' (RCMD).
- Defines 2 subtypes of RAEB: RAEB-1 (5–9% BM blasts) and RAEB-2 (10–19% BM blasts) reflecting worse clinical outcomes with ≥10% blasts.
- Recognizes the '5q– syndrome' as a distinct narrowly defined entity.
- Removes CMML to a newly created disease group: MDS/MPD.

📖 See Table 6.2 for a comparison of FAB and WHO classifications.

Table 6.1 WHO classification system[3]

Condition	PB finding	BM findings
Refractory anaemia (RA)	Anaemia No or rare blasts	Erythroid dysplasia only <5% blasts <15% ringed sideroblasts
Refractory anaemia with ringed sideroblasts (RARS)	Anaemia No blasts	≥15% ringed sideroblasts erythroid dysplasia only <5% blasts
Refractory cytopenia with multilineage dysplasia (RCMD)	Cytopenias (bi- or pan-) No or rare blasts No Auer rods $<1 \times 10^9$/L monocytes	Dysplasia in ≥10% cells in ≥2 myeloid cell lines <5%blasts No Auer rods <15% ringed sideroblasts
Refractory cytopenia with multilineage dysplasia and ringed sideroblasts (RCMD-RS)	Cytopenias (bi- or pan-) No or rare blasts No Auer rods $<1 \times 10^9$/L monocytes	Dysplasia in ≥10% cells in ≥2 myeloid cell lines ≥15% ringed sideroblasts <5% blasts No Auer rods
Refractory anaemia with excess blasts (RAEB-1)	Cytopenias <5% blasts No Auer rods $<1 \times 10^9$/L monocytes	Unilineage or multilineage dysplasia 5–9% blasts No Auer rods
Refractory anaemia with excess blasts (RAEB-2)	Cytopenias 5–19% blasts Auer rods ± $<1 \times 10^9$/L monocytes	Unilineage or multilineage dysplasia 10–19% blasts Auer rods ±
MDS associated with isolated del(5q)	Anaemia <5% blasts Platelets ↔ or ↑	↔ to ↑ megakaryocytes with hypolobated nuclei <5% blasts No Auer rods Isolated del(5q)

Reproduced from reference 3, with permission. Copyright American Society of Hematology.

Table 6.2 Comparison of FAB and WHO classifications

FAB	WHO
RA	RA (unilineage)
	5q– syndrome
	RCMD
RARS	RARS (unilineage)
	RCMD-RS
RAEB	RAEB-1
	RAEB-2
RAEB-t	AML
CMML	MDS/MPD
	MDS-U

References

1. NCCN Practice Guidelines in Oncology: Myelodysplastic Syndromes V.2.2008. www.nccn.org/professionals/physician_gls/PDF/mds.pdf
2. Bennett, J.M. *et al.* (1982). Proposals for the classification of the myelodysplastic syndromes. *Br J Haematol*, **51**, 189–99.
3. Vardiman, J.W. *et al.* (2002). The World Health Organization (WHO) classification of the myeloid neoplasms. *Blood*, **100**, 2292–302.
4. Germing, U. *et al.* (2000). Validation of the WHO proposals for a new classification of primary myelodysplastic syndromes: a retrospective analysis of 1600 patients. *Leukaemia Res*, **24**, 983–92.
5. Malcovati, L. *et al.* (2005). Prognostic factors and life expectancy in myelodysplastic syndromes classified according to WHO criteria: a basis for clinical decision making. *J Clin Oncol*, **23**, 7594–603.
6. Bowen, D. *et al.* (2006). Prospective validation of the WHO proposals for the classification of myelodysplastic syndromes. *Haematologica*, **91**, 1596–604.

Clinical features of MDS

- Presentation ranges from mild anaemia to profound pancytopenia.
- May be asymptomatic with mild anaemia identified on routine FBC.
- Macrocytic or normocytic anaemia usual (60–80%) ± neutropenia (50–60%) ± thrombocytopenia (40–60%).
- Isolated thrombocytopenia is an unusual presentation for MDS.
- Symptoms of underlying cytopenias and cellular dysfunction may develop:
  - Anaemia—fatigue, shortness of breath, exacerbation of cardiac symptoms.
  - Neutropenia and dysfunctional granulocytes—recurrent infection.
  - Thrombocytopenia and dysfunctional platelets—spontaneous bruising, purpura, bleeding gums.
- Constitutional symptoms including anorexia, weight loss, fevers, and sweats usually features of more 'advanced' subgroups; may be due to cytokine release.
- Splenomegaly commonly occurs in CMML and may cause abdominal pain and easy satiety.

Investigation and diagnosis

- ***History:*** prior exposure to chemotherapy/radiation; FH of MDS/AML; symptoms of anaemia, recurrent infection, bleeding or bruising; timing, severity and tempo of cytopenias; previous transfusion; medication and co-morbidities.
- ***Examination:*** pallor; infection; bruising; splenomegaly.
- ***FBC:*** macrocytic/normocytic anaemia ± neutropenia ± thrombocytopenia ± neutrophilia ± monocytosis ± thrombocytosis.
- ***Blood film:*** may demonstrate dimorphic red cells ± Pappenheimer bodies in RARS/RCMD-RS; basophilic stippling in RBCs; dysplastic granulocytes: pseudo-Pelger forms (Fig. 6.1), hypersegmented neutrophils, hypogranular neutrophils, dysmorphic monocytes ± blasts; platelets may be large or hypogranular.
- ***Reticulocyte count:*** not ↑.
- ***U&E, LFTs, ECG, and CXR:*** to assess comorbidity.
- ***Serum ferritin, vitamin B12, and RBC folate:*** usually ↔ levels; ferritin may be elevated in RARS/RCMD-RS.
- ***Serum EPO level:*** **(prior to transfusion)** indicates potential for response to EPO.
- ***BM aspirate:*** report cellularity, M:E ratio and blast %; demonstrates >10% dysplastic cells in ≥1 lineage (FAB ≥2): megaloblastoid erythropoiesis, nuclear-cytoplasmic asynchrony in myeloid/erythroid precursors, dysmorphic megakaryocytes or micro-megakaryocytes; ↑ monocytes (CMML); Perl's stain: normal/ ↑ storage Fe; ≥15% ringed sideroblasts (RARS/RCMD-RS).
- ***BM trephine biopsy:*** assess cellularity, usually ↑/↔ but NB hypocellular variant; may show multifocal accumulation of immature (CD34+) progenitors (formerly termed 'abnormal localization of immature myeloid precursors' (ALIPs) centrally in interstitium)[1], megakaryocyte dysplasia, ↑ angiogenesis, ↑ mast cells; ↑ reticulin or fibrosis; ↑ storage Fe; excludes occult neoplasia.

- ***Immunohistochemistry:*** minimum of CD34 (progenitors), CD31, 42, or 61 (megakaryocytes) and tryptase (mast cells) recommended in all cases; CD3/15/20/25/117 in selected cases.[1]
- ***BM cytogenetic analysis:*** may demonstrate clonal chromosome abnormality(s) confirming diagnosis and providing prognostic information; karyotype evolution is associated with progression; exclude Fanconi and dyskeratosis congenita in familial cytopenia; FISH (5q31, CEP7, 7q31, CEP8, 20q, CEPY, *p53* probes) useful if low metaphase yield or difficult case.
- ***HLA-typing and CMV serology:*** for patients eligible for allogeneic SCT.
- ***HIV serology:*** in selected cases.
- ***Flow cytometry:*** **in selected cases to exclude PNH (**hypoplastic marrow) and LGLL.
- ***HLA-DR15 screening:*** in younger patients with hypoplastic marrow and normal cytogenetics (possible response to immunosuppression).
- ***Clonality studies:*** used in some centres to establish diagnosis in difficult cases; flow cytometry for clonal BM blasts expressing phenotypic deviations; molecular analysis (X-inactivation based human androgen receptor locus (HUMARA) assay; gene chip profiling or point mutation (e.g. *RAS*) analysis) and colony (CFU) assays.[1]

Definitive diagnosis of early MDS (e.g. isolated cytopenia) may be difficult; regular review with repeat blood count and film assessment is recommended; in all cases a measure of the tempo of the disease over several weeks is of prognostic value.

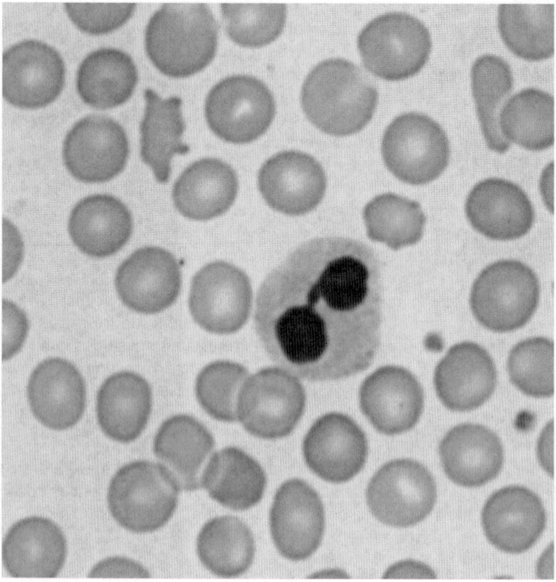

Fig. 6.1 Blood film in MDS showing bilobed pseudo-Pelger neutrophil (see Plate 23).

1. Valent, P. et *al.* (2007). Definitions and standards in the diagnosis and treatment of the myelodysplastic syndromes: Consensus statements and report from a working conference. *Leukaemia Res*, **31**, 727–36.

Cytogenetic analysis

- Cytogenetic analysis yields 3 patterns: (i) normal karyotype; (ii) balanced abnormalities producing fusion oncogenes; (iii) complex karyotypes (≥3 abnormalities).
- Cytogenetic abnormalities found in BM in 40–70% de novo MDS and 80–90% 2° MDS.
- Single or complex abnormalities at diagnosis may evolve during course of disease.
- More complex abnormalities associated with more aggressive subtypes and higher % blasts and with 2° MDS.
- Most frequent abnormalities involve chromosomes 5, 7, 8, 11, 12, 13, 17, and 20; most typical are 8+, 7– or 7q–, 5– or 5q–.
- Complex karyotypes occur in 30% de novo MDS and 50% 2° MDS.
- Prognostic value—isolated 5q–, 20q–, and normal karyotype favourable; complex karyotypes (≥3 abnormalities), 7– ,or 7q– unfavourable.

Diagnostic criteria of MDS

Minimal diagnostic criteria have been recommended by an International Consensus Working Group[1] and comprise two 'pre-requisite-type criteria' (both required) plus at least 1 (out of 3) MDS-related (decisive) criteria and several co-criteria (Table 6.2).

Table 6.3 Minimal diagnostic criteria in MDS[a]

(A) Prerequisite criteria
- Constant cytopenia in ≥1 of the following cell lineages:
  - Erythroid (Hb <11g/dL).
  - Neutrophilic (ANC $<1.5 \times 10^9$/L) **or**
  - Megakaryocytic (plates $<100 \times 10^9$/L).
- Exclusion of all other haematopoietic or non-haematopoietic disorders as 1° reason for cytopenia/dysplasia.[b]

(B) MDS-related criteria
- Dysplasia in ≥10% of all cells in 1 of the following lineages in BM smear:
  - Erythroid, neutrophil, or megakaryocytic **or**
  - >15% ringed sideroblasts on Fe stain.
- 5–19% blast cells in BM smears.
- Typical chromosomal abnormality (by conventional karyotype or FISH).[c]

(C) Co-criteria[d] (for patients fulfilling 'A' but not 'B' and otherwise typical clinical features)
- Abnormal phenotype of BM cells clearly indicative of monoclonal population of erythroid or/and myeloid cells by flow cytometry.
- Clear molecular signs of monoclonal cell population in HUMARA assay, gene chip profiling, or point mutation analysis (e.g. *RAS* mutations).
- Markedly and persistently reduced colony (± cluster) formation of BM or/and circulating progenitor cells (CFU-assay).

[a] The diagnosis can be established when both prerequisite criteria and at least 1 decisive criterion are fulfilled. Co-criteria should be applied if no decisive criteria are fulfilled but the patient is likely to suffer from a clonal myeloid disease and may help in reaching the conclusion that the patient has MDS or a condition 'highly suspicious of MDS'.
[b] MDS can be diagnosed even if another co-existing disease potentially causing cytopenia was detected.
[c] Typical abnormalities are those recurrently found in MDS (+8, −7, 5q−, 20q−, etc). [d] Co-criteria not considered standard assays in all centres. If not available, questionable cases should be monitored and tests repeated to establish the diagnosis of MDS.

The diagnosis of ***'idiopathic cytopenia of uncertain (undetermined) significance'*** (ICUS) was introduced to describe cases with cytopenia in ≥1 lineage for ≥6 months but that do not meet the minimal criteria for MDS and cannot be explained by another diagnosis. These patients should be monitored with repeat FBC, differential and serum chemistry at 1–6-month intervals and a repeat BM if MDS is suspected.

Differential diagnosis

Exclude:
- Other causes of anaemia—haematinic deficiency, haemolysis, blood loss, renal failure.

- Other causes of neutropenia—drugs, viral infection.
- Other causes of thrombocytopenia—drugs, ITP.
- Other causes of bi-/pancytopenia—drugs, infection, aplastic anaemia.
- Other causes of monocytosis—infection, AML; or neutrophilia—infection, CML.
- Reactive causes of BM dysplasia—megaloblastic anaemia, HIV infection, alcoholism, recent cytotoxic therapy, severe intercurrent illness.
- Other causes of marrow hypoplasia in hypoplastic MDS—aplastic anaemia, PNH.

1. Valent, P. *et al.* (2007). Definitions and standards in the diagnosis and treatment of the myelodysplastic syndromes: Consensus statements and report from a working conference. *Leukaemia Res*, **31**, 727–36.

Prognostic factors in MDS

Table 6.4[1] Prognosis by FAB classification

FAB classification	RA	RARS	RAEB	RAEB-t	CMML
Proportion of patients	25%	15%	12%	15%	10%
Median survival (months)	43	73	12	5	20
Transformation to AML	15%	5%	40%	50%	35%
Transformed at 1 year	5%	0	25%	55%	np
Transformed at 2 years	10%	0	35%	65%	np

np: data not provided

CMML median survival <5% blasts 53 months; 5–20% blasts16 months.

International Prognostic Scoring System (IPSS)

- Uses % BM blasts, BM cytogenetics, and number of cytopenias to compute a risk score and stratify patients into 4 distinct groups (Tables 6.5 and 6.6)
- Improved prognostic power for both survival and evolution into AML compared with earlier systems.
- Analysis excluded CMML with a WBC $>12 \times 10^9$/L as this was considered myeloproliferative rather than MDS.
- IPSS score should be calculated during a stable clinical state and not, for example, during florid infection at initial presentation.
- IPSS score is the 'gold standard' for risk assessment in patients with *de novo* MDS and may be used to assist management decisions.

Table 6.5 Calculation of IPSS Score

Prognostic variable	Score value				
	0	0.5	1.0	1.5	2.0
BM blast %	<5	5–10	–	11–20	21–30
Karyotype	Good	Intermediate		Poor	
Cytopenias	0/1		2/3		

Karyotype: Good: normal, –Y alone, del(5q) alone, del(20q) alone. Poor: complex (≥ 3 abnormalities) or chromosome 7 anomalies. Intermediate: other abnormalities.
Cytopenias: Hb <10g/dL; neutrophils $<1.8 \times 10^9$/L; platelets $<100 \times 10^9$/L.

Table 6.6[2] Prognosis by IPSS Score

IPSS risk group (% patienss)	Combined score	Median survival	25% AML evolution
Low (33)	0	5.7 years	9.4 years
Intermediate–1 (38)	0.5–1.0	3.5 years	3.3 years
Intermediate–2 (22)	1.5–2.0	1.2 years	1.1 years
High (7)	>2.5	0.4 years	0.2 years

Other prognostic factors

- Serum LDH has been proposed as a refinement of the IPSS that splits each risk group into 2 prognostically distinct sub-groups.[3]
- Flow cytometric characterization of BM blast maturation stages has prognostic value and immature markers (e.g. CD7)[4] and a scoring systems reflecting the complexity of the findings[5] correlate with poor risk features, IPSS score, and OS. Further multicentre studies are required to standardize methods and define applicability.
- Development of transfusion dependence significantly worsens OS and development of 2° Fe overload (serum ferritin >1000mg/L) further worsens OS.[6] Survival has been shown to be inversely related to serum ferritin in low risk MDS.[7]

References

1. Greenberg, P.L. (2000). In: Hoffman, R. *et al.* eds *Hematology: Basic Principles & Practice.* 3rd ed. New York, NY: Churchill Livingstone, pp.1106–29.
2. Greenberg, P. *et al.* (1997). International scoring system for evaluating prognosis in myelodysplastic syndromes. *Blood,* **89**, 2079–88.
3. Germing, U. *et al.* (2005). Refinement of the international prognostic scoring system (IPSS) by including LDH as an additional prognostic variable to improve risk assessment in patients with primary myelodysplastic syndromes (MDS) *Leukaemia,* **19**, 2223–31.
4. Ogata, K. *et al.* (2002). Clinical significance of phenotype features of blasts in patients with myelodysplastic syndrome. *Blood,* **100**, 3887–96.
5. Wells, D.A. *et al.* (2003). Myeloid and monocytic dyspoiesis as determined by flow cytometric scoring in myelodysplastic syndrome correlates with the IPSS and with outcome after haemopoietic stem cell transplantation. *Blood,* **102**, 394–403.
6. Malcovati, L. *et al.* (2005). Prognostic factors and life expectancy in myelodysplastic syndromes classified according to WHO criteria: a basis for clinical decision making. *J Clin Oncol,* **23**, 7594–603.
7. Malcovati, L. *et al.* (2006). Predicting survival and leukaemic evolution in patients with myelodysplastic syndrome. *Haematologica,* **91**, 1588–90.

Clinical variants of MDS

These variants were recognized before the development of the FAB and WHO classifications because of their distinctive clinical characteristics. It is now even more important to identify several of these because of new therapeutic options.

5q– syndrome

Separately defined in WHO classification; characterized by ♀ preponderance; more indolent clinical course; lower rate of evolution to AML (10%); severe anaemia; pronounced macrocytosis; ↔ or moderate ↓ WBC; ↔ or moderate ↑ platelets; dysplastic megakaryocytes; no blast excess; high response rate to lenalidomide.

Pure sideroblastic anaemia (PSA)

Defined as sideroblastic anaemia with dysplasia confined to erythropoietic cells (RARS in WHO classification); survival better (77% OS at 3 years) than when dysplastic features are also present in myeloid or megakaryocytic lineages (WHO classification RCMD-RS; 56% OS at 3 years) and very low risk of AML. High risk of transfusion siderosis.

2° MDS

Incidence ↑ due to successful chemotherapy and ↑ pollution; multiple chromosomal abnormalities in almost all patients; poorer prognosis than *de novo* MDS.

Hypoplastic MDS

<15% of cases of MDS have hypocellular BM on biopsy (<30% cellularity age <60 years; <20% aged ≥60 years); dysplastic megakaryocytes ± myeloid cells or excess blasts may be difficult to see; may be difficult to distinguish from aplastic anaemia in which pancytopenia usually more severe: cytogenetic findings typical of MDS may be necessary for diagnosis; ↔ or ↑ %CD34+ cells suggests MDS; no particular age range, FAB type and no difference in prognosis but may respond to immunosuppressive therapy.

MDS with myelofibrosis (MDS-F)

Up to 50% of cases have ↑ BM fibrosis but <15% have marked fibrosis; all FAB types; more common in 2° MDS; BM hypercellular with MF, diffuse coarse reticulin fibrosis and dysplasia in at least 2 cell lineages; PB shows pancytopenia and dysplastic features and sometimes leucoerythroblastic picture; organomegaly unusual; rapid deterioration usual; must distinguish from acute megakaryocytic leukaemia, acute panmyelosis with fibrosis and chronic myeloproliferative disorders, metastatic cancer, lymphoma and HCL.

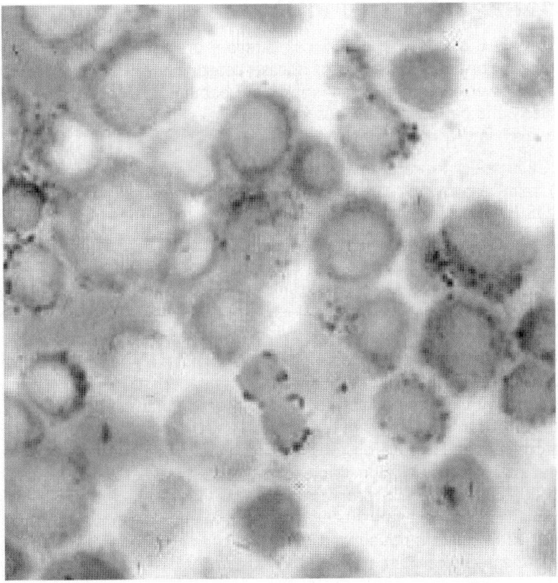

Fig. 6.2 BM in RARS stained for Fe: note Fe granules round the nucleus of the erythroblast (see Plate 24).

Management of MDS

WHO/FAB diagnosis and IPSS risk category are used in deciding therapeutic priorities. The tempo of disease determined by observation over several weeks/months is an important parameter. Most patients are elderly and performance status and individual patient preferences should be taken into consideration.

NCCN guidelines recommend stratifying patients into 2 major risk groups: (i) relatively low risk patients with IPSS low/intermediate-1(int-1) risk MDS in whom haematological improvement is the therapeutic aim and (ii) higher risk patients with int-2/high risk MDS in whom alteration of the natural history is the priority.[1]

For patients with *low risk MDS*, a 'watch and wait' approach may be adopted prior to the introduction of therapy. Supportive care may be the only treatment indicated. Patients with *low/int-1 MDS* should be treated with low intensity therapy. However, development of transfusion-dependence significantly worsens OS[2] and a delayed transplantation strategy for selected patients with low/int-1 MDS with disease progression has been suggested.[3] Intensive therapy is indicated for patients with *int-2/high risk MDS* who can tolerate it. Palliative or investigational therapy is indicated for patients with int-2/high risk MDS ineligible for intensive therapy, to maintain quality of life (QoL) and delay progression. Diagnosis of AML with multilineage dysplasia in a patient with 20–29% blasts (FAB RAEB-t) or indeed AML-MD with ≥30% blasts, is not a mandate for use of a regimen for *de novo* AML.[4] Treatment choice must be based on age, prior history of MDS, clinical features, performance status, and MDS evolution.

Supportive care

Supportive care is administered with the aim of reducing morbidity and maintaining QoL. For many patients this will be the mainstay of management. It involves monitoring, psychosocial support, and QoL assessment.

Red cell transfusion

Should be administered only for symptomatic anaemia; symptomatology rather than a 'trigger' Hb level should initiate red cell support. Some patients with minimal requirements have better QoL on EPO (📖 see EPO ± G-CSF, p.239).

Fe chelation therapy

Should be considered once a patient has received 20–25 units of RBCs if long-term transfusion is required e.g. RA, RARS, or 5q– syndrome, those with serum ferritin >2500mg/L, and those with concurrent cardiac or hepatic dysfunction. Effects of Fe overload may become apparent after 20–40 units of red cells and serum ferritin of 1500–2000mg/L and is a significant cause of morbidity and mortality in low risk patients with isolated erythroid dysplasia.[2]

- *Desferrioxamine* has been underutilized in elderly patients particularly with co-morbidities and with limited survival expectation due to its inconvenient administration and toxicity; dose 20–40mg/kg by 12h SC infusion 5–7 nights/week reduced to 25mg/kg when ferritin <2000mg/L; vitamin C 100–200mg/day PO may be added after 1 month; bolus administration is not effective in chronic Fe overload; aim for serum ferritin <1000mg/L; monitor renal function; audiometric and ophthalmological assessments prior to therapy and annually.

- *Deferasirox* is approved by FDA and in UK for treatment of Fe overload; 20–30mg/kg PO od; comparable efficacy to desferrioxamine;[5] monitor renal and hepatic function monthly and eyes and ears pre-therapy and annually.
- *Deferiprone* is another approved orally active chelator; dose 25mg/kg tds; agranulocytosis has been reported.

Platelet transfusion

Should be administered for patients with haemorrhagic problems and those with severe thrombocytopenia with the aim of maintaining a platelet count $>10 \times 10^9$/L. Tranexamic acid 0.5–1g tds may be useful in patients with bleeding refractory to platelets or with profound thrombocytopenia.

Anti-infective therapy

Empirical broad spectrum antibiotics and/or antifungals should be administered promptly for neutropenic sepsis; no evidence to support routine use of prophylactic anti-infectives in neutropenic patients; prophylactic anti-infective agents may be useful in neutropenic patients with recurrent infection.

Low intensity therapy

Erythropoietin (EPO) ± G-CSF

Considered 1st-choice therapy for transfusion-dependent low risk/int-1 MDS and low serum EPO levels with low transfusion frequency.[1,6,7] Maintenance of stable augmented Hb may provide better QoL than the cyclical fluctuations of transfusion programmes.[8] No effect on progression to AML,[8] but may improve OS.[9] 20–30% respond to EPO alone, 40–60% to Epo+G-CSF; synergistic effect most evident in RARS or patients with serum EPO <500IU/L.[9] A study of 403 patients achieved 50% responses by IWG 2006 criteria (📖 p.244) with serum EPO <200 IU/L, absence of transfusion requirement, IPSS low/int-1 and interval from diagnosis to EPO therapy <6 months as predictors of response.[10] Responses generally occur within 6–8 weeks; median response 1–2 years, longer responses associated with lower % BM blasts, low/int-1 IPSS, and major erythroid response. A validated predictive model for response based on serum EPO and transfusion history has been developed.[8,9] Check Fe stores and replete if necessary.

- For patients with RA/RAEB with symptomatic anaemia, transfusion requirement <2U/month and a basal EPO level of <200IU/L consider trial of EPO (10,000U/d or 40–60,000U 1–3 × /week for 6 weeks); in non-responders consider adding daily G-CSF (1–2mg/kg/d or 1–3 × /week) SC or double dose EPO or both for further 6 weeks; no response after 2–3 months = treatment failure; in responders, reduce G-CSF to 3-weekly and EPO in steps to lowest dose retaining response.
- For patients with RARS with symptomatic anaemia, transfusion requirement < 2U/month and basal EPO levels <500U/L combined therapy should be used from outset; consider EPO dose escalation if no response after 6 weeks; no response after 2–3 months = treatment failure; in responders titrate doses and frequency as tolerated.

- A hyperglycosylated long-acting EPO derivative (darbepoetin alfa 150-300mcg/week) is a convenient and effective alternative with response in up to 60%; some patients only require maintenance every 2–4 weeks.[11]

G-CSF

- Useful for patients with neutropenia and recurrent or antibiotic resistant infections; not recommended simply for chronic prophylaxis.

Lenalidomide

- Achieves major clinical responses and cytogenetic responses in most patients with 5q– syndrome.[12–14] Mode of action appears to be direct cytotoxic effect suppressing 5q– clone. Long-term follow-up suggests it may alter natural history of MDS with durable responses (median 2.2 years), improved OS (10-year estimate of 78% for cytogenetic responders *vs.* 4% in non-responders) and reduced AML transformation (15% at 10 years in responders *vs.* 67%) at 10 years.[15]
- At 10mg/day for 21d every 4 weeks, 66% transfusion dependent patients with low/int1 and 52% with higher IPSS 5q– MDS achieved transfusion-independence (TI) at 24 weeks with 76% cytogenetic response (55% complete); median duration of major responses >2 years. Similar but less durable responses in MDS with 5q– plus additional abnormalities where it also normalized % BM blasts in 75%. Less effective in MDS without 5q– (26% TI, median duration 41 weeks; 19% cytogenetic response).[16] Optimal dose and duration of therapy not established.
- Therapy interrupted in ~50% for grade 3/4 neutropenia or thrombocytopenia; generally transient and improves after first 6–8 weeks in parallel with erythroid response.
- Monitor patients with renal dysfunction carefully. FDA approved for MDS with 5q–. Not NICE assessed in UK.

Epigenetic therapy (hypo-methylating agents)

- azacitidine 5-azacytidine (Aza-C) and decitabine (5-aza -2-deoxycytidine) inhibit DNA methyl transferase, reduce DNA methylation, and reactivate abnormally suppressed gene expression. In a subset of MDS patients they ameliorate anaemia, decrease the risk of leukaemic transformation, and improve OS.
- *Aza-C* achieved haematological responses, delayed AML transformation, and improved QoL (47% OR 10% CR; 36% haematological improvement (HI)) with a trend to ↑ OS.[17] Usual dose 75mg/m^2/d SC 7d monthly × 4–6 courses. Most responses observed between courses 4 and 6. Addition of G-CSF and shortened 5d administration may improve response rates as does addition of valproic acid which also speeds response rates.[18] Early maintenance studies are encouraging. An oral formulation is in clinical trial.
- *Decitabine* early trials at 45mg/m^2/d IV achieved 17% OR (9% CR) plus 13% HI;[19] myelosuppressive; required hospitalization. Lower doses (20mg/m^2/d IV for 5d monthly) effective (up to 39% CR) and more tolerable and may be administered in outpatients.[20] In higher risk MDS, 31% major cytogenetic responses and predicts for ↑ OS (24 *vs.* 11 months).[21] Addition of valproic acid improves and accelerates response rates.[18]

- *Aza-C* and *decitabine* approved by FDA for MDS. Not NICE assessed in UK. Consider in int-2/high-risk MDS patients not candidates for intensive therapy or who require therapy prior to SCT.[1] Optimum dose and duration of therapy of both agents not yet established. Low dose, high dose-intensity regimens may be best. Both cause myelosuppression but low treatment-related mortality. Rash and vomiting more frequent with Aza-C. Response often only after several months; minimum 3 cycles required before evaluating response. Response duration generally <1 year for both.

Immunosuppression

May produce trilineage responses notably in hypoplastic MDS but also in other patients with low risk MDS (RA; IPSS ≤ int-1).

- *ATG* 40mg/kg/d × 4d achieved transfusion independence in ~33% patients (median response >2 years); erythroid improvement in up to 66%, and sustained neutrophil and platelet responses in up to 50%; response associated with significant survival benefit.[22,23]
- *Ciclosporin A* has achieved transfusion independence in a high proportion of patients with RA in small clinical trials; improved Hb (34% HI-E) neutrophils (22%) and platelets (16%) also.[24]
- *ATG+ciclosporin A* may be used in combination as in aplastic anaemia (📖 see p.98).[25]
- Younger age, shorter duration of transfusion dependence, HLA-DR15, hypoplastic BM, and presence of a PNH clone associated with response to immunosuppression.

Non-intensive chemotherapy

May be tolerated by elderly patients with transformed or 'transforming' MDS; but transient reductions in blast counts may be at the price of ↑ cytopenia and transfusion dependence.

- *Hydroxycarbamide* is used to control monocytosis in CMML; titrate dose to achieve optimum control of myeloproliferation with minimum additional cytopenia; preferable to oral etoposide.
- *Low dose melphalan* (2mg/d): small trials show 40% response rate in patients with RAEB or RAEB-t without severe side effects and prolonged survival in responders; best responses in hypoplastic MDS.

Other agents

Thalidomide (13% HI-E (📖 see p.246) at 100–400mg/d),[26] arsenic trioxide (11% HI-E),[27] valproic acid (11% HI-E),[28] the FTI, tipifarnib (12% OR, 7% CR),[29] and the anti-TNF analogue etanercept have shown efficacy in Phase I/II trials.[30]

Intensive therapy

Chemotherapy

AML induction chemotherapy should be considered in patients <60 years with int-2/high risk MDS and good performance status; lower responses (40–50%) and higher treatment related morbidity and mortality than in *de novo* AML; age >50 and karyotypic abnormalities associated with poor response. No clearly superior regimen.[31] Prolonged DFS rare. Without SCT option, benefit marginal and survival not prolonged in most patients.[32] Consolidate with SCT where possible.

High dose therapy and SCT

- Sibling allogeneic SCT offers the best prospect of prolonged survival and curative therapy (35–40% 3-year DFS); few eligible but treatment of choice for patients aged <50 years with ≥IPSS int-1 and sibling donor. In selected younger patients with fully matched sibling donors 60–70% long-term DFS achievable.[33]
- Statistical analysis suggests that IPSS int-2/high risk patients 60 years should proceed to HLA-matched sibling SCT at diagnosis for best OS but SCT should be delayed in low/int-1 MDS patients until progression.[3]
- Age, co-morbidity, disease-stage, non-transplant chemotherapy, type of donor, source of stem cells, and conditioning regimen all influence the decision to transplant and the outcome.[33]
- Need for remission induction chemotherapy pre-transplant unclear.
- High treatment related mortality (~40%); relapse rate up to 40%; relapse risk relates to IPSS score—low risk <5%, high risk >25% as does 5-year DFS—IPSS low/int-1 60%, int-2 36% and high risk 28%; favourable outcome associated with younger age, shorter disease duration, compatible graft, 1° MDS, <10% blasts, good risk cytogenetics.
- Conditioning regimens not incorporating total body irradiation appear to have a lower treatment-related mortality.[33]
- RIC regimens reduce toxicity (100d TRM as low as 7% and 1-year DFS up to 77%) and increase eligible age range for SCT.[34] Longer follow-up needed to assess value fully.
- MUD allogeneic SCT associated with lower DFS (<30% at 2 years), higher treatment related mortality (>50%) but lower relapse rates (<15%); high mortality associated with patient age;[35] this option should be discussed with patients ≤40 years with ≥IPSS intermediate-1 who lack a sibling donor.
- Autologous SCT remains investigational for patients in CR after AML regimens; poor mobilization, adequate stem cell numbers achieved in only 40–60% patients; lower TRM but higher relapse rate (>60%) than allograft; 15% long-term DFS has been reported.[36] Consider in younger patients in CR after chemotherapy if no donor available.

References

1. NCCN Practice Guidelines in Oncology: Myelodysplastic Syndromes V.2.2008 www.nccn.org/professionals/physician_gls/PDF/mds.pdf
2. Malcovati, L. *et al.* (2005). Prognostic factors and life expectancy in myelodysplastic syndromes classified according to WHO criteria: a basis for clinical decision making. *J Clin Oncol*, **23**, 7594-7603.
3. Cutler, C.S. *et al.* (2004). A decision analysis of allogeneic bone marrow transplantation for the myelodysplastic syndromes. Delayed transplantation for low risk myelodysplasia is associated with improved outcome. *Blood*, **104**, 579–85.
4. Brunning, R.D. *et al.* (2001). Myelodysplastic syndromes. In Jaffe, E.S. *et al.* (eds) *World Health Organization classification of tumours. Pathology and genetics. Tumours of haematopoietic and lymphoid tissues, vol 1*. Lyon: IARC Press, pp.62–73.
5. Cazzola, M. *et al.* (2005). ICL670, a once daily iron chelator, is effective and well tolerated in patients with myelodysplastic syndrome (MDS) and iron overload. *Haematologica*, **90**(Suppl 2), 306 (Abst 0769).
6. Valent, P. *et al.* (2007). Definitions and standards in the diagnosis and treatment of the myelodysplastic syndromes: Consensus statements and report from a working conference. *Leukaemia Res*, **31**, 727–36.
7. Bowen, D. *et al.* (2003). Guidelines for the diagnosis and therapy of adult myelodysplastic syndromes. *Br J Haematol*, **120**, 187–200. www.bcshguidelines.com/pdf/BJH120_02_187.pdf
8. Hellstrom-Lindberg, E. *et al.* (2003). A validated decision model for treating MDS with erythropoietin and GCSF: significant effects on quality of life. *Br J Haematol*, **120**, 1037–46.
9. Hellstrom-Lindberg, E. *et al.* (1997). Erythroid response to treatment with G-CSF plus erythropoietin for the anemia of patients with myelodysplastic syndromes: proposal for a predictive model. *Br J Haematol*, **99**, 344–51.

10. Park, S. *et al.* (2008). Predictive factors of response and survival in myelodysplastic syndrome treated with erythropoietin and G-CSF: the GFM experience. *Blood,* **111**, 574–82.
11. Musto, P. *et al.* (2005). Darbepoietin-alpha for the treatment of anaemia in low-intermediate risk myelodysplastic syndromes. *Br J Haematol,* **128**, 204–9.
12. List, A. *et al.* (2005). Efficacy of lenalidomide in myelodysplastic syndromes. *N Engl J Med,* **352**, 549–57.
13. List, A. *et al.* (2006). Lenalidomide in the myelodysplastic syndrome with chromosome 5q deletion. *N Engl J Med,* **355**, 1456–65.
14. Nimer, S.D. *et al.* (2006). Clinical management of myelodysplastic syndromes with interstitial deletion of chromosome 5q. *J Clin Oncol,* **24**, 2576–82.
15. Melchert, M. and List, A. (2007). Management of RBC-transfusion dependence. *Hematology 2007*, 398–404.
16. Raza, A. *et al.* (2008). Phase 2 study of lenalidomide in transfusion-dependent, low-risk, and intermediate 1-risk myelodysplastic syndromes with karyotypes other than deletion 5q. *Blood,* **111**, 86–93.
17. Silverman, L.R. *et al.* (2006). Further analysis of trials with azacitidine in patients with myelodysplastic syndrome: studies 8421, 8921 and 9221 by the Cancer and Leukemia Group B. *J Clin Oncol,* **24**, 3895–903.
18. Garcia-Manero, G. (2007). Modifying the epigenome as a therapeutic strategy in myelodysplasia. *Hematology 2007*. 405–11.
19. Kantarjian, H. *et al.* (2006). Decitabine improves patient outcomes in myelodysplastic syndromes: results of a phase III randomized study. *Cancer,* **106**, 1794–80.
20. Kantarjian, H. *et al.* (2007). Results of a randomized study of 3 schedules of low-dose decitabine in higher-risk myelodysplastic syndrome and chronic myelomonocytic leukaemia. *Blood,* **109**, 52–7.
21. Lubbert, M. *et al.* (2001). Cytogenetic responses in high risk myelodysplastic syndrome following low-dose treatment with the DNA methylation inhibitor 5-aza-2'-deoxycytidine. *Br J Haematol,* **114**, 349–57.
22. Killick, S.B. *et al.* (2003). A pilot study of antithymocyte globulin (ATG) in the treatment of patients with 'low-risk' myelodysplasia. *Br J Haematol,* **120**, 6769–684.
23. Lim, Z. *et al.* (2005). European multi-centre study on the use of anti-thymocyte globulin in the treatment of myelodysplastic syndromes. *Blood,* **1056**, 707a.
24 Shimamoto, T. *et al.* (2003). Cyclosporin A therapy for patients with myelodysplastic syndrome: multicentre pilot studies in Japan. *Leuk Res,* **27**, 783–8.
25. Broliden, P. *et al.* (2006). Antithymocyte globulin and cyclosporin A as combination therapy for low-risk non-sideroblastic myelodysplastic syndromes. *Haematologica,* **91**, 667–70.
26. Raza, A. *et al.* (2001). Thalidomide produces transfusion independence in long-standing refractory anaemias of patients with myelodysplastic syndromes. *Blood,* **98**, 958–65.
27. Vey, N. *et al.* (2004). Trisenox (arsenic trioxide) in patients with myelodysplastic syndrome (MDS): preliminary results of a phase i/ii study. *Blood,* **104**, 401a–2a.
28. Kuendgen, A. *et al.* (2004). Treatment of myelodysplastic syndromes with valproic acid alone or in combination with all-trans retinoic acid. *Blood,* **104**, 1266–9.
29. Kurzrock, R. *et al.* (2004). High risk myelodysplastic syndrome(MDS): first results of international phase 2 study with oral farnesyltransferase inhibitor R115777 (ZARNESTRA) *Blood,* **104**, 23a.
30. Deeg, H.J. *et al.* (2002). Soluble TNF receptor fusion protein (etanercept) for the treatment of myelodysplastic syndrome. *Leukaemia,* **16**, 162–4.
31. Estey, E.H. *et al.* (2001). Comparison of idarubicin + ara-C, fludarabine + ara-C and topotecan + ara-C-based regimens in treatment of newly diagnosed acute myeloid leukemia, refractory anemia with excess blasts in transformation or refractory anemia with excess blasts. *Blood,* **98**, 3575–83.
32. Oosterveld, M. *et al.* (2003). The impact of intensive antileukaemic treatment strategies on prognosis of myelodysplastic syndrome patients aged less than 61 years according to International Prognostic Scoring System risk groups. *Br J Haematol,* **123**, 81–9.
33. Deeg, H.J. (2005). Optimization of transplant regimens for patients with myelodysplastic syndromes. *Hematology 2005*, 167–73.
34. Ingram, W. *et al.* (2007). Allogeneic transplantation for myelodysplastic syndrome (MDS). *Blood Reviews,* **21**, 61–71.
35. Castro-Malaspina, H. *et al.* (2002). Unrelated donor marrow transplantation for myelodysplastic syndromes: outcome analysis in 510 transplants facilitated by the National Marrow Donor Program. *Blood,* **99**, 1943–51.
36. de Witte, T. *et al.* (2007). Autologous stem cell transplantation in myelodysplastic syndromes. *Semin Hematol,* **44**, 274–7.

Response criteria

An International Working Group proposed[1] and subsequently modified[2] response criteria to standardize assessment of clinical trials of therapy, to identify risk-based treatment goals and to identify clinically meaningful responses. 4 aspects of response were defined:

- Altering the natural history of MDS— 📖 see definitions in Table 6.6.
- Cytogenetic response—requires examination of 20 metaphases.
- Haematological improvement (Table 6.7)—pre-therapy baseline is average of ≥2 *measurements over at least 1 week, not affected by transfusion.*
- QoL—correlation with Hb level.[3] QoL assessment should be an integral part of MDS management.

Treatment strategy[4,5]

- ***MDS with 5q–:*** if symptomatic cytopenia, lenalidomide therapy; offer non-responders supportive care, clinical trial, or azacytidine or decitabine, if available.
- ***IPSS low/int-1 ≤60 + HLA-DR15, PNH clone or hypoplastic MDS:*** if symptomatic anaemia, trial of immunosuppressive therapy; offer non-responders supportive therapy, clinical trial, or azacytidine or decitabine, if available.
- ***IPSS low:*** high intensity therapy inappropriate; for symptomatic anaemia in RA and serum EPO <200U/L (BCSH guideline[5]; <500 NCN guideline[4]) or RARS <500U/L, consider trial of EPO (or darbepoietin) ±G-CSF; if serum EPO >500U/L or non-response to EPO offer supportive care, clinical trial, or azacytidine or decitabine, if available.
- ***IPSS int-1:*** offer allograft to patients <50 years with sibling donor; consider patients 50–65 years with good performance status and sibling donor for RIC and allograft within clinical trial; offer allograft within clinical trial (standard or RIC) to patients ≤40 years with MUD donor; *Note*: pre-transplant cytoreductive chemotherapy not recommended for IPSS int-1; offer patients ≥65 or <65 years without donors supportive care, EPO ± G-CSF (if eligible), clinical trial, or azacytidine or decitabine, if available.
- ***IPSS int-2/high:*** determine whether patient is candidate for intensive therapy; consider patients <65 years for AML cytoreductive chemotherapy; those achieving CR or good PR after induction ± consolidation chemotherapy should receive sibling or MUD allograft; those in CR or good PR without a donor but with good performance status and adequate harvest may receive autologous SCT within clinical trial; azacytidine or decitabine may be considered to reduce blast count prior to SCT; if ineligible for intensive therapy, supportive care, consider azacytidine or decitabine, if available, clinical trial, or non-intensive chemotherapy.

Table 6.7 Modified IWG response criteria: altering MDS natural history[2]

Category	Response criteria (must last ≥4 weeks)
Complete remission (CR)	• BM ≤5% myeloblasts • ± persistent dysplasia • FBC: Hb ≥11g/dL; platelets ≥100 x 109/L; neutrophils ≥1.0 x 109/L; blasts 0%
Partial remission (PR)	All CR criteria if abnormal pre-treatment except BM blasts ↓ ≥50% but still >5%
Marrow CR	• BM ≤5% blasts and ↓ ≥50%. • FBC: if HI responses, to be noted in addition
Stable disease	Failure to achieve ≥PR but no evidence of progression for >8 weeks
Failure	Death during treatment or worsening cytopenia, ↑ % BM blasts or progression to more advanced subtype
Relapse after CR/PR	At least 1 of: • Return to pre-therapy % BM blasts • ↓ ≥50% from max. neutrophil/platelet counts • Hb ↓ ≥1.5g/dL or transfusion dependence
Cytogenetic response	• Complete: disappearance of abnormality without new one • Partial: ≥50% reduction of abnormality
Disease progression	If: • <5% blasts: ≥50% ↑ to >5%. • 5–10% blasts: ≥50% ↑ to >10%. • 10–20%blasts: ≥50% ↑ to >20%. • 20–30%blasts: ≥50% ↑ to >30%. Or any of: • ≥50% ↓ max. neutrophils / platelets. • ↓ Hb ≥2g/dL. • Transfusion dependence.
Survival	• Endpoints: OS death from any cause. • EFS: failure /death from any cause. • PFS: disease progression/death from MDS. • DFS: time to relapse. • Cause-specific death: death related to MDS.

Table 6.8 Modified IWG response criteria for haematological improvement[2]

Haematological improvement (HI)	Response criteria (must last ≥8 weeks)
Erythroid response (pre-treatment <11g/dL) HI-E	Hb ↑ by ≥1.5g/dL or ↓ of RBC transfusions (for Hb ≤9g/dL) by ≥4U/ 8 weeks compared to previous 8 weeks
Platelet response (pre-treatment <100 x 10^9/L) HI-P	↑ of ≥ 30 x 10^9/L for patients starting >20 x 10^9/L; ↑ from <20 to >20 x 10^9/L and by at least 100%
Neutrophil response (pre-treatment <1.0 x 10^9/L) HI-N	At least 100% ↑ and absolute ↑ >0.5 x 10^9/L
Progression or relapse after HI	At least 1 of: • ≥ 50% ↓ from max. response in neutrophils or platelets. • ↓ Hb by ≥ 1.5g/dL • Transfusion dependence

References

1. Cheson, B. *et al.* (2000). Report of an international working group to standardize response criteria for myelodysplastic syndromes. *Blood*, **96**, 3671–4.
2. Cheson, B. *et al.* (2006). Clinical application and proposal for modification of the International Working Group (IWG) response criteria in myelodysplasia. *Blood*, **108**, 419–25.
3. Jansen, A.J.G. *et al.* (2003). Quality of life measurement in patients with transfusion-dependent myelodysplastic syndromes. *Br J Haematol*, **121,** 270–4.
4. NCCN Practice Guidelines in Oncology: Myelodysplastic Syndromes V.2.2008 www.nccn.org/professionals/physician_gls/PDF/mds.pdf
5. Bowen, D. *et al.* (2003). Guidelines for the diagnosis and therapy of adult myelodysplastic syndromes. *Br J Haematol*, **120,** 187–200. www.bcshguidelines.com/pdf/BJH120_02_187.pdf.

Myelodysplastic/myeloproliferative diseases (MDS/MPD)

This category was created in the WHO classification of myeloid neoplasms for a group of disorders that have both dysplastic and proliferative features at diagnosis and are difficult to assign to either myelodysplastic or myeloproliferative groups.[1]

WHO classification of MDS/MPD diseases

- Chronic myelomonocytic leukaemia (CMML)
- Atypical chronic myeloid leukaemia (aCML).
- Juvenile myelomonocytic leukaemia (JMML).
- MDS/MPD unclassifiable (MDS/MPD-U).

CMML

Myeloproliferative element in CMML formerly recognized by sub-classification into MDS-like or MPD-like on the basis of WBC at presentation; MPD-like CMML associated with WBC >12 × 10^9/L, splenomegaly and constitutional symptoms; not a distinct condition as many patients who present with low WBC count and minimal splenomegaly ultimately progress to meet 'proliferative' criteria.

Clinical features

- Predominantly presents in >60 years age group, median 65–75 years;
- ♂:♀ ratio ~2:1.
- Often asymptomatic and found on routine FBC.
- Weight loss, fatigue, night sweats may occur.
- Skin and gum infiltration may occur.
- Splenomegaly (50%) and hepatomegaly (up to 20%) usually only in cases with leucocytosis and symptoms.
- Serous effusions (pericardial, pleural, ascetic, and synovial) associated with high PB monocytosis.

Investigations and diagnosis

- Investigations as for MDS.
- Variable leucocytosis; marked in 50%; neutrophilia in some patients.
- Monocyte count >1.0 × 10^9/L is diagnostic minimum.
- Variable anaemia; platelets usually ↔ or ↓.
- Marrow typically hypercellular; blasts and promyelocytes <20%.
- Immunophenotype of PB and BM: CD13+, CD33+, CD14±, CD64±, CD68±; ↑ % CD34 may be associated with early AML transformation.
- Karyotypic abnormalities associated with MDS found in 20–40% (8+, 7–, 7q–, abnormal 12p); none specific for CMML apart from rarity of 5q–;
  - Exclude 5q31–33 translocation and/or *PDGFRβ* gene re-arrangement; occurs in <1–2% of CMMLs, usually with marked eosinophilia; may be a unique entity; these patients may respond to imatinib.[2]
- Lysozyme raised in serum and urine.
- Hypokalaemia may be present.
- Reactive causes of monocytosis must be excluded (📖 see p.117).

WHO diagnostic criteria for CMML

- Persistent peripheral blood monocytosis $>1.0 \times 10^9$/L.
- No Ph chromosome or *BCR-ABL* fusion gene.
- <20% myeloblasts, monoblasts, and promyelocytes in PB or BM.
- Dysplasia in ≥1 myeloid lineages or if myelodysplasia absent or minimal, CMML may be diagnosed if above criteria met, and:
  - An acquired clonal cytogenetic abnormality is present in BM cells.

  or
  - Monocytosis has been persistent for ≥3 months ***and***
  - All other causes of monocytosis have been excluded.

3 subcategories have been defined:

- *CMML-1:* <5% PB blasts and <10% BM blasts.
- *CMML-2:* 5–19% PB blasts **or** 10–19% BM blasts **or** when Auer rods present with <20% BM or PB blasts.
- *CMML-1 or CMML-2 with eosinophilia:* above criteria met plus PB eosinophil count $>1.5 \times 10^9$/L; associated with complications related to eosinophil degranulation: fever, fatigue, cough, angioedema, muscle pains, pruritus, diarrhoea, endomyocardial fibrosis, pulmonary infiltrates.

Prognostic factors

BM blasts: median survival for CMML with <5% BM blasts 53 months *vs.* 16 months for those with 5–20%.

Management

- Asymptomatic cases with near ↔ haematology apart from a monocytosis of $>1.0 \times 10^9$/L require no intervention and should simply be monitored. Therapy otherwise supportive.
- Patients with symptoms, organomegaly, and/or ↑↑ WBC may respond to oral chemotherapy; hydroxycarbamide performed better than oral etoposide in a randomized study.[3]
- Infrequent younger patients may be treated with high dose therapy and allogeneic SCT which offers only curative option. EBMT reported 5-year estimated OS 21% and DFS 18% and 52% TRM.[4]

Natural history

Prognosis for asymptomatic patients is favourable (several years). For those requiring therapy, median survival is 6–12 months. Median survival overall is 20–40 months. AML (usually FAB M4/M5) develops in ~20% after median of 1.5–2 years; poorly responsive to intensive chemotherapy.

aCML[5]

- Heterogeneous group of patients with Ph chromosome and *BCR-ABL* fusion gene –ve CML.
- Rare; 1–2 cases per 100 cases of CML.
- Occurs in elderly; median age in 7th or 8th decade
- Most have symptoms related to anaemia; splenomegaly frequent.
- FBC: ↑ WBC due to dysplastic immature (>10–20%) and mature neutrophils; generally $35–96 \times 10^9$/L though sometimes $>300 \times 10^9$/L; PB monocytes rarely >10%; PB blasts usually <5%, always <20%; anaemia and thrombocytopenia common; no or minimal basophilia (<2%) (*cf.* CML).

- BM: hypercellular due to ↑ and dysplastic myeloid series; M:E ratio usually >10; often multilineage dysplasia; blasts <20%
- Cytogenetic abnormalities frequent: 8+, 13+, 20q–, i(17q), 12p–.
- Short median survival (11–18 months).
- Hydroxycarbamide may control the leucocytosis and ↓ splenomegaly.
- Evolution to AML in 20–40%; others die of BM failure.

JMML[6]

- Clonal disorder arising in pluripotent stem cell causing selective hypersensitivity to GM-CSF due to dysregulated signal transduction through RAS/MAPK pathway.
- Affects infants and young children (75% <3 years); ♂:♀ ratio ~2:1; 10% of cases occur in children with neurofibromatosis type 1.
- Most present with malaise, pallor, fever infection, or bleeding. Maculopapular rash in 40–50%.
- Hepatosplenomegaly almost universal; due to leukaemic infiltration.
- FBC: ↑ WBC (usually 25–35 × 10^9/L; >100 × 10^9/L in 5–10%) due to neutrophilia (with promyelocytes and myelocytes) and monocytosis; eosinophilia and basophilia in a minority; anaemia and thrombocytopenia usual; nucleated RBCs frequent.
- Polyclonal hypergammaglobulinaemia and ↑ LDH in majority.
- BM: hypercellular with myeloid proliferation; monocytes usually 5–10%.
- Abnormal karyotype in 30–40%; none specific.
- 33% carry *PTPN11* mutations, 15–20% without evidence of neurofibromatosis *NF1* mutations and 15–20% *RAS* mutations.

Diagnostic criteria

- PB monocytosis >1 × 10^9/L.
- Blasts (including promonocytes) <20% in PB and BM.
- No Ph chromosome or *BCR-ABL* fusion gene.
- *Plus* ≥2 of the following:
  - Haemoglobin F ↑ for age.
  - Immature granulocytes in PB
  - WBC >10 × 10^9/L
  - Clonal chromosomal abnormality (e.g. 7–)
  - GM-CSF hypersensitivity of myeloid progenitors *in vitro*.

Management

No consistently effective therapy including allogeneic SCT which is treatment of choice (up to 55% relapse). 5-year OS ~50%.[7] Untreated, 30% progress rapidly and die within 1 year of diagnosis.

MDS/MPD-U[8]

Applied to patients with both myelodysplastic and myeloproliferative features but who do not meet the criteria for the 3 conditions above.

Diagnostic criteria

- Clinical, laboratory, and morphological features of one of the categories of MDS with <20% blasts in PB & BM ***and***
- Prominent myeloproliferative features e.g. plates ≥600 × 10^9/L or WBC ≥13x10^9/L ± prominent splenomegaly ***and***

- Has no prior history of MPD or MPS, cytotoxic, or growth factor therapy and no Ph chromosome or *BCR-ABL* fusion gene, 5q-, t(3;3)(q21;q26) or inv3(q21;q26) ***or***
- Patient has mixed features of MPD and MDS and cannot be assigned to any other category of MDS, MPD, or MDS/MPD.
- JAK2^{V617F} mutation found in 25%.[9]

Management

- Manage as in patients with MDS or atypical MPD.

References

1. Vardiman, J.W. *et al.* (2001). Myelodysplastic / myeloproliferative diseases. In Jaffe, E.S. *et al.* (eds.) *World Health Organization classification of tumours. Pathology and genetics. Tumours of haematopoietic and lymphoid tissues, vol 1.* Lyon: IARC Press, pp.46–59.
2. Apperley, J.F. *et al.* (2002). Response to imatinib mesylate in patients with chronic myeloproliferative diseases with rearrangements of the platelet-derived growth factor receptor beta. *N Engl J Med,* **347**, 481–7.
3. Wattel, E. *et al.* (1996). A randomized trial of hydroxyurea versus VP16 in adult chronic myelomonocytic leukemia. *Blood,* **88**, 2480–7.
4. Kroger, N. *et al.* (2002). Allogeneic stem cell transplantation of adult chronic myelomonocytic leukaemia: a report on behalf of the Chronic Leukaemia Working Party of the European Group for Blood and Marrow Transplantation (EBMT). *Br J Haematol,* **118**, 67–73.
5. Costello, R. *et al.* (1997). Clinical and biological aspects of Philadelphia-negative/BCR-negative chronic myeloid leukemia. *Leuk Lymphoma,* **25**, 225–32.
6. Vardiman, J.W. *et al.* (2001). Juvenile myelomonocytic leukaemia. In Jaffe, E.S. *et al.* (eds.) *World Health Organization classification of tumours. Pathology and genetics. Tumours of haematopoietic and lymphoid tissues, vol 1.* Lyon: IARC Press, pp.55–7.
7. Locatelli, F. *et al.* (2005). Hematopoietic stem cell transplantation (HSCT) in children with juvenile myelomonocytic leukemia (JMML): results of the EWOG-MDS/EBMT trial. *Blood,* **105**, 410–19.
8. Bain, B. *et al.* (2001). Myelodysplastic / myeloproliferative disease, unclassifiable. In Jaffe, E.S. *et al.* (eds.) *World Health Organization classification of tumours. Pathology and genetics. Tumours of haematopoietic and lymphoid tissues, vol 1.* Lyon: IARC Press, pp.46–59.
9. Jones, A.V. *et al.* (2005). Widespread occurrence of the JAK2 V617F mutation in chronic myeloproliferative disorders. *Blood,* **106**, 2162–8.

Chapter 7

Myeloproliferative neoplasms

Myeloproliferative neoplasms (MPNs)

The term 'myeloproliferative neoplasm' replaces the term 'chronic myeloproliferative disorder' in the 2008 revision of the WHO classification.[1] This revision reflects information on molecular pathogenesis not available in 2001.[2] The MPNs are a heterogeneous group of clonal haemopoietic stem cell neoplasms with excessive proliferation of one or more of the erythroid, megakaryocytic, or myeloid lineages and relatively normal maturation resulting in ↑ numbers of red cells, platelets, and/or granulocytes in the peripheral blood. Constitutive tyrosine kinase activation appears to be a common pathogenetic mechanism. Phenotypic diversity is a result of different mutations affecting protein kinases or related molecules causing different signal transduction abnormalities.[3] MPNs are characterized by effective haematopoiesis devoid of dyserythropoiesis, granulocytic dysplasia, or monocytosis. Splenomegaly and hepatomegaly are common. The MPNs share a potential to progress to myelofibrosis, ineffective haematopoiesis or blastic transformation.

2008 WHO classification[1]

MPNs

- Chronic myelogenous leukaemia (CML, 📖 see p.140).
- Polycythaemia vera (PV).
- Essential thrombocythaemia (ET).
- 1° myelofibrosis (MF).
- Chronic neutrophilic leukaemia.
- Chronic eosinophilic leukaemia (CEL), not otherwise categorized (📖 see p.300).
- Hypereosinophilic syndrome (HES).
- Mast cell disease.
- MPNs, unclassifiable.

1 Tefferi, A. and Vardiman, J.W. (2008). Classification and diagnosis of myeloproliferative neoplasms: The 2008 World Health Organization criteria and point-of-care diagnostic algorithms. *Leukemia*, **22**, 14–22.

2 Vardiman, J.W. *et al.* (2002). The World Health Organization (WHO) classification of the myeloid neoplasms. *Blood*, **100**, 2292–2302.

3 Tefferin, A. and Gilliland, D.G. (2007). Oncogenes in myeloproferative disorders. *Cell Cycle* **6**: 550–66.

Pathogenesis of the MPNs

*Although included in the WHO Classification of MPNs, CML is widely regarded as a separate entity characterized by the presence of BCR-ABL which is a consequence of t(9;22) and has a clear role in pathogenesis (**📖 p.140**).*

Mutations of a number of protein kinases have now been described in the *BCR-ABL*-–ve MPNs.

The *JAK2*-V617F mutation was detected by 4 groups using different methods (reviewed in references 1 and 2). This G>T transversion in exon 14 is found in up to 95% of patients with PV.[3] Several different activating mutations have been found in *JAK2* exon 12 in *JAK2*-V617F-–ve patients with PV with isolated erythropoiesis without leucocytosis or thrombocytosis.[4] Thus 98% of patients with PV have a *JAK2* mutation.

This point mutation in the –ve regulatory pseudokinase domain of *JAK2* leads to constitutive activation of the JAK (Janus kinase)-STAT (signal transducers and activators of transcription) signalling pathway involved in regulation of cell growth and differentiation. Cytokines and growth factors (e.g. EPO) activate this pathway by binding to cell surface receptors. JAKs bound to the cytoplasmic domain of the receptor are activated by binding of ligand. These activate STAT proteins which dimerize, translocate to the nucleus and activate transcription of target genes. *JAK2* is the sole JAK kinase involved in EPO-receptor signalling.[1,2] The mutation has been found in different lineages including B and T lymphocytes.

Expression of *JAK2*-V617F (or an exon 12 mutant) confers cytokine hypersensitivity and cytokine-independent growth to haemopoietic cells [1,2] and in a mouse model results in erythrocytosis and marrow fibrosis but not thrombocytosis.[5] Constitutive activation of the JAK-STAT pathway causes excessive erythropoiesis in PV though its relationship to thrombotic complications and progression to myelofibrosis is unclear.[1] However leucocytosis appears to be a risk factor for thrombosis in PV and ET and *JAK2*-V617F-mediated granulocyte activation may contribute to thrombosis.[6,7]

The finding of *JAK2*-V617F –ve but clonal AML transformation in PV suggests that a prior abnormality may be present as appears to occur in familial clonal MPN.[1,8] Rare families have an ↑ incidence of MPN with clonal haematopoiesis and most affected members carry a somatic mutation of *JAK2*. It is suggested that this low penetrance, late onset familial clonal MPN is due to an inherited predisposition to somatic mutations.[1,8]

The *JAK2*-V617F mutation has also been found in 58% of patients with PMF, 50% with ET[3] and 50% with refractory anaemia with ringed sideroblasts associated with thrombocytosis (RARS-T),[9] a provisional 'MDS/MPD unclassifiable' entity, and much less commonly in 5q– MDS (5%) and other myeloid neoplasms.

The reason why this mutation is associated with three different MPN clinical phenotypes remains unclear. Additional genetic factors clearly contribute to the clinical phenotype of *JAK2*-V617F +ve MPN. Homozygosity for *JAK2*-V617F resulting from mitotic recombination and duplication of the mutant allele (acquired uniparental disomy; UPD) is common in PV (30%), rare in ET, and occurs occasionally in PMF (13%)[10] Duplication may be important to pathogenesis of PV. Other differences are (i) the proportion of chromosomes expressing the mutation (gene dosage) is higher in PV and PMF than in ET; (ii) the allelic frequency of *JAK2*-V617F remained stable over time in ET but ↑ slightly in PV and (iii) in PV the allelic frequency is identical in neutrophils and platelets, in ET it is higher in platelets[11]

It has been suggested that *JAK2*-V617F +ve ET is a *forme-fruste* of PV and may have a different clinical course from *JAK2*-V617F –ve ET.[12] Evidence has been contradictory (reviewed in references 1 and 8). Many patients with ET display low allelic ratios of *JAK2*-V617F (less common in PV) and evidence of another larger clone by X-chromosome inactivation pattern or del(20q) suggesting events that may precede the acquisition of *JAK2*-V617F[8]

Presence of *JAK2*-V617F may correlate with poorer survival in PMF[13]

Clonal haematopoiesis is found in *JAK2*-V617F –ve MPN suggesting that other alleles cause myeloproliferation in these patients.[14]

Somatic mutations of codon 515 at the transmembrane–juxtamembrane junction of the thrombopoietin receptor gene (*MPL*), *MPL*-W515L or *MPL*-W515K have been detected in ~10% of patients with *JAK2*-V617F –ve PMF and a smaller proportion of patients with *JAK2*-V617F –ve ET[15] Expression of MPL-W515L transforms haematopoietic cells to factor-independent growth and activates STAT, MAPK, and P13K-Act signalling pathways in a manner similar to *JAK2*-V617F but *in vivo* results in thrombocytosis and myelofibrosis.[1]

A *KIT*-D816F allele has been detected in systemic mastocytosis (SM)[16] and an interstitial deletion producing a fusion protein *FIP1L1.PDGFRA* involving platelet derived growth factor-α has been detected in patients with a diagnosis of chronic eosinophilic leukaemia (CEL) or SM.[17]

References

1. Levine, R.L. *et al.* (2007). Role of JAK2 in the pathogenesis and therapy of myeloproliferative disorders. *Nat Rev Cancer*, **7**, 673–83.
2. Campbell, P.J. and Green, A.R. (2006). The myeloproliferative disorders. *N Engl J Med*, **355**, 2452–66.
3. Baxter, E.J. *et al.* (2005). Acquired mutation of the tyrosine kinase JAK2 in human myeloproliferative disorders. *Lancet*, **365**, 1054–61.
4. Scott, L.M. *et al.* (2007). JAK2 exon 12 mutations in polycythaemia vera and idiopathic erythrocytosis. *N Engl J Med*, **356**. 459–68.
5. Wernig, G. *et al.* (2006). Expression of Jak2V617F causes a polycythemia vera–like disease with associated myelofibrosis in a murine bone marrow transplant model. *Blood*, **107**, 4274–81.
6. Landolfi, R. *et al.* (2007). Leukocytosis as a major thrombotic risk factor in patients with polycythemia vera. *Blood*, **109**, 2446–52.
7. Carobbio, A. *et al.* (2007). Leukocytosis is a risk factor for thrombosis in essential thrombocythemia: interaction with treatment, standard risk factors, and Jak2 mutation status. *Blood*, **109**, 2310–13.
8. Skoda, R. (2007). The genetic basis of myeloproliferative disorders. *Hematology 2007*, 1–10.

9. Szpurka, H. *et al.* (2006). Refractory anemia with ringed sideroblasts associated with marked thrombocytosis (RARS-T), another myeloproliferative condition characterized by JAK2 V617F mutation. *Blood,* **108**, 2173–81.
10. Scott, L.M. *et al.* (2006). Progenitors homozygous for the V617F JAK2 mutation occur in most patients with polycythemia vera, but not essential thrombocythemia. *Blood,* **108**, 2435–7.
11. Moliterno, A.R. *et al.* (2006). Molecular mimicry in the chronic myeloproliferative disorders: reciprocity between quantitative JAK2 V617F and Mpl expression. *Blood,* **108**, 3913–5.
12. Campbell, P.J. *et al.* (2005). Definition of subtypes of essential thrombocythaemia and relation to polycythaemia vera based on JAK2 V617F mutation status: a prospective study. *Lancet,* **366**,1945–53.
13. Campbell, P.J. *et al.* (2006). V617F mutation in JAK2 is associated with poorer survival in idiopathic myelofibrosis. *Blood,* **107**, 2098–2100.
14. Levine, R.L. *et al.* (2006). X-inactivation based clonality analysis and quantitative JAK2V617F assessment reveal an association between clonality and JAK2V617F in PV but not ET/MMM, and identifies a subset of JAK2V617F–negative ET and MMM patients with clonal haematopoiesis. *Blood,* **107**, 4039–41.
15. Pardanani, A.D. *et al.* (2006). MPL515 mutations in myeloproliferative and other myeloid disorders: a study of 118 patients. *Blood,* **108**, 3472–6.
16. Buttner, C. *et al.* (1998). Identification of activating c-kit mutations in adult-, but not in childhood-onset indolent mastocytosis: a possible explanation for divergent clinical behaviour. *J Invest Dermatol,* **111**, 1227–31.
17. Cools, J. *et al.* (2003). A tyrosine kinase created by fusion of the *PDGFRA* and *FIP1L1* genes as a therapeutic target of imatinib in idiopathic eosinophilic syndrome. *N Engl J Med,* **348**, 1201–14.

Polycythaemia vera (PV)

Erythrocytosis is defined as an increase in total red cell mass (RCM). The term 'polycythaemia' is widely used synonymously but lacks precision and can lead to confusion. It is suspected by finding a raised haematocrit (Hct) (packed cell volume, PCV).

Persistent elevation of Hct >0.48 in adult ♀ and >0.51 in adult ♂ is abnormal. *Note*: an elevated Hct can occur with a ↔ RCM (in the absence of erythrocytosis) if the plasma volume is reduced ('relative' erythrocytosis (RE)).

PV is a neoplastic clonal disorder of the BM stem cell causing excessive proliferation of the erythroid, myeloid, and megakaryocyte lineages and carries a risk of thrombotic complications. PV was traditionally diagnosed using the criteria of the Polycythaemia Vera Study Group by the presence of an ↑ red cell mass. The detection of *JAK2* mutations in most patients with PV[1] has revolutionized diagnostic procedures.

Incidence

PV is the most common MPN with an incidence of up to 3 per 100,000 per annum. It occurs in all races but is 10 × less frequent in Japan. Median age at diagnosis is 60 years. PV occurs at all ages but is very rare below 30 years. It occurs extremely rarely in childhood. The ♂:♀ ratio is 1.2:1.

Aetiology

Mutation of the cytoplasmic tyrosine kinase *JAK2* has a clear pathogenetic role (see p.256). Incidence of PV is ↑ in populations exposed to radiation (including Japan) and petroleum refinery and chemical workers.

Differential diagnosis of erythrocytosis

Table 7.1 Differential diagnosis of erythrocytosis

1°erythrocytosis	***Congenital***	1° familial and congenital polycythaemia (PFCP): gain-of-function mutation of *EPO* receptor gene → truncated receptor; 10 different alleles described; autosomal dominant; high penetrance; early age of onset; ↑ RCM, low sEPO, polyclonal haematopoiesis, ↔ WBC and platelet counts.
		Familial clonal MPD: low penetrance, late onset, often *JAK2*-V617F +ve
	Acquired	PV (*syn.* polycythaemia rubra vera (PRV); 1° proliferative polycythaemia(PPP)).
2°erythrocytosis (SE) due to ↑ endogenous EPO production	***Congenital***	High O_2-affinity haemoglobinopathy

Table 7.1 Differential diagnosis of erythrocytosis (*continued*)

		Congenital 2,3-DPG deficincy
		Autonomous high EPO production; autosomal recessive mutation of von Hippel-Lindau (*VHL*) gene; Chuvash polycythaemia (VHL-598C>T) resulting in ↑ levels of hypoxia-induced transcription factor (*HIF1*) and ↑ expression of *EPO* gene; other alleles described.
	Acquired	
	Hypoxaemia	Chronic lung disease
		Cyanotic congenital heart disease with right→left shunt
		Living at high altitude
		Chronic alveolar hypoventilation e.g. gross obesity
		Sleep apnoea syndromes
	Other causes of impaired tissue O_2 delivery	Smoking (↑ COHb)
	Renal disease (EPO mediated)	Polycystic kidneys
		Renal tumours
		Renal artery stenosis
		Post-renal transplantation
	Tumours causing pathological EPO production	Hepatoma
		Cerebellar haemangioblastoma
		Uterine leiomyoma
		Bronchial carcinoma
		Adrenal tumours
		Parathyroid carcinoma
	Liver disease	Cirrhosis
		Hepatitis
	Drugs	EPO doping
		Androgens
Idiopathic erythrocytosis (IE)		Persistent ↑ RCM, no cause found but no evidence of MPN or clear cause of 2° erythrocytosis.
Relative erythrocytosis (RE). *Syns.* apparent polycythaemia, spurious erythrocytosis, pseudo-polycythaemia		Normal RCM and ↓ plasma volume; Diuretic therapy or dehydration; Gaisbock's syndrome (📖 see p.273); smoking, alcohol, hypertension, obesity.

Clinical evaluation of a patient with suspected erythrocytosis

A patient with erythrocytosis may be asymptomatic or may present with thrombosis (up to 40% with PV), haemorrhage (up to 20% with PV), or vague symptoms (~40% with PV) of headache, dizziness, weakness, excessive sweating, tinnitus, visual upset, or gout.

Take a detailed history with attention to smoking habits, alcohol consumption, diuretic therapy, dyspepsia, and thrombosis. A history of pruritus (especially after bathing) suggests PV (occurs in ~50%). A burning sensation in fingers and toes with erythema, pallor, or cyanosis (erythromelalgia) is typical of PV.

Physical examination may identify facial plethora or abnormalities associated with 2° erythrocytosis such as gross obesity, hypertension, evidence of obstructive airways disease or cyanotic cardiac conditions. Splenomegaly and hepatomegaly occur in 67% and 40% of patients with PV at diagnosis, respectively.

Investigations

- ***FBC and film:*** ↑↑ RCC and ↓ or ↔ MCV and MCH (may be evidence of Fe deficiency) in PV; neutrophils and platelets frequently ↑ in PV (rare in other causes of erythrocytosis).
- ***JAK2 mutation analysis:*** screen for *JAK2*-V617F mutation; found in 95% of patients with PV; differentiates PV from SE and RE but not from PMF or ET (58% and 50% *JAK2*-V617F +ve)[1]; several *JAK2* exon 12 mutations described in patients with *JAK2*-V617F –ve PV;[2] bear in mind false-+ve results due to highly sensitive allele specific assays and false negatives due to low mutant allele burden.[3]
- ***Serum erythropoietin (sEPO):*** include in initial work-up; usually ↓ but can be normal in PV, extremely unlikely to be ↑; ↑ sEPO suggests 2° erythrocytosis; may be ↓ in RE and idiopathic erythrocytosis.
- ***BM examination:*** trephine may be diagnostic in PV; typically hypercellular for age due to trilineage hyperplasia (mainly erythroid and megakaryocytic); megakaryocytes conspicuous, pleomorphic (small to giant) and clustered round sinusoids or near trabeculae with deeply lobulated nuclei; usually ↓ Fe stores (95%); ↑ reticulin fibrosis present in 30%; normal BM histology does not exclude PV but is more usual in SE; late in the disease collagen fibrosis may supervene with clusters of dysmorphic megakaryocytes.
- ***Serum ferritin:*** ↓ (esp. PV) or ↔; occasionally overt Fe deficiency.
- ***Serum chemistry:*** U and E (to exclude renal disease); uric acid (often ↑ in MPNs); LFTs (to exclude liver disease).
- ***Urinalysis:*** haematuria or proteinuria should prompt further renal investigations.
- ***Arterial oxygen saturation:*** pulse oximetry most convenient to detect chronic hypoxia. SaO_2 <92% suggests causal relationship with absolute erythrocytosis.
- ***CXR:*** to exclude pulmonary disease and congenital cardiac abnormalities.

Additional investigations useful in selected patients

- Abdominal USS: for hepatosplenomegaly, renal or pelvic abnormalities.
- NAP score: ↑ score usually present in PV (but not diagnostic in isolation).

- BM cytogenetics: not routine; up to 30% have abnormalities, typically 20q–. +8, +9, 7–, and 10–.
- BFU-E culture: not routine; PV progenitors show ↑ sensitivity to growth factors and develop 'endogenous erythroid colonies' (EEC) without added EPO.
- Haematinic assays: serum vitamin B12: levels commonly ↑ in PV due to ↑ transcobalamin release reflecting associated granulocytosis. Folate deficiency may occur.
- Sleep studies may be indicated by history of snoring, waking unrefreshed, and somnolence.
- Pulmonary function tests are indicated if lung disease is suspected.
- O_2 dissociation curve to determine the p50 in a patient with erythrocytosis and suspected high affinity haemoglobin.
- *EPOR* or *VHL* gene analysis if congenital erythrocytosis suspected.
- RCM and plasma volume: former mainstay of diagnostic process; no longer routine; patient red cells labelled with ^{51}Cr and re-injected; simultaneous plasma volume measurement using ^{131}I-labelled albumin. RCM ↑ >25% above mean predicted value is diagnostic of absolute erythrocytosis. Plasma volume also ↑ (if marked splenomegaly present.

Table 7.2 Red cell mass and plasma volume studies in erythrocytosis

	PV	SE	RE
RCM	↑	↑	↑ within NR or ↔
Plasma volume	N or ↑	N	↓ within NR or ↔

PV, polycythaemia vera; SE, 2° erythrocytosis; RE, relative erythrocytosis

Diagnostic algorithm for suspected PV

In a patient with suspected PV, Tefferi and Vardiman[3] recommend the following diagnostic algorithm based on the 2008 WHO criteria (Table 7.3).

Screen blood for JAK2-V617F mutation and measure serum EPO.

- V617F +ve and sEPO ↓: PV highly likely → BM biopsy encouraged but not essential.
- V617F +ve but sEPO ↔ or ↑: PV likely → BM biopsy recommended for confirmation
- V617F –ve ***but*** sEPO ↓: *PV possible* → BM biopsy and *JAK2* exon 12 mutation screening → if results still not consistent with PV, consider congenital polycythaemia with EPO receptor mutation
- V617F –ve and sEPO ↔ or ↑: *PV unlikely* → consider SE including congenital polycythaemia with *VHL* mutation.

Table 7.3 2008 WHO diagnostic criteria for PV[3]

Major criteria	1. Hgb >18.5g/dL (♂), > 16.5g/dL (♀) *or* Hgb or Hct >99th percentile of reference range for age, sex, or altitude of residence *or* Hgb >17g/dl (men). >15g/dl (women) if associated with sustained increase ≥ 2g/dl from baseline that cannot be attributed to correction of iron deficiency *or* Elevated RCM >25% above mean ↔ predicted value. 2. Presence of *JAK2*-V617F or similar mutation
Minor criteria	1. BM trilineage myeloproliferation 2. Subnormal serum EPO level 3. EEC growth *in vitro*

Diagnosis of PV requires that the patient meets both major criteria plus 1 minor criterion or the first major criterion and 2 minor criteria.

1. Baxter, E.J. *et al.* (2005). Acquired mutation of the tyrosine kinase JAK2 in human myeloproliferative disorders. *Lancet*, **365**, 1054–61.

2. Levine, R.L. *et al.* (2007). Role of JAK2 in the pathogenesis and therapy of myeloproliferative disorders. *Nat Rev Cancer*, **7**, 673–83.

3. Tefferi, A. and Vardiman, J.W. (2008). Classification and diagnosis of myeloproliferative neoplasms: The 2008 World Health Organization criteria and point-of-care diagnostic algorithms. *Leukemia*, **22**, 14–22.

Natural history of PV

Untreated PV carries a significant risk of early thrombotic complications and a further long-term risk of transformation into myelofibrosis or less commonly AML. There is also an ↑ risk of bleeding notably from peptic ulcers. The life expectancy of untreated patients is ~18 months from diagnosis. The aim of treatment is to reduce the risk of thrombotic complications and to prevent progression to myelofibrosis (MF) or leukaemia. Current treatments improve median survival to >15 years but some myelosuppressive treatments (notably chlorambucill and ^{32}P) have been associated with an ↑ risk of AML.

A large study records a death rate pf 3.7 per 100 patients per annum, an excess over controls of 2.1 times.[1] Cardiovascular complications notably MI, stroke, and VTE were the most common causes of death (41%). The rate of non-fatal thrombosis was 3.8 per 100 patients per annum. Major and fatal haemorrhage was rare (0.8 and 0.15 per 100 patients per annum). Age and thrombotic history are the most important risk factors for thrombosis.

PV characteristically presents during a proliferative phase when control of erythrocytosis and prevention of thrombotic complications is often an urgent priority. This is often followed by a stable phase of variable (but often short) duration where near ↔ counts are maintained without therapy as a result of ↓ proliferative capacity due to early myelofibrosis. Subsequently an advanced or 'spent phase' develops which is due to extensive myelofibrosis and associated with progressive hepatosplenomegaly, pancytopenia, and systemic symptoms (fever and weight loss). Incidence 10–15% after 10 years rising to >30% at 20 years; median survival <18 months. The incidence of AML is estimated at 2% in the absence of therapy but is over 14% after myelosuppressive therapy.

Risk stratification

Age and thrombotic history are predictive for vascular events in PV (and ET) and are used for risk stratification to inform treatment decisions (Table 7.4).

- Platelet count >1500 × 10^9/L is a risk factor for bleeding but not for thrombosis.[2]
- ↑ leukocyte count (>15 × 10^9/L)[3] and the quantitation of *JAK2* mutant allele (*JAK2*-V617F/ *JAK2* wild type ratio >75%)[4] are possible additional risk factors for thrombosis but these findings need confirmation.

Table 7.4 Risk stratification in PV[2]

Risk category	Age >60 years or history of thrombosis	Cardiovascular risk factors*
Low	No	No
Intermediate	No	Yes
High	Yes	Not applicable

*hypertension, hypercholesterolaemia, diabetes, smoking.

. Marchioli, R. *et al.* (2005) Vascular and neoplastic risk in a large cohort of patients with olycythemia vera. *J Clin Oncol,* **23**, 2224–32.

. Finazzi, G. and Barbui, T. (2007). How I treat patients with polycythemia vera. *Blood,* **09**, 5104–11.

. Landolfi, R. *et al.* (2007). Leukocytosis as a major thrombotic risk factor in patients with olycythemia vera. *Blood,* **109**, 2446–52.

Vannucchi, A.M. *et al.* (2007). Prospective identification of high risk polycythemia vera patients ased on *JAK2* allele burden. *Leukemia,* **21**, 1952–9.

Management of PV

Modifiable factors and lifestyle

In all PV patients, identify and treat any additional risk factors (e.g. hyper tension) and encourage the patient to adopt a healthy lifestyle (e.g. stop smoking, take exercise).

Patients with a low risk of thrombosis

Venesection

↓ RCM to ↔ as rapidly as possible to prevent complications (target Hct <0.45 (♂), <0.42 (♀)). No firm data exist to support these targets. Removal of RBCs by venesection is the quickest way of reducing RCM 450mL blood (± isovolaemic replacement with 0.9% saline) removed safel from younger adults every 2–3d (↓ volume to 200–300mL and frequenc to twice weekly in elderly or patients with cardiovascular disease). If Hc very high (>0.60) venesection may be technically difficult due to extrem viscosity.

Maintenance therapy

Venesection alone can be used to maintain the Hct at 0.42–0.45. Once target achieved monitor 4–8-weekly to establish the requirement fo further venesection. Individual requirements are variable (e.g. 2 proce dures per year to monthly venesection). Fe supplements should not b given. Early studies showed ↑ risk of thrombosis in first 3 years after treat ment with venesection alone thus additional cytoreductive treatment i required in patients with a higher risk of thrombosis.

Aspirin

75–100mg daily is recommended in all PV patients without a history c major bleeding or gastric intolerance. Higher doses (900mg/d) were assoc ated with haemorrhage in early studies. The ECLAP study randomized 51 mainly asymptomatic low-risk PV patients to aspirin 100mg/d or placebo Aspirin significantly reduced the risk of the combined endpoint of nor fatal MI, nonfatal stroke, pulmonary embolism, major venous thrombosi or death from cardiovascular causes (RR 0.40; CI 0.18–0.91; p=0.03). Th incidence of major bleeding was not significantly ↑ (RR 1.62; CI 0.27–9.71 It has been argued that the risks and benefits of aspirin should be carefull considered in very low risk patients e.g. <55 years with no additional ris factors as benefits are proportional to vascular risk and below a certai level bleeding events due to aspirin may exceed vascular events prevente by it.[3]

Patients with an intermediate risk of thrombosis

Treatment of these patients must be individualized. Most may be manage as for low-risk patients but cytoreductive therapy may be required i some. Poor compliance to venesection or progressive myeloproliferatic (splenomegaly, leukocytosis, and thrombocytosis) would be an indicatic for cytoreductive therapy.[4] Interferon-α may be preferred to hydroxyca bamide in younger patients <40 years).

Additional treatment for patients with a high risk of thrombosis

Hydroxycarbamide (HC)

HC (formerly hydroxyurea) an antimetabolite (ribonucleotide reductase inhibitor), is cytoreductive treatment of choice. Onset of myelosuppression with HC is rapid, and overdosage is quickly corrected by temporary withdrawal. Start at 15–20mg/kg/day until Hct <0.45, then adjust to a maintenance dose to preserve response without WCC $<3 \times 10^9$/L. Review every 2 weeks initially and in steady-state monitor FBC every 3 months. Randomized trials in ET[5,6] have demonstrated the antithrombotic effect of HC but similar trials have not been reported in PV. However HC has been shown to be effective and safe in PV and is the most widely used agent.[4] Continuous treatment is required and some patients find the need for follow-up difficult. Lower incidence of leukaemia than ^{32}P or alkylator therapy. Longstanding concerns that HC may still carry a risk are not supported by a large observational study[7] and >10 years use in sickle cell disease. Nonetheless use HC cautiously in younger patients. Some patients experience GI upset, skin pigmentation and leg ulcers. Leg ulcers occur in up to 10% and do not heal until HC is discontinued. In the 'spent' phase HC may cause anaemia. The anti-thrombotic effect of HC may be due to more than myelosuppression including qualitative changes in leukocytes, ↓ expression of endothelial adhesion molecules, and ↑ NO generation.[1]

IFN-α

IFN-α can control erythrocytosis and ↓ leucocytosis, thrombocytosis, and modest splenomegaly. IFN-α directly inhibits fibroblast progenitors and antagonizes PDGF, TGF-β, and other cytokines that may be involved in myelofibrosis. Commence 3 million units SC daily and when Hct <0.45 achieved reduce to lowest dose that maintains response.[1] Monitor patients frequently initially. Side effects (fever, flu-like symptoms, weakness, myalgia, depression) can reduce compliance. A review of 16 studies suggests that 50% achieve target Hct without venesections, 77% have ↓ splenomegaly and 75% have ↓ severity of pruritus but ~33% discontinue it due to toxicity.[8] Long-term follow-up in 55 patients (median 13 years) shows ↓ thrombotic and haemorrhagic events and confirms the absence of leukaemogenesis.[9] Pegylated-IFN may be better tolerated; begin at 0.5mcg/kg/week, double dose if response not achieved after 12 weeks then reduce to maintenance dose. IFN is treatment of choice in patients <40 years, women of child-bearing age, and pregnant women with ET.[1,10]

Radioactive phosphorus (^{32}P) and busulfan

These are early treatments for PV. Produce ↓ in RCM 6–12 weeks after administration (^{32}P 2.3 mCi/m^2 by IV injection every 12 weeks as necessary; busulfan by single oral dose 0.5–1mg/kg). Either agent may be repeated after 3–6 months if further myelosuppression is required. Both individually ↓ thrombosis and myelofibrosis but markedly ↑ the risk of AML. The incidence of AML after ^{32}P alone is 2.5–15%.[10] The use of ^{32}P with either busulfan or hydroxycarbamide in an individual carries a very high risk of AML. Neither is recommended for patients ≤75 years who should receive hydroxycarbamide. However, in patients >75 in whom compliance or regular monitoring of hydroxycarbamide dose is a problem, busulfan or ^{32}P can be considered as both offer intermittent therapy rather than long term maintenance.[10]

Anagrelide

Oral imidazoquinazoline with anti-cyclic AMP phosphodiesterase activity and profound effect on megakaryocyte maturation resulting in ↓ platelet production. Useful for control of thrombocytosis in PV patients who do not tolerate or fail to respond to HC or IFN. More useful in ET as no effect on progression of PV: erythrocytosis or splenomegaly. Commence at 500mcg bd, adjusting according to response with weekly increments of 500mcg/d; usual therapeutic dose 2–3mg/d. Therapeutic effect usually within 14–21 days. No evidence of mutagenic activity. Side effects may reduce long-term tolerance—headache (50%), forceful heartbeat, fluid retention, dizziness, arrhythmia (<10%), CCF (2%), and diarrhoea. Use cautiously in patients with known or suspected cardiac disease. May be used in combination with HC or IFN to achieve disease control with reduced side effects.

Supportive treatment

- Maintain adequate fluid intake and avoid dehydration.
- Give allopurinol (300mg/d) to minimize risks of hyperuricaemia.
- Acute gout is managed by standard therapies.

New treatments for PV

Several pharmaceutical companies have developed small molecule inhibitors of JAK2 that are in phase 2 studies.

Continued care and follow-up

Patients with PV and idiopathic erythrocytosis should have long-term haematological follow-up. Measure Hct at least 3-monthly. For patients on cytotoxic therapy with hydroxycarbamide the FBC should be checked every 8–12 weeks.

Treatment of advanced phase PV

Symptomatic management should be prioritized. Patients often require blood product support. Splenectomy is often considered due to discomfort, recurrent infarction, or hypersplenism but often followed by massive hepatomegaly due to extramedullary haematopoiesis.

Complications of PV

Pruritus: typically aquagenic, a troublesome complication for some patients. Unfortunately there is no satisfactory treatment. Sometime abates when excess myeloproliferation controlled and Hct reduced but may persist despite adequate control. Worth trying antihistamines (e.g. cyproheptadine 4–16mg/d), H_2-antagonists (cimetidine 400mg bd), IFN-α (3 million units 3 × weekly), the selective serotonin re-uptake inhibitor (SSRI) paroxetine (20mg/d), or phototherapy with psoralen and UV light.

Erythromelalgia: due to microvascular disturbance. Aspirin (loading dose 300–500mg/d then 75 or 100mg/d maintenance) is usually effective.

Thrombosis: manage venous thromboembolic events according to current guidelines. Follow LMW heparin with warfarin (INR 2.0–3.0) for 3–6 months. Low-dose aspirin (75–100mg/d) is recommended following ischaemic stroke, TIA, peripheral arterial occlusion, MI, unstable angina, or in patients with evidence of coronary artery disease.[1] Role of clopidogrel unclear. Cytoreduction recommended in all patients with acute vascular events.

Haemorrhage: major haemorrhage uncommon. Most frequent from skin, mucous membranes and GI tract. May be precipitated by antithrombotic therapy: avoid in patients with history of haemorrhagic events, gastric ulcers, or varices. Associated with platelet count >1500 × 10^9/L. May be related to acquired von Willebrand disease due to loss of large vWF multimers resulting in a functional defect. Normalization of the platelet count corrects the coagulopathy.[11] Treat by withdrawal of any antithrombotic therapy and correction of thrombocytosis with HC. Consider antifibrinolytic therapy and /or vWF containing concentrates.[12]

Surgery in PV patients

Relatively contraindicated in uncorrected PV. Defer surgery until Hct and platelets normalized for ≥2 months due to risk of thrombotic and haemorrhagic complications; if emergency surgery necessary perform venesection and cytapheresis.

PV in pregnancy

Rare. Assess risk of thrombosis and complications of pregnancy. Pre-plan conception when possible with cessation of any teratogenic agents and control of Hct. Administer low dose aspirin throughout pregnancy and prophylactic LMW heparin for 6 weeks post-partum. When cytoreduction is necessary for uncontrolled Hct or progressive myeloproliferation, IFN-α is recommended.[1,10,13]

References

1. Finazzi, G. and Barbui, T. (2007). How I treat patients with polycythemia vera. *Blood*, **109**, 5104–11.
2. Landolfi, R. *et al.* (2004). Efficacy and safety of low dose aspirin in polycythemia vera. *N Engl J Med*, **350**, 114–24.
3. Landolfi, R. and Di Gennaro, L. (2008). Prevention of thrombosis in polycythemia vera and essential thrombocythemia. *Haematologica*, **93**, 331–5.
4. Finazzi, G. and Barbui, T, (2005). Risk-adapted therapy in essential thrombocythemia and polycythemia vera. *Blood Rev*, **19**, 243–52.
5. Cortelazzo, S. *et al.* (1995). Hydroxyurea in the treatment of patients with essential thrombocythemia at high risk of thrombosis: a prospective randomized trial. *N Engl J Med*, **332**, 1132–6.
6. Harrison, C.N. *et al.* (2005). Hydroxyurea compared with anagrelide in high-risk essential thrombocythemia. *N Engl J Med*, **353**, 33–45.
7. Finazzi, G. *et al.* (2005). Acute leukemia in polycythaemia vera: an analysis of 1638 patients enrolled in a prospective observational study. *Blood*, **105**, 2664–70.
8. Lengfelder, E. *et al.* (2000). Interferon alpha in the treatment of polycythemia vera. *Ann Hematol*, **79**, 103–9.
9. Silver, R.T. (2006). Long-term effects of the treatment of polycytemia vera with recombinant interferon alpha. *Cancer*, **107**, 451–8.
10. McMullin, M.F. *et al.* (2005). Guidelines for the diagnosis, investigation and management of polycythemia/erythrocytosis. *Brit J Haematol*, **130**, 174–95. http://www.bcshguidelines.com/pdf/polycythaemia.pdf
11. Budde, U. and van Genderen, P.J. (1997). Acquired von Willebrand disease in patients with high platelet counts. *SeminThromb Hemost*, **23**, 425–31.
12. Landolfi, R. *et al.* (2006). Thrombosis and bleeding in polycythemia vera and essential thrombocythemia: pathogenetic mechanisms and prevention. *Best Pract Res Clin Hematol*, **19**, 617–33.
13. Robinson, S. *et al.* (2005). The management and outcome of 18 pregnancies in women with polycythemia vera. *Haematologica*, **90**, 1477–83.

Secondary erythrocytosis

📖 Causes of 2° erythrocytosis are listed in Table 7.1, p.261.

Effects of the ↑ red cell mass

- ↑ peripheral vascular resistance.
- ↓ cardiac output.
- ↓ systemic O_2 transport resulting in e.g. ↓ cerebral blood flow and O_2 and glucose delivery to the brain.
- Thromboembolic complications also occur. Thus 'compensatory' erythrocytosis is a pathological rather than physiological condition.

Symptoms and signs are non-specific and those of the underlying cause (particularly if cardiac or pulmonary) may predominate. Pruritus, splenomegaly, or the presence of leucocytosis or thrombocytosis suggest the alternative diagnosis of PV.

Investigation as listed under PV (📖 Investigations, p.262), notably *JAK2* mutation analysis, serum EPO, arterial O_2 saturation, renal and hepatic function, urinalysis, renal ultrasound and, if necessary, abdominal CT.

The aim of therapy must be correction of the underlying cause where possible and reduction of the RCM. Venesection is the treatment of choice and if possible should be continued until a target Hct is achieved.

The indications for venesection and recommended target Hct vary with the underlying cause.[1]

- High O_2 affinity haemoglobins:
  - Indications—dizziness, dyspnoea or angina, thrombosis, comparable family member with thrombosis; target Hct <0.60 or if thrombosis or symptoms with Hct <0.60, target <0.52.
- Hypoxic pulmonary disease:
  - Indications—symptoms of hyperviscosity or Hct >0.56; target Hct 0.50–0.52.
- Cyanotic congenital heart disease:
  - Indications—isovolemic venesection for symptoms of hyperviscosity (chest and abdominal pain, myalgia and weakness, fatigue, headache, blurred vision, amaurosis fugax, paraesthesiae, slow mentation) and ↑ viscosity; target individualized; avoid Fe deficiency which may compromise O_2 delivery.
- Post renal transplant erythrocytosis:
  - Indication—failure to respond to ACE inhibitor or angiotensin II receptor antagonist; target Hct <0.45.

In patients with cyanotic congenital heart disease, pulmonary disease or high O_2 affinity haemoglobin, the benefit of venesection can be determined by symptomatic response or by using the serum EPO level as a measure of tissue hypoxia.

Myelosuppressive therapy is not indicated in any of these disorders.

1. McMullin, M.F. *et al.* (2005). Guidelines for the diagnosis, investigation and management of polycythemia/erythrocytosis. *Brit J Haematol*, **130**, 174–95.

🖫 http://www.bcshguidelines.com/pdf/polycythaemia.pdf

Relative erythrocytosis (RE)

Elevation of Hb and Hct with ↔ or minimally ↑ RBC mass and ↔ or ↓ plasma volume defines RE. Apparent polycythaemia, spurious polycythaemia, pseudopolycythaemia, stress erythrocytosis and Gaisbock's syndrome (RE associated with hypertension and nephropathy) are synonymous terms for this disorder. However the existence of chronic plasma contraction is contentious.

Aetiology

Unclear. Some cases may represent extreme ends of ↔ ranges for red cell and plasma volumes, but in most obesity, cigarette smoking, and hypertension are present singly or in combination. Haemoconcentration from dehydration or diuretic therapy should be excluded.

Investigations

- FBC generally shows only modest ↑ Hct. Confirm persistence with at least 2 measurements over a 3-month period. Further investigations should be undertaken as appropriate for persistent erythrocytosis but, by definition, fail to reveal any other abnormality.
- Serum EPO usually ↔; may be ↓
- *JAK2*-V617F mutation –ve.
- RCM studies now rarely performed as PV excluded by sEPO and *JAK2* analysis; demonstrate ↔ RCM and ↓ plasma volume in ~33%; most have high ↔ RCM and low ↔ plasma volume.
- Important to exclude renal disease and arterial hypoxaemia.
- BM biopsy not usually necessary but ↔ when carried out.

Management

- Involves dealing with reversible associated features, i.e. weight reduction, cessation of smoking, control of ↑ BP (without thiazide diuretic), reduction of alcohol intake, and reduction in stress (where possible). Correction of these factors may result in spontaneous improvement.
- Venesection is not standard management; however, it is suggested that patients with recent thrombosis or Hct levels chronically >0.54 should be considered for venesection.[1]
- Monitor untreated patients to exclude further ↑ in Hct.

Natural history and treatment

- Not clear. Retrospective analysis appears to suggest an ↑ incidence of vaso-occlusive episodes that may relate to associated risk factors in the lifestyle of the patients under observation (rather than the ↑ PCV).
- Low-dose aspirin (75mg/d) advisable for patients with overt thrombotic risks and no GI contraindication.
- No role for myelosuppressive therapy.
- Many patients improve with the simple measures specified. In ~33% the Hct returns to the ↔ range. In a further 33% the Hct oscillates between minimal elevation and the ↔ range. In the remaining 33% the Hct remains elevated and these patients should receive long-term follow-up. In a minority absolute erythrocytosis may develop.

1. McMullin, M.F. *et al.* (2005). Guidelines for the diagnosis, investigation and management of polycythemia/erythrocytosis. *Brit J Haematol*, **130**, 174–95.

http://www.bcshguidelines.com/pdf/polycythaemia.pdf

Idiopathic erythrocytosis (IE)

Heterogeneous group with absolute erythrocytosis (↑ RCM) but no clear cause of 1° or 2° erythrocytosis. Some patients formerly given this diagnosis have been shown to have *JAK2* exon 12 mutations.

- May be physiological variant: extreme 'high-normal' values
- 5–10% showed definite features of PV after several years follow-up.
- Others develop clear evidence of SE, e.g. sleep apnoea.
- Long-term follow-up is required in these patients.
- Venesection to a Hct <0.45 has been recommended because of an incidence of fatal thrombo-embolic and haemorrhagic events similar to PV.[1]
- Myelosuppressive therapy is contraindicated.

1. McMullin, M.F. *et al.* (2005). Guidelines for the diagnosis, investigation and management of polycythemia/erythrocytosis. *Brit J Haematol*, **130**, 174–95.

http://www.bcshguidelines.com/pdf/polycythaemia.pdf

Essential thrombocythaemia (ET)

ET (*syn.* 1° or idiopathic thrombocythaemia) is characterized by persistent thrombocytosis that is neither reactive (i.e. 2° to another condition; 📖 p.285) nor due to another myeloproliferative neoplasm or a myelodysplastic disorder. It is a diagnosis of exclusion and is biologically heterogeneous.

Incidence

True incidence unknown but probably up to 3 per 100,000 annually[1]; slight excess in ♀; median age at diagnosis 60 years; frequently occurs <40 years; very rare <20 years.

Pathogenesis

Aetiology unknown. No association with radiation, drugs, chemicals, or viral infection. Pathogenetically heterogeneous. The *JAK2*-V617F mutation is found in approximately 50% of patients with ET,[2] though it is not clear how this mutation produces 3 different clinical phenotypes of MPN. The mutation load in ET is lower than in PV and IMF and very rarely shows homozygous *JAK2* mutation.[3, 4] Further differences are lower gene dosage in ET, generally stable frequency of the *JAK2*-V617F mutant allele over time, and higher expression in platelets than in neutrophils.[5]

There is evidence of clonality in some patients with *JAK2*-V617F –ve ET including the presence of a mutation of the thrombopoietin (TPO) receptor (MPL). Somatic mutations of codon 515 at the transmembrane–juxtamembrane junction of MPL (*MPLW515L* or *MPLW515K*) have been identified in about 10% of *JAK2*-V617F –ve PMF patients and 1% with *JAK2*-V617F –ve ET.[6] Hereditary thrombocytosis has been described due to mutations causing hypersensitivity of MPL to TPO[7] or ↑ translation of TPO from mRNA.[8]

ET patients with the *JAK2*-V617F mutation may have a higher frequency of thrombotic complications and it has been suggested that they have a clinical phenotype similar to PV and a different clinical course from ET patients without the mutation.[9]

Platelets in ET are often functionally abnormal showing impaired aggregation *in vitro*. High platelet counts ($>1000 \times 10^9$/L) are associated with an acquired von Willebrand syndrome.[10] the mechanism may be ↑ catabolism of large molecular weight multimers; reduction in the platelet count corrects the abnormality and reduces haemorrhagic episodes.[10,11]

Clinical features

- Diagnosis often follows detection of thrombocytosis on a routine FBC; up to 50% patients asymptomatic. Others may present with 'vasomotor', thrombotic, and/or haemorrhagic symptoms.
- Vasomotor symptoms occur in 40%: headache, light-headedness, syncope, atypical chest pain, visual upset, paraesthesiae, livedo reticularis, and erythromelalgia (erythema and burning discomfort in hands or feet due to digital microvascular occlusion).

- Haemorrhagic symptoms occur in 25% (major <5%): easy bruising, mucosal or GI bleeding, or unexplained or prolonged bleeding after trauma or surgery.
- Thrombosis occurs in ~20% (major <10%): arterial > venous, e.g. MI, CVA, splenic or hepatic vein thrombosis.
- Splenomegaly found in <40% (less common and less marked than in other myeloproliferative disorders).
- Splenic atrophy may occur from repeated microvascular infarction.
- Recurrent abortions and fetal growth retardation due to multiple placental infarctions may occur in young women with ET.

Differential diagnosis

Most cases of isolated thrombocytosis are reactive and <10% are due to a 1° haematological disorder. The overlapping clinical phenotypes of ET, PV. PMF, and CML can also make diagnosis difficult. Before a diagnosis of ET is made, causes of RT (📖 Reactive thrombocytosis, p.285) must be excluded by detailed history and examination and investigation, as must PV, CML, PMF, and MDS with a predominant thrombocytosis which can all mimic ET.

Investigations

- FBC:
  - Platelets persistently >450 × 10^9/L (may be as high as 5000 × 10^9/L); the degree of thrombocytosis is not a criterion for differentiating ET from RT.
  - Hb usually ↔; may be ↓ with ↓ MCV due to chronic blood loss; WBC usually ↔.
  - Mean platelet volume (MPV) usually ↔; raised platelet distribution width (PDW).
  - Automated FBC may give erroneous data in severe cases as giant platelets may be counted as RBCs.
- Blood film:
  - Thrombocytosis, variable shapes and sizes (platelet anisocytosis), giant platelets, and platelet clumps; megakaryocyte fragments; basophilia may be present; variable degree of RBC abnormality: may be hypochromic and microcytic if Fe deficient; may be changes of hyposplenism, e.g. Howell–Jolly bodies.
- Peripheral blood mutation screening for *JAK2*-V617F mutation:
  - Detected in approximately 50% of patients with ET; presence excludes reactive thrombocytosis; absence does not exclude ET.
  - Bear in mind false-+ve results due to highly sensitive allele-specific assays and false –ve due to low mutant allele burden especially in ET.[12]
- BM examination:
  - Required to help differentiate ET from RT in *JAK2*-V617F –ve patients and to differentiate ET from other MPNs, notably pre-fibrotic PMF, and from MDS.
  - Aspirate: may show ↑ platelet clumps, ↑ large megakaryocytes with 'hypermature' appearances, ↑ nuclear lobation, and large cytoplasm; little or no granulocyte or erythroid hyperplasia. Fe stores present in 40–70%.

    - Trephine biopsy: ↑ megakaryocytes, dispersed throughout the marrow or with loose clustering; large, 'hypermature' with deeply lobated and hyperlobated nuclei; bizarre atypical forms seen in PMF not usual; little or no granulocyte or erythroid hyperplasia. Reticulin normal or minimal ↑ (up to 25%); no fibrosis. No dysplastic features.
    - Cytogenetics: abnormal in 5%; no specific diagnostic abnormalities; most frequent: 20q–, +1, +8, +9, or der(1;7); always Ph–ve.
- Other tests:
    - Uric acid: ↑ in 25%.
    - Pseudohyperkalaemia: in 25%.
    - ESR and acute phase proteins (CRP and fibrinogen) usually ↔ in ET, often raised in RT but not discriminatory as inflammation can also occur in patients with ET.
    - Serum ferritin: if low Fe replacement therapy should fail to ↑ Hb to the PV range.

2008 WHO diagnostic criteria for ET[12]

Availability of the *JAK2*-V617F clonal marker and an ↑ use of BM histology has resulted in a recommended lower platelet count threshold for the diagnosis of ET from 600 to 450 × 10^9/L. Diagnosis of ET requires that all 4 of these criteria are met (Table 7.5).

Table 7.5 WHO diagnostic criteria for ET (2008)[12]

1	Persistent elevation of the platelet count ≥450 × 10^9/L.
2	Megakaryocyte proliferation with large and mature morphology; no or little granulocyte or erythroid proliferation.
3	Not meeting WHO criteria for CML, PV, PMF, MDS, or other myeloid neoplasm.
4	Demonstration of *JAK2*-V617F or other clonal marker or in the absence of a clonal marker, no evidence of reactive thrombocytosis.

Diagnostic algorithm for suspected ET

Once RT has been excluded by history and examination, the diagnostic algorithm recommended by Tefferi and Vardiman[12] and based on the 2008 WHO criteria may be used in a patient with suspected ET.

- Peripheral blood mutation screening for *JAK2*-V617F:
    - V617F+ve: *ET, PV, or PMF highly likely* → BM biopsy and cytogenetics
    - V617F–ve: *ET and PMF still possible and CML should also be considered* → BM biopsy and cytogenetics
- BM biopsy and cytogenetics → *use 2008 WHO criteria for specific diagnosis.*
    - *Consider FISH for BCR-ABL in the absence of Ph chromosome but presence of dwarf megakaryocytes.*

Risk factors in ET

- Thrombosis associated with previous thrombosis and age >60 years; no clear relationship between marked thrombocytosis and thrombotic risk; potential novel risk factors are leukocytosis[13], *JAK2*-V617F mutation +ve, JAK2-V617F homozygosity (reviewed in reference 7).
- Haemorrhage associated with extreme thrombocytosis (>1500 × 10^9/L) and anti-platelet therapy.

Risk stratification in ET[14]

Low risk

- Age < 60 years *and*
- No history of thrombosis *and*
- Platelet count <1500 × 10^9/L *and*
- No cardiovascular risk factors (smoking, obesity, hypertension, hyperlipidaemia, diabetes mellitus)

Intermediate risk

- Neither low risk nor high risk.

High risk

- Age ≥ 60 years *or*
- Previous history of thrombosis.

Natural history

ET is usually associated with a more favourable prognosis than the other MPNs. It generally follows an indolent course and life expectancy is near ↔. The risk of life-threatening complications or of leukaemic transformation is very low. However, the risk of AML has in the past been ↑ by cytotoxic therapy (busulfan and ^{32}P) though the risk is much less with hydroxycarbamide. Need for therapy must be individualized, balancing the risk of therapy against risk of thrombosis or haemorrhage, FBC results, co-morbidity, and age. Risk of transformation is low for a patient with ET in the absence of busulfan or ^{32}P therapy: 2% leukaemic transformation and 4% evolution to myelofibrosis at 15 years.[15] Death due to thrombosis is reported in 11–25% with a cumulative rate of cardiovascular events of 2–3% per patient year with arterial thrombosis accounting for 60–70% of events (reviewed in reference 16).

Management

Aim is to alleviate symptoms of microvascular disturbance (e.g. headache, lightheadedness, atypical chest pain, or erythromelalgia) and ↓ risks and incidence of thrombotic and haemorrhagic complications by use of aspirin and normalization of platelet count (target <400 × 10^9/L); balance these risks against the short and long-term risks of therapy.

- All patients with ET should be advised to make lifestyle changes (smoking, exercise, obesity) to reduce their risk of thrombosis and atherosclerosis and reversible cardiovascular risk factors should be treated (hypertension, hypercholesterolaemia).
- NSAIDs and standard dose aspirin should be avoided due to risk of haemorrhage.

- *Note*: acquired von Willebrand syndrome (AvWS) occurs in some patients with ET with >1000 × 10^9/L platelets; use aspirin cautiously and consider screening for AvWS and cytoreduction prior to aspirin therapy; in symptomatic patients cytoreductive therapy usually corrects the clinical symptoms and laboratory abnormality; cytoreduction is advised in asymptomatic patients with AvWS only if RiCoF <30%; low-dose aspirin may be used if the RiCoF remains >50%.[10]

Low risk patients
- These patients have no ↑ risk of thrombosis (<2/100 patient years) or haemorrhage (~1/100 patient years) compared to age- and sex-matched controls;[17] thrombotic deaths are rare; a 'watch and wait' policy is recommended.[14]
- No added risk with pregnancy or surgery.
- Cytoreductive therapy should be avoided unless complications occur.
- Observation ± aspirin 75mg/d (if no contraindication).
- Although the anti-thrombotic benefit of low-dose aspirin was demonstrated in the ECLAP study in PV[18] there is no evidence to support 1° prophylaxis in asymptomatic low risk ET; the Italian guidelines do not recommend it[19] though others do in the absence of a contraindication;[20,21] the risks and benefits of low-dose aspirin should be carefully balanced in the individual patient.[22]
- Microvascular symptoms (e.g. erythromelalgia) are an indication for low-dose aspirin and usually respond promptly (commence with loading dose 300–500mg/day followed by 75–100mg/day maintenance).[23]

Intermediate risk patients
- Individualize therapy.
- Many patients in this group may simply be treated with low-dose aspirin (if no contraindication: previous GI haemorrhage, symptomatic AvWS, or RiCoF >50%) and observation.
- Smokers should be encouraged to stop smoking and obese patients to lose weight to reduce their risks of thrombosis.
- Cytoreductive therapy for patients with marked thrombocytosis (>1500 ×10^9/L) associated with a bleeding diathesis, or who are at ↑ risk of haemorrhage, or have cardiovascular risk factors; many would choose anagrelide or interferon-α in younger patients.[19]
- Aim for platelet count providing symptom relief or control of bleeding rather than necessarily <400 × 10^9/L.[20]

High risk patients
- *Aspirin*: 75–100mg/d recommended for patients with previous thrombotic event or at high risk of thrombosis; ↑ risk of haemorrhage (safest when platelets <1000 ×10^9/L; delay until cytoreduction of platelets >1500); quickly relieves erythromelalgia (2–4d); extreme caution in patients with marked thrombocytosis, haemorrhagic complications or history of peptic ulceration; H_2-antagonist or PPIs may be needed; markedly ↑ bleeding risk with higher aspirin doses. *Dipyridamole* is an alternative for patients unable to tolerate aspirin. No data on the use of clopidogrel.

- *Hydroxycarbamide (HC):* established as treatment of choice in combination with aspirin (when not contraindicated) for patients >60 years (0.5–1.5g/d maintenance after higher initial doses aiming to bring platelets <400 × 10^9/L).
  - Control of thrombocytosis with HC reduces risk of thrombosis in high risk patients (3.6% *vs.* 24% after 27 months in randomized study vs observation[24]);
  - HC + aspirin superior to anagrelide + aspirin in the UK MRC PT-1 randomized trial in 809 patients with high risk ET: despite similar ↓ in platelets, ↓ rates of arterial thrombosis, major haemorrhage, transformation to myelofibrosis (3 ×) and treatment withdrawal though ↑ rate of venous thrombosis.[25]
  - Use in symptomatic patients <60 years intolerant of anagrelide and IFN-α; some patients require HC in combination with anagrelide or IFN-α to achieve a ↔ platelet count;
  - Side effects: myelosuppression, oral ulceration, rash; contraindicated in pregnancy and breast feeding; risk of leukaemia not ↑ by HC.[10,25,26]
  - Up to 10% of patients do not achieve the desired reduction in platelets; others develop unacceptable side effects, e.g. leg ulcers, cytopenias, or fever; a working group has developed criteria to define clinical resistance and intolerance to HC in ET to facilitate analysis of trials and management of individual patients.[27]
    —Platelets >600 × 10^9/L after 3 months of at least 2g/day HC (2.5g/d if weight >80kg) *or*
    —Platelets >400 × 10^9/L and WBC count <2.5×10^9/L at any dose of HC *or*
    —Platelets >400 × 10^9/L and Hb <10g/dL at any dose of HC *or*
    —Presence of leg ulcers or other unacceptable mucocutaneous manifestations at any dose of HC *or*
    —HC-related fever.
- *Interferon-α:* (start at 3 million units, 3 × weekly; usual maintenance 1–5 million units, 3 × weekly) can control thrombocytosis due to ET; useful in younger patients intolerant of anagrelide or older patients intolerant of HC; no risk of leukaemogenesis; 85% response rate with 54% achieving ↔ platelet counts; reduction in splenomegaly in 66% with 17% normalization of spleen size;[19] rarely used due to inconvenience of SC administration and poor tolerance; drug of choice in pregnancy; pegylated IFN has equal efficacy and a more convenient once weekly dose schedule.
- *Anagrelide:* (commence 500mcg bd, adjust according to response with weekly increments of 500mcg/d to usual therapeutic dose of 2–3mg/d) has been preferred in younger patients <60 years (especially those of childbearing potential); interferes with megakaryocyte differentiation; therapeutic effect usually seen within 14–21d; side effects: headache (>50%), palpitations (>50%), fluid retention, diarrhoea (15–20%); contraindicated in pregnancy and patients with CCF or known cardiac disease.
- *Busulfan*: alkylating agent; produces prolonged control of platelet count; ↑ risk of AML; restricted to patients >75 years unable to comply with regular HC therapy; administer intermittently at 4–6mg/d for 2–6 weeks until response or as single dose of 0.5–1mg/kg repeated if necessary after 2–3 months.

- *Radioactive phosphorus (^{32}P)*: may be considered in elderly patients (>75 years) unable to comply with regular HC therapy; side effects: myelosuppression, long-term risk of AML (10%); 2.3mCi/m^2 IV; may be repeated after 3–6 months.

Table 7.6 Treatment for ET[20]

Risk group	Age <60 years	Age ≥60 years	Women of childbearing age
Low risk	?Low-dose aspirin*	Not applicable	?Low-dose aspirin*
Intermediate risk**	Low-dose aspirin*	Not applicable	Low-dose aspirin*
High risk	Hydroxycarbamide/ IFN-α/anagrelide*** + low-dose aspirin	Hydroxycarbamide + low-dose aspirin	IFN-α + low-dose aspirin

* In the absence of a contraindication, including a RiCoF <50%. ** Decision to use cytoreductive agents in intermediate risk ET should be made on individual patient basis. *** The Nordic MPD Study Group Guidelines[28] recommend IFN-α and anagrelide as 1st and 2nd choice treatments for patients aged <60 years with hydroxycarbamide 3rd line unless leucocyte reduction or constitutional symptom control is required when it is 2nd line to IFN-α Adapted from reference 20.

ET in pregnancy

- 1st trimester abortion occurs frequently in young women with ET (25–40%) with late pregnancy loss in 10%; abruptio placentae occurs in 3.6% and intrauterine growth retardation (IUGR) in 4–5%.[29]
- Maternal thrombosis and haemorrhage are uncommon.
- ↑ risk in women with a history of severe complications in a previous pregnancy.
- Patients with the *JAK2*-V617F mutation have a higher risk of developing complications in pregnancy; aspirin did not prevent these and may worsen the outcome in mutation –ve mothers.[30]
- If possible, stop potentially teratogenic drugs (hydroxycarbamide, anagrelide) at least 3 months before conception.
- Low-dose aspirin is recommended by the Italian Guidelines[19] for pregnant women with ET with a history of microvascular symptoms or a previous adverse pregnancy event; Harrison recommends low-dose aspirin throughout pregnancy and for at least 6 weeks after delivery for all women with ET and PV without contraindications;[31] if possible, aspirin should be commenced before conception.
- LMW heparin is recommended for prophylaxis and treatment of DVT in selected high-risk pregnant women with ET and a history of late fetal loss, pre-term delivery and IUGR (enoxaparin 40mg od, then bd from 16 weeks then od for 6 weeks post-partum).[29]
- IFN-α is cytoreductive treatment of choice when indicated: previous history of major thrombosis or haemorrhage; platelet count >1000–1500 × 10^9/L; familial thrombophilia or cardiovascular risk factors.[29]
- Successful pregnancy reported following 1st trimester treatment with hydroxycarbamide.

Life-threatening haemorrhage in ET

- Main sites: skin, mucous membranes, and GI tract.
- Most frequent in patients with platelet counts >1000–1500 × 10^9/L.
- Stop anti-platelet agents.
- Identify site of bleeding.
- Hydroxycarbamide 2–4g/d × 3–5d to ↓ platelets (takes 3–5d for effect).
- Plateletpheresis if persistent life-threatening haemorrhage.
- Antifibrinolytic agents e.g. tranexamic acid may be used.
- DDAVP/Factor VIII concentrate of limited value if evidence of AvWS.[10]
- Platelet transfusion may be helpful if no evidence of AvWS.

Arterial thrombosis in ET

- Commence aspirin 75mg/d (rapid response in TIA and erythromelalgia) if no major contraindication.
- Hydroxycarbamide to normalize platelet count.
- Plateletpheresis if life threatening.

Venous thrombosis in ET

- Commence heparin followed by oral anticoagulant therapy (target INR 2.0–3.0) according to standard protocols.
- Commence concomitant hydroxycarbamide to reduce risk of recurrence.
- Monitor platelet count and INR closely because of greater bleeding risk.

Surgery in ET

- ↑ morbidity and mortality risk if surgery undertaken with poor control.
- Withhold aspirin for at least 1 week before elective surgery with high bleeding risk or if elective anticoagulation required peri-operatively.
- Commence/adjust hydroxycarbamide to achieve platelet count <400 × 10^9/L; especially if splenectomy planned.
- Resume oral cytoreductive therapy as soon as possible post-operatively; resume aspirin 24h after surgery if no excessive bleeding.
- Plateletpheresis may be required for extreme post-operative thrombocytosis.
- Surgical procedures may require specific antithrombotic strategies e.g. heparin. Monitor patient with ET carefully for haemorrhage or thrombosis.
- Thrombotic risks ↓ if platelet count reduced to ↔.

References

1. Johansson, P. *et al.* (2004). Trends in the incidence of chronic Philadelphia chromosome negative (Ph–) myeloproliferative disorders in the city of Gothenberg, Sweden, during 1983–99. *J Intern Med*, **256**, 161–5.
2. Baxter, E.J. *et al.* (2005). Acquired mutation of the tyrosine kinase JAK2 in human myeloproliferative disorders. *Lancet*, **365**, 1054–61.
3. Scott, L.M. *et al.* (2006). Progenitors homozygous for the V617F JAK2 mutation occur in most patients with polycythemia vera, but not essential thrombocythemia. *Blood*, **108**, 2435–7.
4. Kralovics, R. *et al.* (2006). Acquisition of the V617F mutation of JAK2 is a late genetic event in a subset of patients with myeloproliferative disorders. *Blood*, **108**, 1377–80.
5. Moliterno, A.R. *et al.* (2006) Molecular mimicry in the chronic myeloproliferative disorders: reciprocity between quantitative JAK2 V617F and Mpl expression. *Blood*, **108**, 3913–15.
6. Pardanani, A.D. *et al.* (2006). MPL515 mutations in myeloproliferative and other myeloid disorders: a study of 118 patients. *Blood*, **108**, 3472–6.

7. Ding, J. *et al.* (2004). Familial essential thrombocythemia associated with a dominant-positive activating mutation of the *c-MPL* gene, which encodes for the receptor for thrombopoietin. *Blood,* **103**, 4198–200.
8. Wiestner, A. *et al.* (1998). An activating splice donor mutation in the thrombopoietin gene causes hereditary thrombocythemia. *Nat Genet,* **18**, 49–52.
9. Campbell, P.J. *et al.* (2005). Definition of subtypes of essential thrombocythaemia and relation to polycythaemia vera based on JAK2 V617F mutation status: a prospective study. *Lancet,* **366**, 1945–53.
10. Elliot, M.A. and Tefferi, A. (2005). Thrombosis and haemorrhage in polycythemia vera and essential thrombocythaemia. *Br J Haematol,* **128**, 275–90.
11. Budde, U. and van Genderen, P.J. (1997). Acquired von Willebrand disease in patients with high platelet counts. *SeminThromb Hemost,* **23**, 425–31.
12. Tefferi, A. and Vardiman, J.W. (2008). Classification and diagnosis of myeloproliferative neoplasms: The 2008 World Health Organization criteria and point-of-care diagnostic algorithms. *Leukemia,* **22**, 14–22.
13. Carobbio, A. *et al.* (2007). Leukocytosis is a risk factor for thrombosis in essential thrombocythemia: interaction with treatment, standard risk factors, and Jak2 mutation status. *Blood,* **109**, 2310–13.
14. Finazzi, G. and Barbui, T. (2005). Risk-adapted therapy in essential thrombocythemia and polycythemia vera. *Blood Rev,* **19**, 243–52.
15. Passamonti, F. *et al.* (2004). Life expectancy and prognostic factors for survival in patients with polycythemia vera and essential thrombocythemia. *Am J Med,* **117**, 755–61.
16. Vannucchi, A.M. and Barbui, T. (2007). Thrombocytosis and thrombosis *Hematology 2007,* 363–70.
17. Ruggeri, M. *et al.* (1998). No treatment for low risk thrombocythaemia: results from a prospective study. *Br J Haematol,* **103**, 772–7.
18. Landolfi, R. *et al.* (2004). Efficacy and safety of low dose aspirin in poilycythemia vera. *N Engl J Med,* **350**, 114–24.
19. Barbui, T. *et al.* (2004). Practice guidelines for the therapy of essential thrombocythemia. A statement from the Italian Society of Hematology, the Italian Society of Experimental Hematology and the Italian Group for Bone Marrow Transplantation. *Haematologica,* **89**, 215–32.
20. Tefferi, A. and Barbui, T. (2005). *bcr/abl*–negative, classic myeloproliferative disorders: diagnosis and treatment. *Mayo Clin Proc,* **80**, 1220–32.
21. Campbell, P.J. and Green, A.R. (2005). Management of polycythemia vera and essential thrombocythemia. *Hematology2005,* 201–8.
22. Landolfi, R. and Di Gennaro, L. (2008). Prevention of thrombosis in polycythemia vera and essential thrombocythemia. *Haematologica,* **93**, 331–5.
23. McCarthy, L. *et al.* (2002). Erythromelalgia due to essential thrombocthemia. *Transfusion,* **42**, 1245.
24. Cortelazzo, S. *et al.* (1995). Hydroxyurea for patients with essential thrombocythemia and a high risk of thrombosis. *N Engl J Med,* **332**, 1132–6.
25. Harrison, C.N. *et al.* (2005). Hydroxyurea compared with anagrelide in high-risk essential thrombocythemia. *N Engl J Med,* **353**, 33–45.
26. Finazzi, G. *et al.* (2005). Acute leukemia in polycythaemia vera: an analysis of 1638 patients enrolled in a prospective observational study. *Blood,* **105**, 2664–70.
27. Barosi, G. *et al.* (2007). A unified definition of clinical resistance/intolerance to hydroxyurea in essential thrombocythemia: results of a consensus process by an international working group. *Leukemia,* **21**, 277–80 plus corrigenda **21**, 1135.
28. Nordic MPD Study Group (2007). Guidelines for the diagnosis and treatment of patients with polycythemia vera, essential thrombocythemia and idiopathic myelofibrosis. www.sfhem.se/filarkiv/files/vardprogram/NMPDGuidelines2007.pdf
29. Barbui, T. and Finazzi, G. (2006). Myeloproliferative disease in pregnancy and other management issues. *Hematology 2006,* 246–52.
30. Passamonti, F. *et al.* (2007). Increased risk of pregnancy complications in patients with essential thrombocythemia carrying the *JAK2* (617V>F) mutation. *Blood,* **110**, 485–9.
31. Harrison, C. (2005). Pregnancy and its management in the Philadelphia-negative myeloproliferative diseases. *Br J Haematol,* **129**, 293–306.

Reactive thrombocytosis (RT)

Platelet counts of >450 × 10^9/L occur as a reactive phenomenon and maybe seen in:

- Infection.
- Following surgery.
- Post splenectomy or functional asplenia
- Malignancy e.g. occult carcinoma.
- Trauma.
- Chronic inflammatory states e.g. collagen disorders.
- Blood loss
- Fe deficiency.
- Haemolytic anaemia.
- Rebound in response to haematinics and/or chemotherapy.
- Any severely ill patient on ITU.

Raised platelet count in clonal haematological disorders occurs in CML, ET, PV, PMF, and also in MDS (esp. 5q– syndrome).

In RT platelets are usually <1000 × 10^9/L but levels of 1500 × 10^9/L may occur. Platelet morphology usually ↔ but differentiation from ET relies on full clinical evaluation. BM examination reveals ↑ megakaryocytes with ↔ morphology.

RT is generally not associated with an ↑ risk of thrombosis or haemorrhage and no specific treatment is required. However, short term anticoagulant or antiplatelet therapy is advised for marked thrombocytosis occurring in the immediate post-splenectomy period as an ↑ incidence of thrombosis has been described in this situation.

Improvement or resolution of the underlying cause usually results in normalization of the platelet count in RT.

Primary myelofibrosis (PMF)

1° myelofibrosis (*syns.* idiopathic myelofibrosis, myelofibrosis with myeloid metaplasia, agnogenic myeloid metaplasia) is a MPN characterized by marrow fibrosis, splenomegaly, extramedullary haematopoiesis, and tear drop poikilocytes and leucoerythroblastosis in the peripheral blood film. Cases of myelofibrosis (MF) that evolve from PV (10–15% evolve into MF) or ET (~2% evolve to MF) are designated post-PV myelofibrosis and post-ET myelofibrosis respectively. The term PMF is reserved for *de novo* cases.

Incidence

Rare disorder; ~5 cases per million per annum; predominantly elderly patients (median 65 years); affects ♂ and ♀ equally.

Pathogenesis

- PMF is a clonal neoplastic proliferation arising from an early haematopoietic stem cell that leads to marked hyperplasia of morphologically abnormal megakaryocytes and clonal monocytes that stimulate reactive fibrosis of the BM.
- The *JAK2*-V617F mutation has been found in up to 58% of patients with PMF[1]; it is homozygous in 13% of patients with PMF compared to 30% with PV and rare in ET;[2, 3] in a murine model the *JAK2*-V617F mutation caused erythrocytosis, extrameduallary haematopoiesis, and marrow fibrosis.[4]
- Presence of *JAK2*-V617F may correlate with poorer survival in PMF;[5] homozygosity is associated with more frequent unfavourable cytogenetic abnormalities.[6]
- The *MPL*-W515L or *MPL*-W515K mutation of the transmembrane domain of the thrombopoietin receptor (cMPL) has been detected in 9% of patients with *JAK2*-V617F –ve PMF; these mutations can co-exist in the same patient; 30% of patients with a cMPL mutation also have the *JAK2*-V617F mutation;[7] the burden of each mutation appears to remain constant over time;[8] in a murine model the *MPL*-W515L mutation results in thrombocytosis and marrow fibrosis.[9]
- Patients with *MPL*-W515L/K mutations may be older, have more severe anaemia, and be more likely to require transfusion support.[10]
- ~50% of patients with clinically similar PMF have no detectable mutation of JAK2 or cMPL, so these mutations cannot be the only cause of PMF; other genetic events clearly contribute to the development of PMF; gains of genetic material occur in >50% of patients, most commonly 9p, 2q. 3p. 4, 12q, and 13q.[11]
- PMF fibroblasts are non-clonal; fibrosis is a reactive process in response to cytokines released by clonal megakaryocytes and monocytes, notably TGF-β;[12] PDGF, IL-1, EGF, calmodulin, and bFGF may also play a role.
- Exaggeration of normal BM reticulin pattern progresses to intense collagen fibrosis that disrupts and finally obliterates normal marrow architecture; ultimately osteosclerosis may develop.
- High levels of endothelial progenitors appear in PB in the prefibrotic phase and haematopoietic progenitors (CD34 cells) increase as PMF advances which facilitates seeding of extramedullary haematopoiesis.[13]

- Extramedullary haematopoiesis develops in spleen and/or liver, and occasionally other sites, e.g. lymph nodes, skin, and serosal surfaces.
- Marrow fibrosis can also be 2° to other disorders: a minority may follow chemotherapy or radiotherapy; can develop in response to chronic myeloproliferative disorders, myelodysplasia, and 2° carcinoma.

Clinical features and presentation

- ~20% may be asymptomatic at diagnosis: mild abnormalities identified on routine FBC or splenomegaly on clinical examination.
- 70–80% are diagnosed in the fibrotic stage; most present with symptoms of progressive anaemia and hepatosplenomegaly associated with hypercatabolic features of fatigue, weight loss, night sweats, and low grade fever.
- Abdominal discomfort (heavy sensation in left upper quadrant) and/or dyspepsia from pressure effects of splenic enlargement may prompt presentation.
- Symptoms and signs of marrow failure: lethargy, infections, bleeding.
- Splenomegaly is almost universal (>90%): moderate-to-massive (35%) enlargement; variable hepatomegaly (up to 70%); lymphadenopathy is uncommon (<10%).
- Gout in ~5%; portal hypertension, pleural effusion, and ascites (due to portal hypertension or peritoneal seeding) also occur.
- 20–30% of patients with PMF are diagnosed in pre-fibrotic stage which may clinically mimic ET; it evolves from hyperproliferation of megakaryocytes with moderate-to-marked thrombocytosis (88% $\geq 500 \times 10^9$/L), occasionally with thrombosis or bleeding, mild anaemia, mild-to-moderate leucocytosis, and no or modest splenomegaly (15%) to classical fibrotic PMF.[14]

Investigations and diagnosis

- FBC: Hb usually ↓ or ↔ (<10g/dL in 60%); normochromic normocytic indices; WBC may be ↓, ↔ or ↑ (~30%; rarely >100 × 10^9/L); basophilia and eosinophilia in 10–30%; platelets usually ↓ or ↔; occasionally ↑.
- Blood film:
  - Prefibrotic stage: thrombocytosis and mild leucocytosis but no or minimal red cell poikilocytosis, tear drops, or leukoerythroblastosis.
  - Fibrotic stage: leucoerythroblastic anaemia (nucleated red cells, myelocytes) with tear drop poikilocytes (96%) and polychromasia; giant platelets and megakaryocyte fragments;
- BM aspirate: usually unsuccessful ('dry tap').
- BM trephine biopsy: essential for diagnosis:
  - Characteristically shows patchy haemopoietic cellularity (often focally hypercellular) ↑ numbers of small-to-large irregular megakaryocytes with aberrant nuclear–cytoplasmic ratio and hyperchromatic, bulbuous, or irregularly folded nuclei and dense clustering; bare megakaryocyte nuclei common; usually reticulin fibrosis (often coarse and branching) and/or collagen fibrosis; distended marrow sinusoids with intravascular haematopoiesis (Fig. 7.1).
  - Prefibrotic stage: minimal or absent reticulin fibrosis, ↑ cellularity due to granulocyte proliferation and often ↓ erythropoiesis; differentiate from ET by ↑ atypical megakaryocytes.

- *JAK2* mutation analysis: +ve in 58%.
- Coagulation screen: features of DIC in 15%; usually occult but causes problems at surgery (e.g. splenectomy); defective platelet aggregation common.
- Cytogenetics: abnormalities in up to 50%: 13q–, 20q–, +8, +9, t(1;7), der(6), t(1;6),(q21~23;p21.3), 12p–, 7–, 7q–, and 1q+ most frequent; exclude Ph chromosome by FISH on PB if dry tap on BM.
- Serum chemistry: bilirubin ↑ in 40%; alkaline phosphatase and ALT ↑ in 50%; urate ↑ in 60%.
- LDH ↑ due to ineffective erythropoiesis and haemolysis; ↑ in 20% of prefibrotic MF.
- Serum ferritin: to assess Fe stores; ↓ by occult GI blood loss in sub-clinical PV.
- Serum EPO: patients with level <125 U/L respond more readily to EPO therapy.
- Skeletal radiology: to assess osteomyelosclerosis.
- MRI: readily distinguishes fibrotic BM from cellular BM.

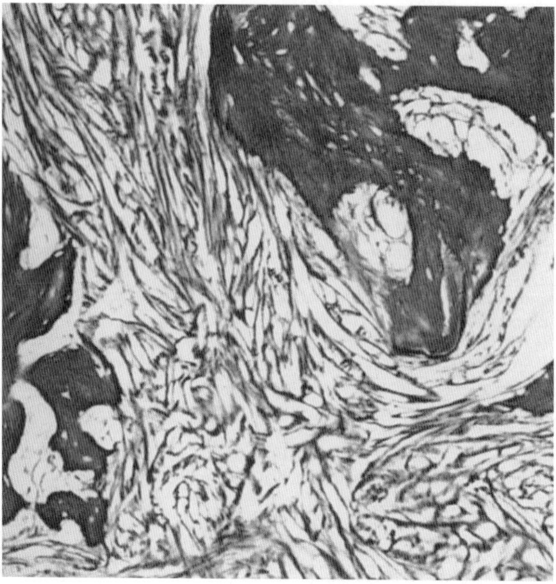

Fig. 7.1 BM trephine in myelofibrosis: note streaming effect caused by intense fibrosis (📖 Plate 25).

Differential diagnosis

- Exclude other myeloproliferative neoplasms (CML, PV, ET) M7 AML (acute MF), myelodysplasia, lymphoproliferative disorders (particularly HCL), metastatic cancer (esp. breast, lung, prostate, gastric), tuberculosis, histoplasmosis and SLE.
- IMF is –ve for Ph chromosome and *BCR-ABL* fusion gene.
- Metastatic cancer in marrow, especially breast, prostate, and thyroid, can give similar FBC features but without splenomegaly; metastatic carcinoma cells are usually apparent on marrow biopsy and/or aspirate.
- Prefibrotic stage may be difficult to distinguish from PV/ET; prominent neutrophil proliferation, ↓ erythroid precursors and particularly the markedly abnormal megakaryocytes assist in correct diagnosis.

Table 7.7 Conditions associated with BM fibrosis[15]

Haematological disorders	Non-haematological disorders
• PMF • PV • CML • ET • AMF (AML-M7) • Other AML • Myelodysplastic syndromes • Chronic myelomonocytic leukaemia • ALL • HCL • Hodgkin lymphoma • Non-Hodgkin lymphoma • MM • CEL • Mast cell disease • Malignant histiocytosis	• Metastatic cancer (breast, lung, prostate, gastric) • Autoimmune myelofibrosis • Systemic lupus erythematosis • Kala-azar (leishmaniasis) • Tuberculosis • Histoplasmosis • Paget's disease • HIV infection • Vitamin D-resistant rickets • Renal osteodystrophy • Hyperparathyroidism • Gray platelet syndrome • Familial infantile myelofibrosis • Radiation exposure • Osteopetrosis

Adapted from reference 15.

Diagnostic criteria

The 2008 revised WHO diagnostic criteria for PMF define 3 major and 4 minor criteria and require all 3 major criteria plus 2 minor criteria for the diagnosis of PMF (📖 Table 7.8).[16]

Table 7.8 2008 WHO diagnostic criteria for PMF[16]

Major criteria	1. Megakaryocyte proliferation and atypia* accompanied by either retuculin and/or collagen fibrosis, *or* In the absence of reticulin fibrosis, the megakaryocyte changes must be accompanied by ↑ marrow cellularity, granulocytic proliferation, and often ↑ erythropoiesis (i.e. pre-fibrotic PMF)
	2. Not meeting WHO criteria for CML, PV, MDS, or other myeloid neoplasm.
	3. Demonstration of *JAK2*-V617F or other clonal marker *or* No evidence of reactive marrow fibrosis
Minor criteria	1. Leukoerythroblastosis
	2. ↑ serum LDH
	3. Anaemia
	4. Palpable splenomegaly

* Small-to-large megakaryocytes with an aberrant nuclear/cytoplasmic ratio and hyperchromatic and irregularly folded nuclei and dense clustering.

Diagnostic algorithm for PMF

Tefferi and Vardiman[16] suggest a diagnostic algorithm based on the 2008 WHO diagnostic criteria.

- BM biopsy, reticulin stain, cytogenetic studies and mutation screening for *JAK2*-V617F:
  - Ph chromosome +ve → *CML.*
  - V617F +ve or del(13q) → *PMF likely* **but** *use histology to exclude other myeloid neoplasm.*
  - Other cytogenetic abnormalities → *Could be PMF* **but also** *MDS or other myeloid neoplasm.*
  - Normal cytogenetics and V617F –ve → *If megakaryocytes dwarf* **consider** *FISH for BCR-ABL* **otherwise** *use histology for specific diagnosis.*

Prognostic factors

Adverse prognosis is associated with:

- Marked anaemia—degree of anaemia appears to be the most important prognostic factor for a patient with PMF.
- Older age.
- WBC count.
- Number of blasts in peripheral blood.
- Constitutional symptoms.
- Abnormal karyotype (other than 13q– or 20q–); strongest predictor of poor survival in post-PV MF and post-ET MF.[17]
- High CD34+ cell count.
- Presence of *JAK2*-V617F mutation.

Risk assessment

Risk assessment has become important to identify patients for whom the risks of SCT are appropriate. A number of systems have been developed but none is clearly superior.

The simple Lille scoring system based on 2 adverse prognostic factors has been widely used in both PMF and post-PV/ET MF.[18]

Adverse factors

- Hb <10 g/dL.
- WBC $<4 \times 10^9$/L or $>30 \times 10^9$/L

Table 7.9 Lille prognostic scoring system for MF

Number of factors	Risk group	Cases (%)	Median survival (months)
0	Low	47	93
1	Intermediate	45	26
2	High	8	13

An expanded scoring system has been developed[15] to incorporate 3 additional independent risk factors (📖 Table 7.10):

- Hb <10 g/dL.
- WBC $<4 \times 10^9$/L or $>30 \times 10^9$/L.
- Constitutional symptoms.[19]
- ≥1% blasts in PB.[19]
- Cytogenetic abnormalities other than 13q– or 20q–.[20]

Table 7.10 Expanded prognostic scoring system for MF

Number of factors	Risk group	Expected median survival (years)
0	Low	>10
1	Intermediate	5–10
≥2	High	<5

A system using 3 adverse prognostic factors has been developed for younger patients with PMF based on analysis of 121 patients aged ≤55 years with a median survival of 10.6 years (double that for PMF patients in general at 3.5–5 years)[21] (📖 Table 7.11):

- Hb ≤10 g/dL.
- Constitutional symptoms (fevers, sweats, weight loss).
- ≥1% blasts in PB.[19]

Table 7.11 Prognostic scoring system for younger patients with PMF

Number of factors	Risk group	Median survival (years)
≤1	Low	>14
2–3	High	<3

A further system based on the analysis of 160 younger (<60 years) transplant-eligible patients uses 3 parameters from the FBC; it is simple and has strong discriminative value (Table 7.12):[22]

- Hb <10g/dL.
- WBC <4 ×10⁹/L or >30 ×10⁹/L.
- Platelets <100 ×10⁹/L.

Table 7.12 FBC-based prognostic scoring system for transplant-eligible patients with PMF

Number of factors	Risk group	Median survival (months)
0	Low	155
1	Intermediate	69
≥2	High	23.5

Management

- MF is incurable except by allogeneic SCT but few patients are eligible; no other treatment alters disease course, prevents leukaemic transformation, or prolongs survival.
- Treatment is largely palliative; aims to improve anaemia, alleviate symptomatic organomegaly, and hypercatabolic symptoms.
- Asymptomatic cases with minimal FBC abnormalities and splenic enlargement should simply be observed with regular follow-up.
- *Allopurinol* should be commenced to treat or prevent hyperuricaemia.

Treatment of anaemia

- Treatment for anaemia should be considered at Hb <11g/dL, in symptomatic patients and those with reduced functional capacity.[23]
- *Red cell transfusion* for symptomatic anaemia; transfuse on basis of symptoms not at a specific Hb level; Fe chelation therapy should be initiated when long-term transfusion therapy is commenced.
- *Androgen therapy:* semi-synthetic androgen danazol commenced at a dose of 200mg tds, tapering to minimum effective dose in responders after 6 months improves Hb in ~40%[24]; median time to response 5 months; most respond within 2–3 months, some later (6–9 months); response usually transient; fewer side effects than other androgens e.g. oxymetholone; frequent slight ↑ in LFTs and androgenic effects in ♀; monitor LFTs; may have synergistic effect with EPO[25]; recommended 1st-line treatment of anaemia in PMF by the Nordic Guidelines.[23]
- *Corticosteroids*: prednisolone (1mg/kg/d) primarily indicated for PMF patients with DAGT+ haemolysis but may be effective in others.[23]

- *EPO*: rHuEPO at initial dose of 10,000 units 3 × weekly achieves responses in 40–50% of patients which may be maintained >12 months in half [25, 26]; Darbepoetin alfa at initial dose 150mcg/week rising to 300mcg/week if no response after 4–8 weeks achieves similar response rate[27]; serum EPO level <125 U/L increases the probability of response; EPO recommended in treatment of PMF-associated anaemia in patients unresponsive to danazol or in whom it is inappropriate[23]; alternatively if serum EPO inadequate give trial of rHuEPO/darbepoetin for 3 months and continue in responders; if serum EPO adequate or non-reponder to EPO, give trial of danazol. [28]

Anti-angiogenic agents

- *Thalidomide*: at low dose (50mg/d) in combination with prednisolone (0.5mg/kg/d) can improve anaemia (in up to 70%), thrombocytopenia (in up to 75%), and reduce speen size (in 19%) [29]; higher doses of thalidomide are poorly tolerated and benefit has been difficult to demonstrate; low dose thalidomide +prednisolone is recommended in non-responders to danazol and EPO. [23]
- *Lenalidomide*: (10mg/d for 3–4 months) can improve anaemia (22%), thrombocytopenia (50%), and splenomegaly (33%) [30] and reduce cells bearing marker chromosomes and *JAK2*-V617F. [31]

Cytoreductive therapy

- Controls proliferative features (leucocytosis, thrombocytosis, splenomegaly, and constitutional symptoms); no effect on disease course; generally worsens anaemia.
- *Hydroxycarbamide (HC)*: cytoreductive therapy of choice[23]; usually promptly reduces leucocytosis, thrombocytosis and hypercatabolic symptoms; splenomegaly response may take several months; commence at 15–20mg/kg/d and titrate to maintain ↔ counts; generally well tolerated apart from worsening anaemia.
- *Cytotoxic alternatives to HC*: low-dose *melphalan* (2.5mg tiw) and *busulfan* (2mg/d for 1–2 monthss at 3–6-month intervals) can normalize counts and reduce splenomegaly but are associated with rates of leukaemic transformation up to 30% (reviewed in references 23 and 32).
- *Cladribine (2-CDA):* recommended in symptomatic patients refractory to other therapies[23]; also useful for management of thrombocytosis, leucocytosis, and progressive hepatomegaly after splenectomy[33]; dose 0.05–0.1mg/kg for 7d per month for up to 5 cycles.
- *IFN-α:* 5 million units tiw controls hyperproliferative features but poor tolerance limits its utility (reviewed in reference 32); has been recommended for younger patients due to concerns about leukaemogenesis risk with HC. [23]
- *Anagrelide*: may control thrombocytosis in patients intolerant of other cytoreductive therapy but no impact on myelofibrosis.

Splenectomy

- Palliative measure indicated for massive or symptomatic splenomegaly, excessive transfusion requirements, refractory thrombocytopenia, hypercatabolic symptoms unresponsive to cytoreduction, uncontrollable haemolysis, and portal hypertension;

- Evaluate coagulation system pre-operatively; contra-indicated in patients with thrombocytosis—control pre-operatively.
- A review of 314 patients treated from 1976–2004 reports 7% operative mortality, 28% peri-operative morbidity (infection, thrombosis, bleeding), 76% symptomatic improvement, 50% improvement in anaemia, and 19-month median overall survival; survival was ↓ in patients with pre-operative thrombocytopenia $<100 \times 10^9$/L; postsplenectomy thrombocytosis occurred in 29% and accelerated hepatomegaly in 10%; peri-operative thrombo-haemorrhagic complications were ↓ by platelet apheresis and prompt use of cytoreductive agents.[34]
- No evidence that splenectomy is followed by an ↑ risk of leukaemic transformation.

Radiotherapy

- *Splenic irradiation* may be used to reduce spleen size and discomfort in patients unfit for splenectomy (3–6-month benefit)[35]; due to transient benefit and the risk of severe pancytopenia (~45%), not recommended for most patients; irradiation pre-splenectomy increases risk of post-op bleeding.
- Hepatic irradiation contraindicated due to same problems.
- Low dose involved field irradiation is useful treatment for extramedullary haemopoietic (EMH) infiltrates at other sites e.g. paraspinal, pericardium, pleural, or peritoneal cavities (causing effusion or ascites) and whole lung irradiation is effective when pulmonary EMH causes pulmonary hypertension.[15,32]

Allogeneic SCT

- Only therapy for PMF with curative potential; consider in all patients ≤65 years with high-risk features at diagnosis or later in the disease course.
- Myeloablative conditioning regimens have been associated with high transplant-related mortality (25–48%; reviewed in reference 36).
- Advanced age is an important prognostic factor in myeloablative SCT: 14% patients ≥45 years survived at 5 years *vs.* 62% younger patients.[37]
- Cyclophosphamide + busulfan appears to give better outcomes than TBI-based conditioning regimens due to lower toxicity.
- Myeloablative SCT may be expected to achieve 33–53% CR rate, 27–48% TRM at 1 year and 41–64% OS between 2.8–5 years (reviewed in reference 36)
- Reduced-intensity conditioning (RIC) reduces toxicity in older patients including those with unrelated donors; the 2 largest studies (reviewed in reference 36) each with 21 patients with median age ~54 years, reported CR in ~75%, 10–16% TRM at 1 year, and ~85% OS between 2.2–2.7 years.
- The optimum RIC regimen has not been established.
- The place of splenectomy before SCT is unclear though it may be associated with more rapid haematological reconstitution.
- Responses to donor lymphocyte infusions (DLI) in patients who have relapsed after allo-SCT have been reported.[32]
- Myeloablative or RIC SCT is indicated in patients with high risk PMF aged <45 years; RIC SCT should be considered in patients suitable for

intensive therapy with high risk PMF aged 45–65 years; RIC SCT should be considered in patients with intermediate risk PMF on an individual basis.

Novel therapies[36]

- Small molecule inhibitors of *JAK2*-V617F are in early phase clinical trials; encouraging clinical activity in PMF with partial or complete resolution of splenomegaly and reduction in constitutional symptoms.
- Bortezomib, the proteasome inhibitor that inhibits NFκB is in early phase trials in PMF.
- Azacitidine and decitabine are hypomethylating agents in early phase studies as single agents or in combination with a histone deacetylase inhibitor.
- Inhibitors of vascular endothelial growth factor (VEGF) are in early phase trials.

Prognosis

- Worst prognosis of the Ph –ve MPNs: median survival 3.5–5 years (range 1–30 years).
- Morbidity and mortality commonly due to leukaemic transformation, portal hypertension, infection, haemorrhage, and thrombosis.
- Hypersplenism often develops as the spleen enlarges.
- Progressive cachexia occurs due to hypercatabolic state in advanced PMF.
- Death in symptomatic cases usually due to infection or haemorrhage.
- Up to 20% transform to AML refractory to intensive chemotherapy.

References

1. Baxter, E.J. *et al.* (2005). Acquired mutation of the tyrosine kinase JAK2 in human myeloproliferative disorders. *Lancet*, **365**, 1054–61.
2. Scott, L.M. *et al.* (2006). Progenitors homozygous for the V617F JAK2 mutation occur in most patients with polycythemia vera, but not essential thrombocythemia. *Blood*. **108**, 2435–7.
3. Mesa, R. *et al.* (2006). A longitudinal study of the JAK2V617F mutation in myelofibrosis with myeloid metaplasia: analysis at two time points. *Haematologica*, **91**, 415–6.
4. Wernig, G. *et al.* (2006). Expression of Jak2V617F causes a polycythemia vera-like disease with associated myelofibrosis in a murine bone marrow transplant model. *Blood*. **107**, 4274–81.
5. Campbell, P.J. *et al* (2006). V617F mutation in JAK2 is associated with poorer survival in idiopathic myelofibrosis. *Blood*, **107**, 2098–100.
6. Tefferi, A. *et al.* (2006). Respective clustering of unfavorable and favorable cytogenetic clones in myelofibrosis with myeloid metaplasia with homozygosity for JAK2V617F and response to erythropoietin therapy. *Cancer*, **106**, 1739–43.
7. Pardanani, A.D. *et al.* (2006). MPL515 mutations in myeloproliferative and other myeloid disorders: a study of 118 patients. *Blood*. **108**, 3472–6.
8. Lasho, T.L. *et al.* (2006). Concurrent MPL515 and JAK2V617F mutations in myelofibrosis: chronology of clonal emergence and changes in mutant allele burden over time. *Br J Haematol*, **135**, 683–7.
9. Levine, R.L. *et al.* (2007). Role of JAK2 in the pathogenesis and therapy of myeloproliferative disorders. *Nat Rev Cancer*, 7, 673–83.
10. Guglielmelli, P. *et al.* (2007). GIMEMA –Italian Registry of Myelofibrosis; MPD Research Consortium. Anaemia characterizes patients with myelofibrosis harbouring Mpl mutation. *Br J Haematol*, **137**, 244–7.
11. Al-Assar, O. *et al.* (2005). Gains on 9p are common genomic aberrations in idiopathic myelofibrosis: a comparative genomic hybridization study. *Br J Haematol*, **129**, 66–71.
12. Dong, M. and Blobe, G.C. (2006). Role of transforming growth factor-beta in hematologic malignancies. *Blood*, **107**, 4589–96.

13. Massa, M. *et al.* (2005). Circulating CD34+, CD133+ and vascular endothelial growth factor receptor 2-positive endothelial progenitor cells in myelofibrosis with myeloid metaplasia. *J Clin Oncol*, **23**, 5688–95.
14. Thiele, J. *et al.* (2001). Clinical and morphological criteria for the diagnosis of prefibrotic idiopathic (primary) myelofibrosis. *Ann Hematol*, **80**, 160–5.
15. Tefferi, A. and Barbui, T. (2005). *bcr/abl*–negative, classic myeloproliferative disorders: diagnosis and treatment. *Mayo Clin Proc*, **80**, 1220–32.
16. Tefferi, A. and Vardiman, J.W. (2008). Classification and diagnosis of myeloproliferative neoplasms: The 2008 World Health Organization criteria and point-of-care diagnostic algorithms. *Leukemia*. **22**, 14–22.
17. Dingli, D. *et al.* (2006). Presence of unfavorable cytogenetic abnormalities is the strongest predictor of poor survival in secondary myelofibrosis. *Cancer*, **106**, 1985–9.
18. Dupriez, B. *et al.* (1996). Prognostic factors in agnogenic myeloid metaplasia: a report on 195 cases with a new scoring system. *Blood*, **88**, 1013–8.
19. Cervantes, F. *et al.* (1997). Identification of 'short-lived' and 'long-lived' patients at presentation of idiopathic myelofibrosis. *Br J Haematol*, **97**, 635–40.
20. Tefferi, A. *et al.* (2001). Cytogenetic findings and their clinical relevance in myelofibrosis wioth myeloid metaplasia. *Br J Haematol*, **113**, 763–71.
21. Ahmed, A. and Chang, C.C. (2006). Chronic idiopathic myelofibrosis: clinicopathologic features, pathogenesis and prognosis. *Arch Pathol Lab Med*, **130**, 1133–43.
22. Dingli, D. *et al.* (2006). Prognosis in transplant eligible patients with agnogenic myeloid metaplasia: a simple CBC-based scoring system. *Cancer* **106**, 623–30.
23. Nordic MPD Study Group (2007). Guidelines for the diagnosis and treatment of patients with polycythemia vera, essential thrombocythemia and idiopathic myelofibrosis. www.sfhem.se/filarkiv/files/vardprogram/NMPDGuidelines2007.pdf
24. Cervantes, F. *et al.* (2005). Efficacy and tolerability of danazol as a treatment for the anaemia of myelofibrosis with myeloid metaplasia: long-term results in 30 patients. *Br J Haematol*, **129**, 771–5.
25. Hasselbalch, H.C. *et al.* (2002). Successful treatment of anaemia in idiopathic myelofibrosis with recombinant human erythropoietin. *Am J Hematol*, **70**, 92–9.
26. Cervantes, F. *et al.* (2004). Erythropoietin treatment of the anaemia of myelofibrosis with myeloid metaplasia: results in 20 patients and review of the literature. *Br J Haematol*, **127**, 399–403.
27. Cervantes, F, *et al.* (2006), Darbepoetin-alpha for the anaemia of myelofibrosis with myeloid metaplasia. *Br J Haematol*, 134, 184–6.
28. Cervantes, F. (2007). Myelofibrosis: biology and treatment. *Eur J Haematol*, **79** (68), 13–17.
29. Mesa, R.A. *et al.* (2003). A phase 2 trial of combination low-dose thalidomide and prednisone for the treatment of myelofibrosis with myeloid metaplasia. *Blood*, **101**, 2534–41.
30. Tefferi, A. *et al.* (2006). Lenalidomide therapy in myelofibrosis with myeloid metaplasia. *Blood*, **108**, 1158–64.
31. Tefferi, A. *et al.* (2007). Lenalidomide therapy in del(5)(q31)-associated myelofibrosis: cytogenetic and JAK2v617F molecular remissions. *Leukemia*, **108**, 1158–64.
32. Arana-Yi, C. *et al.* (2006). Advances in the therapy of chronic idiopathic myelofibrosis. *Oncologist*, **11**, 929–43.
33. Faoro, L.N. *et al.* (2005). Long-term analysis of the palliative benefit of 2-chlorodeoxyadenosine for myelofibrosis with myeloid metaplasia. *Eur J Haematol*, **74**, 117–20.
34. Mesa, R.A. *et al.* (2006). Palliative goals, patient selection and perioperative platelet management: outcomes and lessons from 3 decades of splenectomy for myelofibrosis with myeloid metaplasia at the Mayo Clinic. *Cancer*, **107**, 361–70.
35. Elliot, M.A. *et al.* (1998). Splenic irradiation for symptomatic splenomegaly associated with myelofibrosis with myeloid metaplasia. *Br J Haematol*, **103**, 505–11.
36. Hoffman, R. and Rondelli, D. (2007). Biology and treatment of primary myelofibrosis. *Hematology 2007*, 346–354.
37. Guardiola, P. *et al.* (2000). Myelofibrosis with myeloid metaplasia. *N Engl J Med*, **343**, 659.

Chronic neutrophilic leukaemia (CNL)

- Characterised by peripheral blood mature neutrophilia ($\geq 25 \times 10^9$/L) without significant left shift, monocytosis, eosinophilia, or basophilia.[1]
- Monoclonality of neutrophil proliferation in CNL demonstrated by human androgen receptor gene assay (HUMARA) in ♀ patients.[2]
- Before considering a diagnosis of CNL, must exclude:
  - Leukaemoid reaction due to underlying chronic infection or occult neoplasia esp. myeloma (a high proportion of reported cases of 'CNL' associated with a plasma cell disorder[3]) or carcinoma.
  - CML.
  - MDS.
- Very rare; although ~150 cases reported,[2] a critical review suggests minority fulfil criteria for 'true' CNL and this diagnosis has encompassed a number of distinct pathological entities.[3]
- Median age ~65 years, range 15–86; ♂:♀ ratio 2:1.[3]
- Usually asymptomatic at diagnosis; fatigue commonest symptom.[4]
- Modest splenomegaly usual ± hepatomegaly; both due to neutrophil infiltration.
- Usually no anaemia or thrombocytopenia at presentation.
- Mean WBC 54 × 10^9/L (>80% segmented neutrophils and bands; <10% (usually <5%) immature granulocytes; <1% blasts); toxic granulation frequent; NAP usually ↑; no dysplastic features; both CML and reactive leucocytosis usually associated with more marked 'left shift'.
- ↑ serum B_{12} and ↑ uric acid (and history of gout) common.
- Marrow hypercellular due to neutrophil proliferation; M:E ratio may be ≥ 20:1; blasts <5%; normal megakaryocytes; no dysplasia or significantly ↑ reticulin; no evidence of other MPN or MDS.
- BM cytogenetics usually normal; abnormalities described in up to 37%[3]; none specific; del(20q), +8, +9, and del(11q) reported but may be 2°[5]; no Ph chromosome or *BCR-ABL* fusion gene.
- Variable prognosis described for patients with 'CNL' with survival up to 20 years.[1] 'True' CNL may have median OS of 30 months with only 28% 5-year OS,[3,4] death due to blast transformation, progression without transformation, bleeding, and infection.[4]
- Progressive neutrophilia with anaemia and thrombocytopenia common; a significant proportion of patients with CNL progress to AML.
- Disease acceleration heralded by progressive treatment-refractory neutrophilia, marked splenomegaly, anaemia, thrombocytopenia, and the appearance of immature myeloid progenitors including blasts in the peripheral blood.[4]
- No standard treatment recommendation; optimum therapy undefined.
- Treatment may be unnecessary if asymptomatic.
- Hydroxycarbamide (HC) may control progessive neutrophilia and splenomegaly and maintain a prolonged stable phase; recommended 1st-line therapy with median response of 12 months;[4] busulfan can achieve the same effect; IFN-α is option as 2nd-line therapy[4] though responses to 2nd-line therapy often short-lived.[5]
- AML-type induction therapy is ineffective.[5]

- Splenic irradiation and splenectomy can reduce tumour bulk and relieve abdominal discomfort; splenectomy may aggravate leucocytosis.[6]
- Allogeneic SCT is potentially curative [6,7] and in view of the poor prognosis of patients with 'true' CNL, should be considered in eligible patients.

References

1. Imbert, M. *et al.* (2001). Chronic neutrophilic leukaemia. In Jaffe, E.S. *et al.* (eds.) *World Health Organization classification of tumours. Pathology and genetics. Tumours of haematopoietic and lymphoid tissues, vol 1*. Lyon: IARC Press, pp.27–8.
2. Bohm, J. *et al.* (2003). Evidence of clonality in chronic neutrophilic leukaemia. *J Clin Pathol,* **56**, 292–5.
3. Reilly, J.T. (2002). Chronic neutrophilic leukaemia: a distinct clinical entity? *Br J Haematol,* **116**, 10–18.
4. Tefferi, A. *et al.* (2006). Atypical myeloproliferative disorders: diagnosis and treatment. *Mayo Clin Proc,* **81**, 553–63.
5. Elliot, M.A. *et al.* (2001). Chronic neutrophilic leukemia (CNL): a clinical, pathologic and cytogenetic study. *Leukemia*, **15**, 35–40.
6. Hasle, H. *et al.* (1996). Chronic neutrophilic leukaemia in adolesence and young adulthood. *Br J Haematol,* **9**, 628–30.
7. Pilotis, E. *et al.* (2002). Allogeneic bone marrow transplantation in the management of chronic neutrophilic leukemia *Leuk Lymphoma,* **43**, 2051–4.

Chronic eosinophilic leukaemia (CEL) and idiopathic hypereosinophilic syndrome (HES)

Eosinophilia in the peripheral blood and tissues may occur in a heterogeneous group of conditions. Diagnosis of CEL or HES requires exclusion of conditions associated with 2° eosinophilia, molecularly defined myeloid neoplasms associated with eosinophilia, and phenotypically abnormal and/or clonal T-lymphocytes.

Conditions associated with 2° eosinophilia should be excluded (📖 see p. 115):

- Allergic: asthma, allergic broncopulmomary aspergillosis, drug reactions.
- Infectious and parasitic: helminths, ectoparasites (scabies), protozoa, fungi (coccidiomycosis), mycobacteria, and viruses (HIV, HSV).
- Inflammatory: Loeffler's syndrome, collagen vascular disorders (Wegener's granulomatosis, PAN, SLE), sarcoid.
- Neoplastic: CML, AML with inv(16), ALL, angioimmunoblastic lymphoma, chronic MPNs, Hodgkin and non-Hodgkin lymphoma, adenocarcinoma.
- Immune dysregulation: Wiskott–Aldrich syndrome, phenotypically aberrant T lymphocytes with abnormal release of cytokines.
- Metabolic: hypoadrenalism.

The 2008 WHO classification[1] has redefined myeloid neoplasms with molecularly characterized clonal eosinophilia, previously classified under CEL/HES, as a new category of their own and removed them from the MPN category (📖 p.254).

Myeloid neoplasms associated with molecularly characterized eosinophilia

- Myeloid neoplasms associated with platelet derived growth factor α (*PDGFRA*) rearrangement.
- Myeloid neoplasms associated with platelet derived growth factor β (*PDGFRB*) rearrangement.
- Myeloid neoplasms associated with fibroblast growth factor receptor 1 (*FGFR1*) rearrangement (8p11 myeloproliferative syndrome).

Myeloid neoplasms associated with PDGFRA rearrangement

- Rare disorder. Karyotype usually normal.
- Activating mutation of the gene for *PDGFRA* due to interstitial deletion at 4q12 producing a *FIP1L1-PDGFRA* fusion gene[2] associated with HES, CEL, and systemic mastocytosis (SM).[2–4]
- t(4;22)(q12;q11) producing *BCR-PDGFRA* fusion gene also described associated with atypical CML.[5]
- *FIP1L1-PDGFRA* detected by FISH in 14% of patients with '1° eosinophilia'; also detectable by RT-PCR; almost all classified histologically as SM due to mast cell infiltrates in the BM.[4] SM-CEL has been suggested as nomenclature.[6]

- Occurs almost exclusively in ♂; associated with eosinophil-related tissue damage, elevated serum tryptase, splenomegaly, BM hypercellularity with reticulin fibrosis, and atypical mast cells.
- Extremely sensitive to imatinib therapy: 100mg/d achieved 100% durable clinical and haematological CR in 8 patients;[7] if clinical or molecular relapse occurs, the dose should be ↑ to 400mg/d;[8] concomitant prednisolone therapy (1mg/kg/d) is recommended for initial 1–2 weeks to reduce risk of drug-induced cardiogenic shock.[6]

Myeloid neoplasms associated with PDGFRB rearrangement

- Rare disorder.
- Activating mutation of *PDGFRB* gene at 5q33 associated with eosinophilia sometimes accompanied by monocytosis.[9]
- Usually involves translocation e.g. t(5;12)(q33;p13) and karyotype usually abnormal.
- Detected in patients previously diagnosed with CEL or CMML.[10]
- Rarely affects ♀; also responds to imatinib.

Myeloid neoplasms associated with FGFR1 rearrangement

- Rare aggressive disorder also known as 8p11 myeloproliferative syndrome (EMS)/stem cell leukemia-lymphoma syndrome causing eosinophilia associated with myeloproliferative and myelodysplastic features and T-cell ALL with progression to AML.[11]
- Translocations involving 8p11 and multiple partners result in constitutive activation of a fusion tyrosine kinase involving *FGFR1*.[11]
- Unresponsive to imatinib; only allogeneic SCT is effective at suppressing the malignant clone.[11]

Eosinophilia associated with aberrant T-lymphocytes

- Eosinophilia may result from the presence of immunophenotypically aberrant, often demonstratively clonal, IL-5-secreting T-lymphocytes.[12]
- A study of 60 patients, recruited mainly from dermatology clinics reported 16 with circulating T-cells with aberrant phenotype of whom 8 had clonal T-cell receptor (TCR) rearrangement; 4 patients subsequently developed T-cell lymphoma.[13]
- Aberrant phenotype includes absent, reduced, or ↑ expression of several antigens (e.g. CD2, CD3, CD4, CD5, CD6, CD7, or CD95), usually CD3–,CD4+,CD8–, or expression of activation markers (CD25 or HLA-DR).
- Elevated serum IgE may be further evidence of Th2 activation.
- Equal frequency in ♂ and ♀; dermatological involvement in majority; GI symptoms and obstructive lung disease also common but endomyocardial fibrosis and myelofibrosis rare; CD3–CD4+CD8– and del(6q) associated with ↑ risk of progrssion to T-cell lymphoma.[14]
- In a patient with skin abnormalities, lymphocytosis, or abnormal lymphocytes, immunophenotype and TCR gene analysis are recommended.[12]
- Prednisolone as a single agent or in combination with IFN-α is usually effective; mepolizumab (monoclonal antibody to IL-5) may have a role.

CEL, not otherwise categorized (CEL-NOC)

Uncommon clonal proliferation of eosinophil precursors causing persistent ↑ in mature and immature eosinophils in PB (≥1.5 × 10^9/L) and in BM.

Diagnosis of CEL-NOC[1, 15] requires:

- Persistent peripheral blood eosinophilia ≥1.5 × 10^9/L.
- Exclusion of 2° eosinophilia.
- Exclusion of molecularly characterized myeloid neoplasms associated with eosinophilia.
- Exclusion of other acute or chronic myeloid neoplasm.
- No evidence of phenotypically abnormal and/or clonal T-lymphocytes.
- Evidence of another clonal cytogenetic abnormality (e.g. +8, i(17q)), *or* >2% PB blasts *or* >5% (but <20%) BM blasts.

Marked ♂ predominance; usually age 20–50 years; incidental finding or short history of fever, malaise, fatigue, sweats, weight loss, skin rash, angio-edema, muscle pains, pruritus, diarrhoea, and ↑ susceptibility to infection; splenomegaly in 30–50%.

PB eosinophils mainly mature with few eosinophilic myelocytes or pro-myelocytes; some show abnormalities: sparse granulation, vacuolation, hypersegmentation, hyposegmentation, or large forms; neutrophilia with left shift frequent; platelets may be ↔, ↓, or ↑.

BM hypercellular; usually 10–30% eosinophils; often >5% blasts; no specific cytogenetic or molecular abnormality; no dysplastic features, Ph chromosome or *BCR-ABL* fusion gene.

Associated with tissue infiltration by immature eosinophils, anaemia, and thrombocytopenia; end-organ damage may occur due to leukaemic infiltration or release of eosinophil cytokines or enzymes: scarring of mitral/tricuspid valves, peripheral neuropathy, CNS dysfunction, pulmonary symptoms, and arthritis.

Eosinophilia may be controlled by hydroxycarbamide (up to 2g/d); does not generally respond to imatinib. In younger patients consider sibling allogeneic SCT.

HES

Characterized by PB eosinophilia ≥1.5 × 10^9/L for >6 months for which no underlying cause can be found and by end-organ damage. Diagnosis of HES is by exclusion and requires the first 5 criteria listed for CEL-NOC[1, 15] but in addition:

- **NO** evidence of a clonal cytogenetic abnormality *and* ≤2% PB blasts *and* ≤5% BM blasts.

Incidental finding or symptoms as per CEL-NOC; ♂:♀ ratio ~9:1 (N.B. 20–50% of patients previously diagnosed with HES had *FIP1L1-PDGFR* abnormality which occurs almost exclusively in ♂[13]); peak incidence in 4th decade.

PB eosinophils indistinguishable from CEL-NOC; neutrophilia with left shift frequent; platelets may be ↔, ↓, or ↑; polyclonal increase in immunoglobulins including IgE common; splenomegaly 40%, anaemia 50%; BM hypercellular with 25–75% eosinophils with left shift.

An episodic form associated with angioedema, urticaria, weight gain, fever, and a polyclonal gammopathy including elevated levels of IgE that follows a relatively benign course and is steroid responsive has been described (Gleich's syndrome).[16]

Endomyocardial fibrosis progressing to restrictive cardiomyopathy, skin lesions (angioedema, urticaria), thrombo-embolic disease, pulmonary lesions, arthritis, and CNS dysfunction occur commonly due to infiltration and release of enzymes.

Eosinophilia may be rapidly controlled by prednisolone (1mg/kg/d) tailing slowly to a maintenance dose (70% respond); HC (starting dose 500mg bd, titrating up to 2g/d as necessary) may be added in patients with tissue damage,[6] IFN-α (starting dose 1 million units tiw) is 2nd-line treatment of choice[6,17] and may maintain prolonged remissions associated with improved clinical symptoms and organ disease;[114,17]; IFN-α + HC allows dose reduction and better control than with either agent alone;[18] vincristine, cyclophosphamide, 6-thioguanine and cytarabine have been used with variable results; mepolizumab (monoclonal antibody to IL-5) and alemtuzumab (anti-CD52) may have a role;[14] a trial of imatinib may be effective in some *FIP1L1-PDGFRA* –ve patients;[17] allogeneic SCT may be curative in younger patients.[17]

Investigation of a patient with eosinophilia

All patients with eosinophilia should be assessed with a detailed history including drugs and travel, a full physical examination, blood count and film, routine chemistry, serum IgE, serum B_{12}, ECG, echocardiogram, CXR, pulmonary function tests, and CT chest and abdomen. Further investigations may be indicated by the findings, e.g. parasite screen, HIV serology. If eosinophilia remains unexplained, the diagnostic algorithm recommended by Tefferi and Vardiman[1] and based on the 2008 WHO criteria should be used:

- Perform BM biopsy, tryptase stain, T-cell clonality studies (immunophenotyping and TCR gene rearrangement studies), cytogenetic studies, and FISH or RT-PCR for *FIP1L1-PDGFRA*
  - *FIP1L1-PDGFRA* +ve → *PDGFRA rearranged myeloid neoplasm with eosinophilia*
  - 5q33 translocations → *PDGFRB rearranged myeloid neoplasm with eosinophilia*
  - 8p11 translocations → *FGFR1 rearranged myeloid neoplasm with eosinophilia*
  - BM histology shows abnormalities other than eosinophilia → *Use histology to make specific diagnosis*
  - BM histology unremarkable other than eosinophilia and no clonal T cells → *PB blasts >2% or BM blasts >5% or abnormal cytogenetics*
    —→ Yes → CEL-NOC
    —→ No → HES

Prognosis of CEL-NOC and HES

Variable survival; up to 80% at 5 years decreasing to 42% at 15 years in a series including 40 patients with both diagnoses; in this cohort poor prognostic factors included presence of a concurrent myeloproliferative disorder, lack of response to steroids, cardiac disease, ♂ sex, and degree of eosinophilia.[18] The WHO review identified marked splenomegaly PB blasts, BM blasts, cytogenetic abnormalities and myeloid lineage dysplasia as unfavourable features.[15]

References

1. Tefferi, A. and Vardiman, J.W. (2008). Classification and diagnosis of myeloproliferative neoplasms: The 2008 World Health Organization criteria and point-of-care diagnostic algorithms. *Leukemia,* **22**, 14–22.
2. Cools, J. *et al.* (2003). A tyrosine kinase created by fusion of the *PDGFRA* and *FIP1L1* genes as a therapeutic target of imatinib in idiopathic eosinophilic syndrome. *N Engl J Med,* **348**, 1201–14.
3. Vandenberghe P *et al.* (2004). Clinical and molecular features of FIP1L1-PDGFRA (+) chronic eosinophilic leukemias. *Leukemia,* **18**, 734–42.
4. Pardanani, A. *et al.* (2004). FIP1L1-PDGFRA fusion: prevalence and clinicopathologic correlatesin 89 consecutive patients with moderate to severe eosinophilia. *Blood,* **104**, 3038–45.
5. Trempat, P. *et al.* (2003). Chronic myeloproliferative disorders with rearrangement of the platelet-derived growth factor alpha receptor: a new clinical target for STI571/Glivec. *Oncogene,* **22**, 5702–6.
6. Tefferi, A. *et al.* (2006). Atypical myeloproliferative disorders: diagnosis and treatment. *Mayo Clin Proc,* **81**, 553–63.
7. Elliot, M.A. *et al.* (2004). Immmunophenotypic normalization of aberrant mast cells accompanies histological remission in imatinib-treated patients with eosinophilia-associated mastocytosis. *Leukemia,* **18**, 1027–9.
8. Klion, A.D. *et al.* (2003). Molecular remission and reversal of myelofibrosis in response to imatinib mesylate treatment in patients with the myeloproliferative variant of hypereosinophilic syndrome. *Blood,* **103**, 473–8.
9. Steer, E.J. and Cross, N.C. (2002). Myeloproliferative disorders with translocations of chromosome 5q31–35: role of the platelet-derived growth factor beta. *Acta Haematol,* **107**,113–22.
10. Apperley, J.F. *et al.* (2002). Response to imatinib mesylate in patients with chronic myeloproliferative diseases with rearrangements of the platelet-derived growth factor receptor beta. *N Engl J Med,* **347**, 481–7.
11. Macdonald, D. *et al.* (2002). The 8p11 myeloproliferative syndrome: a distinct clinical entity caused by constitutive activation of FGFR1. *Acta Haematol,* **107**, 101–7.
12. Bain, B. (2004). The idiopathic hypereosinophilic syndrome and eosinophilic leukemias. *Haematologica,* **89**, 133–7.
13. Simon, H.U. *et al.* (1999). Abnormal clones of interleukin-5-producing T cells in idiopathic eosinophilia. *N Engl J Med,* **341**, 1112–20.
14. Klion, A.D. (2005). Recent advances in the diagnosis and treatment of hypereosinophilic syndromes. *Hematology 2005,* 209–14.
15. Bain, B. *et al.* (2001). Chronic eosinophilic leukaemia and the hypereosinophilic syndrome In Jaffe, E.S. *et al.* (eds.) *World Health Organization classification of tumours. Pathology and genetics. Tumours of haematopoietic and lymphoid tissues, vol 1.* Lyon: IARC Press, pp.29–31.
16. Gleich, G.J. *et al.* (1984). Episodic angioedema associated with eosinbophilia. *N Engl J Med* **310**: 1621–6.
17. Gotlib, J. *et al.* (2004). The FIP1L1-PDGFRα fusion tyrosine kinase in hypereosinophilic syndrome and chronic eosinophilic leukemia: implications for diagnosis, classification and management. *Blood,* **103**, 2879–91.
18. Butterfield, J.H. (2005). Interferon treatment for hypereosinophilic syndromes and systemic mastocytosis. *Acta Haematol,* **114**, 26–40.

Mast cell disease (mastocytosis)

Mastocytosis is a heterogeneous group of diseases characterized by abnormal proliferation of mast cells in one or more organ systems including skin, BM, liver, spleen, and lymph nodes. They range from skin lesions that may spontaneously regress to aggressive multi-system disease with a poor prognosis (Table 7.13).

Table 7.13 WHO classification of mastocytosis [1,2]

Variant	Subvariants
Cutaneous mastocytosis (CM)	• Maculopapular CM (MPCM)/ urticaria pigmentosa (UP) • Diffuse CM (DCM) • Mastocytoma of skin
Indolent systemic mastocytosis (ISM)	• Smouldering SM (SSM) • Isolated bone marrow mastocytosis (BMM)
Systemic mastocytosis with an associated clonal haematological non-mast cell lineage disease (SM-AHNMD)*	• SM-AML • SM-MDS • SM-MPN • SM-CMML • SM-NHL • SM-CEL • SM-HES
Aggressive systemic mastocytosis. (ASM)	• Lymphadenopathic SM with eosinophilia**
Mast cell leukaemia (MCL)	• Typical MCL • Aleukaemic MCL***
(Extracutaneous) mast cell sarcoma (MCS)	
Extracutaneous mastocytoma	

* The non-mast cell lineage disease must also be defined by WHO criteria; ** in a subgroup of these patients the *FIP1L1/PDGFRA*-fusion gene is detectable; *** circulating mast cells <10%.

Epidemiology

Occurs at any age; median age of SM 50–60 years; range 5–88; CM most common in children: median age 2.5 months, may be present at birth, usually evident by 6 months;[2] after age 10 years median age of CM 26 years.

Pathogenesis

Mast cells are derived from pluripotential haemopoietic cells and are the effector cells of the immediate allergic reaction via high affinity receptors for IgE. Most variants of SM are clonal and a somatic mutation of c-*KIT* (usually D816V on exon 17), the proto-oncogene, located at 4q12, that encodes the transmembrane tyrosine kinase receptor for stem cell factor (SCF), is present in >80%.[3–5] Other mutations described in ~25% of cases lacking the D816V mutation but each individually rare.[5–7] Several other KIT mutations described in familial SM.[5] These mutations lead to constitutive activation of KIT protein independent of SCF binding, causing mast cell proliferation and suppressing apoptosis. In paediatric mastocytosis and CM *KIT*-activating mutations are rare.

KIT mutations are frequently observed in other neoplasms. The D816V mutation is rarely found in AML with inv(16) or t(8;21), seminoma, germinoma while exon 11 mutations of *KIT* are found in gastrointestinal stromal tumours (GIST).[5]

Clinical symptoms in mastocytosis are due (1) to the release of mast cell granules containing pro-inflammatory and vasoactive mediators (including histamine, tryptase, heparin, TNF-α, PGD2, cytokines, and chemokines) that have both local and systemic effects, and (2) to organ infiltration.

In CM mast cell proliferation is confined to skin; involvement of at least one extracutaneous organ defines SM, whether there is evidence of skin involvement or not.[2]

CM

Clinical features and presentation

- Most cases of CM are seen in infants and children; involvement is generally limited to the skin; commonest form is MCPM/UP with widespread cutaneous involvement with a few or many small lightly pigmented red-brown macules and papules. Intensifies on rubbing (Darier's sign). Usually transient; begins in 1st year and disappears at or shortly after puberty; progression to SM is unusual [6,8]
- Diffuse CM is less frequent, almost exclusive to children and may cause smooth, red, or greatly thickened skin; solitary localized mastocytoma occurs as a tumour; rare; generally occurs in infants; benign course.
- Adult MCPM/UP is associated with small heavily pigmented macular lesions; onset in young adults; lesions remain stable or increase with time though rarely decrease spontaneously;[6,8] often progressive with systemic organ involvement usually BM (46%), lymph nodes (~25% at diagnosis), spleen (~50% at diagnosis), liver, and GI tract.
- Familial mastocytosis causes cutaneous disease in infancy, persists into adult life, and may progress to systemic involvement; rare.

Investigation and diagnosis

- Diagnosis of CM (usually in children) requires demonstration of typical clinical findings with histological evidence of skin infiltration by mast cells and no evidence of systemic involvement, e.g. elevated serum tryptase or organomegaly.
- Adults with rash frequently misdiagnosed as CM, but SM criteria present in most cases. Undertake SM investigations in all adult patients.
- Pre-diagnostic term 'mastocytosis in the skin' (MIS) should be applied until SM excluded.[6]
- Evaluate MIS by:
  - Inspection of lesional skin (plus photography).
  - Skin biopsy with tryptase immunohistochemistry (IHC).
  - *KIT* mutation analysis.
- Proposed minimum diagnostic criteria for MIS are typical exanthema (major criterion) plus ≥1 of the following minor criteria: (i) monomorphic MC infiltrate either large aggregates of tryptase-+ve cells (>15 per

cluster) or scattered MC (>20 per 40 × high power field); (ii) detection of *KIT* mutation at codon 816 in affected skin.[6]

- Most patients with CM have a normal serum tryptase (median 5ng/mL); almost all patients with SM have a level >20 ng/mL.[6,9]
- In children with serum tryptase >100ng/mL or symptoms/signs of SM and in all adults undertake BM examination to exclude SM.
- In children with serum tryptase <20ng/mL diagnosis of CM may be made without marrow examination unless other signs of SM present.
- In children with serum tryptase 20–100ng/mL, without other signs of SM, provisional diagnosis of MIS established and monitored until puberty; if MIS persists at pubety, examine BM.

Grading

- A clinical grading system has been proposed[6] based on the severity of MIS-specific symptoms: pruritus, flushing, blistering and bullae formation (Table 7.14)

Management

- Patients should avoid agents and situations that provoke a reaction.
- Grade 0 patients are usually not treated unless they suffer from significant non-organic symptoms or systemic mediator-related symptoms; grade 4 patients may be hospitalized and require anti-mediator drugs, stabilizing agents and topical therapy; Valent *et al.*[6] propose the following therapeutic approach shown in Table 7.15.
- Response to therapy is scored as complete regression, major regression (>50% reduction in affected skin), partial regression (10–50%) and no regression (<10%).[6]
- Serum tryptase can be used for monitoring patients with CM; a significant increase can be regarded as evidence of an increase in MC burden and an indication for histological re-assessment of the BM to exclude indolent SM.[9]

Table 7.14 Grading of skin-specific symptoms[a] in patients with mastocytosis[6]

Grade	Definition
0 = no symptoms	Prophylaxis[b], but requires no other therapy[c]
1 = mild, infrequent	Prophylaxis ± therapy as required
2 = mild/moderate, frequent	Requires and can be controlled by daily therapy[d]
3 = severe, frequent	Suboptimal or unsatisfactory control with daily and combination therapy[d]
4 = severe adverse event[e]	Requires immediate therapy and hospitalisation

[a] Pruritus, flushing, blistering, bullae formation; [b] all patients with mastocytosis are advised to avoid precipitating factors and events—for most, prophylactic antihistamines (H1 and H2 receptor antagonists) are recommended; [c] unless patient is focused on cosmetic consequences of the disease or suffers from systemic mediator-related symptoms; [d] despite avoidance of precipitating factors; [e] the frequency of severe adverse events should be reported: 4A: <1/year; 4B: >1/year and <1/month; 4C: >1/month.

Table 7.15 Therapeutic options for cutaneous symptoms in patients with mastocytosis[6]

Symptom (variant)	1st-line, grade 1-2	1st-line, grade 3 and 2nd–line grade 2
Pruritus (all)	H_1 antihistamines Topical sodium cromoglicate	UV irradiation, PUVA, H_1 and H_2 antihistamines, leukotriene antagonists, glucocorticoids
Flushing (all)	H_1 antihistamines Leukotriene antagonists	H_1 and H_2 antihistamines UV irradiation, PUVA,
Blistering (all)	Local therapy H_1 antihistamines	H_1 and H_2 antihistamines Systemic glucocorticoids Topical sodium cromoglicate
Bullae (usually DCM and mastocytomas)	Local care, dressing	H_1 and H_2 antihistamines Systemic glucocorticoids Topical sodium cromoglicate
Mastocytoma lesion with symptoms or increasing size	Local immunosuppressants, local UV irradiation and psoralen bath or cream	Excision

References

1. Valent, P. *et al.* (2001). Diagnostic criteria and classification of mastocytosis: a consensus proposal. Conference Report of "Year 2000 Working Confer4ence on Mastocytosis. *Leuk Res*, **25**, 603–25.
2. Valent, P. *et al.* (2001). Mastocytosis (mast cell disease) In Jaffe, E.S. *et al* (eds.) *World Health Organisation classification of tumours. Pathology and genetics. Tumours of haematopoietic and lymphoid tissues, vol 1.* Lyon: IARC Press, pp.291–302.
3. Buttner C *et al* (1998) Identification of activating c-kit mutations in adult-, but not in childhood-onset indolent mastocytosis: a possible explanation for divergent clinical behaviour. *J Invest Dermatol*, **111**, 1227–31.
4. Fritsche-Polanz, R. *et al.* (2001). Mutation analysis of C-KIT in patients with myelodysplastic syndromes without mastocytosis and cases of systemic mastocytosis. *Br J Haematol*, **113**, 357–64. 5. Orfao, A. *et al.* (2007). Recent advances in the understanding of mastocytosis: the role of *KIT* mutations. *Br J Haematol*, **138**, 12–30.
6. Valent, P. *et al.* (2007). Standards and standardization in mastocytosis: Consensus statements on diagnostics, treatment recommendations and response criteria. *Eur J Clin Invest*, **37**, 435–53.
7. Valent, P. and Metcalfe, D.D. (2004). Mast cell proliferative disorders: diagnosis, classification and therapy. *Hematology 2004*, 153–62.
8. Wolff, K. *et al.* (2001). Clinical and histopathological aspects of cutaneous mastocytosis. *Leuk Res*, **25**, 519–28.
9. Horny, H.P. *et al.* (2007). Mastocytosis: state of the art. *Pathobiology*, **74**, 121–32.

Systemic mastocytosis (SM)

Clinical features and presentation

- Patients typically present with symptoms of mediator release which vary in severity (mild to life-treatening) and may be chronic and recurrent or acute lasting minutes or hours:
  - Urticaria, flushing, dermatographism, pruritus, angioedema, anaphylaxis.
  - Paroxysmal hyper- or hypotension.
  - GI symptoms (80%): abdominal cramps, dyspepsia, nausea, diarrhoea, malabsorption, multiple peptic ulcers, haemorrhage; consider aggressive SM if malabsorption or weight loss.
  - Wheezing, dyspnoea, rhinorrhoea.
  - Neuropsychiatric symptoms (headache, fatigue, irritability, cognitive disorganisation, nightmares).
  - Musculoskeletal pain (25%).
- Less often, patients present with an abnormal blood count (~20%), organomegaly, lymphadenopathy, or pathological fracture.
- May present without skin involvement; frequent in ASM and MCL though may have isolated BM involvement subvariant of ISM.
- SM may follow either an indolent or an aggressive course; organomegaly due to mast cell infiltration may occur in patients with an indolent course;[1]; aggressive SM is characterized by progressive mast cell infiltration of organs causing impaired function: BM failure, hepatocellular failure with ascites, severe diarrhoea and malabsorption, pathological fractures, organomegaly, and pancytopenia.
- Clinical features of SM have been classified as 'B-findings' and 'C-findings' and assist in staging, identification of clinical variants, selection of therapy, and assessment of response.[2,3]
  - ***B-findings:*** define spread of disease; indication of high burden of mast cells, and expansion of the disease without impairment of organ function; B = borderline benign.[2, 4]
    —BM biopsy showing >30% infiltration by mast cells (focal, dense aggregates) and/or serum tryptase level >200ng/mL
    —Hypercellular marrow with loss of fat cells, discrete signs of dysmyelopoiesis without substantial cytopenias or WHO criteria for MDS or MPN
    —Organomegaly: palpable hepatomegaly, splenomegaly or lymphadenopathy (on CT or US >2cm) without impaired organ function
  - ***C-findings:*** define aggressiveness of the infiltrate; indication of impaired organ function due to mast cell infiltration (has to be confirmed by biopsy in most cases); C= consider cytoreduction.[2,5]
    —Cytopenia(s): ANC $<1.0 \times 10^9$/L or Hb <10g/dl or Plt $<100 \times 10^9$/L.
    —Hepatomegaly with ascites and impaired liver function.
    —Palpable splenomegaly with hypersplenism.
    —Malabsorption with hypoalbuminaemia and weight loss.
    —Skeletal lesions: large sized osteolyses or/and severe osteoporosis causing pathological fractures
    —Life threatening organopathy in other organ systems that is definitely caused by an infiltration of the tissue by neoplastic mast cells.

Investigations and diagnosis

When SM is suspected or when an adult is diagnosed with 'MIS' (📖 p.307) or a child with MIS has a serum tryptase >100ng/mL. BM should be examined with tryptase stain, flow cytometry for phenotypically abnormal mast cells (CD25+), and, if available, mutation screening for *KIT*-D816V.[6]

BM biopsy

- Usually sharply demarcated mast cell aggregates in perivascular or peritrabecular locations or randomly distributed; often comprise varying proportions of mast cells, lymphocytes, eosinophils, and fibroblasts; frequently significant fibrosis (90%) and thickening of adjacent bone; in advanced SM diffuse infiltration with marked reticulin or collagen fibrosis.[2]
- Exclude a co-existing haematopoietic neoplasm (SM-AHNMD), hypercellularity or dysmyelopoiesis (prognostic value); exclude reactive non-clonal mast cell hyperplasia that may accompany several haematological disorders where mast cells lack atypia and are sprinkled throughout the marrow rather than in aggregates.[2]
- Immunohistochemistry for tryptase, CD117 (KIT) and CD25 to demonstrate infiltrate of tryptase-+ve spindle-shaped mast cells; if tryptase-+ve round cell infiltrate (<5% spindle-shaped +ve cells), co-expression of CD117 and CD25 highly suggestive of SM but if CD25 –ve consider reactive mast cell hyperplasia.[3]
- If isolated infiltrate only or multifocal small aggregates (<15 MCs) consider minor diagnostic criteria (Table 7.15); if sub-diagnostic (n<3), repeat biopsy; if remains subdiagnostic in patient with MIS, diagnosis CM, in patient without MIS or clonal marker (*KIT*-D816V) diagnosis 'reactive mast cell hyperplasia', without MIS but with monoclonal mast cells (*KIT*-D816V+) 'monoclonal MC activation syndrome' (MMAS) if there are mediator symptoms or 'monoclonal MC with undetermined significance' (MMUS) if asymptomatic.[3]

BM aspirate

- ≥5% mast cells suggests an unfavourable prognosis; ≥20% defines MCL; mild myelodysplasia is found in most patients with SM.[3]
- Mast cells in SM show aberrant morphological features.[3]
- *'Atypical mast cell type I'* is predominant cell type in ISM, associated with a good prognosis and defined by any **2** of:
  - Cytoplasmic extensions (spindle shape).
  - Hypogranular cytoplasm, *or*
  - Off-centre oval nucleus.
- *'Atypical mast cell type II'* mostly immature with bi- or polylobed nucleus, frequently seen in MCL and ASM, also in SSM but rarely ISM, associated with poor prognosis if >5% of MCs.
- Metachromatic blasts may predominate in MCL, also seen in ASM or SSM.
- Non-metachromatic myeloblasts suggest AHNMD and dysplasia; >5% SM-MDS and >20% SM-AML.
- Mature mast cells are well granulated, round cells with a round nucleus; usually seen with atypical mast cells type I in ISM; if predominant cell, consider rare sub-variant 'well-differentiated SM' (*KIT*-F522C or other *KIT* mutation).

Flow cytometry

- Neoplastic SM mast cells usually aberrantly express CD25 ± CD2.
- A suspension of BM cells should be analysed; minimum recommended panel includes CD2, CD25, CD45, and CD117; CD34 may be added when CD117 expression low (frequent in *KIT* mutation[7]) to define MC as CD34–/CD117+/CD45+[3]

KIT-D816V and other KIT mutation analysis

- Neoplastic mast cells in >80% adults with SM exhibit activating *KIT* mutation at codon 816; D816V most common (SM 70–90%; CM 10–30%), all others rare.[3]
- *KIT* mutations also found in some patients with germ cell tumours without co-existing SM (D816V in 10–20%, also in <5% AML).[3]
- RT-PCR and RFLP analysis of unfractionated BM cells after RBC-lysis or marrow mononuclear cells; PB is not an acceptable alternative as often –ve in ISM.[3]
- If –ve result with small infiltrate, interpret with caution; if large infiltrate, confirm –ve result in reference laboratory as wt-KIT and certain other mutants confer imatinib-sensitivity.

Serum tryptase

- Almost all patients with SM have serum tryptase level >20ng/mL.
- In severe allergic reactions, tryptase may be markedly elevated so wait 2d after clinical resolution before measuring; if elevated, consider SM.[3]
- Also elevated in myeloid non-mast cell disorders, AML, CML, MPN, and MDS; therefore a minor criterion only in absence of AHNMD.
- Tryptase level higher with high mast cell burden; in ISM level remains reasonably constant over years; in ASM or MCL levels often increase as disease progresses.
- In ASM or MCL, tryptase levels often decrease with successful cytoreduction.[3]

FBC and film

- No characteristic features; circulating mast cells rare (2%) unless very advanced disease or MCL.
- Mild-to-moderate anaemia ~45%; eosinophilia up to 25% but not all have HES or CEL (screen for *FIP1L1*-PDGFRA, if +ve = SM-CEL; if –ve but CEL-related organopathy = SM-HES), many have ASM, SM-AHNMD or ISM[109]; thrombocytopenia ~20%; monocytosis ~15%; pancytopenia may develop due to BM infiltration or hypersplenism.

Other investigations

- Bone scan/skeletal survey shows bone lesions in 60%; generalized osteosclerosis, focal sclerosis, osteopenia, osteoporosis, or osteolysis.
- Bone densitometry (DXA scan) in all patients with SM.
- Ultrasound of abdomen.
- Serum chemistry.
- Coagulation screen.
- Endoscopy in patients with GI symptoms.
- EEG: if necessary.

Table 7.16 WHO diagnostic criteria for SM[2 3]

Major criterion*	Multifocal, dense infiltrates of mast cells (≥15 mast cells per aggregate) in BM and/or other extracutaneous organ(s) confirmed by tryptase immunohistochemistry
Minor criteria*	1. In biopsy sections of BM or other extracutaneous organs >25% of mast cells show an abnormal spindle-shaped morphology or >25% of mast cells in BM aspirate smears are immature or atypical type I 2. Detection of *c-KIT* mutation D816V or other activating mutation at codon 816 in extracutaneous organ(s); marrow is recommended for screening 3. KIT+ MCs in BM or other extracutaneous organs express CD2 or/and CD25 4. Serum tryptase >20ng/mL (does not count in patients who have AHNMD-type disease)

* If at least 1 major and 1 minor criterion or at least 3 minor criteria are fulfilled, the diagnosis of SM can be established.

Variants of SM

- *Indolent SM (ISM):* most common form of SM (~66%); no 'B' or 'C' findings; mast cell burden low; usually involves skin and BM; associated with maculopapular skin lesions (90%); flushing and abdominal cramps frequently reported; slow involvement of organs; prolonged course and good prognosis in almost all with survival >20 years; poor quality of life if inadequate control of mediator symptoms; small number transform into ASM or SM-AHNMD.[2,4,5]
- *BM mastocytosis:* rare subvariant of ISM with isolated marrow involvement and no skin lesions or multi-organ involvement, low MC burden and good prognosis.[2]
- *Smouldering SM (SSM):* as ISM with 2 or more 'B' findings but no 'C' finding; intermediate between ISM and ASM with high degree of tissue infiltration, high serum tryptase (>200ng/mL) and organomegaly; uncertain prognosis and variable clinical course; some have prolonged stable course others develop ASM or AHNMD.[2–5]
- *Well-differentiated SM (WDSM)*: another subclass of ISM; compact infiltrates of round mature-appearing mast cells; CD25 –ve and –ve for D816CV; other exon KIT mutations described; good prognosis.[5,7]
- *Aggressive SM (ASM):* ~5% of all SM patients; ≥1 'C' finding; may present with hepatosplenomegaly and/or generalized lymphadenopathy without typical skin lesions; characterized by impaired organ function due to progressive infiltration of BM, liver, spleen, GI tract, or skeletal system; predisposition to severe mediator release attacks with haemorrhagic complications; median survival 3–5 years.[2,5]
- *Lymphadenopathic mastocytosis with eosinophilia:* rare subvariant of ASM; progressive lymphadenopathy with PB eosinophilia often with extensive bone involvement and hepatosplenomegaly but usually without skin lesions.[2,5]

- *SM with associated haematological non-mast cell disease (SM-AHNMD):* 20–30% of SM patients; <50% have skin lesions; 80–90% myeloid, commonest CMML; 10–20% lymphoid, commonest myeloma; classify using WHO criteria; prognosis poor, largely determined by accompanying disorder and poorer survival than patients without SM.[2,5]
- *Mast cell leukaemia (MCL):* rare; ≥20% MC in BM aspirate and ≥10% in PB (aleukaemic variant <10%); diffuse infiltration on trephine biopsy; no skin lesions, severe peptic ulcer disease, hepatosplenomegaly, anaemia, multiorgan failure; poor response to chemotherapy and short survival (most <1 year).[2,4,5]
- *Mast cell sarcoma (MCS):* extremely rare (<5 published cases); unifocal tumour consisting of atypical mast cells; high grade cytology; locally destructive growth; no skin or systemic involvement at diagnosis; prognosis grave; rapid progression with terminal phase resembling MCL.[2,5]
- *Extracutaneous mastocytoma:* extremely rare; most reported cases involve lung; unifocal tumour; low-grade cytology; non-destructive growth pattern; no skin or systemic involvement.[2,5]

Differential diagnosis

Diagnosis often delayed due to protean clinical features. Exclude reactive mast cell hyperplasia, mast cell activation syndromes, MPNs with ↑ mast cells, carcinoid syndrome, phaeochromocytoma, liver disease, and lymphoma. Not all patients with SM and eosinophilia have CES or HES; organ damage due to ASM (C-findings) can clearly be distinguished from CEL-related organ damage (cardiomyopathy, lung fibrosis).[3]

Management

- No curative therapy; management consists of prevention of mediator effects, an attempt to control organ infiltration by mast cells by cytoreductive therapy where appropriate, and treatment of accompanying haematological disease where present.
- Selection of intensive therapy should be based on signs and symptoms of aggressive disease, C-findings.[3]
- B-findings: borderline benign—be careful, wait and watch if progrssion occurs; C-findings: consider cytoreduction with chemotherapy or with targeted drugs.[3]
- Patients should avoid factors triggering acute mediator release: extremes of temperature, pressure, friction, aspirin, NSAIDs, opiates, alcohol, specific allergies.
- Treatment of *acute* mast cell mediator release:
  - Anaphylaxis: epinephrine (adrenaline) 0.3mL of 1:1000 dilution (adult dose) every 10–15min as needed.
  - Refractory hypotension and shock: fluid resuscitation and epinephrine (adrenaline) IV bolus plus infusion of 1:10,000 dilution (up to 4–10mg/min); add inotropes if unresponsive.
  - Patients at risk of severe hypotension should be advised to carry 2 or more epinephrine self-injectors.[3]
  - Commence H_1 plus H_2 receptor antagonists and steroids.

- Treatment of *chronic* mast cell mediator release:
  - H_1 plus H_2 receptor antagonists: H_1 antihistamines: diphenhydramine (25–50mg PO 4–6 hourly; 10–50mg IM/IV), hydroxyzine (25mg PO tid or qid; 25–100 mg IM/IV) or loratadine (non-sedating; 10mg PO od); H2 antihistamines: ranitidine (150mg PO bd; 50mg IV) or cimetidine (400–1600mg/day PO in divided doses; 300mg IV). Titrate doses for individual patient requirements.
  - GI symptoms unresponsive to H_1 and H_2 antagonists may respond to sodium cromoglicate or short term corticosteroids; prednisolone 40–60 mg/d PO for malabsorption, tailing dose.
  - Bisphosphonates for osteoporosis; analgesia for bone pain, radiotherapy in severe cases; osteolysis is a sign of advanced disease and an indication for IFN-α or cytoreductive therapy.[3]
  - PUVA for urticaria pigmentosa.
  - A small number of patients gain symptomatic relief from IFN-α or ciclosporin-A for refractory symptoms.
- In SM-AHNMD, treat associated haematological disorder as for cases without SM and treat SM component as required.[3] Generally achieve short partial remission at best; splenectomy may help pancytopenic patients. SCT should be considered in appropriate patients. SM-CEL with *FIP1L1-PDGFRA* fusion gene will respond to imatinib.
- Cytoreductive treatment:[3,4]
  - First establish diagnosis of ASM, MCL, or MCS and *KIT* mutation status.
  - ISM or SSM: cytoreductive treatment generally not required, but in SSM with rapidly progressive B-findings, consider IFN-α (3 million units SC tiw) ± corticosteroids (50–75mg/d, commence before IFN-α and monitor carefully during initial days of treatment[4]) or 2CdA (5mg/m^2/d by infusion for 5d every 4 weeks × 4–6 cycles); CR or prolonged remission uncommon.[8]
  - *KIT*-D816V –ve (wild type or other mutation) ASM or MCL: consider imatinib (FDA approved); N.B. *KIT*-D816V+ SM is imatinib resistant.
  - ASM with slow progression: IFN-α (15–20% major clinical responses in ASM/MCL[5]) ± corticosteroids; if IFN-α intolerant, or no response, 2CdA.
  - ASM with rapid progression: polychemotherapy e.g. daunorubicin and cytarabine ± IFN-α; consider SCT in selected cases who respond to polychemotherapy; 2CdA; splenectomy for hypersplenism; hydroxycarbamide as palliation.
  - MCL: AML-type polychemotherapy ± 2CdA ± IFN-α; consider SCT; splenectomy for hypersplenism; hydroxycarbamide as palliation.
- Novel therapies: nilotinib, dasatinib, and midostaurin are under evaluation in clinical trials and NF-κB inhibitors, heat shock protein 90 inhibitors, geldanamycin, alemtuzumab, and mylotarg are being studied.[7] Thalidomide has achieved durable major responses in 2 patients with advanced SM.[9]

Response assessment

Response criteria for patients receiving cytoreductive drugs have been agreed and relate to C-findings.[3]

- ***Major response:*** Complete resolution of ≥1 C-finding *and* no progression in other C-findings.
  - Complete remission: disappearance of mast cell infiltrates in affected organs *and* decrease of serum tryptase to <20ng/mL *and* disappearance of SM-associated organomegaly
  - Incomplete remission: decrease in mast cell infiltrates in affected organs and/or substantial decrease of serum tryptase level and/or visible regression of splenomegaly.
  - Pure clinical response: without decrease in mast cell infiltrates, without decrease in tryptase levels and without regression of splenomegaly.
- ***Partial response:*** incomplete regression of ≥1 C-finding without complete regression and without progression.
  - Good partial response: >50% regression; no progression in other C-findings.
  - Minor response; <50% regression; no progression in other C-findings.
- ***No response:*** C-finding(s) persistent or progressive.
  - Stable disease: C-finding parameters show constant range.
  - Progressive disease: ≥1 C-finding shows progression.

Prognosis

Most patients with SM have only slowly progressive disease and many survive several decades. The life expectancy of patients with pure CM, ISM, BMM and WDSM is similar to that of individuals without mastocytosis.[7] ~33% of patients with SM evolve into a haematological malignancy, frequently leukaemia. Mast cell leukaemia is resistant to intensive chemotherapy and has a survival of only a few months.

References

1. Valent, P. and Metcalfe, D.D. (2004). Mast cell proliferative disorders: diagnosis, classification and therapy. *Hematology 2004*, 153–62.
2. Valent, P. *et al.* (2001). Mastocytosis (mast cell disease). In Jaffe, E.S. *et al.* (eds.) *World Health Organization classification of tumours. Pathology and genetics. Tumours of haematopoietic and lymphoid tissues, vol 1*. Lyon: IARC Press, pp.291–302.
3. Valent, P. *et al.* (2007). Standards and standardization in mastocytosis: Consensus statements on diagnostics, treatment recommendations and response criteria. *Eur J Clin Invest*, **37**, 435–53.
4. Valent, P. and Metcalfe, D.D. (2004). Mast cell proliferative disorders: diagnosis, classification and therapy. *Hematology 2004*, 153–62.
5. Horny, H.P. *et al.* (2007). Mastocytosis: state of the art. *Pathobiology* **74**, 121–32.
6. Tefferi, A. and Vardiman, J.W. (2008). Classification and diagnosis of myeloproliferative neoplasms: The 2008 World Health Organization criteria and point-of-care diagnostic algorithms. *Leukemia*, **22**, 14–22.
7. Orfao, A. *et al.* (2007). Recent advances in the understanding of mastocytosis: the role of KIT mutations. *Br J Haematol*, **138**, 12–30.
8. Kluin-Nelemans, H.C. *et al.* (2003). Cladribine therapy for systemic mastocytosis. *Blood*, **102**, 4270–6.
9. Damaj, G. et al. (2008). Thalidomide in advanced mastocytosis. *Brit J Haematol*, **141**, 249–53.

MPNs-unclassifiable (MPN-U)

This is a group of MPN-like disorders that do not meet the diagnostic criteria for either the classic or non-classic MPNs and may account for 10–20% of MPNs.[1] Most cases fall into 2 groups: (i) initial stages of PV, PMF, or ET presenting before characteristic features have developed and (ii) advanced MPN where marked myelofibrosis, osteosclerosis, or transformation obscures the underlying disorder. The former should be screened for MPN-associated mutations and monitored until a clear diagnosis can be determined. The latter have advanced disease and should be treated appropriately.

1. Thiele, J. *et al.* (2001). Chronic myeloproliferative disease, unclassifiable. In Jaffe ES *et al.* (eds.) *World Health Organization classification of tumours. Pathology and genetics. Tumours of haematopoietic and lymphoid tissues, vol 1*. Lyon: IARC Press, pp.42–4.

Chapter 8

Paraproteinaemias

Paraproteinaemias

A heterogeneous group of disorders characterized by deranged proliferation of a single clone of plasma cells or B lymphocytes and usually associated with detectable monoclonal immunoglobulin (paraprotein or M-protein) in serum and/or urine.

Conditions associated with paraprotein production

Stable production

- Monoclonal gammopathy of undetermined significance (MGUS).
- Smouldering myeloma (*syn.* asymptomatic myeloma).
- Cryoglobulinaemia

Progressive production

- Multiple myeloma (MM).
  - Complete immunoglobulins: IgG, IgA, or IgD; very rarely IgM or IgE.
  - Free light chains (LCs): κ or λ (Bence Jones proteinuria).
  - 'Non-secretory'.
- Plasma cell leukaemia (PCL).
- Solitary plasmacytoma of bone (SPB).
- Extramedullary plasmacytoma (SEP).
- POEMS syndrome
- Waldenström macroglobulinaemia (WM).
- Chronic lymphocytic leukaemia.
- Malignant lymphoma.
- Heavy chain disease (HCD).
- 1° amyloidosis (AL).

Monoclonal gammopathy of undetermined significance (MGUS)

MGUS describes an asymptomatic premalignant disorder characterized by limited monoclonal plasma cell proliferation and the presence of a stable monoclonal paraprotein in serum or less commonly in urine in the absence of clinicopathological evidence of multiple myeloma (MM), Waldenström macroglobulinaemia (WM), amyloidosis (AL), or another lymphoproliferative disorder (LPD).

Epidemiology

Prevalence 3.2% ≥50 years in large population-based study. Slight ♂ excess (1.3 ×). Prevalence rises with age: 1.7% age 50–59; 3% 60–69; 4.6% 70–79; 6.6% ≥85 years. In USA, >2 × more frequent in African Americans than Caucasians. Median age 72 years; 2% <40; 59% ≥70 years. MGUS diagnosed ~4 × as frequently as MM.

Pathophysiology

MGUS appears to arise from a pre-germinal centre cell whose progeny pass through the germinal centre and undergo mutation. Antigenic stimulation related to autoimmune, infectious, or inflammatory disorders (but not allergies) may be an initiating event. Mutation probably occurs during Ig heavy chain (IgH) gene switch recombination or somatic hypermutation.

There is genomic instability on molecular analysis and 90% of patients have abnormalities. Chromosomal translocation involving the IgH gene at 14q32 is found by FISH in 50% of patients with MGUS usually in association with dysregulation of a gene on 1 of 7 recurrent partner chromosomes (📖 see Multiple myeloma, p.330). The prevalence of these abnormalities differs between MGUS and MM. These probably have an important pathogenetic role. A further 40% have hyperdiploidy. Hyperdiploidy appears to be mutually exclusive with 14q32 translocation. Other or unknown abnormalities occur in ~10%.

Progression to MM may be due to outgrowth of a single clone but the precise trigger is unclear. There is a continuing rate of progression to MM, WM, AL, or other LPDs. This constant rate suggests a random 2nd hit. Second triggers may be further genetic abnormalities, e.g. *ras* or *p53* mutations, 1q21 amplification, p16 methylation, myc abnormalities, and further translocatons. FISH demonstrates the same MM cytogenetic abnormalities in MGUS often acquired over time e.g. –13 (in 50% MGUS). Expression microarrays show MGUS much closer to MM than to ↔ plasma cells.

The BM microenvironment also changes at progression with ↑ angiogenesis, suppression of cell mediated immunity, and paracrine loops involving IL-6 and VEGF.

Natural history

- >50% die of unrelated causes after >25-year follow-up.
- ~1% per annum progress to MM, WM, AL, or other LPD, usually NHL or CLL.

- Actuarial rate of progression 17% at 10 years; 39% at 25 years but true probability is lower when other causes of death are taken into account.
- 69% who progress develop MM, 12% AL, 11% WM, and 8% LPD.
- ~5% patients do not progress.
- Some may show an ↑ in paraprotein ≥30g/L or BM PC >10% without developing symptomatic MM or WM or requiring therapy.

Clinical features

- Typically asymptomatic and an incidental finding on investigation of ↑ ESR/PV or ↑ globulin on routine LFTs.
- No abnormal physical findings (end-organ damage) except due to unrelated pathology.
- Lack of progression and absence of additional evidence of progressive plasma cell or B-cell lymphoproliferative malignancy.

Investigations and diagnosis (Table 8.1)

- Check FBC, renal biochemistry, serum calcium, serum immunoglobulins, serum protein electrophoresis and paraprotein quantitation, serum free light chains (SFLC) (and/or urine for Bence Jones proteinuria), and skeletal survey.
- BM aspirate and trephine biopsy indicated if paraprotein ≥15g/L or non-IgG paraprotein present or abnormal FBC, serum creatinine, serum calcium, SFLC ratio, or skeletal survey.
- FBC: no anaemia or other cytopenia except due to unrelated causes.
- Serum chemistry: no hypercalcaemia or otherwise unexplained renal impairment.
- Serum protein electrophoresis with immunofixation and densitometry to detect, characterize, and quantitate paraprotein levels:
  - IgG 70%; IgM 15%; IgA 12%; biclonal 3%; LC <1%.
  - Median quantitation 5g/L; ~10% too small to quantify; 64% <10g/L; ~30% 10–20g/L; <5% ≥20g/L.
- Immunoglobulin quantitation: by nephelometry; up to 40% have immuneparesis of uninvolved Ig classes (*cf.* myeloma).
- SFLCs: ~30% have abnormal κ:λ ratio.
- Urine electrophoresis: identifies low levels of Bence Jones proteinuria in up to 30%; ~60% κ, ~40% λ; generally <1g/24h, ~15% >150mg/24h.
- Skeletal radiology: no evidence of lytic lesions or pathological fracture; osteoporosis may co-exist from other causes e.g. post menopausal ♀.
- Serum β_2-microglobulin levels ↔ (unless renal impairment).
- BM aspirate: <10% plasma cells in BM; median ~5%.
- BM cytogenetics: ↔ by conventional techniques but all abnormalities in MM described in MGUS by FISH; del(13), t(4;14), *ras* mutations, *p16* and *p53* inactivation less common.
- BM trephine biopsy: no evidence of diffuse plasma cell infiltration or osteoclast erosion of trabeculae.
- Other radiological imaging not routine; MRI of the spine; FDG-PET and ^{99m}Tc-MIBI scan are –ve in MGUS.
- *N.B.* Patients with MGUS should have stable paraprotein and other parameters on prolonged observation.

Differential diagnosis

- Exclude conditions listed on p.320 notably MM, WM, and AL.
- Bone pain/damage, unexplained anaemia, or impaired renal function suggests MM.
- Lymphadenopathy or splenomegaly with an IgM paraprotein suggests WM.
- The presence of neuropathy attributable to the monoclonal gammopathy would be termed '*monoclonal gammopathy associated with neuropathy*'.

Risk factors for progression

No specific features at initial presentation predict the patients who will progress but risk of progression ↑ by:

- Paraprotein level: progression rate at 20 years: 10g/L=16%; 15g/L=25%; 20g/L=41%; 25g/L=49%.
- Paraprotein type: IgM > IgA > IgG.
- Abnormal SFLC ratio (<0.26 or >1.65)
- BM plasma cells >5% (2 × risk of <5%).
- Circulating plasma cells by immunofluorescence.
- Other possible risk factors: immuneparesis, presence of urinary paraprotein, BM angiogenesis.

Risk stratification

A scoring system has been developed using 3 parameters (Table 8.2)

- Quantity of paraprotein (<15g/L *vs.* ≥15g/L).
- Isotype of paraprotein (IgG *vs.* any other subtype).
- SFLC ratio (↔ *vs.* abnormal).

Management

- No treatment; observation with long term follow-up and review of clinical and laboratory features required due to risk of progression.
- Clinical and laboratory (FBC, PV, renal function, serum Ca^{2+}, serum Igs, paraprotein quantitation, SFLC, and urine electrophoresis) re-evaluation at 6 months then annually.
- Less frequent follow-up (e.g. every 2 years) may be appropriate in low-risk patients.
- Where diagnosis in doubt (e.g. elderly woman with paraprotein <30g/L and osteoporosis) review over 3–6 months usually differentiates MGUS from MM.
- Advise patients to seek early assessment if relevant or unexplained symptoms develop.

Table 8.1 Diagnostic criteria for MGUS: all 4 criteria must be met[1]

1	Serum monoclonal protein <30g/L
2	Bone marrow plasma cells <10% (IgM MGUS—lymphoplasmacytic cells <10%)
3	No evidence of other B-cell lymphoproliferative disorder
4	No myeloma-related end-organ or tissue impairment, e.g. lytic bone lesions, anaemia, hypercalcaemia, or renal failure (IgM MGUS—no anaemia, constitutional symptoms, hyperviscosity, lymphadenopathy or hepatosplenomegaly)

Reproduced with permission of Wiley-Blackwell publishing© 2003

Table 8.2[2] Risk stratification system for MGUS

Risk group	Number of patients	Relative risk	Absolute risk of progression at 20 years (%)	20-year progression risk with death as competing risk (%)
Low-risk: M-band <15g/L; IgG isotype; normal SFLC ratio (0.26–1.65)	449	1	5	2
Low–intermediate risk (any 1 factor: M-band ≥15glP, non-IgG-isotype, or abnormal SFLC ratio)	420	5.4	21	10
High–intermediate risk (any 2 factors)	226	10.1	37	18
High risk (all 3 factors)	53	20.8	58	27

Reproduced with permission, copyright. American Society of Hematology

References

1. International Myeloma Working Group (2003). Criteria for the classification of monoclonal gammopathies, multiple myeloma and related disorders: a report of the International Myeloma Working Group. *Brit J Haematol*, **121**, 749–57.
2. Rajkumar, S.V. *et al.* (2005). Serum free light chain ratio is an independent risk factor for progression in monoclonal gammopathy of undetermined significance (MGUS). *Blood*, **106**, 812–7.
3. Kyle, R.A. and Rajkumar, S.V. (2007). Epidemiology of the plasma cell disorders. *Best Pract Res Clin Haematol*, **20**, 637–64.
4. Kyle, R.A. et *al.* (2006). Prevalence of monoclonal gammopathy of undetermined significance. *N Engl J Med*, **354**, 1362–9.
5. Kyle, R.A. et *al.* (2002). A long-term study of prognosis in monoclonal gammopathy of undetermined significance. *N Engl J Med*, **346**, 564–69.
6. Kyle, R.A. *et al* (2004). Long-term follow-up of 241 patients with monoclonal gammopathy of undetermined significance: the original Mayo Clinic series 25 years later. *Mayo Clinic Proceedings*, **79**, 859–66.
7. Morris Brown, L. *et al.* (2007). Risk of multiple myeloma and monoclonal gammopathy of undetermined significance among white and black male United States veterans with prior autoimmune, infectious, inflammatory and allergic disorders. *Blood*, **111**, 3388–94.
8. Chng, W.J. *et al.* (2007). Genetic events in the pathogenesis of multiple myeloma. *Best Practice and Res Clin Haematol*, **20**, 571–96.
9. Rajkumar, S.V. *et al.* (2007). Monoclonal gammopathy of undetermined significance and smoldering multiple myeloma. *Blood Reviews*, **21**, 255–65.

Smouldering multiple myeloma (*syn.* asymptomatic myeloma)

Smouldering or asymptomatic MM identifies patients with a paraprotein >30g/dL and/or >10% plasma cells in the BM but in whom the natural history is that of MGUS rather than MM, i.e. no clinical evidence of complications associated with MM or progression.

Incidence

- Accounts for ~15% of all new cases of myeloma.

Pathogenesis

- Almost all have either translocation involving IgH (50%) or hyperdiploidy (~40%).
- BM angiogenesis is greater than in MGUS but less than in MM.

Prognosis

- Clinical stability may persist for months or years but most patients eventually progress to symptomatic MM.
- Risk of progression is higher than MGUS and time dependent: 10% per annum for first 5 years, ~3% per annum for next 5 years, and 1% per annum for next 10 years.
- Cumulative probability of progression 73% at 15 years.
- Median time to progression ~5 years.
- Important to recognize because there is no survival advantage from chemotherapy before progressive or symptomatic disease develops.
- Survival is same as for newly diagnosed myeloma from the time chemotherapy is started.

Clinical and laboratory features

- Absence of symptoms or physical signs attributable to myeloma.
- Performance status >50%.
- Perform investigations listed for MM (📖 Multiple myeloma, p.333).
- FBC: pre-transfusion haemoglobin >10g/dL.
- Serum chemistry: post-rehydration creatinine <130 micromol/L; ↔ serum Ca^{2+}.
- β2-microglobulin: ↔ or minimally raised.
- BM aspirate: plasmacytosis >10% but normally <25%.
- BM cytogenetics: FISH identifies the abnormalities associated with MM; some patients have detectable chromosomal abnormalities by standard karyotype analysis.
- Skeletal radiology: should be ↔.
- Other imaging: not yet routine; CT, MRI of spine FDG-PET and ^{99m}Tc MIBI scan identify bone lesions in ~25% of patients with normal conventional radiology.
- BM plasma cell labelling index: (when measured) <1%.
- Stable paraprotein and other parameters on prolonged observation.

Table 8.3 Diagnostic criteria for smouldering (asymptomatic) multiple myeloma[1]

1	Serum monoclonal protein ≥30g/L *and/or* bone marrow plasma cells ≥10%
2	No evidence of other B-cell LPD
3	No myeloma-related end-organ or tissue impairment, e.g. lytic bone lesions, anaemia, hypercalcaemia, or renal failure (see Myeloma-related organ or tissue impairment p334)

Differential diagnosis

- Exclude MGUS, MM, WM, and AL.
- Bone pain/damage, unexplained anaemia or impaired renal function suggests MM.

Risk factors for early progression of asymptomatic MM

Shorter time to progression associated with:

- Serum paraprotein >30g/L.
- IgA protein type.
- Urinary Bence Jones proteinuria >50mg/d.
- BM plasmacytosis >25%.
- Suppression of uninvolved Igs.
- SFLC ratio <0.125 or >8.
- Abnormal MRI (median 1.5 years *vs.* 5 years).

These risk factors have no impact on survival after progression. Other possible risk factors for progression are high plasma cell labelling index, circulating plasma cells, β2-microglobulin >2.5mg/L, and karyotype abnormalities on conventional cytogenetics.

Risk stratification

- A scoring system has been developed using 2 parameters (Table 8.4):
  - Quantity of paraprotein (<30g/L *vs.* >30g/L).
  - Isotype of paraprotein (IgG *vs.* IgA).
- Another scoring system has been devised using 3 parameters, with one point awarded for each (Table 8.5):
  - BM plasmacytosis ≥10%.
  - Serum M protein ≥30g/L.
  - SFLC ratio <0.125 or >8.

Management

- Chemotherapy is not indicated for these patients until there is evidence of clinical progression; 2 small, randomized trials show no benefit for therapy before symptomatic disease develops.
- Review clinical and laboratory features as for MGUS but more frequently: every 3–4 months recommended.
- Median survival following chemotherapy 3–5 years, i.e. identical to that of *de novo* symptomatic myeloma.

- Clinical trials evaluating the value of early therapy with bisphosphonates, thalidomide and lenalidomide to delay progression are underway.

References

1. International Myeloma Working Group (2003). Criteria for the classification of monoclonal gammopathies, multiple myeloma and related disorders: a report of the International Myeloma Working Group. *Brit J Haematol*, **121**, 749–57.
2. Weber, D. *et al.* (2003). Risk factors for early progression of asymptomatic multiple myeloma. *The Hematology Journal*, **4**(1), S31–2.
3. Dispenzieri, A. *et al.* (2008). Immunoglobulin free light chain ratio is an independent risk factor for progression of smoldering (asaymptomatic) multiple myeloma. *Blood*, **111**, 785–9.
4. Rajkumar, S.V. *et al.* (2007). Monoclonal gammopathy of undetermined significance and smoldering multiple myeloma. *Blood Reviews*, **21**, 255–65.
5. Kyle, R.A. *et al.* (2007). Clinical course and prognosis of smoldering (asymptomatic) multiple myeloma. *N Engl J Med*, **356**, 2582–90.

Table 8.4 Risk stratification scoring system in SMM (see text)[2]

Risk group	Factors	Proportion of patients	Median time to progression
Low-risk	M-band ≤30g/L **and** IgG isotype	~45%	>4 years
Intermediate-risk	M-band >30g/L **or** IgA isotype	~45%	~2 years
High-risk	M-band >30g/L **and** IgA isotype	<10%	9 months

Reproduced with permission

Table 8.5 Risk stratification scoring system in SMM (see text)[3]

Risk group	Number of factors	Number of patients (%)	Relative risk (95%CI)	Absolute risk at 5 years	Absolute risk at 10 years
Low-risk	1	81 (28%)	1	25%	50%
Intermediate-risk	2	114 (42%)	1.9 (1.2–2.9)	51%	65%
High-risk	3	78 (30%)	4.0 (2.6–6.1)	76%	84%

Originally published in *Blood*. Reproduced with permission© American Society of Hematology

Multiple myeloma (MM)

MM (*syn.* symptomatic MM, myelomatosis) is a clonal B-cell malignancy characterized by proliferation of plasma cells that accumulate mainly within BM and usually secrete monoclonal Ig or Ig LCs, (*syn.* paraprotein, M-protein). MM may be associated with lytic bone lesions, diffuse osteoporosis or pathological fracture. Normal Ig production is usually impaired (immuneparesis; hypogammaglobulinaemia). Uncommon cases are 'non-secretory' with no detectable serum or urine paraprotein.

Epidemiology

MM accounts for 1% of all malignancies; 10% of haematological malignancies. Incidence ~4 per 100,000 per annum, 2500 new cases/year in UK. Median age 66 years; <3% <40 years. ♂:♀ ratio 1.5. Incidence in Afro-Caribbeans >2 × Caucasians; lowest in Asians. Most present *de novo* but some documented as arising from MGUS (most cases of MM may follow undetected MGUS). Weak associations have been reported with farm working and exposure to radiation, benzene, or pesticides. Familial clusters have been reported, suggesting a possible genetic element. The apparent ↑ incidence of MM is due to improved diagnosis and ageing populations.[1]

Pathophysiology[2,3]

MM arises from a post germinal centre B-cell (probably in LN or spleen) that has undergone antigen selection, VDJ recombination, somatic hypermutation of V regions, and switch-recombination of IgH genes.

2 mutually exclusive pathogenetic pathways have been postulated:

- Hyperdiploid (48–75 chromosomes): ~ 50%; typically with multiple trisomies involving chromosomes 3, 5, 7, 9, 11, 15, 19, and 21; rarely with a recurrent IgH translocation (usually t(4;14)).
- Non-hyperdiploid (<48 or >75 chromosomes): aberrant class-switch recombination or somatic hypermutation may contribute to neoplastic transformation; IgH translocations at 14q32, usually within or near switch regions, detected by FISH in 55–70% of MM; usually associated with dysregulation of a gene in 1 of 7 recurrent partner chromosomes grouped by gene affected:
    1. *Cyclin D*: 11q13 (cyclin D1), 20%; 12p13 (cyclin D2), <1%; 6p21 (cyclin D3), 2%.
    2. *MAF*: 16q23 (c-MAF), 5%; 20q11 (MAFB), 2%; 8q24.3 (MAFA), <1%.
    3. *MMSET/FGFR3*: 4p16.3 (MMSET and usually FGFR3), 15%.

2 other early events have been described:

- Loss of chromosome 13 or 13q14 deletion: occurs in ~50% MM and 40–50% MGUS; concurrent 13/13q– occurs in both pathogenetic pathways; much more prevalent (80–90%) in t(4;14) or t(14;16) than others (30–40%); low incidence in hyperdiploid MM.
- Dysregulation of a *Cyclin D* gene: ↑ levels of cyclin D1 (less commonly cyclin D2) are expressed by almost all MM tumours: 25% due to IgH translocation; in others mechanism unclear; may make cells more susceptible to proliferative stimuli e.g. IL-6.

Other genetic abnormalities, likely to be late progression events, occur with similar prevalence in both pathways:

- 17p– or *p53* mutations: rare in newly diagnosed MM (5%); frequency rises as disease progresses to 30% in PCL.
- *ras* mutations: found in <5% MGUS but 30–40% newly diagnosed MM; may mark the MGUS → MM transition; mutually exclusive with *FGFR3* mutation.
- 2° Ig translocations: occur in 10–20%; breakpoints distant from IgH switch or VDJ regions, unbalanced or complex structures; similar frequency in both pathways.
- Translocations involving a *myc* gene: 25–60% involve Ig locus; usually complex rearrangements; rare in MGUS, occur in ~15% newly diagnosed MM, 44% advanced MM, and 90% of human myeloma cell lines; probably represent very late progression event associated with ↓ stroma-dependence and ↑ proliferation.
- Gain of sequences and gene expression at 1q21 occurs in 30–40%; associated with t(4;14) or t(14;16), high proliferation index, progression and ↑ proliferative capacity.
- Constitutive activation of the NFκB pathway due to a number of mutations has been described in 20% of MM patients; 50% of MM patients have an expression signature of NFκB target genes.

Novel classification systems have been described, based on (i) translocations, cyclin D gene overexpression, and clinical features or (ii) co-expression of unique gene clusters on molecular analysis. These identify 7 and 8 subgroups respectively which show significant overlap and may have prognostic and therapeutic implications.

↔ plasmablasts generated from post-GC B cells, migrate to the BM where they differentiate into long-lived plasma cells. The BM microenvironment is also critical to MM clonal expansion. Adhesion to stromal cells enhances MM-cell growth and survival and confers protection against drug-induced apoptosis. MM-cells activate the stroma, triggering paracrine and autocrine secretion of a range of cytokines and growth factors including IL-6, IGF-1, VEGF, TNF-α, bFGF, MIP-1α, SCF, HGF, and IL-1β. IL-6 is the major growth and survival factor in MM and confers resistance to dexamethasone. VEGF induces MM-cell growth, migration, and survival as does IGF-1 which also confers drug resistance. Angiogenesis is altered (VEGF is main angiogenic factor) and ↑ BM microvascular density correlates with disease progression and poor prognosis.

Bone disease in MM is due to osteoclast (OC) activation and osteoblast (OB) inhibition causing the characteristic 'punched-out' lytic lesions and hypercalcaemia associated with normal alkaline phosphatase. OC proliferation and activation is triggered by a variety of OC-activating factors (OAFs) produced by MM-cells and stroma, including MIP-1α, RANK-ligand, VEGF, TNF-α,, IL-1β, PTHrP, HGF, and IL-6. Production of the RANK-L antagonist, osteoprotogerin (OPG) is down-regulated. OC activation in turn modulates MM-cell growth and survival. In addition there are ↓ numbers of OBs and ↓ bone formation due to dysregulation of Runx2/Cbfal, Wnt, and IL-3.

BM infiltration by the neoplastic clone causes anaemia. Immuneparesis of normal Ig production predisposes to infection. The physico-chemical properties of the paraprotein determine whether amyloid deposition, renal damage, or hyperviscosity (IgA > IgG) occur.

Clinical features and presentation

- Spectrum from asymptomatic paraproteinaemia detected on routine testing (~20%) to a rapidly progressive illness with extensive, destructive bone disease.
- Most patients present with bone (usually back) pain (~75%) or pathological fracture; kyphosis and loss of height may occur from vertebral compression fractures.
- Weakness and fatigue (>50%), recurrent infection (10%) and thirst, polyuria, nocturia or oedema due to renal impairment (~10%) are also common presenting symptoms.
- Acute hypercalcaemia, symptomatic hyperviscosity (mental slowing, visual upset, purpura, haemorrhage), neuropathy, spinal cord compression, amyloidosis, and coagulopathy are less frequent at presentation.

Investigations and diagnosis

A full history and physical examination should be undertaken in all patients with suspected MM. The investigations detailed in Table 8.6 should be performed to confirm or exclude the diagnosis and if confirmed, to establish tumour burden and prognosis. Further investigations that are not routine, may be necessary in individual patients, e.g. MRI (see Plates 28–31). Diagnostic criteria are listed in Table 8.7.

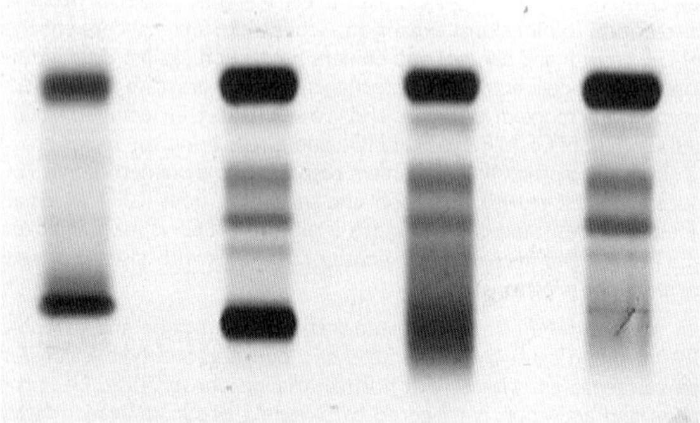

Fig. 8.1 Electrophoresis: from L → R: urine with BJP and generalized proteinuria (albumin band at top of strip, BJP near foot); serum M band in myeloma; polyclonal gammopathy; normal sample, showing albumin, α, β, and γ globulins (see Plate 26).

Table 8.6 Investigation of patients with suspected myeloma[4–7]

Screening tests	
FBC and film	Normochromic normocytic anaemia in 60%; film may show rouleaux
ESR or PV	↑ in 90% ; not in LC or non-secretory (NS) MM
Serum urea, creatinine, and electrolytes	May identify renal impairment (~25%)
Uric acid	May be ↑
Serum albumin, calcium, phosphate, alk phos	May reveal low albumin or hypercalcaemia (~20%) with normal alk phos
Serum protein electrophoresis with immunofixation	To detect serum paraprotein (80%)
Serum immunoglobulins	To detect immuneparesis
SFLC	To detect LC MM (22%); useful response parameter in LC MM, amyloidosis and 75% of 'NS' MM
Routine urinalysis	To detect proteinuria (~70%)
Urine electrophoresis with immunofixation:	To detect Bence Jones proteinuria: (22% have BJP only and no serum M-band: LC MM)
24h urine collection	For creatinine clearance and 24h proteinuria —to assess renal damage
X-ray sites of bone pain	May reveal pathological fracture(s) or lytic lesion(s)
Diagnostic tests	
BM aspirate	Demonstrates plasma cell infiltration—may be only way to diagnose NS MM
Radiological skeletal survey	Identifies lytic lesions, fractures, and osteoporosis (80%; 5–10% osteoporosis only; 20% ↔)
Paraprotein immunofixation and densitometry	Characterizes and quantifies paraprotein; IgG ~55%; IgA ~22% IgD ~2%; IgM 0.5%; IgE <0.01%; LC ~22%; *Note*: serum and urine EPS –ve in NS ~1% but SFLC abnormal in 75% of NS MM
Tests to establish tumour burden and prognosis	
Serum β2-microglobulin	Measure of tumour burden
Serum C-reactive protein	Surrogate measure of IL-6 which correlates with tumour aggression
Serum LDH	Measure of tumour aggression; ↑ in plasmablastic MM
Serum albumin	Hypoalbuminaemia correlates with poor prognosis
BM cytogenetics and FISH	Clear prognostic value, esp. t(4;14) and del(17p) (📖 Cytogenetics, p.335)
BM trephine biopsy with immunohistochemistry	Shows LC restriction, extent of infiltration and haematopoietic reserve

(*continued*)

Table 8.6 Investigation of patients with suspected myeloma[4–7] (*continued*)

Tests which may be useful in some patients	
MRI	Urgent in patients with suspected cord compression; MRI whole spine important in staging solitary plasmacytoma of bone to exclude occult disease; useful to clarify ambiguous CT findings; abnormal in ~25% of MM patients with ↔ skeletal survey
CT	For detailed evaluation of localized sites of disease, e.g. extraosseous plasmacytoma, including CT-guided biopsy; urgent CT indicated in suspected cord compression where MRI contra-indicated or unavailable; useful to clarify ambiguous radiographic findings; may identify lesions that are –ve on radiography
FDG-PET scan	Not recommended as routine but may clarify extent of extramedullary disease if other imaging techniques do not do so; identifies focal recurrent disease and focal extramedullary disease; abnormal in ~25% with ↔ skeletal survey; persistent +ve post-therapy may predict early relapse
PET/CT	May be useful in solitary plasmacytoma of bone
BM flow cytometry	Confirms monoclonal PC infiltration and aberrant phenotype; useful when BM PC <10%
Plasma cell labelling index	Provides prognostic information but not widely available
Fat pad biopsy for amyloid and SAP scan	When amyloid suspected (📖 p.380)
Tissue biopsy	To diagnose solitary plasmacytoma of bone or extraosseous plasmacytoma
Bone densitometry	Provides baseline in patients with osteoporosis but not recommended as routine
^{99m}Tc-MIBI scan	Not recommended; may identify extensive BM involvement

Table 8.7 Diagnostic criteria for MM[8]

- Monoclonal protein in serum and/or urine (*Note*: no minimum level).
- Clonal BM plasma cells (*Note*: no minimum level; 5% have <5% plasma cells) or plasmacytoma.
- Myeloma-related organ or tissue impairment (end-organ damage, *acronym* 'CRAB')
  - Elevated Ca^{2+} levels: serum Ca^{2+} >0.25mmol/L (>1mg/dL) above upper limit of ↔ or corrected serum Ca^{2+} >2.75mmol/L (>11mg/dL).
  - Renal insufficiency: (creatinine >173 micromol/L or >2mg/dL).
  - Anaemia: Hb 2g/dL below ↔ range or Hb <10g/dL.
  - Bone lesions: lytic lesions or osteoporosis with compression fractures recognized by conventional radiology.
  - Others: symptoms of hyperviscosity; amyloidosis; recurrent bacterial infection.

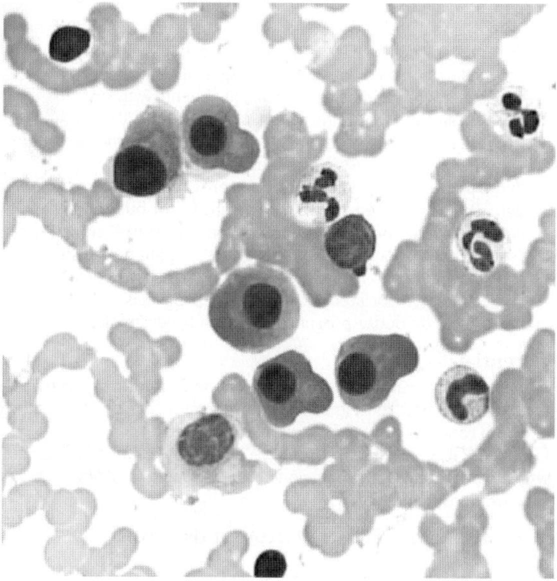

Fig. 8.2 BM aspirate in myeloma showing numerous plasma cells (see Plate 27).

Cytogenetics[2,9]

- Conventional techniques demonstrate abnormal karyotypes in only 30–50% due to the low proliferative rate of MM-cells and low proportion within samples for cytogenetic analysis; heterogeneous pattern and complex abnormalities common.
- High-density comparative genetic hybridization arrays show abnormalities in almost 100%.
- Interphase FISH on sorted or labelled MM-cells demonstrates aneuploidy in nearly all patients:
  - Hyperdiploidy in ~50%; median 54 chromosomes; commonly involves trisomy 3, 5, 7, 9, 11, 15, 19, and 21.
  - Abnormalities involving 14q32 (IgH locus) in ~60% (esp. non-hyperdiploid karyotypes): t(11;14)(q13;q32) ~20%, t(4;14)(p16;q32) ~15%, t(14;16)(q32;q23) ~5% and non-recurrent abnormalities.
  - Monosomies in vast majority, especially 8, 13, 14, 16, and 22.
  - del(13): ~50%; usually monosomy 13, less often del(13q14).
  - del(17p;13.1): ~10%; loss of *p53* tumour suppressor gene.
  - Gain of 1q21 in ~30%.

- Prognostic value of cytogenetic findings:
  - t(4;14): associated with poor prognosis after conventional or high-dose therapy due to early relapse; bortezomib overcomes poor prognosis associated with t(4;14) in both newly diagnosed and relapsed MM; should be assessed in all patients with MM.
  - t(14;16): also associated with poor prognosis.
  - t(11;14): newly diagnosed MM may have better prognosis than those with t(4;14) or t(14;16); inferior survival at relapse.
  - del(17p): powerful independent poor prognostic factor.
  - del(13): was regarded as poor prognostic factor but not an independent factor effect due to concomitant t(4;14) or del(17p).
  - Gain of 1q21: poor prognostic factor in some but not all studies; probably due to close association with poor-risk genetics.
  - Hypodiploidy: associated with very poor prognosis.
  - Hyperdiploidy: better prognosis than non-hyperdiploid.

Differential diagnosis

- Suspect MM in a patient >50 years with bone pain, lethargy, anaemia, recurrent infection, renal impairment, hypercalcaemia, or neuropathy or in whom rouleaux or an ↑ ESR or PV is detected.
- Exclude MGUS, smouldering myeloma and other conditions associated with a paraprotein (📖 p.320), notably solitary plasmacytoma, systemic AL amyloidosis and LPDs.

Prognostic factors: adverse factors at diagnosis

- Age >65 years.
- Performance status 3 or 4.
- High paraprotein levels (IgG >70g/L; IgA >50g/L; BJP >12g/24h).
- Low haemoglobin (<10g/dL).
- Hypercalcaemia.
- Advanced lytic bone lesions.
- Abnormal renal function (creatinine >180 micromol/L).
- Low serum albumin (<30g/L).
- High β2-microglobulin (≥6mg/mL).
- High C-reactive protein (≥6mg/mL).
- High serum LDH.
- High % BM plasma cells (>33%).
- Plasmablast morphology.
- Adverse cytogenetics.
- Circulating plasma cells in PB.
- High serum IL-6 (measured in only a few centres).
- High plasma cell labelling index (measured in only a few centres).
- Gene-expression-defined high-risk molecular signature

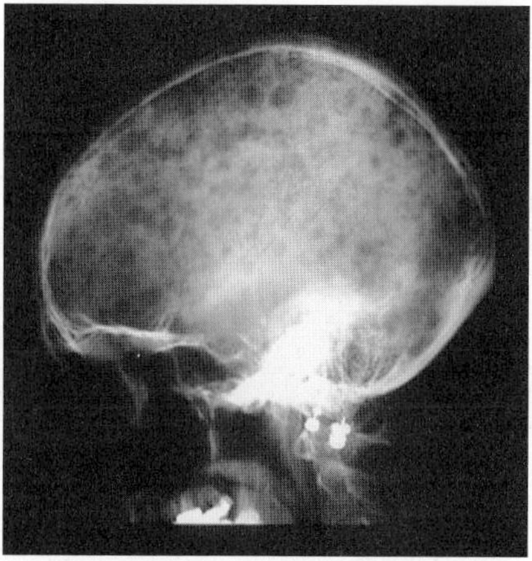

Fig. 8.3 Skull x-ray in a patient with myeloma: multiple lytic lesions.

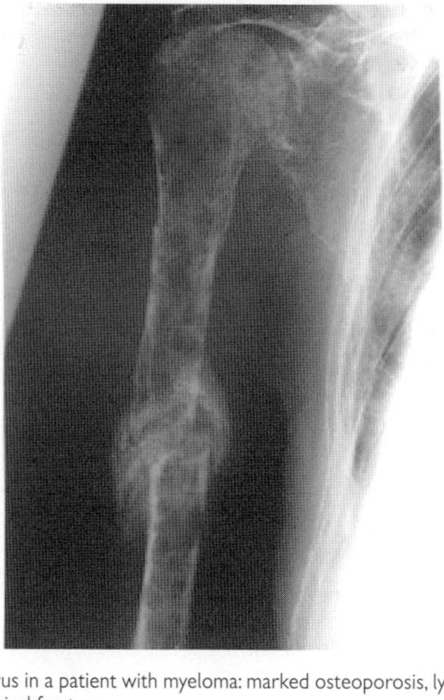

Fig. 8.4 Humerus in a patient with myeloma: marked osteoporosis, lytic lesions, and healing pathological fracture.

Staging systems

The Durie–Salmon staging system (Table 8.8) has been widely used since 1975.[10] It attempts to assess tumour bulk but may not provide as good prognostic discrimination as more recent systems:

Table 8.8 Durie–Salmon staging system[10]
Patients staged as I, II, or III and A or B; stage represents tumour burden

	Stage I	**Stage II**	**Stage III**
Tumour cell mass	*Low* All of the following:	*Medium* Not fitting stage I or III	*High* One or more of the following:
Monoclonal IgG (g/L)	<50		>70
Monoclonal IgA (g/L)	<30		>50
BJP excretion (g/24h)	<4		>12
Hb (g/dL)	>10		<8.5
Serum Ca^{2+} (mmol/L)	≤2.6 (≤12mg/dL)		>2.6 (>12mg/dL)
Lytic lesions	None or one		Advanced
Stage A: serum creatinine	<175 micromol/L (<2.0mg/dL)		
Stage B: serum creatinine	≥175 micromol/L (≥2.0mg/dL)		

Serum β2-microglobulin (β2-M) is the most powerful prognostic factor (measure of tumour bulk) and was used with serum C-reactive protein (CRP), a surrogate measure for serum IL-6, as a measure of tumour aggression to assess prognosis (Table 8.9).[11]

Table 8.9 Bataille Staging System

Low risk	**Both**	β_2-M <6mg/L and CRP <6mg/L	Median survival 54 months
Intermediate risk	**Either**	β_2-M or CRP ≥6mg/L	Median survival 27 months
High risk	**Both**	β_2-M ≥ 6mg/L and CRP ≥6mg/L	Median survival 6 months

The International Staging System (ISS)[12] was devised using data from 10,750 untreated patients from America, Europe, and Asia. It uses serum β_2-M and serum albumin to define 3 stages (Table 8.10).

Table 8.10 International Staging System (ISS)[12]

Stage I	Serum β_2-M <3.5mg/L and serum albumin ≥35g/L	Median survival 62 months
Stage II	Serum β_2-M <3.5mg/L and serum albumin <35g/L ***or*** Serum β_2-M 3.5 – <5.5mg/L	Median survival 44 months
Stage III	Serum β_2-M ≥5.5mg/L	Median survival 29 months

ISS provides useful prognostic groupings in patients <65 and ≥65 years and conventional or high-dose therapy. Cytogenetic data was available in only a subset of patients and was therefore not fully assessed. Reproduced with permission of Dowden Health media© 2007

Intergroupe Francophone du Myelome (IFM)[13] identified t(4;14), del(17p), and β2-M >4mg/L as independent predictors of overall survival on multivariate analysis of patients treated by double transplantation. Patients lacking any of these factors made up 36% of the series and had an excellent prognosis (expected 4-year OS 83%). Patients with either t(4;14) or del(17p) plus β2-M >4mg/L had median OS of only 19 months. Others made up an intermediate group. These genetic parameters were also shown to markedly improve the survival prediction power of each ISS stage.

Mayo Stratification of Myeloma and Risk-Adapted Therapy (mSMART)[14] defines a high-risk group based on cytogenetic and proliferation data (including using conventional cytogenetics to correlate with a high MM-cell proliferative rate) to identify patients who should be managed differently from standard-risk patients:

Table 8.11 Mayo Stratification of Myeloma and Risk-Adapted Therapy[14]

High risk	**Standard risk**
~25% of patients	*~75% of patients*
Presence of any of the following: • FISH del(17p) • FISH t(4;14) • FISH t(14;16) • Cytogenetic del(13q) • Cytogenetic hypodiploidy • PC labelling index ≥3%	All other FISH or cytogenetic abnormalities, including: • Hyperdiploidy • FISH t(11;14) • FISH t(6;14)

Gene expression profile analysis[15] defines a high-risk molecular signature using the ratio of the mean expression levels of 51 up-regulated genes to 19 down-regulated genes to generate a high-risk score present in 13% of patients with shorter event-free and overall survival and a hazard ratio >4.5. A 17 gene subset (12 up-regulated) predicts outcome as well as the 70 gene model but may be difficult to transfer into routine practice.

Response assessment

2 systems are in current use. The system initially developed by the European Group for Blood and Marrow Transplant (EBMT)[16] for patients treated with SCT has been widely used (Table 8.12) but may be superceded by the more recently published but not yet validated system developed by the International Myeloma Working Group[17] (Table 8.13). Although primarily designed for clinical trials, these criteria are useful in clinical practice.

Table 8.12 EBMT response criteria for MM[16]

Response category	Definition
Complete response (CR)	All of the following: • Absence of paraprotein in serum and urine by immunofixation, maintained for ≥6 weeks • <5% plasma cells (PC) in BM and trephine biopsy, if performed; if absent paraprotein sustained 6 weeks, no need to repeat BM • No increase in size or number of lytic bone lesions (development of a compression fracture does not exclude CR) • Disappearance of soft tissue plasmacytomas.
Partial response (PR)	All of the following: • ≥50% ↓ in serum paraprotein, maintained for ≥6 weeks • ↓ in 24h urinary LC excretion by either ≥90% or to <200mg, maintained for ≥6 weeks • For patients with NS myeloma only, ≥50% ↓ in PC in BM aspirate and trephine biopsy, if performed, maintained ≥6 weeks • ≥50% ↓ in size of soft tissue plasmacytomas (by radiology or clinical examination) • No ↑ in size or number of lytic bone lesions (development of a compression fracture does not exclude PR)
Minimal response (MR)	All of the following: • 25–49% ↓ in serum paraprotein level maintained for ≥6 weeks • 50–89% ↓ in 24h urinary LC excretion, which still exceeds 200mg/24h, maintained for ≥6 weeks • For patients with NS myeloma only, 25—49% ↓ in PC in BM aspirate and trephine biopsy, if performed, maintained ≥6 weeks • 25–49% ↓ in size of soft tissue plasmacytomas (by radiology or clinical examination) • No ↑ in size or number of lytic bone lesions (development of a compression fracture does not exclude MR)
No change	Not meeting the criteria of either MR or progressive disease
Plateau	Stable values (within ±25% value at the time response is assessed), maintained for ≥3 months
Relapse from CR	At least one of the following: • Reappearance of serum or urine paraprotein on immunofixation or electrophoresis, confirmed by at least 1 other study • ≥5% PC in BM aspirate or trephine biopsy • Development of new lytic bone lesions or soft tissue plasmacytomas or definite ↑ in size of residual bone lesions • Development of hypercalcaemia not attributable to other cause

Table 8.12 EBMT response criteria for MM[16] (*continued*)

Response category	Definition
Progressive disease	One or more of the following: • >25% ↑ in serum paraprotein, which must also be an absolute ↑ of ≥5g/L, confirmed by ≥1 repeated study • >25% ↑ in 24h LC excretion, which must also be an absolute ↑ of ≥200mg/24h, confirmed by ≥1 repeated study • >25% ↑ in PC in BM aspirate or trephine biopsy, which must also be an absolute ↑ of at least 10% • Definite ↑ in size of existing bone lesions or soft tissue plasmacytomas • Development of new bone lesions or soft tissue plasmacytomas • Development of hypercalcaemia not attributable to other cause

Table 8.13 International Myeloma Working Group uniform response criteria[17]

Response subcategory	Response criteria[a]
Stringent complete response (sCR)	CR as defined below, plus: • ↔ SFLC ratio • Absence of clonal cells in BM[b] by immunohistochemistry or immunofluorescence[c]
Complete response (CR)	All of the following: • –ve immunofixation on the serum and urine • Disappearance of any soft tissue plasmacytomas • ≤5% PC in BM[b]
Very good partial response (VGPR)	One of the following: • Serum and urine M-protein detectable by immunofixation but not on electrophoresis • ≥90% ↓ in serum M-protein plus urine M-protein level <200mg/24h
Partial response (PR)	• ≥50% ↓ of serum M-protein and ↓ in urinary M-protein by ≥90% or to <200mg/24h • If the serum and urine M-protein are unmeasurable, a ≥50% ↓ in the difference between involved and uninvolved SFLC levels is required in place of the M-protein criteria. • If serum and urine M-protein are unmeasurable , and SFLC assay is also unmeasurable, ≥50% ↓ in PC is required in place of M-protein, provided baseline BM PC percentage was ≥30%. In adition to the above listed criteria, if present at baseline, ≥50% ↓ in size of soft tissue plasmacytomas is also required.

(*continued*)

Table 8.13 International Myeloma Working Group uniform response criteria[17] *(continued)*

Response subcategory	**Response criteria**[a]
Stable disease (SD) *Not recommended for use as an indicator of response; stability of disease is best described by providing the time to progression estimates.*	Not meeting criteria for CR, VGPR, PR, or progressive disease

Progressive disease
To be used for calculation of time to progression and progression-free survival end-points for all patients including those in CR (includes primary progressive disease and disease progression on or off therapy).
	Any one or more of the following:
	• ↑ of ≥25% from baseline in:
	  • Serum M-component and/or (absolute ↑ must be ≥5g/L)[d]
	  • Urine M-component and/or (absolute ↑ must be ≥200mg/24h)
	  • Only in patients without measurable serum and urine M-protein levels: the difference between involved and uninvolved SFLC levels (absolute ↑ must be >100mg/L)
	  • BM PC percentage (absolute % must be ≥10%)[e]
	• Definite development of new bone lesions or soft tissue plasmacytomas or definite ↑ in size of existing bone lesions or tissue plasmacytomas
	• Development of hypercalcaemia (corrected serum calcium > 2.65mmol/L (>11.5mg/dL)) solely attributable to the PC proliferative disorder

Clinical relapse *Not used in calculation of time to progression or progression-free survival but is listed as something that can be reported optionally or used in clinical practice.*	Any one or more of the following direct indicators of increasing disease and/or end organ dysfunction (CRAB features)[d]: • Development of new soft tissue plasmacytomas or bone lesions • Definite ↑ in size of existing plasmacytomas or bone lesions; definite ↑ is defined as a 50% (and ≥1cm) ↑ as measured serially by sum of the products of the cross-diameters of measured lesion • Hypercalcaemia (>2.65mmol/L (≥11.5mg/dL)) • Decrease in haemoglobin of ≥2g/dL • Rise in serum creatinine by ≥177 micromol/L (≥2mg/dL)

Table 8.13 International Myeloma Working Group uniform response criteria[17] (*continued*)

Response subcategory	**Response criteria**[a]
Relapse from CR *To be used only if the end-point studied is DFS*[f]	Any one or more of the following: • Reappearance of serum or urine M-protein by immunofixation or electrophoresis • Development of ≥5% PC in the BM • Appearance of any other sign of progression (i.e. new plasmacytoma, lytic bone lesion, or hypercalcaemia)

[a] All response categories require 2 consecutive assessments made at anytime before the institution of any new therapy; all categories also require no new evidence of progressive or new bone lesions if radiographic studies were performed. Radiographic studies are not required to satisfy these response requirements.

[b] Confirmation with repeat BM not needed.

[c] Presence/absence of clonal cells is based upon the κ/λ ratio. An abnormal κ/λ ratio by immunohistochemistry and/or immunofluorescence requires a minimum of 100 plasma cells for analysis. An abnormal ratio reflecting the presence of an abnormal clone is κ/λ of >4:1 or <1:2. [d] For progressive disease, serum M-component increases of ≥ 10g/L are sufficient to define relapse if starting M-component is ≥50g/L. [e] Relapse from CR has the 5% cut-off versus 10% for other categories of relapse. [f] For purposes of calculating time to progression and progression-free survival, CR patients should also be evaluated using criteria listed above for progressive disease. Reproduced with permission from Macmillan Publishers Ltd.© 2007

Management

Partial and complete responses are achieved in a high proportion of patients with MM using a range of chemotherapeutic regimens but these responses are transient. Further responses are commonly achieved with the same or alternative regimens. MM is not curable with conventional regimens and only a small number of patients may have been cured by allogeneic SCT. The recent introduction of novel agents has changed the treatment options in MM and risk-adapted therapy may now be feasible as new prognostic factors more clearly define risk groups.

Initial management of a patient with newly diagnosed MM often requires attention to general aspects of care prior to initiation of cytotoxic therapy.

Initial management considerations and general aspects

Pain control

- Titrate simple analgesia (e.g. paracetamol 1g 4–6-hourly) for mild-to-moderate pain, weak opioids (co-codamol 2 tabs 6-hourly or dihydrocodeine 30–60mg up to 4-hourly) for moderate pain and strong opioids (oramorph 5–10mg 4-hourly converting to slow release preparation, e.g. MST® or fentanyl patch when daily requirement established with 5–10mg morphine sulfate solution prn for 'breakthrough' pain) for moderate-to-severe pain; commence simple laxative with opioids.
- Avoid NSAIDs (if essential, use caution and monitor renal function).
- Local radiotherapy (8–30Gy) often extremely effective.
- A spinal support corset often helpful for severe back pain.
- Neuropathic pain may be relieved by non-analgesic adjuvants, e.g. amitryptiline, carbamazepine, or gabapentin.

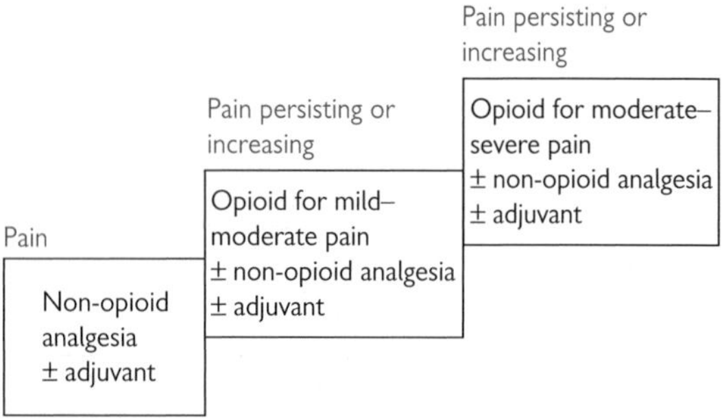

Fig. 8.5 WHO pain treatment ladder. Reproduced with permission from the World Health Organization, *Palliative Care*: symptom management and end of life care, p.12.

Renal impairment

- All patients should be instructed to maintain a high fluid intake (≥3L/d); use caution with nephrotoxic drugs, including NSAIDs.
- Prompt intervention to correct early renal impairment may prevent long-term renal damage.
- Vigorous rehydration with high fluid input (3–4L/d) aiming for urine output >3L/d, and rapid treatment of hypercalcaemia, infection and hyperuricaemia may improve renal function.
- Seek advice of nephrologist if renal failure does not improve within 48h; peritoneal or haemodialysis may be required (<5%).
- Plasmapheresis may have a role in established renal failure due to cast nephropathy.
- Dexamethasone-based regimens were treatment of choice after response to rehydration or in established CRF (Thal/Dex and Vel/Dex regimens now preferred); follow by PBSC harvest (mobilized by G-CSF alone) and HDM (140mg/m^2) with autologous SCT in younger patients; after response EFS and OS same as other patients; allo-SCT not recommended for patients undergoing haemodialysis.

Hypercalcaemia

- Vigorous rehydration with IV saline (3–6L/day IV) with close monitoring of fluid balance and renal function.
- Loop diuretics (furosemide) increase Ca^{2+} excretion and maintain fluid balance.
- IV bisphosphonate (pamidronate 30–90mg IVI over 2h or zoledronic acid 4mg IV over 5min; ↓ dose and infusion rate in renal impairment); zoledronic acid gives higher CR rate (50% by day 4) and duration of effect; repeat if necessary.
- IVcorticosteroids or calcitonin if refractory; chemotherapy.

Bone disease

- Local radiotherapy for localized pain (8–20Gy).
- Fixation of fractures/potential fractures followed by radiotherapy.
- Vertebroplasty or kyphoplasty may be considered in patients with persistent back pain.
- Long term bisphosphonate prophylaxis of further damage.

Infection

- Prompt and vigorous broad spectrum antibiotic therapy; IV antibiotics for severe systemic infection; avoid aminoglycosides if possible.
- Prophylactic trimethoprim-sulfamethoxazole given during the first 2 months of therapy may reduce risk of infection.
- Annual influenza immunization and immunization against *S. pneumonia* and *H. influenza* is recommended.

Anaemia

- Blood transfusion for symptomatic anaemia; use caution if high paraprotein due to risk of hyperviscosity.
- EPO for Hb persistently ≤10g/dL (10,000IU tiw or 30,000IU once weekly ~70% response rate with ≥2g/dL rise in Hb); not recommended until response to chemotherapy assessed then consider 6–8 week trial in patients with symptomatic anaemia on chemotherapy; discontinue if Hb has not risen by 1–2g/dL after 6–8 weeks.

Hyperviscosity

- May develop in patients with high serum paraprotein levels, IgA > IgG causing cerebral, pulmonary, and renal manifestations and bleeding.
- Symptomatic patients should be treated by plasmapheresis (3L exchange) followed by prompt chemotherapy.

Cord compression

- Medical emergency; requires treatment within 24h.
- Commonly presents with sensory loss, paraesthesiae, limb weakness, difficulty walking, and sphincter disturbance.
- Urgent MRI scan to define lesion (CT if MRI unavailable).
- Commence oral dexamethasone stat (8–16mg/d).
- Local radiotherapy should be commenced within 24h.
- Surgery is indicated if there is spinal instability.

Haemorrhage

- Uncommon; several possible mechanisms: direct inhibition of fibrin polymerization, heparin-like anticoagulants, acquired von Willebrand's syndrome and, in the presence of AL amyloid, factor X deficiency; treatment must be individualized.

Specific treatment of MM[5,14]

The aim of treatment is (i) to control disease, (ii) to maximize quality of life, and (iii) to prolong survival. Chemotherapy and good supportive care are both essential to these aims. It is important that, wherever possible, patients are treated within clinical trials to determine the optimum combination and sequence of the effective new agents that have radically altered treatment options in recent years.

An early decision must be whether the patient is a candidate for high dose therapy (HDT) and SCT, based on age, co-morbidities, and risk-assessment. Advanced age and renal dysfunction are not absolute contraindications to SCT. An initial regimen that minimizes stem cell toxicity must be selected for potential candidates for SCT. Alkylating agents remain the mainstay of therapy for patients ineligible for SCT.

Initial therapy for patients ineligible for SCT

Melphalan and prednisolone (MP)[19]

- Until recently, standard initial therapy for elderly patients with MM since 1960; (M 6–9mg/m^2/d PO; P 40–100mg/d PO for 4 days every 4–6 weeks) achieves ≥50% reduction of paraprotein in 50–60% patients; response often slow; continue to maximum response (9–12 months); CR uncommon (<5%); well tolerated; side effects myelosuppression and steroid toxicity (add PPI/H2 antagonist).
- Patients with ≥50% response may achieve plateau phase (stable paraprotein without treatment); median duration 12–18 months.
- Monitor paraprotein 6–8-weekly to detect progression; at progression after durable plateau, may get further response to MP.
- Melphalan resistance ultimately develops in all patients.
- Median survival ~36 months.
- Option for patients unable or unwilling to tolerate thalidomide.

Melphalan, prednisolone, and thalidomide (MPT)[20, 21]

- Thalidomide is an immunomodulatory agent with multiple actions on MM-cells and the microenvironment: inhibition of angiogenesis, inhibition of growth and survival of MM cells, altered cytokine production, altered expression of adhesion molecules and T-lymphocyte stimulation; side effects: constipation, sedation, rash, dizziness, and peripheral neuropathy; VTE is a risk when used in combination and patients at high risk of, or with a history of VTE should receive full-dose anticoagulation therapy; pregnancy prevention programme mandatory.
- MPT (MP +T 100–400mg/d) shows superior response (OR 76% *vs.* 48%; CR+nCR 28% *vs.* 7%) and progression-free survival (PFS: 54% *vs.* 27% at 2 years) *vs.* MP in 2 randomized trials; 1 also demonstrated superior median OS (52 months *vs.* 33 months) and 3-year OS (48% *vs.* 25%).
- MPT has higher toxicity (48% *vs.* 25%): thrombo-embolism 12% *vs.* 2%; neuropathy 10% *vs.* 1%; infections 10% *vs.* 2%; GI events 6% *vs.* 1%; thrombo-embolic events markedly reduced by introduction of LMW heparin prophylaxis.
- Doses and administration differ; optimum schedule unclear:
  - Palumbo *et al.* (2006)[20]—6 × 28d cycles, M 4mg/m^2 and P 40mg/m^2 x 7d ± T 100mg to progression (i.e. T maintenance).
  - Facon *et al.* (2007)[21]—12 × 6 week cycles, M 0.25mg/kg and P 2mg/kg x 4d ± T 200–400mg/d for median 11 months.
- MPT has been approved by the FDA and European Medicines Agency (EMEA) for 1st-line treatment of MM in patients ineligible for SCT; category 1 recommendation in NCCN Guidelines.[5]

Cyclophosphamide, thalidomide, and dexamethasone (CTDa)

- Attenuated dose CTD (C 500mg po/IV once weekly; T 50–200mg/d; D 20mg po days 1–4 and 15–18; 28-d cycle) used in UK Myeloma IX trial; effective and well tolerated initial therapy in elderly patients; results of the randomization *vs.* MP awaited; antithrombotic therapy recommended; pregnancy prevention programme mandatory.

Velcade® (bortezomib), melphalan, and prednisone (VMP)[14,22,23]

- Vel 1.3mg/m^2 IV 2 × weekly (weeks 1, 2, 4, and 5) for four 6-week cycles then weekly (weeks 1, 2, 4, and 5) for five 6-week cycles plus M 9mg/m^2 and P 60mg/m^2 on d1–4 of each cycle.

- A small phase 1/2 study shows an advantage for VMP over MP in RR (89% *vs.* 42%), 16 months EFS (83% *vs.* 51%), and 16 months OS (90% *vs.* 62%); a phase 3 study in 680 patients was terminated early when VMP showed superiority over MP in all measures: CR 35% *vs.* 5%; duration of CR 24 months vs. 13 months, median time to progression 24 months vs. 13 months; similar adverse effects.
- Mayo Clinic (sMART) guidelines suggest that a Vel-containing regimen is considered in patients with high risk features (e.g. t(4;14), t(14;16), or del(17p)) as it may overcome adverse impact.

Melphalan, prednisolone, and Revlimid® (lenalidomide) (MPR)[24]

- M 0.18mg/kg/d and P 2mg/kg/d, R days 1–4, 10mg/d, days 1–21 every 28 days for 9 cycles.
- Several trials are in progress; promising phase 2 data in trial of 54 patients with 81% PR or better, 48% VGPR, 24% CR, and 1 year EFS and OS of 92% and 100%; grade 3+4 toxcity: 52% neutropenia, 24% thrombocytopenia; 5% VTE.

Cyclophosphamide[25]

- 'C-weekly' (300–500mg PO/IV once weekly) may be used as a single agent for patients intolerant of melphalan due to persistent cytopenia and thalidomide; durable plateau phases achieved.

Initial therapy for patients eligible for SCT

Non-alkylator regimens are administered for 4–6 cycles prior to stem cell mobilization, high dose therapy, and SCT. No regimen is clearly superior. VAD, formerly widely used, has been superceded.

High dose dexamethasone (Dex)[26,27]

- Single agent Dex (40mg/d PO on days 1–4, 9–12, and 17–20; 28-d cycle) obviates need for indwelling IV catheter required for VAD (vincristine and doxorubicin by infusion days 1–4 plus Dex; previously widely used but no longer recommended) and reduces thrombotic, neurotoxic, and infective complications; responses ≥ PR achieved in 43–63%.

Thalidomide and dexamethasone (ThalDex)[28,29]

- Addition of thalidomide (200mg/d PO) to Dex (📖 for dose see High dose dexamethasone (Dex)), in a randomized study of 207 patients improved RRs (63% *vs.* 41%) but added toxicity (45% *vs.* 21%), in particular DVT (17% *vs.* 3%), also rash, bradycardia, and neuropathy; superiority to VAD demonstrated plus advantage of oral administration; prophylactic anticoagulation recommended; pregnancy prevention programme mandatory.
- Thal/Dex approved in USA as first-line therapy by FDA in 2006.

Cyclophosphamide, thalidomide and dexamethasone (CTD) (📖 p.727)

- CTD (C 500mg PO/IV once weekly; T 100–200mg/d; D 40mg PO d1–4 and 15–18; 21-d cycle) × 4–6 courses in UK Myeloma IX trial; effective and well tolerated initial therapy pre-HDT; results of randomization *vs.* C-VAD awaited; prophylactic anticoagulation recommended; pregnancy prevention programme mandatory.

Lenalidomide (Revlimid®) and dexamethasone (Rev/Dex)

- Lenalidomide is a thalidomide analogue, immunomodulatory drug (IMiD); multiple effects on both MM-cells and the microenvironment and different side effect profile; main side effects—constipation, cytopenia, VTE, and possible birth defects.
- Rev/Dex (Len 25mg/d PO days 1–21 and Dex 40mg/d PO days 1–4, 9–12, and 17–20; 28-d cycle) is FDA and EMEA approved as therapy for relapsed/refractory MM; not yet reviewed by NICE in UK.
- Phase II study of Rev/Dex initial therapy achieved 91% RR with 6% CR and 32% VGPR; prophylactic anticoagulation recommended.[30,31]
- A study of Rev/Dex as initial therapy in 445 patients on Len[30,31] randomized between low dose Dex (40mg/d, days 1, 8, 15, and 22) and high dose Dex was closed early because better 1-year OS in the low dose arm (96% *vs.* 86%) and fewer side effects (VTE 9% *vs.* 25%; febrile neutropenia 8% *vs.* 19%) despite an inferior RR (71% *vs.* 82%); better OS maintained at 2 years (87% *vs.* 75%).
- Rev/low dose Dex with low dose aspirin thromboprophylaxis is recommended by Mayo Clinic (sMART) Guidelines as standard induction therapy in patients eligible for SCT.[14]

Bortezomib (Velcade®) and dexamethasone (Vel/Dex)

- Bortezomib is a 1st-in-class proteasome inhibitor; multiple effects on both MM-cells and the microenvironment; side effects are transient thrombocytopenia, peripheral neuropathy, neuropathic pain, constipation, nausea, vomiting, and neutropenic fever.
- Bortezomib (1.3mg/m^2 IV 2 × weekly (days 1, 4, 8, 11) for 2 weeks in 3-week cycle × 4–8) approved by FDA, EMEA, and NICE in UK as 2nd-line treatment in relapsed/ refractory MM; ~40% OR in newly diagnosed patients.
- Vel/Dex: Dex 40mg/d usually added on day of and day after Vel.
- Long-term follow-up of 50 patients treated with Vel ± Dex (added if <PR after 2 cycles or <CR after 4 cycles) showed high efficacy: ORR 90%, 19% CR, + nCR; rapid response 50% after cycle 2; 75% required Dex, improving response in 64%; manageable toxicities; SC harvest not compromised.[32,33]
- IFM phase 3 randomized trial *vs.* VAD in 482 patients shows superiority of Vel/Dex: response assessed in 208 patients: ≥PR = 89% *vs.* 71%; CR + nCR = 22% *vs.* 9%; the benefit translates into higher CR and VGPR rates after ASCT.[34]

Bortezomib (Velcade®), thalidomide, and dexamethasone (VTD)

- VTD has been compared with Thal/Dex in a randomized trial in 187 patients giving a better CR + nCR rate (38% *vs.* 7%) with similar toxicity apart from ↑ grade 3 skin rashes and was not adversely affected by poor-risk cytogenetic abnormalities; better CR + nCR rate persisted after SCT (57% *vs.* 28%).[35]
- A rapid response rate was demonstrated for VTD in a study of 38 untreated patients with 16% CR and 87% ≥ PR after ≤3 cycles.[36]

Bortezomib (Velcade®), doxorubicin and dexamethasone (PAD)

- Phase 1/2 study of PAD initial therapy (Vel 1.3 (PAD1) or 1.0 (PAD2) mg/m^2 d1, 4, 8, 11, Dox 9mg/m^2 d1-4, Dex 40mg/d d 1-44) in 42 patients achieved CR + VGPR in 62% (PAD1) and 42% (PAD2), translating to 81% and 53% after HDM + SCT, median responses of 29 and 24mo and 2yr OS of 95% and 73% respectively; toxicity lower with PAD2.[37]

Bortezomib (Velcade®), lenalidomide, and dexamethasone (VRD)

- Preliminary data from 42 of 66 patients in a phase 1/2 study show extremely high response rates with 28% CR + nCR and 98%.[38]

Table 8.14 Initial treatment for MM outside a clinical trial

Ineligible for SCT	MPT to plateau phase
	MP or MPR* if thalidomide not tolerated
	Vel/Dex for short response or refractory disease; consider in patients with poor risk cytogenetics**
Eligible for SCT	Dex***, Thal/Dex or Rev*/Dex x 4–6; PBSC mobilization; HDM + SCT
	Vel/Dex for short response or refractory disease

SCT stem cell transplantation; MPT melphalan, prednisolone and thalidomide; MP melphalan and prednisolone; MPR melphalan, prednisolone and lenalidomide; Vel/Dex bortezomib + dexamethasone; Dex high dose dexamethasone; Thal/Dex thalidomide + dexamethasone; Rev/Dex, revlimid + dexamethasone; PBSC peripheral blood stem cells; HDM high dose melphalan.

* If available;

** Suggested by Mayo Clinic Guidelines[14]

*** Suggested for non-high risk patients, withholding Thal unless no response to first 1–2 cycles of Dex in NCCN Clinical Practice Guidelines in Oncology[5]

Other therapy

Bisphosphonates[39–42]

- Inhibit OC activation; patients on long-term therapy experience less bone pain and fewer new bone lesions and fractures; evidence of improved QoL and possible prolonged survival.
- All patients with active MM should receive bisphosphonate therapy.
- No evidence for superiority of either daily clodronate (1600mg or equivalent PO) or monthly pamidronate (90mg IVI) or zoledronate (4mg IV).
- Use with caution in renal impairment: clodronate, 50% dose if creatinine clearance 10–30mL/min, contraindicated if <10mL/min; pamidronate, slow infusion (20mg/h); zoledronate, check creatinine before each infusion, ensure hydration; not recommended if creatinine >265 micromol/L.
- Monitor for osteonecrosis of jaw with zoledronate (risk factor poor dentition).

Thromboprophylaxis[43]

- Risk of VTE in MM is 3–4% in first 4 months after diagnosis in patients treated with Dex montherapy or MP.
- Thal monotherapy also associated with VTE incidence of 3–4%; thromboprophylaxis not indicated unless patient has history of thrombosis or other risk factors.

- Thal combinations ↑ VTE incidence: Thal/Dex (up to 26%), MPT (up to 20%), and anthracycline combinations (up to 58%); median time to VTE, 3 months.
- Rev monotherapy no ↑ risk and thromboprophylaxis not indicated; ↑ incidence with Rev/Dex (up to 23%) and Rev/CTX (14%).
- *Warfarin*: low fixed dose (1mg/d) ineffective; full dose warfarin (target INR 2–3.0) reduces risk with Thal or Rev combinations; risk of haemorrhage with regimens causing severe thrombocytopenia.
- *LMW heparin* (enoxaparin 40mg/d SC or equivalent) reduces VTE frequency in several Thal combinations but not multi-agent chemotherapy; may be preferable due to shorter half-life and lower risk of haemorrhage but not recommended in renal failure.
- *Aspirin* 75–325mg/d reduces VTE risk with several Thal or Rev combinations but not Thal + doxorubicin or multi-agent chemotherapy; convenient and may be useful in lower-risk combinations e.g. Thal or Rev with low dose Dex.
- *Risk factors:* initial therapy, high tumour load, hyperviscosity, high dose Dex, doxorubicin, multi-agent chemotherapy, concurrent EPO; age, obesity, history of VTE, diabetes, infection, renal disease, cardiac disease, surgery, immobility, HRT, thrombophilia.
- Unless contraindicated, prophylaxis for all patients receiving Thal or Rev in combination with other agents especially as initial therapy; continue for 4–6 months or duration of Thal or Rev therapy; consider longer if additional patient- or treatment-related factors.
- Select prophylaxis on individual patient basis, balancing risks of VTE and haemorrhage (📖 see Table 8.15).
- Treat VTE according to standard protocol; Thal or Rev should be briefly discontinued and may be cautiously resumed when full anticoagulation established; ~10% risk of 2nd DVT; continue anticoagulation for duration of Thal or Rev therapy; discontinue 1 month after completion if no further DVT (minimum 3 mo therapy).[43]

Radiotherapy

- Important modality of treatment in myeloma at all stages of disease; local radiotherapy (8–30Gy) often a rapidly effective treatment for bone pain associated with pathological fracture or lytic lesions.
- Urgent radiotherapy is indicated for patients with spinal cord compression.
- Multiple widespread lesions may be palliated with hemibody irradiation: 10Gy for the lower hemibody or 6Gy for the upper hemibody; side effect myelosuppression; sequential hemibody irradiation may be performed after an interval of 6 weeks.

Follow-up

- Monitor response to therapy with serial quantitation of serum paraprotein, SFLC or BJP (+ FBC, renal biochemistry and serum Ca^{2+} group) at 4–6 weekly intervals to plateau (stable values ±25% over 3 months) or SC mobilization.
- Patients in established plateau phase should be monitored for progression at 6–8 week intervals.

Table 8.15 Proposed risk assessment model for VTE management in MM patients treated with thalidomide or lenalidomide[43]

Risk factors	Actions
Individual • Obesity • Previous VTE • Central venous catheter or pacemaker	If no risk factor or any one risk factor present: • Aspirin 75–325mg once daily
Associated disease • Cardiac disease • Chronic renal disease • Diabetes • Acute infection • Immobilization	If ≥2 risk factors present: • LMW heparin (enoxaparin 40mg once daily or equivalent) ***or*** • Full dose warfarin (target INR 2–3)
Surgery • General surgery • Any anaesthesia • Trauma	
Medications • EPO	
Blood clotting disorders	
Myeloma-related factors • Diagnosis • Hyperviscosity	
Myeloma therapy • High dose dexamethasone (>480mg/month) • Doxorubicin • Multi-agent chemotherapy	If any of these therapies used: • LMW heparin (enoxaparin 40mg once daily or equivalent) ***or*** • Full dose warfarin (target INR 2–3)

Autologous stem cell transplantation (ASCT)[44–48]

- ASCT not curative but prolongs median OS by ~12 months; however its role in the era of targeted therapy is not clear.
- High dose melphalan (HDM; 200mg/m^2) + ASCT achieves high CR rates (25–80%) after initial therapy with a VAD-type regimen and PBSC harvest; median response duration 2–3 years; treatment of choice for patients <65 years; best responders have best survival, median >5 years; improved PFS (32 *vs.* 20 months) and OS (54 *vs.* 42 months) *vs.* conventional therapy in randomized study; side effects: myelosuppression, infection, delayed regeneration.
- Addition of TBI to melphalan 140mg/m^2 with ASCT adds toxicity but no benefit; no convincing benefit for 'double/tandem' ASCT but benefit for those converted from PR to CR after 2nd procedure; no benefit from SC purging procedures; same OS whether ASCT early (after induction) or delayed (as salvage after relapse).
- Mayo Clinic (sMART) Guidelines[14] recommend early SCT in eligible standard risk patients with a tandem SCT in those failing to achieve ≥ VGPR; high risk patients do not derive major benefit from ASCT and consolidation by a bortezomib-based regimen e.g. VMP, is

recommended after SC collection so that ASCT is available at relapse; in young high-risk patients allo-SCT should be considered.

Allogeneic stem cell transplantation[49–51]

- Applicable to fit patients ≤50 years; transplant-related mortality with standard conditioning regimens is high (~33%) due to infection and GvHD; 35–45% long-term survival (>5 years); ~33% chance of durable remission and possible cure; ~33% chance of survival with recurrence; evidence of graft *vs.* myeloma effect.
- Reduced-intensity regimens lower toxicity, increase age limit, but reduce response rate.
- Reduced-intensity allogeneic SCT after ASCT has achieved 52–83% CR with 2–3 year OS 62–78% and PFS ~55% and may be a useful approach as either consolidation or salvage therapy; poor OS associated with chemoresistant MM, >1 prior SCT, and no chronic GvHD.
- Allogeneic SCT should be discussed with patients <55 years with a suitable sibling donor or young patients with a matched unrelated donor.

Maintenance therapy

- Maintenance chemotherapy (MP) does not prolong response or survival but adds toxicity (BM suppression); maintenance dexamethasone not convincingly beneficial.
- Maintenance lenalidomide and bortezomib under investigation.

IFN-α[52]

- Formerly widely used as maintenance therapy during plateau phase after standard or HDT at a dose of $3mu/m^2$ SC tiw.
- Improves response duration by median 6 months on meta-analysis and has small effect on survival.
- Side effects reduce patient compliance and cost–utility profile is unfavourable; no longer recommended or widely used.

Thalidomide

- A randomized trial in 597 patients compared maintenance Thal after ASCT (50–400mg/d) with 2 arms without Thal maintenance and showed significantly benefit: 3-year EFS (52% *vs.* 36%/37%) and 4-year OS (87% *vs.* 77%/74%); median duration 15 months; median dose 200mg; 39% discontinued due to toxicity; side effects neuropathy 68%, fatigue 34%; constipation 20%.[53]
- 50–100mg dose recommended; thromboprophylaxis not required unless individual risk factors are present.
- Mayo Clinic (sMART) Guidelines[14] suggest maintenance therapy with Thal and prednisolone should be considered in high risk patients who fail to achieve CR and continued to maximum response.

Treatment of 1° refractory disease[54]

- Bortezomib has been approved by NICE in UK and FDA for treatment of refractory MM; lenalidomide + dexamethasone (Rev/Dex) has also been approved by FDA and EMEA for refractory MM.
- Patients who progress or fail to respond (<25% ↓ in paraprotein) to initial therapy with MP may respond to single agent Dex (20–40mg/d

× 4d weekly × 3 weeks), Thal/Dex, CDT, Vel/Dex, or Rev/Dex; failures on MPT may respond to Vel/Dex or Rev/Dex; failures on Thal/Dex or Rev/Dex may respond to Vel/Dex.
- Consolidate with ASCT if possible as patients with 1° progressive myeloma may achieve good response to ASCT; 1-year PFS of 70% reported and compares to 83% in responders to initial therapy.

Salvage therapy for disease progression

Treatment of disease progression before the development of novel therapies consisted of progressively shorter responses to available agents with the ultimate development of drug resistance and evolution of adverse features. The development of novel agents has significantly improved the outlook for patients with relapsed myeloma.

- Patients who achieve a durable response (≥18 months) to initial therapy may respond to the same regimen (response rate 25–50% to MP).
- Patients who relapse early after initial therapy (<6 months) will require a different regimen to achieve a further response.
- Patients who relapse after prolonged response to HDM and ASCT (>18 months) with a PBSC harvest sufficient for 2 procedures or with a further successful harvest may benefit from 2nd HDM after re-induction with Thal/Dex, Vel/Dex, Dex, or Rev/Dex.
- Allogeneic SCT should be considered for eligible patients with progressive disease after ASCT.
- There is evidence of a graft-versus-myeloma effect; DLI can re-induce responses in patients with recurrence after allogeneic SCT.
- Alternative salvage regimens include VAD, C-VAD, DT-PACE (dexamethasone, thalidomide, cisplatin, doxorubicin, cyclophosphamide, etoposide), ESHAP (etoposide, methylprednisolone, cisplatin, cytarabine) and DCEP (dexamethasone, cyclophosphamide, etoposide, cisplatin).
- Cyclophosphamide (50–100mg/day PO) is well tolerated palliative therapy for patients with advanced refractory disease or cytopenia who are intolerant of thalidomide or dexamethasone or unable to tolerate Vel/Dex or Rev/Dex.

Thalidomide (Thal)[55–62]

- Single agent Thal (50–400mg/day) achieves ~30% responses in chemotherapy-resistant myeloma; addition of Dex (20–40mg/day × 4d/month) ± cyclophosphamide increases response rates.
- Thal/Dex achieved 56% OR at 1st relapse (46% ≥2nd), PFS 17 months and 3-year OS of 60% *vs.* 11 months EFS and 19 months OS with standard therapy.
- CTD achieved 60% OR (5% CR/nCR), TTP 8 months and OS of z17.5 months.
- Thal + pegylated liposomal doxorubicin + Dex achieved 76% OR, (32% CR/nCR) and 22 months PFS.
- Thal side effects cumulative and dose dependent (worse at doses >200mg/d): constipation, somnolence, neuropathy, neutropenia, tremor, headache; thromboembolism risk ↑ in combination with steroids or anthracyclines (📖 p.349 and Table 8.15 for prophylaxis); discontinue if

grade 3 neuropathy develops and restart at lower dose if improves to grade 1; pregnancy prevention programme mandatory.

Bortezomib (Velcade®)[63–67]

- Approved in 2007 as monotherapy in UK by NICE for treatment of first relapse in MM; approved by FDA and EMEA for treatment of relapsed MM; Vel monotherapy is NCCN category 1 recommendation; Vel/Dex is NCCN category 2a recommendation.[5]
- No dose reduction required in renal impairment.
- In a randomized study *vs.* Dex in 669 patients Vel gave better CR+PR (38% *vs.* 18%), TTP (6.2 *vs.* 3.5 months) and 1-year OS (80% *vs.* 66%); updated analysis shows 43% OR, 9%CR, and 6-month OS advantage (30 *vs.* 24 months).
- FDA also approved bortezomib plus pegylated liposomal doxorubicin (PLD 30mg/m^2 d4) for patients with ≥1 prior therapy not including bortezomib; update of phase 3 randomized trial in 646 patients showed better OR (52% *vs.* 44%), median TTP 10 months *vs.* 7 months and OS for Vel/PLD vs. Vel; ↑ neutropenia and thrombocytopenia.
- Addition of Dex to Vel improves OR from 27% to 50%.
- Other combinations evaluated are Vel/Thal/Dex, Vel/Rev/Dex, Vel/CTX/Dex, Vel/M with OR of 47-82%, CR+nCR 10–16% and EFS 8–12 months.

Lenalidomide (Revlimid®)[68,69]

- Lenalidomide achieves responses as monotherapy in ~25% relapsed MM but is more active combined with Dex (Rev/Dex).
- Dose adjustments are required for patients with renal impairment.
- Rev/Dex is FDA and EMEA approved for relapsed/refractory MM after ≥1 prior therapy; Rev/Dex is NCCN category 1 recommendation; single agent Rev is NCCN category 2a recommendation.[5]
- 2 randomized studies of Rev/Dex *vs.* Dex in relapsed MM each with ~350 patients, reported better OR (60/61 *vs.* 24/20%), CR (16/14 *vs.* 3/1%), longer TTP (11/11 *vs.* 3/5 months) and better OS (30 *vs.* 20 months) in the Rev/Dex arm; commonest toxicities were neutropenia, VTE, thrombocytopenia, pneumonia, anaemia, and fatigue.
- Rev/Dex has an ↑ risk of VTE and thromboprophylaxis is required; pregnancy prevention programme mandatory.

Prognosis[70]

The median survival of a patient treated with MP is ~3 years and this ↑ to ~5 years for patients treated with VAD-type induction followed by HDM and ASCT. Analysis of patient outcome at a single institution shows improved median OS from relapse for patients relapsing after 2000 (24 months) compared to those relapsing before 2000 (12 months). Those treated with one or more of Thal, Rev or Vel, had longer OS from relapse (31 months *vs.* 15 months). Patients diagnosed in the last decade had a 50% improvement in overall survival (45 months *vs.* 30 months). The improvements since 2000 are due predominantly to the introduction of novel agents and in part to improved supportive care.

Table 8.16 Salvage treatment options for relapsed MM outside a clinical trial[5]

Relapse after MP	Early <12 months	Vel or Vel/Dex or Thal/Dex or Rev*/Dex or Dex or CTD or VAD
	Late ≥18 months	MP or MPT or CTD or Thal/Dex or Vel or Vel/Dex or Rev*/Dex or Dex
Relapse after MPT	Early <12 months	Vel or Vel/Dex or Rev*/Dex or Dex
	Late ≥18 months	MPT? or Vel or Vel/Dex or Rev*/Dex or Dex or CTD? or Thal/Dex?
Relapse after ASCT	Early <12 months	Vel or Vel/Dex or Rev*/Dex or Dex or Thal/Dex then consider alloSCT
	Late ≥18 months	Vel or Vel/Dex or Rev*/Dex or Dex or Thal/Dex; consider alloSCT or 2nd ASCT
Relapse after allo-SCT		Consider DLI

* If available; MP melphalan and prednisolone; Vel bortezomib monotherapy; Vel/Dex bortezomib + dexamethasone; Thal/Dex thalidomide + dexamethasone; Rev/Dex, revlimid + dexamethasone; Dex high dose dexamethasone; CTD cyclophosphamide, thalidomide and dexamethasone; MPT melphalan, prednisolone and thalidomide; ASCT autologous stem cell transplantation; allo-SCT allogeneic stem cell transplantation; DLI donor lymphocyte infusion.

References

1. Kyle, R.A. and Rajkumar, S.V. (2007). Epidemiology of the plasma cell disorders. *Best Practice & Research Clin Haematol.* **20**, 637–64.
2. Chn,g W.J. *et al.* (2007). Genetic events in the pathogenesis of multiple myeloma. *Best Practice & Res Clin Haematol* **20**, 571–96.
3. Podar, K. *et al.* (2007). The malignant clone and the bone-marrow environment. *Best Practice & Res Clin Haematol* **20**, 597–612.
4. UK Myeloma Forum and Nordic Myeloma Study Group (2005). Guidelines on the diagnosis and management of multiple myeloma 2005. *Br J Haematol*, **132**,410–51. 🖫 http://www.bcshguidelines.com/pdf/multiplemyeloma0206.pdf
5. NCCN Clinical Practice Guidelines in Oncology Multiple Myeloma V.2.2008 🖫 http://www.nccn.org/professionals/physician_gls/PDF/myeloma.pdf
6. D'Sa, S. *et al.* (2007). Guidelines for the use of imaging in the management of myeloma. *Brit J Haematol*, **137**, 49–63. 🖫 http://www.bcshguidelines.com/pdf/myeloma_management_guidelines.pdf
7. Pratt, G. (2008). The evolving use of serum free light chain assays in haematology. *Br J Haematol* **141**, 413–22.
8. International Myeloma Working Group (2003). Criteria for the classification of monoclonal gammopathies, multiple myeloma and related disorders: a report of the International Myeloma Working Group. *Brit J Haematol* **121**, 749–57.
9. Avet-Loiseau, H. (2007). Role of genetics in prognostication in myeloma. *Best Practice and Res Clin Haematol*, **20**, 625–35.
10. Durie, B.G. and Salmon, S.E. (1975). A clinical staging system for multiple myeloma. Correlation of measured myeloma cell mass with presenting clinical features, response to treatment, and survival. *Cancer*, **36**, 842–54.
11. Bataille, R. *et al.* (1992). C-reactive protein and beta-2 microglobulin produce a simple and powerful myeloma staging system. *Blood*, **80**, 733–7.
12. Greipp, PR. *et al.* (2005). International staging system for multiple myeloma. *J Clin Oncol*, **23**, 3412–20.
13. Avet-Loiseau, H. *et al.* (2007). Genetic abnormalities and survival in multiple myeloma: the experience of the Intergroupe Francophone du Myelome. *Blood*, **109**, 3489–95.

14. Dispenzieri, A. *et al.* (2007). Treatment of newly diagnosed multiple myeloma based on Mayo stratification of myeloma and risk-adapted therapy (mSMART): consensus statement. *Mayo Clin Proc*, **82**, 323–41.
15. Shaughnessy, Jr J.D. *et al.* (2006). A validated gene expression model of high-risk multiple myeloma is defined by deregulated expression of genes mapping to chromosome 1. *Blood*, **109**, 2276–84.
16. Bladé, J. *et al.* (1998). Criteria for evaluating disease response and progression in patients with multiple myeloma treated by high dose therapy and haemopoietic stem cell transplantation. *Brit J Haematol*, **102**, 1115–23.
17. Durie, B.G.M. *et al.* (2006). International uniform response criteria for multiple myeloma. *Leukemia*, **20**,1467–73.
18. UK Myeloma Forum and Nordic Myeloma Study Group (2005). Guidelines on the diagnosis and management of multiple myeloma 2005. *Br J Haematol*, **132**, 410–51. http://www.bcshguidelines.com/pdf/multiplemyeloma0206.pdf
19. Bergsagel, D.E. (1995). The role of chemotherapy in the treatment of multiple myeloma. *Baillieres Clin Haematol*, **8**, 783–94.
20. Palumbo, A. *et al.* (2006). Oral melphalan and prednisolone chemotherapy plus thalidomide compared with melphalan and prednisolone alone in elderly patients with multiple myeloma: randomized controlled trial. *Lancet*, **367**, 825–31.
21. Facon, T. *et al.* (2007). Melphalan and prednisolone plus thalidomide versus melphalan and prednisolone alone or reduced-intensity autologous stem cell transplantation in elderly patients with multiple myeloma (IFM 99-06): a randomized trial. *Lancet*, **370**, 1209–18.
22. Mateos, M.V. *et al.* (2006). Bortezomib plus melphalan and prednisolone in elderly untreated patients with multiple myeloma: results of a multicentre phase 1/2 study. *Blood*, *108*, 2165–72.
23. San Miguel, J.F. *et al.* (2007). A phase 3 study comparing bortezomib-melphalan-prednisolone (VMP) with melphalan-prednisolone (MP) in newly diagnosed multiple myeloma. *Blood*, **110**, 31a.
24. Palumbo, A. *et al.* (2007). Melphalan, predsisolone and lenalidomide treatment for newly diagnosed myeloma: a report from the GIMEMA-Italian Multiple Myeloma Network. *J Clin Oncol*, **25**, 4459–65.
25. MacLennan, I.C.M. *et al.* (1992). Combined chemotherapy with ABCM versus melphalan for treatment of myelomatosis. *Lancet*, **339**, 200–5.
26. Alexanian, R. *et al.* (1992). Primary dexamethasone treatment of multiple myeloma. *Blood*, **80**, 887–90.
27. Kumar, S. *et al.* (2002). Single agent dexamethasone for induction in patients with multiple myeloma undergoing autologous stem cell transplants. *Blood*, **100**, 432a.
28. Cavo, M. *et al.* (2005). Superiority of thalidomide and dexamethasone over vincristine-doxorubicin-dexamethasone (VAD) as primary therapy in preparation for autologous transplantation for multiple myeloma. *Blood*, **106**, 35–9.
29. Rajkumar, S.V. *et al.* (2006). Phase III clinical trial of thalidomise plus dexamethasone alone in newly diagnosed multiple myeloma: a clinical trial conducted by the Eastern Cooperative Oncology Group. *J Clin Oncol*, **24**, 431–6.
30. Rajkumar, S.V. *et al.* (2005). Combination therapy with lenalidamide plus dexamethasone (Rev/Dex) for newly diagnosed myeloma. *Blood*, **106**, 3050–3
31. Rajkumar, S.V. *et al.* (2007). A randomized trial of lenalidomide plus high-dose dexamethasone versus lenalidomide plus low-dose dexamethasone in newly diagnosed multiple myeloma: a trial co-ordinated by the Eastern Co-operative Oncology Group. *Blood*, **110**, 31a.
32. Jagannath, S. *et al.* (2006). Long term follow-up of patients treated with bortzomib alone and in combination with dexamethasone as frontline therapy for multiple myeloma. *Blood*, **108**, 238a.
33. Orlowski, R.Z. *et al.* (2007). Randomized phase III study of pegylated liposomal doxorubicin plus bortezomib compared with bortezomib alone in relapsed or refractory multiple myeloma: combination therapy improves time to progression. *J Clin Oncol*, **25**, 3892–901.
34. Harousseau, J.L. *et al.* (2007). Velcade/dexamethasone (Vel/D) versus VAD as induction therapy prior to autologous stem cell transplantation (ASCT) in newly diagnosed multiple myeloma (MM): updated results of the IFM 2005/01 trial. *Blood*, **110**, 139a.
35. Cavo, M. *et al.* (2007). Bortezomib (Velcade)-thalidomide-dexamethasone (VTD) vs thalidomide-dexamethasone (TD) in preparation for autologous stem cell (SC) transplantation (ASCT) in newly diagnosed multiple myeloma. *Blood*, **110**, 30a.
36. Wang, M. *et al.* (2007). Bortezomib in combination with thalidomide-dexamethasone for previously untreated multiple myeloma. *Hematology*, **12**, 235–9.
37. Popat, R. *et al.* (2008). Bortezomib, doxorubicin and dexamethasone (PAD) front-line treatment of multiple myeloma: updated results after long-term follow-up. *Brit J Haematol* ,**141**, 512–16.

38. Richardson, P.G. *et al.* (2008). Safety and efficacy of lenalidomide (len), bortezomib (Bz) and dexamethasone (Dex) in patients with newly diagnosed multiple myeloma: a phase I/II study. *J Clin Oncol* **25**, 459s abstact 8520.
39. McCloskey, E.V. *et al.* (2001). Long-term follow-up of a prospective, ouble-bind, placebo-controlled randomized trial of clodronate in multiple myeloma. *Br J Haematol*, **113**, 1035–43.
40. Berenson, J.R. *et al.* (1998). Long-term pamidronate treatment of advanced multiple myeloma patients reduces skeletal events. *J Clin Oncol*, **16**, 593–602.
41. Berenson, J.R. *et al.* (2001). Zoledronic acid reduces skeletal events in patients with osteolytic metastases. *Cancer*, **91**, 1191–1200.
42. Kyle, R.A. *et al.* (2007). American Society of Clinical Oncology 2007 clinical practice update on the role of bisphosphonates in multiple myeloma. *J Clin Oncol*, **25**, 2464–72.
43. Palumbo, A. *et al.* (2008). Prevention of thalidomide- and lenalidomide-associated thrombosis in myeloma. *Leukemia*, **22**, 414–23.
44. Attal, M. *et al.* (1996). A prospective randomized trial of autologous bone marrow transplantation and chemotherapy in multiple myeloma. Intergroupe Francais du Myelome. *N Engl J Med*, **335**, 91–7.
45. Child, J.A. *et al.* (2003). High-dose chemotherapy with hematopoietic stem-cell rescue for multiple myeloma. *N Engl J Med*, **348**, 1875–83.
46. Moreau, P. *et al.* (2002). Comparison of 200mg/m^2 melphalan and 8Gy total body irradiation plus 140mg/m^2 melphalan as conditioning regimens for peripheral blood stem cell transplantation in patients with newly diagnosed multiple myeloma: final analysis of the Intergroupe Francophone du Myelome 9502 randomized trial. *Blood*, **99**, 731–5.
47. Attal, M. *et al.*. (2003). Single versus double autologous stem cell transplantation for multiple myeloma. *N Engl J Med*, **349**, 2495–2502.
48. Fermand, J.P. *et al.*. (1998). High dose therapy and autologous peripheral blood stem cell transplantation in multiple myeloma: up-front or rescue treatment? Results of a multicenter sequential randomized clinical trial *Blood*, **92**, 3131–6.
49. Garban, F. *et al.* (2006). Prospective comparison of autologous stem cell transplantation followed by dose reduced allograft (IFM99-03 trial) with tandem autologous stem cell transplantation (IFM99-04) in high risk de novo multiple myeloma. *Blood*, **107**, 3474–80.
50. Kröger, N. (2005). Autologous-allogeneic tandem stem cell transplantation in patients with multiple myeloma. *Leuk Lymphoma*, **46**, 813–21.
51. Crawley, C. *et al.* (2005). Outcome for reduced intensity allogeneic transplantation for multiple myeloma: an analysis of prognostic factors for the Chronic Leukemia Working Party of the EBMT. *Blood*, **105**, 4532–9.
52. Myeloma Trialists' Collaborative Group (2001) Interferon as therapy for multiple myeloma: an individual patient data overview of 24 randomised trials and 4012 patients. *Br J Haematol*, **113**, 1020–34.
53. Attal, M. *et al.* (2006). Maintenance therapy with thalidomide improves survival in patients with multiple myeloma. *Blood*, **108**, 3289–94.
54. Kumar, S. *et al.* (2004). High dose therapy and autologous stem cell transplantation for multiple myeloma poorly responsive to initial therapy. *Bone Marrow Transplantation*, **34**, 161–7.
55. Singhal, S. *et al.* (1999). Antitumor activity of thalidomide in refractory multiple myeloma. *N Engl J Med*, **341**, 1565–71.
56. Rajkumar, S.V. *et al.* (2000). Thalidomide in the treatment of relapsed multiple myeloma. *Mayo Clin Proc*, **75**, 897–901.
57. Glasmacher, A. *et al.* (2005). A systematic review of phase-II trials of thalidomide monotherapy in patients with relapsed or refractory multiple myeloma. *Br J Haematol*, **132**, 584–93.
58. Palumbo, A. *et al.* (2004). Efficacy of low-dose thalidomide and dexamethasone as first salvage regimen in multiple myeloma. *Hematol J*, **5**, 318–24.
59. Dimopoulos, M.A. *et al.* (2004). Pulsed cyclophosphamide, thalidomide and dexamethasone: an oral regimen for previously treated patients with multiple myeloma. *Hematol J*, **5**, 112–17.
60. Offidani, M. *et al.* (2006). Low dose thalidomide with pegylated liposomal doxorubicin and high-dose dexamethasone for relapsed/refractory multiple myeloma: a prospective multicenter, phase II study. *Haematologica*, **91**, 133–6.
61. Hussein, M.A. (2006). Thromboembolism risk reduction in multiple myeloma patients treated with immunomodulatory drug combinations. *Thromb Haemost*, **95**, 924–30.
62. Palumbo, A. *et al.* (2008). Thalidomide for treatment of multiple myeloma: 10 years later. *Blood*, **111**, 3968–77.
63. Richardson, P.G. *et al.* (2005). Bortezomib or high dose dexamethasone for relapsed multiple myeloma. *N Engl J Med*, **352**, 2487–98.

Variant forms of myeloma

Non-secretory myeloma

- ~1% of MM cases; no detectable serum or urine paraprotein by immunofixation but SFLC ratio abnormal in 75%; clonal plasma cells ≥10% in BM or plasmacytoma on biopsy; myeloma-related end-organ damage.
- Treatment as above; response rates comparable to secretory MM; SFLC assay provides a sensitive marker for monitoring response and identifying relapse in most patients; alternatives in others are surrogate markers (β_2-M, CRP) and BM assessment.

IgD myeloma

- ~1% of cases of MM; very small or no visible monoclonal spike on routine electrophoresis; younger mean age (50–60 years); high rate of Bence Jones proteinuria and associated higher frequency of acute and chronic renal failure; tendency to present with other poor prognostic features (high β_2-M; low Hb); extramedullary involvement and amyloidosis may be more frequent.
- Treat aggressively when possible.

IgM myeloma

- Very rare; <0.5% of MM; 1% of all IgM gammopathies; plasma cell infiltrate in BM as opposed to lympho-plasmacytoid infiltrate characteristic of WM; aberrant PC phenotype; characterized by CD20 –ve, CD56 –ve, CD117 –ve phenotype and t(11;14).[1]
- Often associated with osteolytic lesions; no lymphadenopathy or splenomegaly.
- Overall outcome not established; may have inferior outcome to IgG or IgA MM.

IgE myeloma

- Rarest form of MM; younger age; high incidence of plasma cell leukaemia; ?shorter survival.

Plasma cell leukaemia

- Defined as PB plasma cells >2 x 10^9/L or 20% of differential count; may occur *de novo* at presentation or in the terminal stages of otherwise typical MM.
- Aggressive disease associated with BM failure and organomegaly; poor response to conventional dose therapy; few survive >6 months; better responses to HDM.

1. Feyler S et al. (2008). IgM myeloma: a rare entity characterized by a CD20– CD56– CD117– immunophenotype and the t(11;14). *Br J Haematol*, **140**, 547–51.

Cryoglobulinaemia

Classification and pathogenesis

- 3 types:
  - Type I (10–15%) single monoclonal Ig (usually IgM, less often IgG, occasionally LC-only), associated with haematological disorders.
  - Type II (50–60%) polyclonal IgG plus monoclonal IgM with rheumatoid factor (RF) activity (i.e. anti-IgG).
  - Type III (25–30%) polyclonal IgG and IgM usually with small monoclonal component on high resolution assay.
- Types II and III referred to as mixed cryoglobulinaemia (MC); ~75% associated with HCV infection; chronic stimulus may initiate multi-step process of B-cell clonal expansion leading to LPDs; serology reflects progression from polyclonal to oligoclonal to monoclonal IgM-RF and clonal expansion.
- Associated with wide range of conditions: lymphoproliferative, haematological, and auto-immune diseases, infections (esp. HCV) and renal and liver disorders.

Clinical features and diagnosis

- Type I rarely associated with vasculitis but with signs of peripheral vessel obstruction and hyperviscosity: purpura, acrocyanosis, Raynaud's phenomenon, dystrophic manifestations, leg ulcers, gangrene; usually clinically indistinguishable from Waldenström macroglobulinaemia (WM), MM, or CLL; rare complication of paraprotein precipitation at low temperature.
- MC characterized by purpura, weakness and arthralgias with multisystem involvement including chronic hepatitis, glomerulonephritis or peripheral neuropathy due to small and medium vessel vasculitis; biopsy of cutaneous lesions shows vasculitis.
- Diagnose by precipitation at 2–4 °C in serum prepared from blood collected and allowed to clot at 37 °C; immunofix for assessment of clonality and typing; exclude underlying LPD in cases with monoclonal IgM with type I or II cryoglobulinaemia; serum immunoglobulins, plasma viscosity, complement levels, and RF activity.

Treatment[1]

- Type I: treat underlying MM, WM or CLL and avoid cold.
- HCV-related MC: IFN-α ± ribavirin to eradicate HCV; may be followed by regression of established lymphoma.
- Non-HCV-related MC: mild–moderate symptoms, low dose prednisolone and analgesia; severe symptoms, CTX ± prednisolone ± plasmapheresis; rituximab may control B-cell clone and also improve renal function in HCV-related disease.

1. Tedeschi, A. *et al.* (2007). Cryoglobulinaemia. *Blood Rev*, **21**, 183–200.

POEMS syndrome

Clinical features

- Polyneuropathy, Organomegaly, Endocrinopathy, Monoclonal gammopathy, Skin changes: rare paraneoplastic syndrome 2° to a plasma cell neoplasm.
- Other features: papilloedema, extravascular fluid overload (oedema, pleural effusions, ascites), lymphadenopathy, diabetes mellitus, male gynaecomastia and impotence, female amenorrhoea, hypertrichosis and hyperpigmentation, sclerotic bone lesions, thrombocytosis, Castleman disease, polycythaemia and clubbing.
- Association of osteosclerotic plasmacytoma with chronic inflammatory demyelinating progressive polyneuropathy causing predominantly motor disability.
- Endocrinopathy occurs in ~84% usually hypogonadism then thyroid abnormalities, diabetes and adrenal insufficiency; majority multiple.
- 11–30% have Castleman disease or Castleman-like disease with angiofollicular lymph node hyperplasia which may be unifocal or multifocal and associated with B-symptoms, auto-immune phenomena, more subtle sensory neuropathy, and polyclonal gammopathy.

Diagnosis

- Confirm diagnosis by demonstrating monoclonal plasma cells in osteosclerotic plasmacytoma (>95% have monoclonal λ plasmacytoma or BM infiltration) and elevated plasma or serum levels of VEGF.
- BM usually <5% plasma cells (almost always monoclonal λ); low level paraprotein, usually IgGλ or IgAλ (median 11g/L, rarely >30g/L); anaemia, hypercalcaemia, and renal impairment rare.
- Differential diagnosis: chronic inflammatory demyelinating polyneuropathy, Guillan–Barré syndrome, monoclonal gammopathy associated peripheral neuropathy and AL amyloidosis.

Treatment

- Treat solitary sclerotic bone lesion with aggressive radiotherapy (45Gy) ± surgery (≥50% response); widespread lesions or diffuse BM involvement requires systemic therapy; ≥40% respond to MP; HDT and ASCT has been increasingly used with ≥90% response but mortality is higher than MM at ~7%.
- Systemic symptoms and skin changes may respond in 1 month, neuropathy may begin to respond at 3—6 months with maximum benefit often taking 2–3 years.
- Prognosis is good with median survival 13.8 years; number of features does not affect survival; respiratory symptoms predict adverse outcome.

Table 8.17 Criteria for the diagnosis of POEMS syndrome[1]

Major criteria	1. Polyneuropathy 2. Monoclonal plasma cell neoplasm (almost always λ) 3. Sclerotic bone lesions 4. Castleman disease 5. VEGF elevation
Minor criteria	1. Organomegaly (splenomegaly, hepatomegaly, or lymphadenopathy) 2. Extravascular volume overload (oedema, pleural effusion, or ascites) 3. Endocrinopathy (adrenal, thyroid,[b] pituitary, gonadal, parathyroid, pancreatic [b]) 4. Skin changes (hyperpigmentation, hypertrichosis, glomeruloid haemangiomata, plethora, acrocyanosis, flushing, white nails) 5. Papilloedema 6. Thrombocytosis/polycythaemia [c]
Other symptoms and signs	Clubbing, weight loss, hyperhidrosis, pulmonary hypertension/restrictive lung disease
Possible associations	Arthralgias, cardiomyopathy (systolic dysfunction) and fever.

[a] Polyneuropathy and monoclonal plasma cell neoplasm present in all patients; diagnosis requires at least 1 other major criterion and 1 minor criterion. [b] Because of high prevalence of diabetes mellitus and thyroid abnormalities, this diagnosis alone insufficient to meet this minor criterion. [c] Anaemia and/or thrombocytopenia are distinctly unusual in POEMS syndrome unless Castleman disease present. Reproduced with permission from Elsevier© 2007

1. Dispenzieri, A. (2007). POEMS syndrome. *Blood Rev*, **21**, 285–99.

Plasmacytoma

Solitary plasmacytoma of bone (SPB)

Clinical features and diagnosis

- Solitary area of lytic bone destruction due to clonal plasma cells in an otherwise asymptomatic patient.
- Generally no serum/urine paraprotein though may be small band.
- BM from uninvolved site contains <5% plasma cells.
- Otherwise ↔ skeletal survey and MRI of spine and pelvis.
- No myeloma-related organ or tissue impairment (end-organ damage).
- ~5% of plasma cell neoplasms: ♂:♀ ratio 2:1; median age 55 years.
- Lesion usually in axial skeleton; 66% in spine.
- Generally presents with bony pain; may cause cord/root compression.
- Diagnosis requires biopsy or FNA, exclusion of MM (📖 p.333) and exclusion of other bone lesions with MRI.
- Serum/urine paraprotein detected in 24–72%; generally low level.
- Adverse prognostic factors for progression to MM include persistence of paraprotein >1 year after radiotherapy, immuneparesis and lesion >5cm.
- –ve MRI of spine is good prognostic feature.

Treatment and prognosis

- Treat with fractionated radical radiotherapy 40Gy (50Gy for lesions >5cm); local control 80–95%; curative in 50% if solitary lesion; DFS ~40% at 5 years.
- Treat non-responders and those with a rising paraprotein or other evidence of symptomatic MM with MM chemotherapy (📖 p.345).
- Patients who meet diagnostic criteria for SPB but with evidence of clonal BM involvement should be treated with radiotherapy then monitored for disease progression as for MGUS (<10% BM PCs or SMM ≥10% BM PCs).
- Require regular follow-up to monitor paraprotein; disappears in 25–50% (often slowly over several years).
- ~75% progress to MM (~50% within 2 years of diagnosis); treat as *de novo* MM (📖. p.345); high response rate; median survival 63 months.
- Some patients develop multiple solitary recurrences; treat each with local radiotherapy.
- Median survival >10 years; DFS 25–50% at 10 years.

Extramedullary plasmacytoma (SEP)

Clinical features and diagnosis

- Extramedullary tumour of clonal plasma cells.
- Rare; may occur anywhere but 90% in head and neck; most in upper airways: tonsils, nasopharynx, or paranasal sinuses.
- Generally no serum/urine paraprotein though may have small band.
- BM from uninvolved site contains <5% plasma cells.
- ↔ skeletal survey and MRI of spine and pelvis.
- No myeloma-related organ or tissue impairment (end-organ damage).
- Diagnosis requires biopsy or FNA of the lesion; exclusion of MM and other lesions.
- <25% have serum or urine paraprotein.

Treatment and prognosis

- Treat with radical radiotherapy (40Gy; 50Gy if lesion >5cm) including regional lymph nodes if possible (e.g. cervical).
- Radical surgery only for SEP outside head and neck, then usually follow with radiotherapy.
- Patients who meet diagnostic criteria for SEP but with evidence of clonal BM involvement should be treated with radiotherapy then monitored for disease progression as for MGUS (<10% BM PCs or SMM ≥10% BM PCs).
- Most cured; <5% local recurrence; relapse <30%; MM, SPB or soft tissue involvement: chemotherapy for refractory or relapsed disease (📖 p.345).
- If monoclonal protein persists or reappears, patient may need further radiotherapy; if plasmacytoma shrinks but does not disappear and/or paraprotein persists, follow closely; persistent or rising paraprotein may indicate progression to MM.
- >70% survival at 10–14 years; DFS 70–80% at 10 years.

References

1. International Myeloma Working Group (2003). Criteria for the classification of monoclonal gammopathies, multiple myeloma and related disorders: a report of the International Myeloma Working Group. *Br J Haematol*, **121**, 749–57.
2. BCSH/UKMF (2004) Guidelines on the diagnosis and management of solitary plasmacytoma of bone and solitary extramedullary plasmacytoma. *Br J Haematol*, **124**, 717–26. 🖫 http://www.bcshguidelines.com/pdf/Plasmacytoma080304.pdf
3. Liebross, R.H. *et al.* (1998). Solitary bone plasmacytoma: outcome and prognostic factors following radiotherapy. *Int J Radiat Oncol Biol Phys*, **41**, 1063–7.
4. Tsang, R.W. *et al.* (2001). Solitary plasmacytoma treated with radiotherapy: impact of tumor size on outcome. *Int J Radiat Oncol Biol Phys*, **50**, 113–20.
5. Alexiou, C. *et al.* (1999). Extramedullary plasmacytoma: tumor occurrence and therapeutic concepts. *Cancer*, **85**, 2305–14.

Waldenström macroglobulinaemia (WM)

WM is an uncommon indolent chronic B-cell LPD characterized by BM infiltration by lymphoplasmacytic cells and an IgM paraproteinaemia. It is classified as a lymphoplasmacytic lymphoma in the WHO classifications (see p.181).

Epidemiology

- Incidence 0.3 per 100,000 per annum; incidence higher in Caucasians; rare in black population.
- Median age 63–68; rare <40; ♂:♀ ~2:1.
- Cause unknown; no clear link to environmental exposures.
- Several familial clusters described; ~20% of patients have at least one 1st degree relative with B-cell disorder; tend to be younger, have higher % BM involvement and higher IgM level at diagnosis.
- Main risk factor for WM is pre-existing IgM MGUS (46 × relative risk).

Pathophysiology

WM appears to arise from a late stage of B-cell differentiation possibly a memory B-cell, arrested after somatic hypermutation in the germinal centre and before terminal differentiation to a plasma cell; suggested by the immunophenotype and Ig somatic hypermutation without intraclonal variation; absence of IgH rearrangements in WM cells due to defective initiation of normal switching process.

Most cases have a normal karyotype; most frequent chromosomal abnormality del(6q21–23); neither an area of minimal deletion nor a putative tumour-supressor gene has been identified. Candidate genes, e.g. *PRDM1* (*BLIMP-1*) have not been found to have inactivating mutations. Presence of del(6q) may be associated with more aggressive disease. Del(6q) has not been found in IgM MGUS and may be associated with disease progression; limited data at present.

IL-6 is upregulated in WM explaining the elevated serum C-reactive protein; high levels of IL-6 may contribute to anaemia.

Slowly progressive accumulation of clonal cells; symptoms may be due to infiltration of BM (BM failure), spleen (splenomegaly), or liver (hepatomegaly), or to hyperviscosity due to ↑ serum levels of pentavalent monoclonal IgM (when IgM >30g/L).

Clinical features and presentation

- Occasional diagnosis following routine ESR/PV/FBC/blood film; otherwise usually insidious onset of weakness and fatigue.
- Patients often present with symptoms of anaemia, epistaxis, recurrent infection, dyspnoea, CCF, and weight loss.
- Usually no bone pain and no evidence of destructive bone disease.
- Symptoms of hyperviscosity (headache, dizziness, visual upset, bleeding, ataxia, CCF and somnolence, stupor, and coma) 15–20%.
- Peripheral neuropathy—usually sensory or sensorimotor (~20%): distal, symmetrical, slowly progressive, usually lower extremities.

- Hepatomegaly (~25%); splenomegaly and lymphadenopathy less frequent.
- Fundoscopy reveals distended sausage-shaped veins, retinal haemorrhage ± papilloedema.
- Cryoglobulinaemia (<5% present with symptoms though detectable in 20%) may cause Raynaud's syndrome, arthralgia, purpura, and skin ulcers.
- Haemorrhagic symptoms (e.g. epistaxis or easy bruising) may develop as a result of abnormalities of platelet function or coagulation due to the paraprotein.
- Amyloidosis may occur (<5%) causing cardiac, renal, hepatic, or pulmonary dysfunction, or macroglossia.
- Autoimmune disorders may also develop due to the paraprotein: cold agglutinin disease, Schnitzler syndrome (IgM monoclonal gammopathy, urticaria, fever, and arthralgia), neuropathy due to anti-myelin associated glycoprotein (MAG) activity, glomerulonephritis, angioedema, and acquired von Willebrand's syndrome.

Investigations and diagnosis

- No disease-defining morphological, immunophenotypic, or chromosomal abnormalities for WM (Table 8.18).
- ***FBC and film:*** normochromic normocytic anaemia 80% (often spuriously low due to ↑ plasma volume); rarely lymphocytosis or pancytopenia; blood film shows rouleaux or agglutination (cold agglutinins ~5%); may see lymphoplasmacytic cells.
- ***ESR/plasma viscosity:*** ↑ in almost all patients (~70% PV >1.8cP), often markedly (ESR commonly >100mm/h); risk of hyperviscosity symptoms when PV >4cP (5–10% at diagnosis); most have symptoms when PV >6cP; most with PV <4cP will not have symptoms of hyperviscosity; PV often correlates well for symptoms in an individual though not between patients.
- ***Biochemistry:*** renal impairment rare; LFTs may be abnormal in advanced disease or cryoglobulinaemia; urate and LDH may be ↑.
- ***Serum β2-microglobulin:*** ↑ in 33%; prognostic factor.
- ***C-reactive protein:*** ↑ in ~66%; due to ↑ IL-6 production.
- ***Hepatitis C serology:*** association with WM
- ***Serum immunoglobulins:*** ↑ IgM; may be mild immuneparesis of IgG (60%) and IgA (20%).
- ***Serum protein electrophoresis, immunofixation and densitometry:*** to characterize and quantify IgM paraprotein.
- ***Urine electrophoresis:*** scanty Bence Jones protein in ~50%.
- ***BM aspirate:*** often hypocellular; may show infiltration by lymphoplasmacytic cells with variable differentiation; mast cells may be ↑.
- ***BM trephine biopsy:*** essential; usually hypercellular; demonstrates intertrabecular infiltrate (diffuse, interstitial, or nodular) of lymphoplasmacytic cells (*N.B.*: paratrabecular infiltrate suggests follicular NHL); immunochemistry demonstrates LC restriction.
- ***BM immunophenotyping:*** useful in differentiating WM from other B-cell disorders; characteristically pan B-cell marker (CD19, CD20, CD22, CD79) +ve (*cf.* myeloma plasma cells); LC restricted surface IgM; CD10 –ve (*cf.* FL), CD23 –ve (*cf.* CLL); 5–20% express CD5 (must differentiate from CLL and MCL); *N.B.* CD5+ does not rule out diagnosis of WM; CD103 and CD138 rarely +ve.

- ***Cytogenetics:*** optional; most have ↔ karyotype; no consistent defect; most commonly del(6q;21–22.1) by FISH in up to 55% patients with WM; +3, +5, and –8 also described; presence of IgH translocations (14q) suggests myeloma; may help rule out NHL.
- ***CT chest abdomen and pelvis:*** to detect organomegaly and lymphadenopathy.
- ***Other potentially useful tests:*** cryoglobulins, cold agglutinins, coagulation screen, Congo red stain for amyloid on BM or fat aspirates, haemolysis screen, ECG, EEG peripheral blood flow cytometry, EMG, or lymph node/organ biopsy may be useful in some patients.
- WM may be divided by the presence or absence of symptoms attributable to either the IgM paraprotein (e.g. hyperviscosity or neuropathy) or tumour infiltration (BM failure or symptomatic organomegaly) into:
  - Symptomatic WM and
  - Asymptomatic (smouldering/indolent) WM (~25%) (📖 see Table 8.19).

Differential diagnosis

- IgM MGUS: IgM monoclonal protein <30g/L; Hb >12g/dL; no BM infiltrate (<10% clonal BM cells); no organomegaly or lymphadenopathy; no end-organ symptoms; 6q– is not seen in IgM MGUS; risk of progression 1.5% per year.
- IgM-related disorders: IgM monoclonal protein; no overt evidence of lymphoma; symptomatic cryoglobulinaemia, peripheral neuropathy, cold agglutinin disease, or amyloidosis; presence of constitutional or hyperviscosity symptoms, lymphadenopathy or organomegaly more suggestive of WM.
- Other B-cell LPDs: IgM monoclonal protein can be demonstrated in CLL/SLL and NHL (MCL, FL, MZL); generally very low levels; no lymphoplasmacytic BM infiltration; hyperviscosity rare; features of other LPD e.g. phenotype, e.g. splenic marginal zone lymphoma (SMZL) associated with splenomegaly, BM infiltration, and IgM paraprotein; SMZL over-expresses CD11c and CD22; CD25 more common in WM; CD103 +40% (always –ve in WM); cytogenetics 7q-, +3q, and +5q.
- IgM myeloma: very rare; BM contains plasma cells (cytoplasmic IgM+, CD20–, CD38+, CD138+) not lymphoplasmacytic cells; myeloma-associated cytogenetic abnormalities (esp. 14q translocations) and lytic bone lesions frequent.

Table 8.18 Diagnostic criteria for WM[1]

• IgM monoclonal gammopathy of any concentration.
• BM infiltration by small lymphocytes, plasmacytoid cells, and plasma cells.
• Intertrabecular pattern of BM infiltration.
• Immunophenotype: monoclonal surface IgM+ (5:1 κ:λ ratio), CD19+, CD20+, CD5±, CD10–, CD19+, CD20+, CD22+, CD23–, CD25+, CD27+, FMC7+

Table 8.19 Mayo Clinic diagnostic criteria for IgM MGUS, smouldering WM, and WM[2]

IgM MGUS	• <30g/L monoclonal serum IgM **and** • <10% lymphoplasmacytic BM infiltrate **and** • No end-organ damage
Smouldering WM (*syn.* indolent/asymptomatic WM)	• ≥30g/L monoclonal serum IgM **and/or** • ≥10% lymphoplasmacytic BM infiltrate (usually intertrabecular) **and** • No end-organ damage resulting from underlying WM (no anaemia, hepatosplenomegaly, hyperviscosity, constitutional symptoms, lymphadenopathy
Waldenström macroglobulinemia	• Any size monoclonal serum IgM **and** • ≥10% lymphoplasmacytic BM infiltrate (usually intertrabecular) • End-organ damage

Prognostic factors

Predictors of early progression in asymptomatic WM

- Hb <11.5g/dL.
- β2-microglobulin ≥3.0mg/L.
- IgM >30g/L.

Predictors of shorter survival in WM

- Age ≥60 years.
- Hb <10g/dL.
- High β2-microglobulin.
- Other less consistently identified factors—cytopenias: WBC <4.0 × 10^9/L; neutrophils <1.8 × 10^9/L; platelets <150 × 10^9/L; ↓ serum albumin; ♂ sex; constitutional symptoms; plasmacytic and polymorphous morphology in BM.

Table 8.20 Proposed International Prognostic Scoring System (IPSS) for WM[3]

Adverse risk factors	• Age >65 years • Serum β2-microglobulin >3mg/L • Monoclonal protein >70g/L • Haemoglobin ≤11.5g/dL • Platelets ≤100 × 10^9/L
Low risk Median 5-year survival 87%	≤1 adverse risk factors, except age
Intermediate risk Median 5-year survival 68%	2 adverse risk factors **or** age >65 years
High risk Median 5-year survival 36%	>2 adverse risk factors

Management

The aims of treatment in WM are to relieve symptoms, reduce the risk of organ damage, and improve QoL and survival duration with minimal adverse effects. Treatment should be reserved for symptomatic patients and continued to maximal response. There is no indication for therapy in asymptomatic WM but regular review (3–6-monthly) of clinical and laboratory features is required. Consistently monitor paraprotein by densitometry (more reliable than IgM nephelometry).

Indications for therapy

Initiation of therapy should not be based simply on IgM level alone as this does not correlate directly with clinical manifestations but for:

- Constitutional symptoms: recurrent fever, night sweats, fatigue due to anaemia, weight loss.
- Progressive symptomatic lymphadenopathy or splenomegaly.
- Haemoglobin ≤10g/dL due to BM infiltration.
- Platelets <100 × 10^9/L due to BM infiltration.
- Symptomatic hyperviscosity.
- Severe peripheral neuropathy.
- Systemic AL.
- Symptomatic cryoglobulinaemia
- Cold agglutinin disease.

N.B. Avoid red cell transfusion simply to correct low Hb (plasma volume ↑ causing spuriously low Hb; low Hb protects against clinical effects of hyperviscosity).

N.B. Although therapy should not be initiated on IgM level alone, serum monoclonal protein >50g/L carries a high risk of hyperviscosity; exclude early symptoms and signs of hyperviscosity by thorough history and examination including fundoscopy; do not postpone therapy.

At this time there are insufficient data to recommend one 1st-line therapy over another. Choice of initial therapy is based on patient age and co-morbidities, need for rapid disease control, cytopenias, and eligibility for SCT. Treatment recommendations and response criteria were updated at the Third International Workshop for WM (📖 see Table 8.21).[4]

Although response rates may be higher with combination regimens these regimens may not be appropriate 1st-line therapies for patients with indolent disease and the long-term benefit has yet to be demonstrated by direct comparison with single agent tnerapy.

Table 8.21 Updated response criteria from the Third International Workshop on WM[4]

Response	Criteria
Complete response (CR)	Disappearance of monoclonal protein by immunofixation; no histological evidence of BM involvement; resolution of any adenopathy/organomegaly (confirmed by CT scan), or signs or symptoms attributable to WM. Reconfirmation of CR status is required at least 6 weeks apart with a 2nd immunofixation.
Partial response (PR)	≥50% ↓ of serum monoclonal IgM concentration on protein electrophoresis and ≥50% ↓ in adenopathy/organomegaly on physical examination or on CT scan. No new symptoms/signs of active disease.
Minor response (MR)	≥25% but <50% ↓ of serum monoclonal IgM on protein electrophoresis No new symptoms/signs of active disease.
Stable disease (SD)	<25% ↓ and <25% ↑ of serum monoclonal IgM by electrophoresis without progression of adenopathy/ organomegaly, cytopenias, or clinically significant symptoms due to disease and/or signs of WM.
Progressive disease (PD)	≥25% ↑ in serum monoclonal IgM by protein electrophoresis confirmed by a 2nd measurement or progression of clinically significant findings due to disease (i.e., anaemia, thrombocytopenia, leucopenia, bulky adenopathy/ organomegaly) or symptoms (unexplained recurrent fever of ≥38.4°C, drenching night sweats, ≥10% body weight loss, or hyperviscosity, neuropathy, symptomatic cryoglobulinaemia, or amyloidosis) attributable to WM.

Plasmapheresis[5]

- Indicated in acute management of patients with symptoms of hyperviscosity; 1–1.5 volume exchange efficiently reduces plasma viscosity (PV) (80% of large IgM molecule is intravascular) with a 60–75% reduction in plasma IgM and 50% reduction in PV; 1–2 procedures will reduce PV to near-↔ and prevents return of paraprotein to pre-treatment levels for several weeks.
- Rarely required on a regular basis in treatment of neuropathic or chemo-intolerant patients.
- In an emergency, if plasmapheresis is unavailable, venesection and exchange transfusion will ↓ plasma viscosity.

Alkylating agents

- *Chlorambucil* most widely used alkylator; range of dosage schedules, from 0.1mg/kg/d continuously to 0.4mg/kg/d × 2d q14d ± prednisolone 60mg/m^2; 6–10mg/d (0.1mg/kg/d) for 7–14 days q28d, widely used in UK; responses usually slow; 31–75% achieve ≥50% reduction in paraprotein; CR uncommon.

- Addition of steroids does not affect response rate or survival; beneficial if associated autoimmune phenomena.
- Continue to maximum response; optimum duration of therapy not established; no evidence that maintenance improves survival.
- Duration of response 2–4 years; median survival ~ 5 years.
- Reinstitute therapy when paraprotein approaches previously symptomatic levels; often effective on several occasions; resistance ultimately develops; side effects; myelosuppression; AML.
- *Cyclophosphamide* ± prednisolone may achieve comparable results; no directly comparative data.
- Risk of myelodysplasia and stem cell toxicity make alkylating agents less attractive in younger patients; tolerability and ease of administration render them appropriate therapy for elderly patients.

Purine analogues[6–8]

- *Fludarabine* most widely used purine analogue (40mg/m^2 PO × 5d or 25mg/m^2 IV × 5d repeated monthly for 4–6 cycles); response rate 40–86% in previously untreated patients; response duration 40–50 months; patients who achieve response >1 year, may respond again at progression; as salvage treatment, 17–50% responses.
- *Cladribine* (0.1mg/kg continuous infusion × 7d) response rate 64–90% with generally 2–4 cycles in previously untreated patients; as salvage treatment, 38–63% responses; recommended limit of 2 cycles due to risk of myelosuppression; autoimmune complications occur as in CLL.
- These agents generally achieve more rapid responses in untreated WM than chlorambucil.
- Some studies found higher response rates in 1° refractory than refractory relapsed WM.
- Fludarabine and cladribine are cross-resistant.
- Side effects: myelosuppression (may be severe: >60% ≥grade 3 neutropenia) and profound immunosuppression; need *P. jirovecii* prophylaxis and irradiated blood products; consider antimicrobial and antiviral prophylaxis.
- Purine analogues are appropriate for initial and subsequent treatment of WM but should be avoided as initial therapy in patients eligible for SCT; no consensus on which agent is superior or optimum duration of therapy.

Rituximab[9–10]

- Monoclonal anti-CD20 antibody (375mg/m^2 IV × 4) achieves ~27% ≥MR in untreated and previously treated WM; improves haematocrit and platelet counts in >50%; useful in patients with marked cytopenia.
- Better responses if paraprotein <40g/L or IgM <60g/L.
- Responses occur at median ~3 months but best response may be delayed for several months.
- Response duration generally 9–16 months; administration of 8 doses over 4 weeks initially, repeated at 12 weeks, improves response rate (44–48%) and may extend duration.
- Abrupt elevation in serum paraprotein and PV may occur after rituximab therapy in up to 50% ('rituximab flare'); patients should be closely monitored and may require plasmapheresis to prevent hyperviscosity.
- May be beneficial for symptomatic neuropathy associated with anti-MAG antibodies.

- Use of rituximab monotherapy discouraged in patients with paraprotein >50g/dL due to risk of 'flare' effect.

Combination regimens[11–16]

- Higher response rates are achieved with combination regimens but ↑ toxicity.
- Small study of R-CHOP × 6 with rituximab maintenance achieved ≥MR in 11/13 and ≥PR in 10/13.
- Fludarabine (30mg/m^2 IV d1–3) + cyclophosphamide (CTX; 300mg/m^2 IV d1–3) (FC) achieved 78% responses ≥MR with median duration >2 years; cladribine + CTX achieved 58% ≥MR but with significant myelosuppression.
- FC + rituximab (FCR) achieved responses ≥MR in 5/9; pentostatin (4mg/m^2 IV) + CTX (600mg/m^2) ± rituximab (375mg/m^2) q21d in 14 patients achieved 65% responses ≥MR, including 12%CR; cladribine, CTX + rituximab achieved 94% ≥PR (18%CR) in 17 untreated patients with no relapse after median follow-up of 21 months.
- Rituximab, dexamethasone, and CTX active (78%≥MR) and well tolerated; response in most patients without myelosuppression or immunosuppression.
- Bortezomib, rituximab, and dexamethasone highly active (100% OR after median 4 cycles) and well tolerated.

New agents[17–18]

- *Bortezomib* is active in relapsed/refractory WM with 23/27 patients (85%) achieving ≥MR; responses prompt (median 1.4 months) with ~8 months median TTP; discordance between BM and serum IgM responses was observed in some patients.
- *Thalidomide* is less active with 5/20 achieving ≥MR with <3 months TTP; may have role ± steroids in 1st-line failures with pancytopenia.
- *Alemtuzumab* achieves responses but with significant toxicity.

High dose therapy and autologous or allogeneic SCT[7,19]

- Limited data due to age of most patients with WM; SCT undertaken in a number of younger patients; generally high dose melphalan ± TBI; high response rates (generally PR) achieved after autograft but relapse rate high; a registry report of 26 allografts showed a similar relapse rate to autografts at 3 years (24% *vs.* 29%) and inferior OS (46% *vs.* 70%).
- HDT and ASCT have a role in 1° refractory or relapsed disease in eligible patients; patients in whom SCT is planned should have limited prior exposure to alkylator and purine analogue therapy.
- Allografts should be performed in a trial context where possible.

Splenectomy

- May be beneficial for patients with evidence of hypersplenism.

Treatment of relapse

- If response of >1 year achieved most patients will respond to same therapy.
- Refractory patients or those relapsing shortly after prior therapy may respond to an alternative listed in Tables 8.22–8.24.

Table 8.22 Options for 1st-line and salvage therapy: updated consensus panel recommendations from the Third International Workshop on WM[20]

1st-line therapy	Salvage therapy
Alkylators* • Chlorambucil	Re-use of initial therapy** or use of an alternative 1st-line agent*
Purine analogues* • Cladribine or • Fludarabine	Monoclonal antibody • Rituximab • Alemtuzumab
Monoclonal antibody • Rituximab	Combination therapy* • Cladribine/fludarabine + CTX • Fludarabine + rituximab • Cladribine, CTX, and rituximab • Fludarabine, CTX, and rituximab • Pentostatin, CTX, and rituximab • R-CHOP • CTX, dexamethasone, and rituximab
Combination therapy* • Cladribine/fludarabine + CTX • Fludarabine + rituximab • Cladribine, CTX, and rituximab • Fludarabine, CTX, and rituximab • Pentostatin, CTX, and rituximab • R-CHOP • CTX, dexamethasone, and rituximab	Autologous SCT
	Thalidomide ± steroids

* Use of alkylators and purine analogues should be limited in patients eligible for ASCT. ** Re-use of frontline single agent or combination reasonable if patient achieved response of >1 year.

Table 8.23 Mayo Clinic consensus for newly diagnosed WM and first relapse[7]

Stage	Management
Asymptomatic • IgM MGUS (<10% BM lymphoplasmacytic infiltration) • Asymptomatic/smouldering WM • Hb ≥11g/dL • Platelets ≥120 x 10^9/L	→ Observation
Newly diagnosed early WM • Hb <11g/dL or symptomatic • Platelets <120 x 10^9/L • Neuropathy (IgM-related) • WM-associated haemolytic anaemia or glomerulonephritis	→ Consider single agent rituximab
Newly diagnosed advanced WM • Bulky disease • Profound cytopenias (Hb ≤10g/dL or platelets <100 x 10^9/L • Constitutional symptoms • Hyperviscosity symptoms	→ Rituximab + alkylator **or** → Rituximab + purine analogue

Table 8.23 Mayo Clinic consensus for newly diagnosed WM and first relapse[7] (*continued*)

Stage	Management
First relapse	→ Repeat original therapy if response from initial therapy was ≥2 years. → Use alternative 1st-line agent if respnse from initial therapy was <2 years.

Table 8.24 NCCN practice guidelines for WM[21]

Initial treatment*	Response	Follow-up treatment**
Alkylating agents: • Chlorambucil	• Progressive disease **or** • Response with relapse ≤6 months	• Purine analogue (fludarabine cat 1 rec) **or** • Rituximab
	• Response with relapse >6 months	• Alkylating agents **or** • Purine analogue (fludarabine cat 1 rec) **or** • Rituximab
Purine analogues: • Cladribine or • Fludarabine	• Progressive disease **or** • Response with relapse ≤6 months	• Alkylating agents **or** • Rituximab
	• Response with relapse >6 months	• Purine analogue **or** • Alkylating agents **or** • Rituximab
• Rituximab	• Progressive disease **or** • Response with relapse ≤6 months	• Alkylating agents **or** • Purine analogue
	• Response with relapse >6 months	• Rituximab **or** • Alkylating agents **or** Purine analogue

* Initial treatment options include clinical trial. ** Progressive disease after follow-up treatment is an indication for either salvage therapy in clinical trial (including studies of SCT) **or** rituximab **or** thalidomide ± dexamethasone.

Follow-up[21]

- Review FBC, quantitative immunoglobulins, and paraprotein quantitation after every 2 treatment cycles with PV in symptomatic patients; repeat CT at 3–6-month intervals if abnormal at diagnosis.
- After response to therapy, patients should be monitored every 2–3 months without mainenance therapy.

Prognosis[6-8,22]

- Median time to progression of asymptomatic WM ~7 years.
- Median survival of patients with WM ~5 years with 10% alive at 15 years.
- Patients who achieve CR with chlorambucil have median survival of ~11 years.
- Up to 20% die of unrelated causes and 33% from infection; others from disease progression, transformation and bleeding.
- Indolent course may be interrupted by transformation to diffuse large B-cell NHL; worsening constitutional symptoms, profound cytopenias, ↑ serum LDH, lymphadenopathy, extramedullary disease, and organomegaly; often poorly responsive to treatment; poor tolerance of aggressive treatment due to poor marrow reserve.

References

1. Owen, R.G. *et al.* (2003). Clinicopathological definition of Waldenström's macroglobulinaemia. *Semin Oncol*, **30**,110–115.
2. Rajkumar, S.V. *et al.* (2006). Monoclonal gammopathy of undetermined significance, Waldenström macroglobulinemia, AL amyloidosis and related plasma cell disorders: diagnosis and treatment. *Mayo Clin Proc*, **81**, 693–703.
3. Morel, P. *et al.* (2006). International prognostic scoring system (IPSS) for Waldenström's macroglobulinaemia (WM) *Blood* **108**, 42a.
4. Kimby, E. *et al.* (2006). Update on recommendations for assessing response from the Third International Workshop on Waldenström's macroglobulinemia. *Clinical Lymphoma and Myeloma*, **6**, 380–3.
5. Buskard, N.A. *et al.* (1977). Plasma exchange in the long-term management of Waldenström's macroglobulinemia. *Can Med Assoc J*, **117**, 135–7.
6. Johnson, .SA. *et al.* (2006). Guidelines on the management of Waldenström macroglobulinaemia. *Br J Haematol*, **132**, 683–97. http://www.bcshguidelines.com/pdf/waldenstroms_151106.pdf
7. Fonseca, R. and Hayman, S. (2007). Waldenström macroglobulinaemia. *Br J Haematol*, **138**, 700–20.
8. Vijay, A. and Gertz, M. (2007). Waldenström macroglobulinemia. *Blood*, **109**, 5096–103.
9. Dimopoulos, M.A. *et al.* (2002). Treatment of Waldenström's macroglobulinemia with rituximab. *J Clin Oncol*, **20**, 2327–33.
10. Treon, S.P. *et al.* (2005). Extended rituximab therapy in Waldenström's macroglobulinemia. *Ann Oncol*, **16**, 132–8.
11. Treon, .SP. *et al.* (2005). CHOP plus rituximab therapy in Waldenström's macroglobulinemia. *Clinical Lymphoma*, **5**, 273–7.
12. Tamburini, J. *et al.* (2005). Fludarabine plus cyclophosphamide in Waldenström's macroglobulinemia: results in 49 patients. *Leukemia*, **19**, 1831–4.
13. Tam, C.S. *et al.* (2006). Fludarabine, cyclophosphamide and rituximab for the treatment of chronic lymphocytic leukemia or indolent non-Hodgkin lymphoma. *Cancer*, **106**, 2412–20.
14. Hensel, M. *et al.* (2005). Pentostatin/cyclophosphamide with or without rituximab: an effective regimen for patients with Waldenström's macroglobulinemia/lymphoplasmacytic lymphoma. *Clin Lymphoma Myeloma*, **6**, 131–5.
15. Weber, D. *et al.* (2003). 2-chlorodeoxyadenosine alone and in combination for previously untreated Waldenström's macroglobulinemia. *Semin Oncol*, **30**, 243–7.

16. Treon, S. *et al.* (2006). Bortezomib, dexamethasone and rituximab (BDR) is a highly active regimen in the primary therapy of Waldenström's macroglobulinemia: planned interim results of WMCTG Clinical Trial 05-180. *Blood*, **108**, abstract 2765.
17. Treon, S.P. *et al.* (2007). Multicentre clinical trial of bortezomib in relapsed/refractory Waldenström's macroglobulinemia: results of WMCTG Trial 03-248. *Clin Cancer Res*, **13**, 3320–5.
18. Dimopoulos, M.A. *et al.* (2003). Treatment of Waldenström's macroglobulinemia with single-agent thalidomide or with the combination of clarithromycin, thalidomide and dexamethasone. *Semin Oncol*, **30**, 265–9.
19. Anagnostopoulos, A. *et al.* (2006). Autologous or allogeneic stem cell transplantation in patients with Waldenström's macroglobulinemia. *Biol Blood Marrow Transplant*, **12**, 845–54.
20. Treon, S.P. *et al.* (2006). Update on treatment recommendations from the Third International Workshop on Waldenström's macroglobulinemia. *Blood*, **107**, 3442–6.
21. NCCN Clinical Practice Guidelines in Oncology Multiple Myeloma V.2.2008. http://www.nccn.org/professionals/physician_gls/PDF/myeloma.pdf
22. Kyle, R.A. *et al.* (2003). Prognostic markers and criteria to initiate therapy in Waldenström's macroglobulinemia: consensus panel recommendations from the Second International Workshop on Waldenström's Macroglobulinemia. *Semin Oncol*, **30**, 116–120.

Heavy chain disease (HCD)

Uncommon lymphoplasmacytic cell neoplasms characterized by production of incomplete immunoglobulins comprising HCs without LCs. α-HCD is most frequent—γ- and μ-HCD also described but rare.

α-HCD

- Usually occurs in residents or immigrants from Mediterranean or Middle East; generally 10–30 years; associated with low socio-economic group, poor hygiene, recurrent infectious diarrhea, and chronic parasitic infection.
- Commonly presents with diarrhoea, steatorrhoea, weight loss, abdominal pain, and vomiting; mild-to-moderate anaemia; low serum albumin; hypokalaemia, and hypocalcaemia (tetany).
- α-HCD protein detectable in serum of most patients, concentration often low; serum protein electrophoresis normal in 50%; monoclonal α chain on immunofixation of serum or sometimes in concentrated urine otherwise diagnose by biopsy.
- Villous atrophy and infiltrative lesions in duodenum and jejunum in most patients; histology ranges from lymphoplasmacytic infiltration of mucosa (Stage A) to immunoblastic lymphoma invading entire intestinal wall.
- Mesenteric lymph nodes sometimes involved but peripheral lymph nodes, liver, spleen, and BM rarely involved.
- Progressive course without treatment; treat Stage A initially with oral metronidazole and tetracycline for 6 months; treat non-responders and Stage B or C with CHOP-type regimen.
- Variable clinical course; some die within 1–2 years, others have long remissions lasting many years.

γ-HCD (Franklin disease)

- Usually elderly ♂, associated with RA, Sjögren's, SLE, hypereosinophilic syndrome and autoimmune haemolytic anaemia.
- Present with palatal oedema, lymphadenopathy, hepatosplenomegaly, fever and recurrent infection; pancytopenia; eosinophilia and atypical lymphocytes/plasma cells in blood ± BM; monoclonal γ chain in serum and/or urine on immunofixation confirms diagnosis.
- Usually behaves as aggressive lymphoma; survival ~1 year.

μ-HCD

- Rare LPD; may resemble CLL; presents with weight loss, fever, anaemia, and recurrent infection.
- Hepatosplenomegaly; abdominal nodes generally involved; osteolytic lesions and pathological fractures in 40%.
- Vacuolated BM plasma cells in 66%; serum protein electrophoresis generally ↔ or shows hypogammaglobulinaemia; BJP 10–15%.
- Variable clinical course; some develop AL; no specific treatment: observation or alkylating agents according to course.

AL (1° systemic) amyloidosis

AL (1° systemic) amyloidosis is a clonal plasma cell disorder in which systemic disease results from organ dysfunction due to extracellular deposition of fibrillar protein. It can also complicate most clonal B-cell lymphoplasmacytic disorders, notably myeloma, Waldenström's macroglobulinaemia, MGUS, and lymphoma.

Incidence

Estimated incidence 0.5–1 per 100,000 per annum; ♂:♀ ratio 2:1; most cases aged 50–70 years; <10% <50 years; ~1% <40 years; 15% of patients with MM develop amyloid (lower % of MGUS and WM).

Pathophysiology

In AL amyloidosis the fibrillar deposits are composed of the variable regions of immunoglobulin LCs (VL) in association with glycosaminoglycans and amyloid P component derived from the ↔ plasma protein serum amyloid P (SAP) component. More commonly λ LCs. Unique amino acid insertions may render the proteins amyloidogenic. The underlying clonal neoplasm is usually small and <20% of patients meet diagnostic criteria for MM at diagnosis. Subsequent progression to MM is rare but may reflect short survival. The t(11;14) IgH translocation occurs more frequently in AL amyloidosis than in MM or MGUS.

Without treatment, amyloid deposition progressively accumulates in viscera, notably kidneys, heart, liver, and peripheral nervous system causing increasingly severe dysfunction. Under favourable circumstances, further amyloid deposition can be prevented, deposits can regress, and improvement in organ dysfunction can occur.

Clinical features and presentation

- Renal involvement is the predominant feature in 33% with nephrotic syndrome (oedema, fatigue, and lethargy) ± renal impairment (usually mild).
- Cardiac symptoms predominate in 20–30%: CCF due to restrictive cardiomyopathy notably with right sided features (↑ JVP, peripheral oedema, and hepatomegaly).
- Peripheral neuropathy occurs in 20%; 10–15% present with isolated neuropathic symptoms; typically painful sensory polyneuropathy; autonomic neuropathy may cause postural hypotension, impotence and disturbed GI motility in ~10%.
- Carpal tunnel syndrome in ~20%.
- GI involvement may be focal or diffuse: malabsorption, perforation, haemorrhage, and obstruction may occur; hepatomegaly 25%; macroglossia 10%.
- Haemorrhage occurs at some time in up to 33% of patients; usually non-thrombocytopenic purpura, often periorbital causing characteristic 'raccoon eyes' appearance.
- Vocal cord infiltration may cause dysphonia; large joint arthropathy; adrenal and thyroid infiltration may cause endocrine dysfunction; cutaneous plaques and nodules usually on face or upper trunk; pulmonary infiltration rarely symptomatic.

Investigations and diagnosis

- High index of suspicion required; consider in patient with nephrotic syndrome, cardiomyopathy, peripheral neuropathy, hepatomegaly, or autonomic neuropathy.
- Confirm diagnosis by histological examination of biopsy of affected organ (Table 8.25) or subcutaneous fat aspirate, rectal biopsy, or labial salivary gland biopsy stained with Congo Red for red–green birefringence under polarized light; confirm AL amyloidosis by immunochemistry for κ or λ LCs (50% are –ve).
- Assess severity of organ involvement:
  - ***FBC***: ↓ Hb suggests probable myeloma.
  - ***Serum chemistry***: to evaluate renal and hepatic function.
  - ***β2-microglobulin:*** prognostic indicator in MM (📖 Multiple myeloma, p.330).
  - ***Coagulation screen;*** may be coagulopathy due to absorption of factor X and sometimes FIX by the amyloid.
  - ***Serum protein electrophoresis, immunofixation and densitometry:*** to detect, type, and quantitate any paraprotein (~70%; usually only modest quantity).
  - ***Serum immunoglobulins:*** immuneparesis suggests MM.
  - ***SFLC assay:*** identifies excess of κ or λ LC in >95%; provides best assessment of response to therapy in most patients.
  - ***Creatinine clearance and 24h quantitative proteinuria:*** to assess renal dysfunction and severity of albuminuria.
  - ***Urine electrophoresis***: to detect, type and quantify paraprotein (85%; 90% have albuminuria).
  - ***BM aspirate and trephine biopsy:*** usually only mild ↑ in % plasma cells; overt MM in <20%; immunohistochemistry for κ and λ LCs; Congo red for amyloid.
  - ***CXR, ECG, and echocardiography:*** low voltage ECG; echo shows concentrically thickened ventricles, normal-to-small cavities and a normal or mild reduction in ejection fraction.
  - ***SAP (serum amyloid protein) scan:*** radiolabelled serum amyloid P component allows detection and quantification of amyloid deposition and assessment of extent of organ involvement by scintigraphy. (In UK contact National Amyloidosis Centre at Royal Free and University College Medical School, London).
  - ***Skeletal survey:*** only if MM suspected.

Table 8.25 Organ involvement: biopsy of affected organ or an alternate site*[1]

Kidney	• 24h urine protein >0.5g/d, predominantly albumin
Heart	• Echo: mean wall thickness >12mm, no other cardiac cause
Liver	• Total liver span >15cm in the absence of heart failure or alk phos >1.5 × ↔ upper limit
Nerve	• Peripheral: clinical; symmetrical lower extremity sensorimotor peripheral neuropathy • Autonomic: gastric emptying disorder, pseudo-obstruction, voiding dysfunction not related to direct organ infiltration

 (continued)

Table 8.25 Organ involvement: biopsy of affected organ or an alternate site*[1] *(continued)*

GI tract	• Direct biopsy verification with symptoms
Lung	• Direct biopsy verification with symptoms • Interstitial radiographic pattern
Soft tissue	• Tongue enlargement, clinical • Arthropathy • Claudication, presumed vascular amyloid • Skin • Myopathy by biopsy or pseudohypertrophy • Lymph node (may be localized) • Carpal tunnel syndrome

* Alternate sites available to confirm histological diagnosis of amyloidosis: fine needle abdominal fat aspirate and/or biopsy of the minor salivary glands, rectum or gingiva.

Differential diagnosis

Exclude MM (📖 p.333), reactive (AA) amyloidosis (history of chronic inflammatory disorder), and familial amyloidosis (family history).

Prognostic factors

Poor prognostic features

- CCF.
- Multisystem involvement.
- Renal failure.
- Jaundice.
- High total body amyloid load on SAP scan.

Management

The current aim of treatment is to suppress underlying plasma cell neoplasia and paraprotein production to reduce further deposition of amyloid and permit regression resulting in improvement in organ dysfunction.

Most treatment regimens have been adapted from those used in MM but patients with AL amyloidosis often experience greater toxicity. In contrast to MM where CR is the goal, a partial clonal response may halt amyloid deposition and even lead to its regression. Thus treatments with a significant risk of severe toxicity or death may be inappropriate. Many patients with AL amyloidosis may not require prolonged treatment schedules and a risk-adapted approach should be adopted. Good supportive care is essential.

Where possible, patients should be treated within a clinical trial because there are insufficient data to identify the optimal treatment of this condition.

Supportive care

- Nephrotic syndrome: loop diuretic + salt ± fluid restriction.
- Renal failure: peritoneal or haemodialysis if required; rigorous control of hypertension.
- CCF: diuretic + ACE inhibitors if tolerated; digoxin hypersensitivity common; Ca^{2+} channel blockers and β-blockers contraindicated; cardiac transplantation should be considered in appropriate patients.

Chemotherapy[3–13]

Table 8.26 Therapeutic options in AL amyloidosis

Oral melphalan + dexamethasone (M-Dex)
Dexamethasone / VAD
Cyclophosphamide, thalidomide and dexamethasone (CTDa)
Modified-dose or high-dose melphalan + ASCT
Best supportive care

- ***Standard melphalan ± prednisolone:*** prolonged median survival in randomized trial *vs.* colchicine (OS only 12–18 months); slow response rate (9–12 months) allows progressive amyloid deposition and deterioration of organ function; no longer recommended as treatment.
- ***M-Dex:*** melphalan + high dose dexamethasone (M 0.22mg/kg/d and Dex 40mg/d d1–4, q28d) effective in trial of 46 patients with 67% haematological responses (33% CR) in median 4.5 months; improved organ function in 48% responsive patients; well tolerated; long-term follow up reported 4.9 year median clonal remission in 9/15 CRs; a multicentre randomized study confirmed that HDM not superior to M-Dex; haematological responses (67% *vs.* 68%) and OS (22.2 *vs.* 56.9 months).
- ***VAD:*** more rapid response than MP; formerly initial therapy in patients eligible for HDT; caution with vincristine in neuropathic patients and adriamycin in those with CCF; dexamethasone alone produces responses and VAD now less widely used.
- ***CTD:*** thalidomide is poorly tolerated in doses used in MM; combination with cyclophosphamide and dexamethasone in risk-adapted CTD (📖 see p.727) achieved 74% haematological responses (21% CR) and median OS 41 months; organ responses 31%; 3 year estimated OS 100% in CRs and 82% in PRs; TRM 4%.
- ***Novel agents:***
  - Bortezomib active in AL amyloid with 77% responses ≥PR in a small study; short PFS (6 months) and 33% discontinuation for toxicity; lower doses may be more tolerable.
  - Lenalidomide active in combination with dexamethasone, achieving 67% ≥ haematological PR; myelosuppression occurred in 35% and VTE in 9%; lower doses were required.
- ***High dose melphalan and autologous SCT:*** limited availability as <20% are genuinely low-risk for treatment-related mortality (TRM); 41% achieve haematological CR (superior to ~20% achieved by best intermediate dose regimen); procedure related mortality ~10–12%; improves organ function in up to 60%; long-term follow-up in 80 patients reported median OS 57 months; median OS exceeds 10 years if in CR after HDT (51% of 63 at 1 year); 23.5% survived >10 years; superior to standard MP but not clearly superior to intermediate regimens such as M-Dex or CTD; HDT better tolerated if ≤2 organ systems involved; younger patients with good performance status and good renal and cardiac function do best; cardiac involvement or

elevated creatinine adverse prognostic indicators; ↓ melphalan dose to 100–140mg/m^2 in high risk patients; GI haemorrhage a frequent complication. HDT should be undertaken in context of a clinical trial.
  - *N.B.* stem cell mobilisation associated with mortality and morbidity due to cardiac complications (avoid cyclophosphamide), oedema and splenic rupture (low doses of G-CSF recommended).
- Careful selection criteria recommended: Mayo Clinic criteria developed to risk-adapt therapy and strict UK trial entry criteria developed to reduce TRM (Tables 8.27 and 8.28).
- ***Allogeneic SCT:*** isolated reports of small numbers of patients treated with allografts with high TRM (40%); reduced-intensity conditioning reduces this figure; best restricted to clinical trials in highly selected patients in experienced centres.

Table 8.27 Mayo Clinic risk stratification model to predict progression of primary amyloidosis[2]

Risk group	Median survival of patients undergoing SCT (months)	Median survival of patients not undergoing SCT (months)
Low risk (cardiac troponin <0.035mcg/L and NT-proBNP <332ng/L)	Not reached at 40 months	26.4
Intermediate risk (any 1 factor abnormal)	Not reached at 40 months	10.5
High risk (cardiac troponin ≥0.035mcg/L and NT-proBNP ≥332ng/L)	8.4	3.5

Adapted with permission of Dowden Health Media© 2006

Table 8.28 Criteria for eligibility for ASCT in UK amyloidosis treatment trial[3]

- ECOG performance status 0 or 1
- No greater than NYHA class I or II heart failure
- No more than 2 organs involved by amyloid by consensus guidelines
- Age ≤65 years
- Creatinine clearance ≥0.8mL/sec (50mL/min)
- Bilirubin ≤1.5 × and alkaline phosphatase ≤2 × upper limit of normal
- Inter-ventricular and left ventricular posterior wall thicknesses ≤15mm by echocardiography
- Absence of clinically important amyloid related autonomic neuropathy
- Absence of clinically important amyloid related gastrointestinal haemorrhage

Follow-up

Response to therapy should be monitored by quantitation of the SFLCs or in the minority with measurable levels, the serum paraprotein; SAP scintigraphy; ECG, echocardiography, and assessment of other organ dysfunction should be reviewed every 6 months.

Response assessment

Consensus response criteria have been published.[1] Separate haematological and organ responses have been defined. The latter occur slowly and are generally dependent on the former which is a strong predictor of survival.

Table 8.29 Haematological response criteria[1]

Complete response (CR)	• Serum and urine –ve for paraprotein by immunofixation • Free LC ratio ↔ • BM plasma cells <5%
Partial response (PR)	• If serum paraprotein >5g/L and 50% ↓ • If urine LC with visible peak and >100mg/d and 50% ↓ • If free LC >100mg/L and 50% ↓
Progression	• From CR, any detectable paraprotein or abnormal free LC ratio (LC must double) • From PR or stable response, 50% ↑ in serum paraprotein to >5g/L or 50% ↑ in urine paraprotein to >200mg/d; a visible peak must be present • Free LC ↑ of 50% to >100mg/L
Stable	• No CR, no PR, no progression

Table 8.30 Organ response criteria[1]

	Response	Progression
Heart	Mean interventricular septal thickness ↓ by 2mm, 20% ↑ in ejection fraction, improvement by 2 NYHA classes without ↑ diuretic use and no ↑ in wall thickness	Interventricular septal thickness ↑ by 2mm compared with baseline, ↑ in NYHA class by 1 grade with a ↓ in ejection fraction ≥10%
Kidney	50% ↓ (≥0.5g/d) of 24h urine protein (must be >0.5g/d pretreatment)	50% ↑ (≥1g/d) of 24h urine protein to >1g/d or 25% worsening of serum creatinine or creatinine clearance
Liver	50% ↓ in abnormal alk phos; ≥2cm ↓ in liver size radiographically	50% ↑ of alk phos above the lowest value
Nerve	Improvement in EMG nerve conduction (rare)	Progressive neuropathy by EMG or nerve conduction velocity

Prognosis[3, 14]

- Median survival 1–2 years; 4–6 months if CCF at diagnosis.
- Most common cause of death cardiac, progressive congestive cardiomyopathy or sudden death due to VF or asystole.
- Others succumb to uraemia or other complications.

Other causes of amyloid[15]

Acquired

- AA amyloid: reactive systemic amyloidosis associated with chronic inflammatory diseases e.g. rheumatoid arthritis, TB; due to AA fibrils derived from serum amyloid A protein (SAA); treat underlying condition.

- Senile systemic amyloidosis due to transthyretin deposition; no therapy.
- Endocrine amyloidosis, associated with APUD-omas.
- Haemodialysis associated amyloidosis, localized to osteoarticular tissues or systemic due to β2-microglobulin deposition.
- Non-familial Alzheimer's disease, Down syndrome due to β-protein.
- Sporadic Creutzfeldt–Jakob disease, kuru due to prion protein deposition.
- Type II diabetes mellitus due to islet amyloid polypeptide.

Hereditary

- Numerous syndromes with characteristic patterns of peripheral or cranial neurological involvement or visceral or cardiac involvement due to a variety of proteins.
- Familial mutant ATTR due to mutant transthyretin; treat with liver transplant or diflunisal
- Familial Alzheimer's disease due to a β-protein.
- Familial Mediterranean fever due to AA derived from SAA; treat with colchicine.

References

1. Gertz, M.A. *et al.* (2005). Definition of organ involvement and treatment response in immunoglobulin light chain amyloidosis (AL): a consensus opinion from the 10th International Symposium on AMyloid and Amyloidosis. *Am J Hematol,* **79**, 319–28.
2. Rajkumar SV *et al.* (2006) Monoclonal gammopathy of undetermined significance, Waldenström macroglobulinemia, AL amyloidosis and related plasma cell disorders: diagnosis and treatment. *Mayo Clin Proc,* **81**, 693–703.
3. Wechalekar, A.D. *et al.* (2008). Perspectives in treatment of AL amyloidosis. *Br J Haematol* **140**, 365–77.
4. Palladini, G. *et al.* (2004). The association of melphlan and high-dose dexamethasone is effective and well tolerated in patients with AL (primary) amyloidosis ineligible for stem cell transplantation. *Blood,* **103**, 2936–8.
5. Palladini, G. *et al.* (2007). Treatment with oral melphalan plus dexamethasone produces long-term resmissions in AL amyloidosis. *Blood,* **110**, 787–8.
6. Jaccard. A. *et al.* (2007). High dose melphalan versus melphalan plus dexamethasone for AL amyloidosis. *N Engl J Med,* **357**, 1083–93.
7. Wechalekar, A.D. *et al.* (2007). Safety and efficacy of risk-adapted cyclophosphamide, thalidomide and dexamethasone in systemic AL amyloidosis. *Blood,* **109**, 457–64.
8. Wechalekar, A.D. *et al.* (2007). Efficacy and safety of bortezomib in systemic AL amyloidosis – a preliminary report. *Blood,* **108**, 129.
9. Sanchorawala, V. *et al.* (2007). Lenalidomide and dexamethasone in the treatment of AL amyloidosis: results of a phase II trial. *Blood,* **109**, 492–6.
10. Commenzo, R.L. and Gertz, M.A. (2002). Autologous stem cell transplantation for primary systemic amyloidosis *Blood,* **99**, 4276–82.
11. Skinner, M. *et al.* (2004) High-dose melphalan and autologous stem-cell transplantation in patients with AL amyloidosis: an 8-year study. *Ann Intern Med* **140**, 85–93.
12. Dispenzieri, A. *et al.* (2004). Superior survival in primary systemic amyloidosis patients undergoing peripheral blood stem cell transplant: a case control study. *Blood,* **103**, 3960–3.
13. Sanchorawala, V. *et al.* (2007). Long-term outcome of patients with AL-amyloidosis treated with high-dose melphalan and stem cell transplantation. *Blood,* **110**, 3561–3.
14. BCSH/UKMF Guideline. Guidelines on the dignosis and management of AL amyloidosis. *Br J Haematol,* **125**, 681–700.
   http://www.bcshguidelines.com/pdf/ALamyloidosis_210604.pdf
15. Rajkumar, S.V. and Gertz, M.A. (2007). Advances in the treatment of amyloidosis. *N Engl J Med,* **356**, 2413–5.

Chapter 9

Haematopoietic stem cell transplantation (SCT)

Haemopoietic stem cell transplantation (SCT)

Haemopoietic SCT achieves reconstitution of haematopoiesis by the transfer of pluripotent haemopoietic stem cells. In allogeneic SCT stem cells are obtained from a donor e.g. a matched sibling or normal volunteer (matched unrelated donor; UD); in syngeneic SCT the donor is a monozygotic (identical) twin. For autologous SCT the patient acts as his/her own source of stem cells. Umbilical cord blood has become a useful source of stem cells for paediatric transplants (but not for adults due to dose of cells available), particularly when there is no HLA-identical or matched peripheral blood or marrow donor or the patient's condition requires prompt transplantation.

The aim of SCT is:

- To permit haemopoietic reconstitution after potentially curative but myeloablative doses of chemotherapy or chemoradiotherapy (high dose therapy; HDT) in the treatment of malignant disease

or

- To replace congenital or acquired life-threatening abnormal BM or immune function with a normal haematopoietic and immune system.

The therapeutic effect of allogeneic SCT is not restricted to the conditioning as there can be an additional graft-versus-leukaemia (GvL) effect mediated by the incoming donor immune system that contributes significantly to the curative potential of the procedure, though is linked to its major toxicity, graft-versus-host disease (GvHD). No GvL effect occurs in syngeneic or autologous SCT and in allogeneic SCT it can be abrogated by intensive efforts to prevent GvHD.

Stem cells may be obtained from BM (BMT) by multiple aspirations under general anaesthesia (BM harvest) or obtained from peripheral blood after 'mobilization' by G-CSF (± chemotherapy in the case of autologous SCT) and collection by apheresis (peripheral blood stem cell transplants, PBSCT). Whether used fresh from donor harvest or thawed after cryopreservation, stem cells are re-infused IV. PBSCT carries the advantages of avoiding general anaesthesia for the donor and more rapid engraftment (~7d) but may be associated with a higher incidence of chronic GvHD (cGvHD). In the autologous setting not all previously treated patients will mobilize adequate numbers of stem cells.

Stem cell collection for autologous SCT with curative intent in diseases involving the BM should be undertaken after a complete response has been achieved by initial therapy. In some settings e.g. myeloma where HDT is being used with the aim of disease control rather than with curative intent, BM involvement up to 30% is often accepted.

Patient receives 'conditioning' comprising high dose chemotherapy or chemo-radiotherapy ± antibodies (e.g. Campath®) which ablates the recipient's BM and immune system. After conditioning is completed, BM or PBSC are infused IV. After a period of profound myelosuppression (7–25d), engraftment occurs with production of WBCs, platelets, and RBCs. Immunosuppression is required after allogeneic transplantation to prevent GvHD and graft rejection.

Table 9.1 Comparison of autologous and allogeneic SCT

Autologous	Allogeneic
Wide age range, generally ≤70 years	Age range generally ≤60 years
No need for donor search if BM clear	Sibs have ~1 in 4 chance of match
Not feasible if BM involved	May be used in patients with BM disease
Risk of tumour cell re-infusion	No tumour contamination of graft
Not all patients can be mobilized	Donor search may impose delay
No GvHD	GvHD mortality and morbidity
No immunosuppression	GvL effect
Low early treatment related mortality (2–5%)	Higher early treatment related mortality from GvHD and infection (10–20%)
Risk of long-term MDS from BM injury	Less risk of late MDS

Table 9.2 Factors influencing outcome of haemopoietic SCT[1]

Time	Patient	Donor
Pre-transplant		
Disease	Diagnosis, subtype, stage	
Individual	Age, sex, ethnicity, organ status, viral status, Karnofsky score	Age, sex, ethnicity, donor/ recipient sex combination, viral status, histocompatibility: • Major histocompatibility antigens: HLA, KIR • Minor histocompatibility antigens • ABO • Cytokine polymorphisms
Environment	Geographical latitude Economic status	
Peri-transplant		
Conditioning	Intensity	
GvHD prevention	Prevention method	
Graft product	Stem cell source, graft composition	
Post-transplant		
Disease	Relapse	
Individual	Immune reconstitution	Availability for DLI or retransplant
Environment	Retreatment possibilities	

1. Gratwohl, A. (2007). Risk assessment in haemopoietic stem cell transplantation. *Best Pract Res Clin Haematol*, **20**, 119–24.

Early complications of the transplant procedure

Chemoradiotherapy

- Nausea/vomiting.
- Reversible alopecia.
- Fatigue.
- Dry skin.
- Mucositis.
- VOD* (📖 Veno-occlusive disease, p.432).

Infection

- Bacterial (Gram –ve and +ve).
- Viral—HZV.
- CMV (particularly pneumonitis).*
- Fungal—*Candida*, *Aspergillus**, *Mucor**.
- Atypical organisms—*Pneumocystis* (PCP)*, *Toxoplasma**, *Mycoplasma**, *Legionella**.

*Low risk in autologous SCT; significant to high risk in allogeneic SCT

GvHD

May occur in recipients of allogeneic SCT due to tissue incompatibility between donor and recipient undetected by standard tissue-typing tests. Acute and chronic forms. Higher incidence of severe GvHD following unrelated donor SCT and mismatched (haploidentical) grafts.

Late complications of transplantation

- Infertility (both sexes).
- Hypothyroidism.
- 2° malignancy.
- Late sepsis due to hyposplenism.
- Cataracts (where TBI used).
- Psychological disturbance.

Follow up and post-transplant surveillance

Lifelong supervision required. The particular risks and monitoring required depend on the type of graft and whether TBI was used. Suitable conditioning regimens are outlined in 📖 Stem cell transplant conditioning regimens, p.410.

Further reading

Apperley, J. *et al.* (eds.) (2008). The EBMT Handbook Haemopoietic Stem Cell Transplantation. EBMT, Paris.

Cant, A.J. *et al.* (eds.) (2007). Practical Haematopoietic Stem Cell Transplantation. Blackwell Publishing, Oxford.

Gratwohl, A. (ed.) (2007). Risk assessment in haematopoietic stem cell transpantation. *Best Pract Res Clin Haematol*, **20**(2). Elsevier, Oxford.

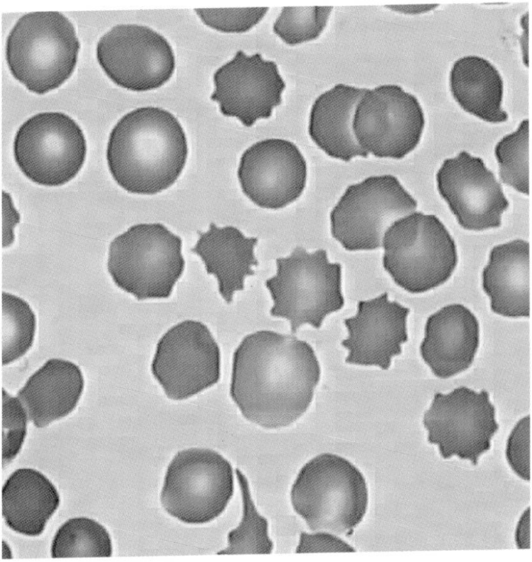

Plate 1 Blood film: chronic renal failure with burr (irregular shaped) cells (📖 see Fig. 2.1 p.35).

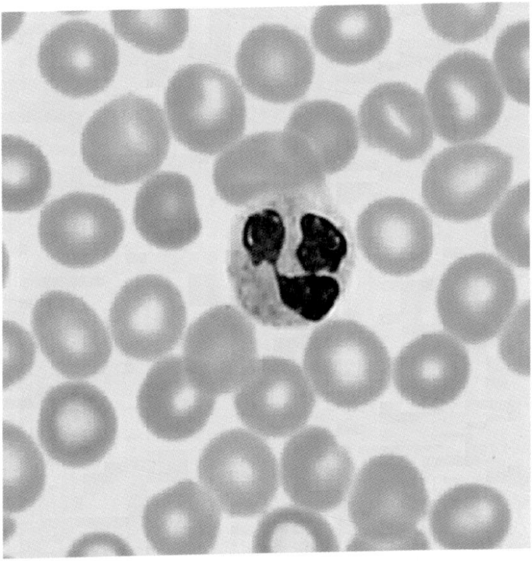

Plate 2 Blood film: normal neutrophil: usually has <5 lobes. This one has 3 lobes (📖 see Fig. 2.3 p.49).

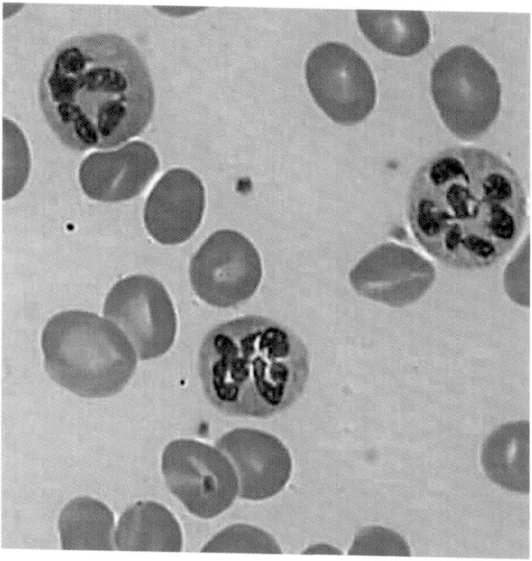

Plate 3 Hypersegmented neutrophils with 7–8 lobes: found in B_{12} or folate deficiency. *Note*: blood films and marrow appearances are identical in B_{12} and folate deficiencies (📖 see Fig. 2.4 p.49).

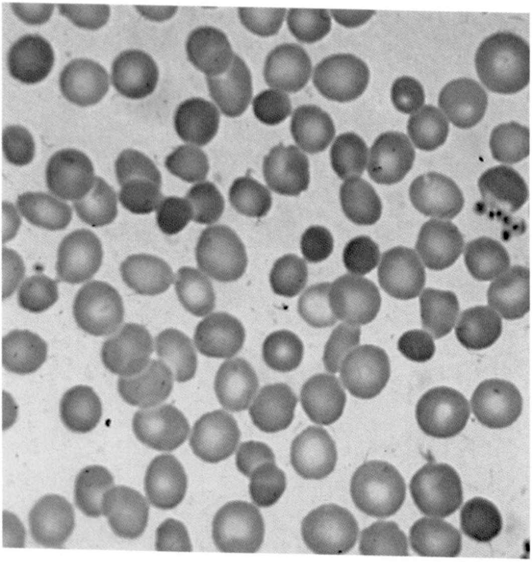

Plate 4 Blood film in hereditary spherocytosis. Note: large numbers of dark spherical red cells (📖 see Fig. 2.11 p.82).

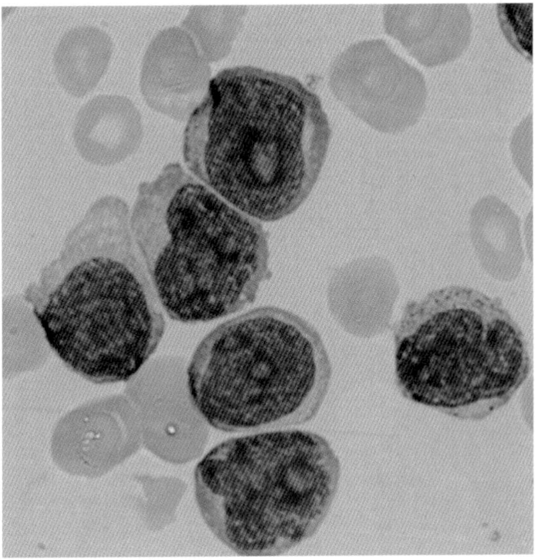

Plate 5 Bone marrow showing myeloblasts in AML (📖 see Fig. 4.1 p.120).

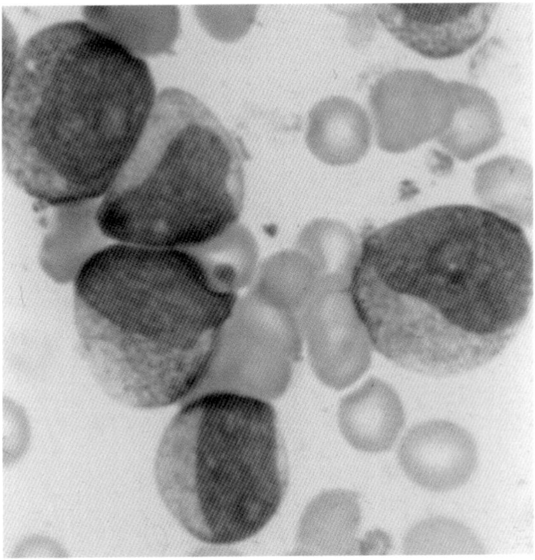

Plate 6 Bone marrow showing myeloblasts in AML (📖 see Fig. 4.2 p. 121).

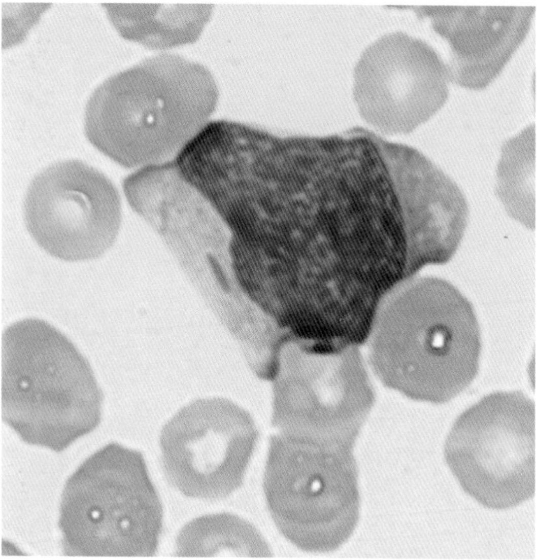

Plate 7 AML: myeloblast with large Auer rod (left) (see Fig. 4.3 p.121).

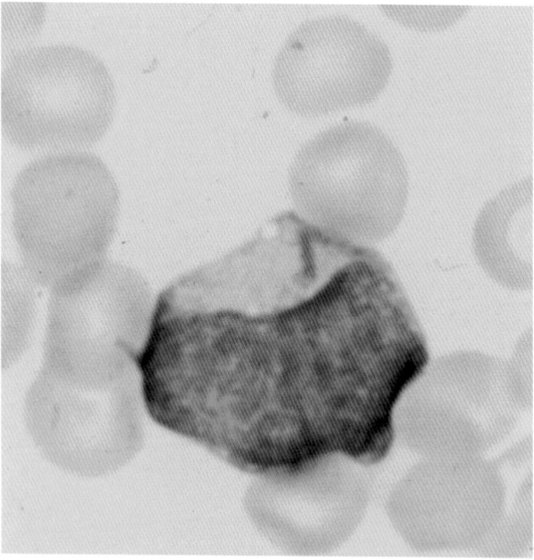

Plate 8 AML: myeloblast with large Auer rod (top of cell) (see Fig. 4.4 p.121).

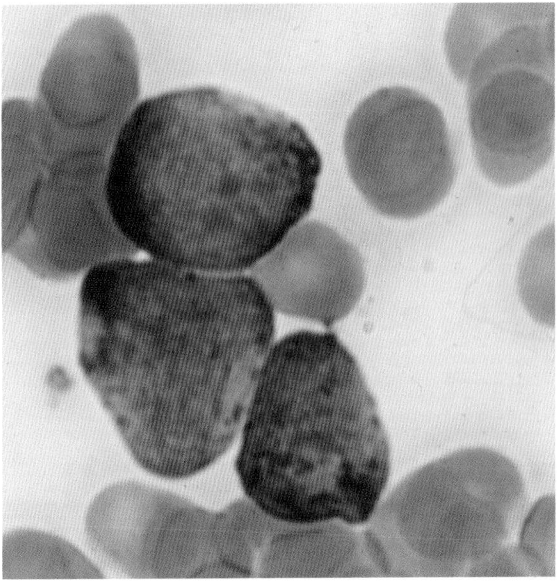

Plate 9 AML: Sudan Black stain (dark granules clearly seen in myeloblasts) (📖 see Fig. 4.5 p.123).

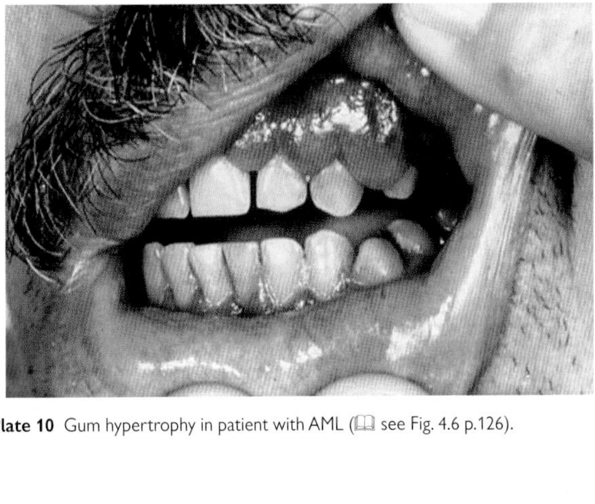

Plate 10 Gum hypertrophy in patient with AML (📖 see Fig. 4.6 p.126).

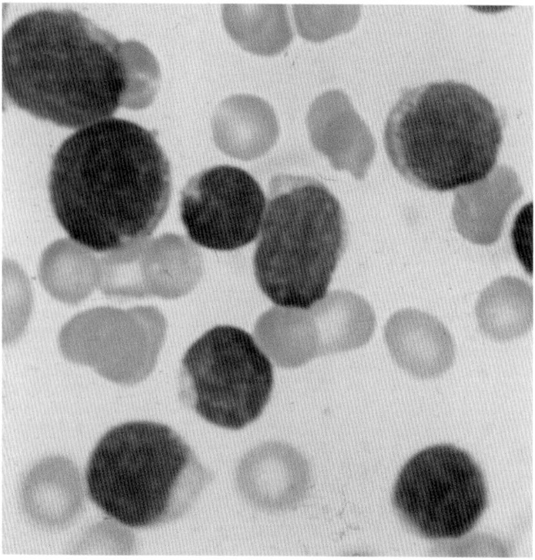

Plate 11 Bone marrow: lymphoblasts in ALL L1 (📖 see Fig. 4.8 p.135).

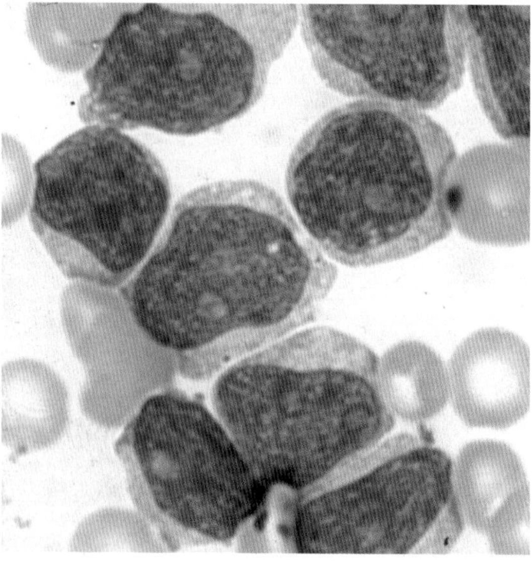

Plate 12 Bone marrow: T-cell ALL showing numerous lymphoblasts (📖 see Fig. 4.9 p.137).

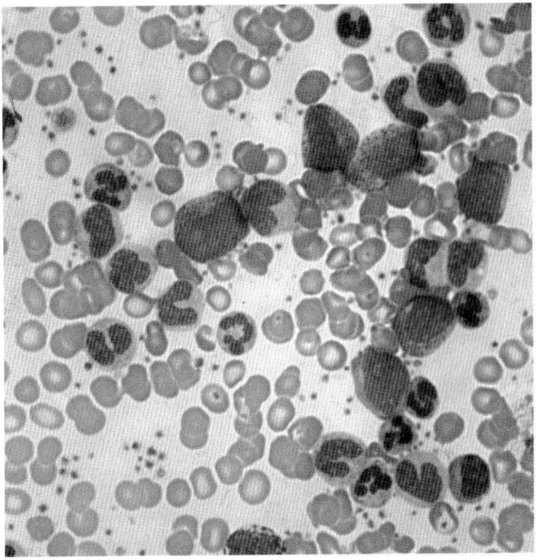

Plate 13 Peripheral blood film in CML: note large numbers of granulocytic cells at all stages of differentiation (low power) (📖 see Fig. 4.10 p.141).

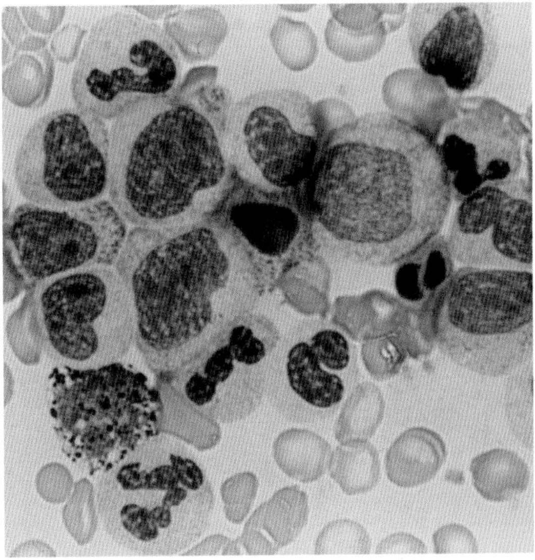

Plate 14 Peripheral blood film in CML: high power (📖 see Fig. 4.11 p.142).

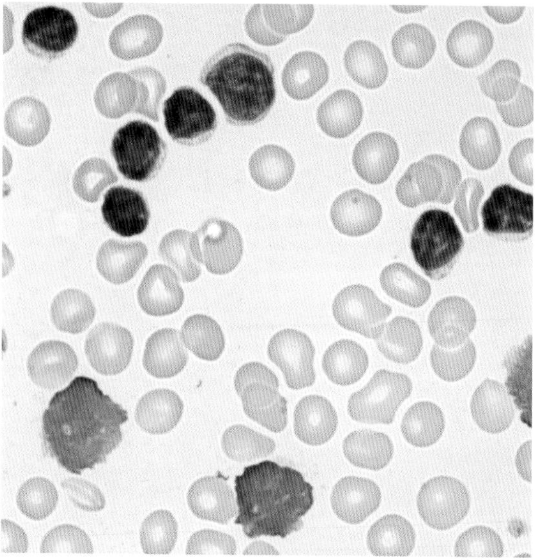

Plate 15 Blood film in CLL showing smear cells (bottom of field) (📖 see Fig. 4.12 p.151).

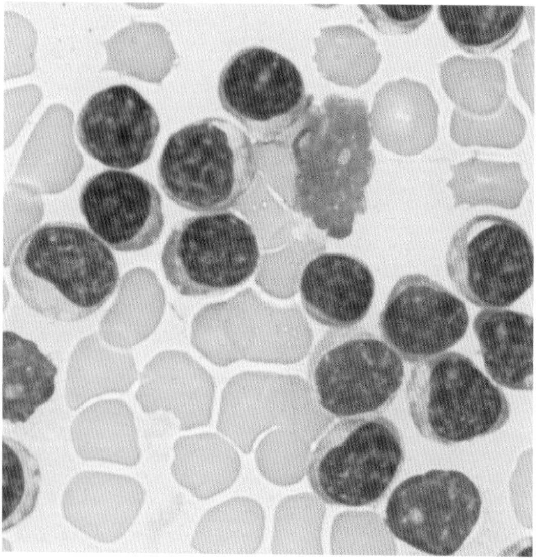

Plate 16 Blood film in PLL: cells are larger than those seen in CLL have large prominent nucleoli and moderate chromatin condensation (📖 see Fig. 4.15 p.160).

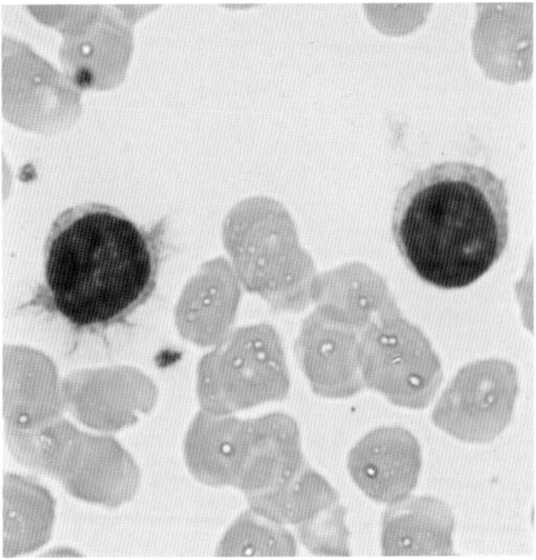

Plate 17 Blood film in HCL showing typical 'hairy' lymphocytes (medium power) (📖 see Fig. 4.16 p.163).

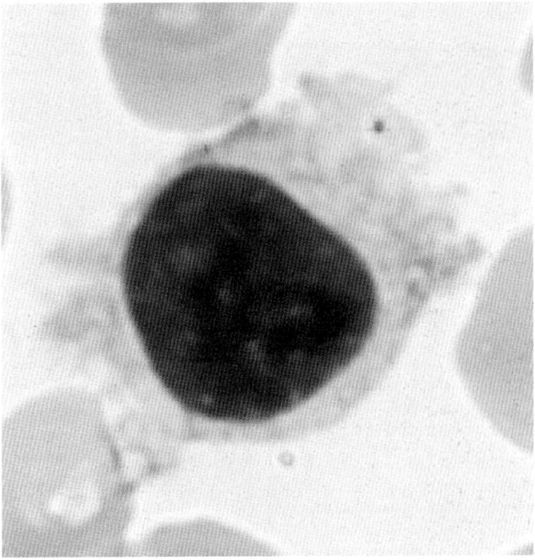

Plate 18 Blood film in HCL showing typical 'hairy' lymphocytes (high power) (📖 see Fig. 4.17 p.163).

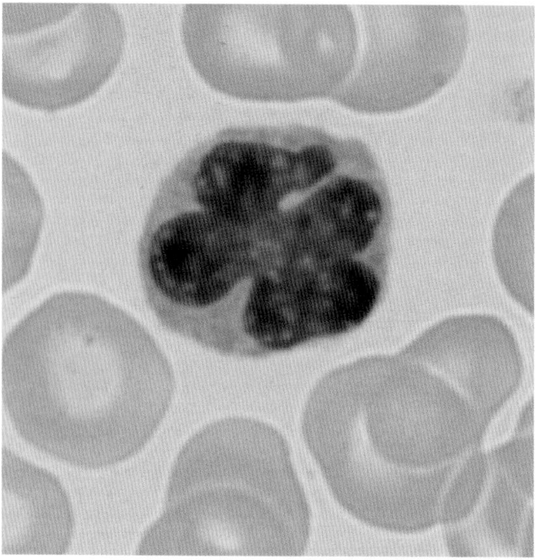

Plate 19 Blood films showing typical ATL cell with lobulated 'clover leaf' nucleus' (📖 see Fig. 4.19(a) p.177).

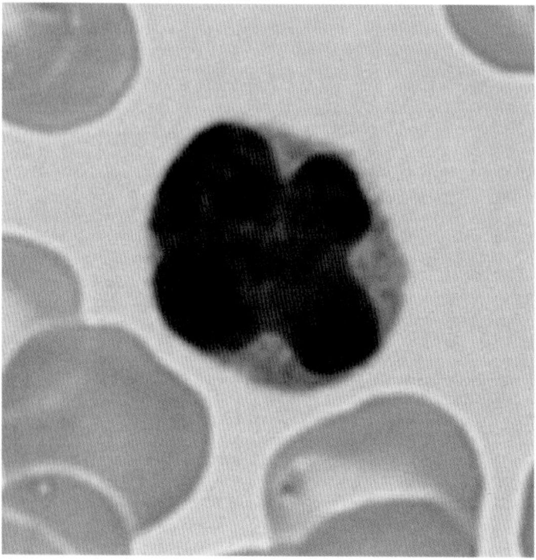

Plate 20 Blood films showing typical ATL cell with lobulated 'clover leaf' nucleus' (📖 see Fig. 4.19(b) p.177).

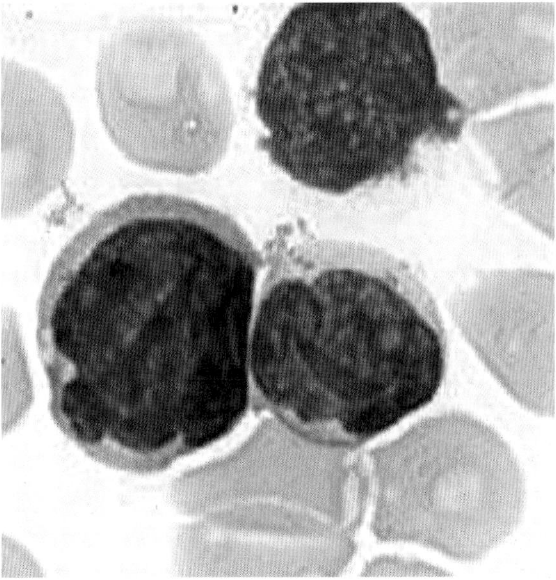

Plate 21 Blood film in Sézary syndrome showing typical cerebriform nuclei (📖 see Fig. 4.20 (a) p.178).

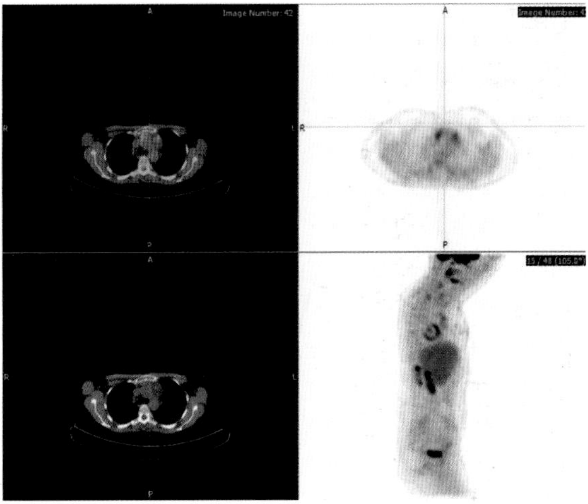

Plate 22 PET and CT scans in patient with nodular sclerosing Hodgkin lymphoma demonstrating active disease (moderate FDG uptake on PET) in residual anterior mediastinal mass on CT after ABVD chemotherapy (📖 see Fig. 5.1 p.209).

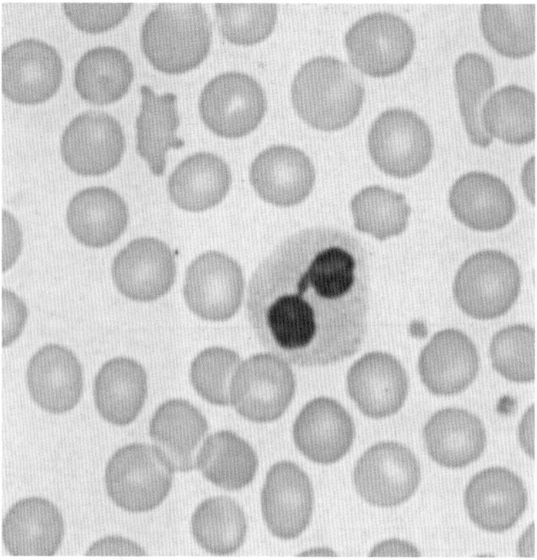

Plate 23 Blood film in MDS showing bilobed pseudo-Pelger neutrophil (📖 see Fig. 6.1 p.230).

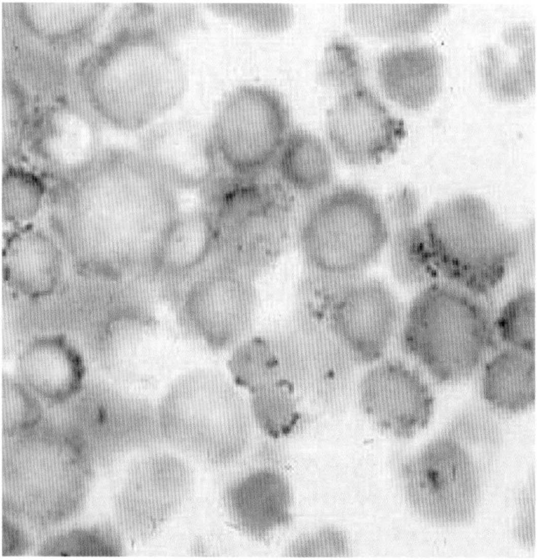

Plate 24 Bone marrow in RARS stained for iron: note iron granules round the nucleus of the erythroblast (📖 see Fig. 6.2 p.237).

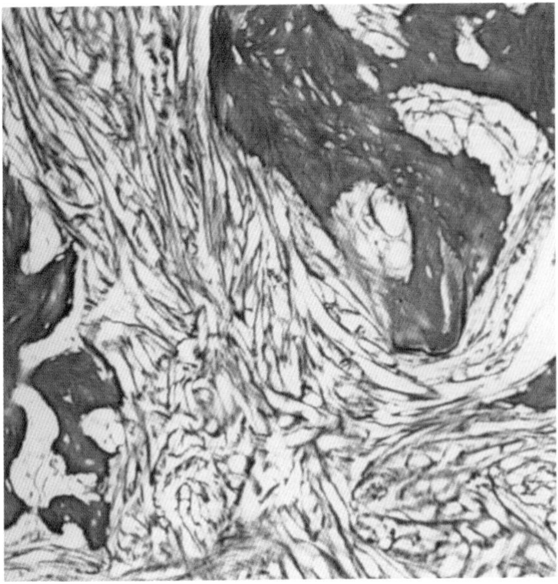

Plate 25 Bone marrow trephine in myelofibrosis: note streaming effect caused by intense fibrosis (see Fig. 7.1 p.288).

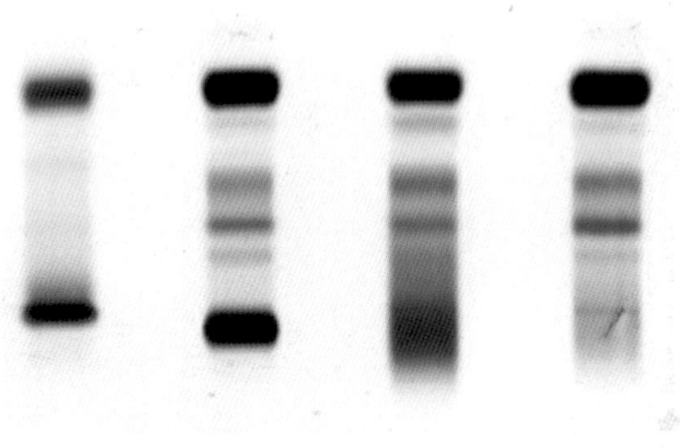

Plate 26 Electrophoresis: from L → R: urine with BJP & generalized proteinuria (albumin band at top of strip, BJP near foot); serum M band in myeloma; polyclonal gammopathy; normal sample, showing albumin, α, β & γ globulins (see Fig. 8.1 p.332).

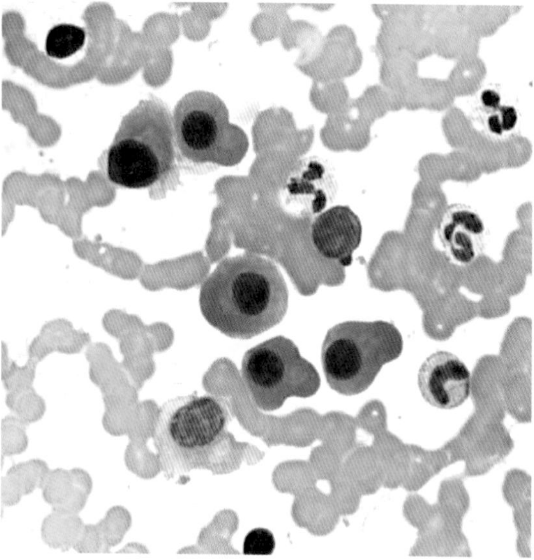

Plate 27 Bone marrow aspirate in myeloma showing numerous plasma cells (📖 see Fig. 8.2 p.335).

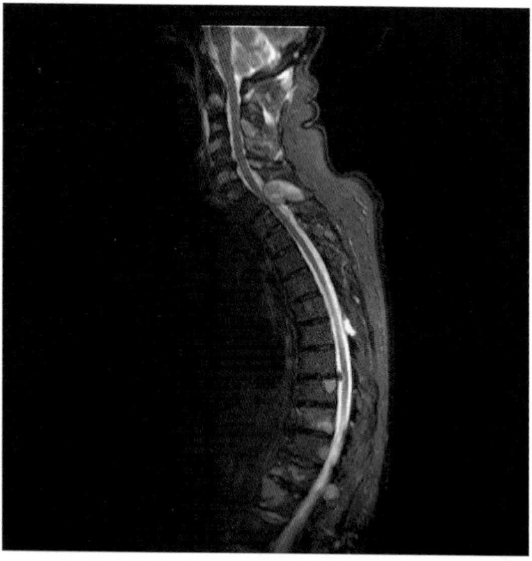

Plate 28 MRI of cervical and thoracic spine in a patient with multiple myeloma: substantial extra-osseous mass at T1 displacing the spinal cord anteriorly & causing some cord compression (📖 see Investigations and diagnosis p.332).

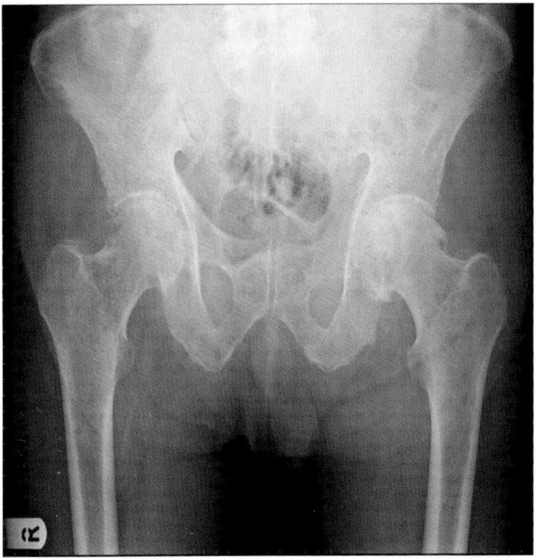

Plate 29 Radiograph of pelvis in a patient with multiple myeloma showing abnormal low density bone texture in the left superior pubic ramus & ischium (📖 see p.332).

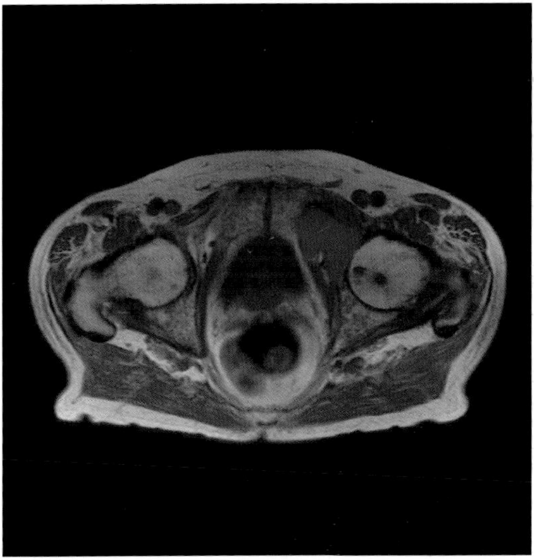

Plate 30 MRI of pelvis in a patient with multiple myeloma (same as Plate 29) showing corresponding soft tissue mass replacing bone & numerous widespread foci of signal change throughout the bony pelvis representing myeloma deposits (📖 see p.332).

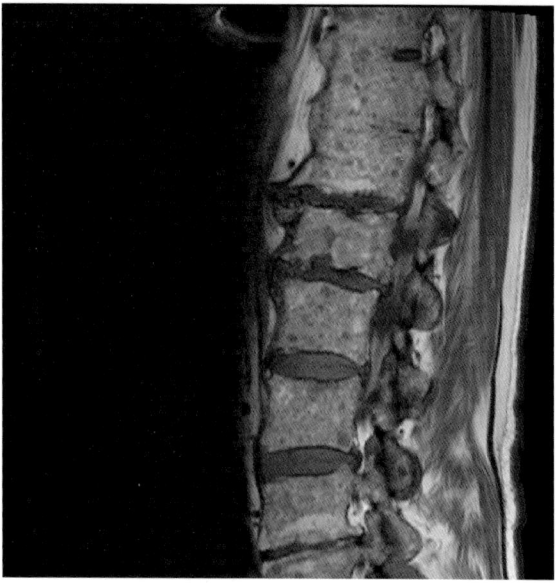

Plate 31 T1 sagittal sequence MRI of thoraco-lumbar spine in a patient with multiple myeloma showing multiple myeloma deposits & partial collapse of one vertebral body (📖 see p.332).

Indications for haemopoietic SCT

The Accreditation Subcommittee of the European Group for Blood & Marrow Transplantation (EBMT) has reported current practice for SCT in Europe (Table 9.3).

Table 9.3 Proposed classification of transplant procedures for adults: 2005[1]

Disease	Disease status	Allo			Auto
		Sibling donor	Well matched unrelated / 1ag mm related	Mismatch unrelated / >1 ag mm related	
AML	CR1 (low risk)	CO	D	NR	CO
	CR1 (intermed/ high risk)	S	CO	D	S
	CR2	S	CO	D	S
	CR3, incipient relapse	S	CO	D	NR
	APML Molecular persistence	S	CO	NR	NR
	APML Molecular CR2	S	CO	NR	S
	Relapse / Refractory	CO	D	NR	NR
ALL	CR1 (low risk)	D	NR	NR	D
	CR1 (high risk)	S	S	CO	NR
	CR2, incipient relapse	S	S	CO	NR
	Relapse / Refractory	CO	NR	NR	NR
CML	Chronic phase	S	S	NR	D
	Accelerated phase	S	S	CO	D
	Blast crisis	NR	NR	NR	NR
Myeloproliferative neoplasms		CO	CO	D	CO
Myelodysplastic syndrome	RA, RAEB	S	S	CO	CO
	RAEBt, sAML CR1/2	S	CO	CO	CO
	More advanced stages	S	CO	D	NR
CLL	Poor risk disease	S	S	D	CO
Diffuse large B-cell NHL	CR1 (intermediate/ high IPI at dx)	NR	NR	NR	CO
	Chemosensitive relapse; ≥CR2	D	D	NR	S
	Refractory	D	D	NR	NR

Table 9.3 Proposed classification of transplant procedures for adults: 2005 (*continued*)

Disease	Disease status		Allo		Auto
Mantle cell lymphoma	CR1	D	D	NR	S
	Chemosensitive relapse; ≥CR2	D	D	NR	S
	Refractory	D	D	NR	NR
Lymphoblastic and Burkitt's	CR1	D	NR	NR	CO
	Chemosensitive relapse; ≥CR2	CO	D	NR	S
	Refractory	D	D	NR	NR
Follicular NHL	CR1 (intermediate/ high IPI at dx)	NR	NR	NR	CO
	Chemosensitive relapse; ≥CR2	D	D	NR	S
	Refractory	D	D	NR	D
T-NHL	CR1	D	R	NR	CO
	Chemosensitive relapse; ≥CR2	D	D	NR	CO
	Refractory	D	D	NR	NR
HL	CR1	NR	NR	NR	NR
	Chemosensitive relapse; ≥CR2	D	D	D	S
	Refractory	D	D	NR	CO
Myeloma		CO	D	NR	S
Amyloidosis (AL)		D	D	NR	CO
Severe aplastic anaemia	Newly diagnosed	S	NR	NR	NR
	Refractory	S	S	CO	NR
PNH		S	CO	CO	NR
Germ-cell tumours	Sensitive relapses	NR	NR	NR	S
	Refractory	NR	NR	NR	CO

S = standard of care , generally indicated in suitable patients; CO = clinical option, can be carried out after careful assessment of risks and benefits; D = developmental, further trials are needed; NR = not recommended.

N.B. This classification does not cover patients for whom a syngeneic donor is available.

Autologous SCT is also a clinical option in suitable patients with immune cytopenias, systemic sclerosis, rheumatoid arthritis, multiple sclerosis, SLE and Crohn's disease. It is a developmental procedure in breast cancer, ovarian cancer and chronic inflammatory deyelinating polyradiculoneuropathy. Allogeneic SCT from a sibling donor is a developmental procedure in metastatic responding breast cancer, refractory ovarian cancer, metastatic renal cell carcinoma, immune cytopenias, systemic sclerosis, multiple sclerosis and SLE.

1. Ljungman, P.J. et al. (2006). Allogeneic and autologous transplantation for haematological diseases, solid tumours and immune disorders: definitions and current practice in Europe. Bone Marrow *Transplan*,t **37**, 439–49.

Table 9.4 Proposed classification of transplant procedures for children: 2005[1]

Disease	Disease status	Allo			Auto
		Sibling donor	Well matched unrelated / 1ag mm related	Mismatch unrelated / >1 ag mm related	
AML	CR1 (low risk)	NR	NR	NR	NR
	CR1 (high risk)	S	CO	NR	S
	CR1 (very high risk)	S	S	CO	NR
	CR2	S	S	S	S
	> CR2	CO	D	D	NR
ALL	CR1 (low risk)	NR	NR	NR	NR
	CR1 (high risk)	S	CO	CO	NR
	CR2	S	S	CO	CO
	> CR2	S	S	CO	CO
CML	Chronic phase	S	S	D	D
	Advanced phase	S	S	D	NR
NHL	CR1 (low risk)	NR	NR	NR	NR
	CR1 (high risk)	CO	CO	NR	CO
	CR2	S	S	CO	CO
HL	CR1	NR	NR	NR	NR
	1st relapse, CR2	CO	D	NR	S
Myelodysplastic syndromes		S	S	D	NR
1° immunodeficiencies		S	S	S	NA
Thalassaemia		S	CO	NR	NA
Sickle cell disease	High risk	S	CO	NR	NA
Aplastic anaemia		S	S	CO	NA
Fanconi anaemia		S	S	CO	NA
Blackfan–Diamond anaemia		S	CO	NR	NA
MPS-1 H Hurler		S	S	CO	NA
MPS-1 H Hurler-Scheie	Severe	NR	NR	NR	NA
MPS-VI Maroteaux–Lamy		CO	CO	CO	NA
Osteopetrosis		S	S	S	NA
Other storage diseases		NR	NR	NR	NR

Table 9.4 Proposed classification of transplant procedures for children: 2005 (*continued*)

Disease	**Disease status**	**Allo**			**Auto**
Autoimmune diseases		NR	NR	NR	CO
Gern cell tumour		NR	NR	NR	CO
Ewing's sarcoma	High risk or >CR1	D	NR	NR	S
Soft tissue sarcoma	High risk or >CR1	D	D	NR	CO
Neuroblastoma	high risk	CO	NR	NR	S
	> CR1	CO	D	D	S
Wilms tumour	> CR1	NR	NR	NR	CO
Osteogenic sarcoma		NR	NR	NR	D
Brain tumours		NR	NR	NR	CO

S = standard of care , generally indicated in suitable patients; CO = clinical option, can be carried out after careful assessment of risks and benefits; D = developmental, further trials are needed; NR = not recommended; NA = not applicable.

N.B. This classification does not cover patients for whom a syngeneic donor is available.

Allogeneic SCT

Patient and donor selection

- Recipients should be in good physical condition and generally ≤55 years old; 'biological' age is more important than chronological age; the development of reduced-intensity conditioning regimens (RIC) associated with less procedure related toxicity, permits an increase in the age-limit for SCT.
- Donor and recipient should be fully or closely HLA-matched to reduce the risk of life threatening GvHD or graft rejection.
- Risk of graft failure and GvHD related to degree of donor–recipient HLA-mismatching; the least mismatched donor should be selected.
- Greatest chance of full HLA match is a sib (small chance of full match with cousin); each sib has ~1:4 chance of full HLA-match.
- Matched-volunteer unrelated donor (UD) may be sought from donor registries e.g. in UK The National Blood Authority and Anthony Nolan panels.
- Haplo-identical sibling or mismatched UD may be considered as a donor for patients in whom no matched sibling or volunteer donor is available (~40%) and the ↑ risks of the procedure are acceptable (e.g. poor risk adult AML, Ph-positive adult ALL); in related SCT graft failure associated with recipient homozygosity at mismatched locus—avoid; in UD SCT risk of graft failure and GvHD higher with antigen mismatch than with allele mismatch; choose allele mismatch if possible.
- Patient and donor CMV status should be considered with +ve donors preferred for +ve patients and -ve donors preferred for –ve patients.
- Male donors are preferred for all recipients; UDs aged ≤40 years preferred to older UDs; ABO-matched donors preferred for heavily pre-transfused patients.

Table 9.5 Proposed HLA hierarchy for best choice of donor

1.	HLA-identical sibling = phenotypically HLA-matched related donor [a] = HLA-identical related donor umbilical cord blood [b]
2.	10/10 molecularly HLA-matched UD = 6/6 HLA-matched umbilical cord blood[b]
3.	9/10 HLA-matched UD = 5/6 HLA-matched related donor = ≥4/6 UD umbilical cord blood [b]
4.	8/10 matched UD = haploidentical related donor [c]

Options 3 and 4 should only be considered in poor risk patients for whom alternative treatment is unavailable. Option 4 usually requires in vitro T-cell depletion. Mismatched related donors may be preferred over UDs in certain disorders.

[a] HLA-matched donor where one haplotype is genetypicaly identical but the other is not.
[b] With nucleated cell dose >3.7 $\times 10^7$/kg recipient weight. [c] Most haploidentical donors for children are parents.

1. Skinner, R. *et al.* (2007). The transplant. In *Practical Haemopoietic Stem Cell Transplantation.* Cant, A.J. et al. (eds) Blackwell Publishing, Oxford., pp.23–40.

Indications for allogeneic SCT

📖 see pp.392–395

Source of stem cells

- Donors should be allowed to choose between donating BM or PBSCs after non-directive counselling.
- From HLA-identical sibling, BM preferred to PB.
- From HLA-matched UD, no preference.
- From HLA-mismatched UD or related donor, PB preferred to BM.

Outline of allogeneic SCT procedure

- Patient receives conditioning therapy with high dose chemoradiotherapy (traditionally, cyclophosphamide (CTX) 120mg/kg + 14Gy fractionated total body irradiation (TBI)) or chemotherapy (e.g. cyclophosphamide 120mg/kg + busulfan 16mg/kg).
- Reduced intensity conditioning regimens (RIC) are increasingly used; moderate doses of chemotherapy and immunosuppression used to achieve engraftment with lower transplant-related mortality and morbidity; shifts balance between risks of transplant-related mortality (TRM) and relapse; lower toxicity allows increased age range for allogeneic SCT (up to 75 years with related donor and 70 with unrelated donor reported); also allows SCT in some patients with comorbidities; permits use of adoptive immunotherapy with donor lymphocyte infusion (DLI) for residual disease post-transplant; encouraging results but full-intensity conditioning treatment of choice in younger patient without co-morbidities; RIC discouraged in patients with progressive or refractory disease.
- In patients receiving UD or haploidentical SCT, Campath®(humanized anti-CD52 monoclonal antibody) is often administered daily for 5d prior to conditioning as an immunosuppressant to the ↓ risk of graft rejection.
- For patients with aplastic anaemia less intensive conditioning is used (200mg/kg CTX combined with anti-thymocyte globulin) and because of sensitivity to alkylating agents in Fanconi anaemia still less intensive conditioning is used.
- In severe combined immunodeficiency (SCID), it is possible to engraft selected cell lineages without conditioning therapy.
- 1d after completing conditioning treatment, BM or PBSC are harvested from donor and infused IV through a central line.
- In UD and haploidentical SCT the graft is usually depleted of T lymphocytes prior to infusion to reduce the risk of severe GvHD.
- After 7–21d of severe myelosuppression, haematopoietic engraftment occurs.
- Reverse barrier nursing in a filtered air environment, prophylactic anti-infectives (ciprofloxacin, itraconazole, aciclovir) reduce the risk of infective complications.
- Immunosuppression is required to prevent GvHD and graft rejection; generally MTX (in the early engraftment phase) + ciclosporin A (for 6 months).

Mechanism of cure: evidence for GvL effect

- ↓ risk of relapse in patients with acute and chronic GvHD.
- ↑ risk of relapse after syngeneic SCT (no GvHD).
- ↑ risk of relapse after T-lymphocyte-depleted SCT.
- Delayed clearance of minimal residual disease detected post SCT.
- Induction of remission by DLI after relapse post-SCT.

Early complications of allogeneic SCT

- Overall transplant related mortality for matched sibling allografts is 15–25%, for volunteer unrelated donors may reach 45%.
- Infection: severe myelosuppression together with immune dysfunction from delayed reconstitution or GvHD predisposes to a wide variety of potentially fatal infections with bacterial (Gram +ve and –ve), viral, fungal, and atypical organisms. Both HSV and HZV infections are common—may present with fulminant extensive lesions. Main causes of infective death post-transplant are: CMV pneumonitis and invasive fungal infections with moulds e.g. *Aspergillus*.
- GvHD: acute GvHD occurs ≤100d of transplant and chronic >100d. (📖 GvHD, pp.424–430)
- Other complications:
  - Endocrine infertility (both sexes), early menopause, and occasionally hypothyroidism.
  - Cataract (TBI induced) >12 months post-transplant.
  - 2° malignancies (esp. skin).
  - EBV associated lymphoma.
  - Mild psychological disturbances common (serious psychoses rare).

Follow-up treatment and post-transplant surveillance

Immunosuppression requires careful monitoring to avoid toxicity. Unlike solid organ transplant recipients, lifelong immunosuppression not required and ciclosporin is usually discontinued at about 6 months post-transplant. Prophylaxis against pneumococcal sepsis 2° to hyposplenism, HZV reactivation and *P. jiroveci* infections required. Despite these complications, most patients return to an active, working life without the need for continuing medication.

Future developments

Molecular HLA gene loci mapping: improved DNA characterization of HLA gene loci should permit greater applicability and success of transplants from volunteer unrelated donors.

Umbilical cord blood transplants: umbilical cord blood donation post-delivery shown to be safe for mother and child. Cord blood stem cells are immunologically immature and may be more permissive of HLA donor/recipient mismatches with less risk of GvHD. Successful grafts in children; cell dose insufficient for adult grafts.

Autologous STC

Patient selection

Patients should be in good physical condition; age range for some procedures can be extended up to ~70 years. BM should be uninvolved or in CR at the time of harvest/mobilization unless disease control rather than cure is the primary intent cf. myeloma.

Indications

📖 see pp.392-395

Outline of autologous SCT procedure

- Haematopoietic stem cells harvested in CR are processed, frozen, and stored in liquid N_2.
- SCT may take place within days of harvest or several years later after treatment for recurrent disease.
- Different conditioning chosen for underlying indication e.g. cyclophosphamide + busulfan for AML or BEAM (📖 p.718) for NHL or HL.
- After completion of conditioning (generally plus 24h to allow clearance of chemotherapeutic agents), the stem cell product is thawed rapidly and infused IV. Bags are thawed by transfer directly from liquid N_2 into water at 37–43°C. Product is infused IV rapidly through indwelling central line.
- There is period of myelosuppression (7–25d) followed by WBC, platelet and RBC engraftment.

Early complications of the transplant procedure

- Overall transplant related mortality is 5–10%.
- Morbidity from conditioning regimens e.g. nausea from chemoradiotherapy and mucositis from the widespread mucosal damage to GIT: oral ulceration, buccal desquamation, oesophagitis, gastritis, abdominal pain, and diarrhoea may all be features.
- Spectrum of infective organisms seen is similar to allografts but severity and mortality are ↓.

Late complications of autologous SCT

- Single commonest long-term complication is relapse of underlying disease.
- Other late complications similar to allografts, but less frequent and less severe.

Follow-up treatment and post-transplant surveillance

- Regular haematological follow-up is mandatory and psychological support from the transplant team, family and friends are important for readjustment to normal life.
- Prophylaxis against specific infections required including *Pneumococcus*, HZV and *P. jiroveci*. Most patients return to an active, working life without continuing medication.

Investigations for BMT/PBSCT

Haematology
- FBC, reticulocytes, ESR.
- Serum B_{12} and red cell folate, ferritin.
- Blood group, antibody screen, and DAT.
- Coagulation screen, PT, APTT, fibrinogen.
- BM aspirate for morphology (cytogenetics if relevant).
- BM trephine biopsy.

Biochemistry
- U&Es, LFTs.
- Ca^{2+}, phosphate, random glucose.
- LDH.
- Thyroid function tests.
- Serum and urine Igs.
- EDTA clearance.

Virology
- Hepatitis BsAg.
- Hepatitis C antibody.
- HIV I and II antibody (counselling and consent required).
- CMV IgG and IgM.
- EBV, HSV and VZV IgG.
- Parvovirus B19 titre (allografts only).
- Toxoplasma titre (allografts only).

Immunology
- Autoantibody screen.
- HLA type, (if not known) in case HLA matched platelets are subsequently required.
- HLA and platelet antibody screen (if previously poor increments to platelet transfusions).
- CRP.

Bacteriology
- Baseline blood cultures (peripheral blood and Hickman line).
- Routine admission swabs: throat, central line site.
- MSU, stool cultures.

Cardiology
- ECG.
- Echocardiogram, to include measurement of systolic ejection fraction.

Respiratory
- Lung function tests.

Radiology
- CXR.
- Sinus x-rays.

Cytogenetics

- Blood for donor/recipient polymorphisms (allografts only).

Other

- Consider semen/embryo storage.
- Dental opinion if caries/gum disease.
- Psychiatric opinion if previous history.

Pretransplant investigation of donors

Haematology

- FBC, reticulocytes, ESR.
- Blood group, antibody screen, and DAT.
- Coagulation screen, PT, APTT, fibrinogen.

Biochemistry

- U&Es.
- LFTs.
- Thyroid function tests.
- Urinalysis: dipstick.

Virology

- Hepatitis BsAg.
- Hepatitis A antibody.
- Hepatitis C antibody.
- HIV I and II antibody (counselling and consent required).
- CMV IgG and IgM.
- EBV, HSV and VZV IgG.
- HTLV III.

Immunology

- Autoantibody screen.
- CRP.

Microbiology

- Syphilis serology.
- Toxoplasma serology.

Cardiology

- BP.
- CXR, ECG if indicated.

Molecular biology

- DNA fingerprinting for chimerism studies.

Bone marrow harvesting

Pre-operative preparations

Important to give advance notice so that theatre time can be booked if necessary and the virological screening results obtained.

Within 30d before the harvest procedure, arrange the following virological investigations

- Hepatitis B surface antigen.
- Hepatitis C antibody.
- HIV 1 and 2.
- HTLV III.
- VDRL.
- Spare serum stored.

Admit patient day before harvest. Clerk patient and arrange:

- U&E.
- FBC.
- X match 2–3U blood (CMV –ve). If harvest is on normal donor, offer autologous blood collection to donor. If declined, arrange for genotyped, CMV –ve and irradiated X-matched blood to be available for the donor. A CXR and ECG may also be arranged, if felt clinically appropriate.

Harvest procedure

1. Give heparin 50U/kg IV at anaesthetic induction.
2. Prepare harvest bag: adding ACD with a dilution factor of 1:10 for the prospective marrow volume; i.e. 100mL of ACD if expected harvest is ~1L.
3. Heparinize aspirate needles/syringes (0.9% saline containing at least 100U heparin/mL).
4. Begin with posterior superior iliac crests, limiting the number of skin entry points, the aspirate needle should be manoeuvred to collect as much marrow as possible with 5–10mL maximum from each penetration of the bone. Each aspirate should be deposited in a sterile harvest bag and syringe rinsed in the heparinized saline prior to re-use. Gently agitate bag at intervals.
5. Midway through harvest (or 500mL) a bag sample should be sent for FBC to determine the adequacy of the harvest. The final total WBC count should be at least 2×10^8 cells/kg of the recipient for autografts and 3×10^8 cells/kg for allografts.

Box 9.1 The volume of marrow required may be calculated as follows:

Total volume required for autograft
= 2.0 × recipient weight (kg) ÷ (bag WBC × 10)

e.g. recip. 100kg and bag WBC 20 $\times 10^9$/L then vol. required
= (2.0 ×100) ÷ (20 ×10) = 1.0L
Volume still needed to be harvested = total volume – volume already taken at time of count + ~10%

Notes:

1. The extra 10% compensates for reduced harvesting efficiency and the ACD.
2. The formula works at whatever volume you choose to do the first WBC but is a more accurate prediction at >500mL.
3. If need to harvest >1L, remember to add additional ACD in the same 1 in 10 ratio.
4. For allograft calculations, substitute 3.0 for 2.0 in the formula.

If yield not adequate from the posterior iliac crests, other sites may be considered (e.g. anterior superior iliac crests and sternum). Review puncture sites the following morning for signs of local infection or continuing bleeding. For normal donors, offer out-patient follow-up appointment as additional safeguard and provide access to counselling services.

Peripheral blood stem cell mobilization and harvesting

Properties of stem cells

- Stem cells are defined as the most primitive haemopoietic precursor cell
- Unique property is capability of both infinite self-renewal and differentiation to form all mature cells of the haemopoietic and immune systems.
- In the resting state almost all stem cells reside in the BM although a tiny minority circulate in peripheral blood.
- Stem cells in marrow can migrate into the blood after treatment with chemotherapy and/or haemopoietic growth factors.
- Once circulating, they can easily be harvested using a cell separator machine.
- Stem cell levels in peripheral blood can be assessed by CD34 immuno-phenotype analysis.
- >1d of apheresis may be necessary to achieve required yield.
- The yield can be assessed for engraftment potential.

Protocols

Mobilization and harvesting protocols differ between diseases. The following illustrate the principal types of schedule:

Mobilization after standard chemotherapy

- No specific additional stimulus given.
- Harvest times determined by WBC and platelet recovery, and CD34 count.
- Yields variable. Improved by addition of G-CSF.

Suitable for:

- NHL post DHAP chemotherapy.
- AML post ADE/DAT chemotherapy.
- ALL post high dose MTX.

Mobilization with chemotherapy and haemopoietic growth factors

The commonest schedule and the best evaluated. Harvest timing and yields more predictable.

Typical protocol for NHL

- Day 0 cyclophosphamide 1.5g/m^2 IVI with Mesna.
- Day +4 to day +10 G-CSF 5mcg/kg/d SC continued until last day of harvesting.
- Harvest ~day +10 when CD34 >10 × 10^6/L and/or WBC >10 × 10^9/L.

Typical protocol for myeloma

- Day 0 cyclophosphamide 4g/m^2 IVI with Mesna.
- Day +1 to day +10–14, G-CSF 5–10mcg/kg/d SC.
- Harvest day +10 to14 when CD34 > 10 × 10^6/L and/or WBC >10 × 10^9/L

Mobilization with haemopoietic growth factor alone

- Suitable for normal volunteers e.g. allograft donors.
- G-CSF 5–10mcg/kg/d SC for 4–5d.
- Harvest d4–5.

Yield evaluation

Common parameters are mononuclear cell counts (MNC); CD34 numbers and haemopoietic colony forming unit assays e.g. CFU-GM. All are a quantitative or functional assessment of engraftment potential expressed per kg of recipient weight.

Typical target yields

Daily apheresis and daily G-CSF continue until the collection exceeds:

- 4×10^8/kg mononuclear cells ***or***
- 10×10^4/kg CFU-GM ***or***
- 3×10^6/kg CD34+ cells.

Microbiological screening for stem cell cryopreservation

Infective agents, particularly viruses, can be transmitted through ster cell preparations as through blood products and may cause significan morbidity and mortality in the recipient. It has been demonstrated tha transmission of hepatitis B virus has occurred following common storag in a liquid nitrogen tank that contained one patient's hepatitis B surfac antigen +ve BM.

The following tests should be performed on all patients in whom it is planned to cryopreserve stem cells

- Hepatitis B surface antigen.
- Hepatitis B surface antibody.
- Hepatitis B core antigen.
- Hepatitis B core antibody.
- Hepatitis C antibody.
- HIV 1 and 2 antibodies.
- HIV 1 and 2 antigen.
- HTLV1 antibody.
- VDRL.
- Additional serum for storage for retrospective analysis.

These results must be available to transplant laboratories before cryop reservation. Since many of these patients will be receiving blood product as part of their ongoing treatment, they must be performed within 30d c cryopreservation to prevent false –ve antibody tests due to the interva between exposure and seroconversion. In practice these constraint dictate that samples should be taken between 7–30d prior to cryopreser vation.

Patient samples shown to be –ve for all the above infectious agents shoul have stem cells stored in a dedicated liquid nitrogen freezer convention ally in the liquid phase.

Patient samples shown to be +ve for any of the above agents should b ***double bagged and stored in a separate liquid nitrogen freezer in th vapour phase*** (to reduce transmissibility). Data on all stem cell produc samples must be registered in a secure environment on a computer ized database with a logical inventory and retrieval system. No materia should be imported to the freezers unless a complete –ve virological audi storage trail can be demonstrated.

Stem cell transplant conditioning regimens

Conditioning is the treatment the patient undergoes immediately prior to a SCT. The purpose is to reduce the burden of residual disease; in allogeneic transplant recipients, it also acts as an immunosuppressant to prevent rejection of the graft. Many different protocols using chemotherapy alone or in combination with total body irradiation (TBI) have been developed. None has proven to be superior. Fractionation of radiation results in less toxicity but the total dose has to be ↑ to achieve similar immunosuppression. Unrelated transplants require immunosuppression with ALG or anti-T-cell monoclonal antibodies or total lymphoid irradiation (TLI). Reduced intensity regimens can reduce transplant-related mortality and offers otherwise ineligible patients a potentially curative treatment.

Examples—Tables 9.6 and 9.7

Table 9.6 Commonly used transplant conditioning regimens by diseases[1]

Disease	Regimen	Total dose	Dose per day	Days
AML and CML	*Cy/TBI*			
	Cyclophosphamide	120mg/kg	60mg/kg	–5, –4
	Total body irradiation	12–14.4 Gy	4-4.8Gy	–3 to –1
	Bu/Cy			
	Busulfan	16mg/kg	4mg/kg	–7 to –4
	Cyclophosphamide	120mg/kg	60mg/kg	–3, –2
ALL	*Cy/TBI*			
	Cyclophosphamide	120mg/kg	60mg/kg	–5, –4
	Total body irradiation	12–14.4 Gy	4-4.8Gy	–3 to –1
	TBI/VP			
	Total body irradiation	12–13.2 Gy	4-5 Gy	–7 to –4
	Etoposide	60mg/kg	60mg/kg	–3
	Cy/VP-16/TBI			
	Cyclophosphamide	120mg/kg	60mg/kg	–6, –5
	Etoposide	30–60 mg/kg	30–60 mg/kg	–4
	Total body irradiation	12–13.2 Gy	4–4.4Gy	–3 to–1
Severe aplastic anaemia	*Cy ± ATG*			
	Cyclophosphamide	200mg/kg	50mg/kg	–5 to –2
	ATG[1]	90mg/kg	30mg/kg	–5 to –3
Thalassaemia	*Bu/Cy*			
	Busulfan	14-16 mg/kg	3.5-4 mg/kg	–9 to –6
	Cyclophosphamide	200mg/kg	50mg/kg	–5 to –2

Table 9.6 Commonly used transplant conditioning regimens by diseases (*continued*)[1]

Disease	Regimen	Total dose	Dose per day	Days
Fanconi anaemia	*Flu/Bu/Cy*			
	Busulfan	6mg/kg	1.5mg/kg	–9 to –6
	Fludarabine	$100mg/m^2$	$25mg/m^2$	–5 to –2
	Cyclophosphamide	40mg/kg	10mg/kg	–5 to –2
	ATG*	6mg/kg	1.5mg/kg	–4 to –1
Myeloma	*High dose melphalan*	$200mg/m^2$	$200mg/m^2$	–1
Lymphoma	*BEAM*			
	Carmustine	$300mg/m^2$	$300mg/m^2$	–6
	Etoposide	$800mg/m^2$	$200mg/m^2$	–5 to –2
	Cytarabine	$1600mg/m^2$	$400mg/m^2$	–5 to –2
	Melphalan	$140mg/m^2$	$140mg/m^2$	–1

*ATG dose depends on specific brand of ATG.

Table 9.7 Examples of reduced intensity conditioning regimens[1]

Regimen	Treatment	Total dose
Flu/TBI	Fludarabine	$90mg/m^2$
	Total body irradiation	2 Gy
*Flu/Bu ± ATG**	Fludarabine	$180mg/m^2$
	Busulphan	8mg/kg
	ATG	40mg/kg
Flu/Mel ± Campath®	Fludarabine	$150mg/m^2$
	Melphalan	100mg
	Campath®-1H	$140–180mg/m^2$
Flu/Cy	Fludarabine	$125mg/m^2$
	Cyclophosphamide	120mg/kg

*ATG dose depends on specific brand of ATG.

1. Aschan, J. (2007). Risk assessment in haematopoietic stem cell transplantation: conditioning. *Best Practice Res Clin Haematol*, **20**, 295–310.

Infusion of cryopreserved stem cells

Equipment

- Dewar containing stem cells in liquid N_2.
- Water bath heated to 37–40°C.
- Tongs.
- Protective gloves.
- Patient's notes.
- Trolley with: syringes, needles, ampoules of 0.9% saline, blood giving sets, sterile dressing towels, chlorhexidine spray, bags of 500mL N/Saline, sterile gloves.

Ensure the patient has had procedure and any possible side effects explained

Method

1. Write up the stem cell infusion on the blood product infusion chart.
2. 30min before re-infusion, ensure water bath is filled and heated to 37°C–40°C and give (chlorphenamine) 10mg IV and paracetamol 1g PO.
3. When ready to return the stem cells take the Dewar and equipment trolley to the patient's bedside.
4. Check the patient's vital signs.
5. Set up a standard blood giving set with microaggregate filter. Never use additional filters. Prime with 500mL 0.9% saline, connect to the patient and ensure good flow before starting to thaw any cells.
6. Check the water bath is 37°C–40°C and using the protective gloves and large tongs remove a bag of cells from liquid nitrogen Dewar and place on the trolley. Carefully remove from the outer sleeve and place in water bath and allow one minute. DMSO cryopreservative is very toxic to cells once thawed so it is important to go straight from rapid thaw to infusion.
7. Remove bag of cells from water bath using the tongs, spray with chlorhexidine and allow to dry. Check patient identification number and DOB with the patient and if correct then connect to the giving set.
8. Cells should be returned as quickly as possible. Each bag contains approximately 100–150mL. Providing the flow is good, start thawing the next bag. Only thaw the next bag if you are able to finish the previous bag within the next minute. Check the patient's details on every bag.
9. Check the patient's observations at 15min intervals.
10. If the patient complains of abdominal pain, nausea or feeling faint, slow down the IVI for a short time. If symptoms persist or patient develops chest tightness or wheezing—stop the infusion. O_2 ± nebulized salbutamol may be required. Anaphylaxis rare.
11. At the end of re-infusion ensure no more bags of stem cells in the Dewar and clear away all equipment.
12. Write the infusion details in the patient's notes in red ink.

Special considerations

► If the bag splits/leaks do not re-infuse—contents will not be sterile. Very rarely, a bag could start to expand rapidly upon thawing if all air not removed from the bag before freezing. A sterile needle may be used to pierce the bag if release of pressure appears essential.

►► Acute anaphylaxis is very rare but epinephrine (adrenaline) (1mL of 1:1000) should be available in the patient's room for SC or IM administration.

Infusion of fresh non-cryopreserved stem cells

Explain procedure and side effects to patient. In general, BM will be in a larger volume than an apheresis product.

Procedure

1. A medical staff member must be available to start the infusion and stay with the patient for the first 30min.
2. Prime blood giving set without an in-line filter with 500mL 0.9% saline and connect to the patient—check there is a good flow.
3. Check BP, pulse, and chest auscultation before the infusion.
4. Give paracetamol 1g PO and chlorphenamine 10mg IV at beginning of infusion.
5. Give stem cells as slowly as possible for the first 15min, then increase the rate to 100mL in 60min. If after 2h the patient is tolerating infusion without problems, increase to 200mL/h until completion.
6. Watch for fluid overload—give diuretic if necessary.
7. Nursing staff should monitor BP and pulse every 15–30min.
8. Write infusion details in the patient's notes in red ink.

Complications of stem cell infusion

- Microemboli occasionally cause dyspnoea and cyanosis. O_2 should be available. Slow down or stop the stem cell infusion if dyspnoea.
- Pyrexia, rash and rigors can occur—treat with hydrocortisone 100mg IV and chlorphenamine 10mg IV.
- Hypertension may occur (especially if patient fluid overloaded). Usually responds to diuretic.

►► Acute anaphylaxis is very rare but adrenalin (1mL of 1:1000) should be available in the patient's room for SC or IM administration.

Daily ward management

Each day check patient for:

- Fever.
- Nausea and vomiting.
- Diarrhoea.
- Bleeding.
- Rashes.
- Fatigue.
- Dyspnoea.
- Pain.
- Weight loss.
- Jaundice.
- Mucositis.
- Skin surveillance needed to observe for signs of acute and chronic GvHD, HSV, HZV, and drug related problems.
- Hickman line infections are common post-transplant. If any signs of infection and fever, line cultures and exit site swab should be taken. Remove line as soon as infusion support no longer needed.

Blood product support for SCT

All cellular blood products, i.e. red cells and platelets, must be irradiated.

Irradiation

- All cellular blood products given to allogeneic and autologous SCT patients must be irradiated to prevent transfusion associated GvHD due to transfused T lymphocytes.
- Transfusion associated GvHD is usually fatal particularly in allografts.
- Fatality can sometimes be avoided by immediate administration of anti-lymphocyte globulin or Campath®.
- Irradiation protocol is standard 2500cGy.
- Commence blood product irradiation 2 weeks prior to allogeneic SCT until 1 year post-SCT or off all immunosuppression whichever is later.
- Commence blood product irradiation 2 weeks prior to autologous SCT until 6 months post-SCT.
- Cell-free blood products e.g. FFP, cryoprecipitate, or albumin do not need to be irradiated.
- Marrow or blood stem cell transplant itself is never irradiated.

CMV status of blood products

- CMV is not destroyed by irradiation.
- All transplant recipients should ideally receive CMV –ve red cells and platelet transfusions regardless of their own CMV status if sufficient CMV –ve blood products available. This is because of good evidence that transfused CMV carried in donor white cells may cause disease post-transplant regardless of the CMV status of the patient. CMV –ve recipients must always have –ve products.
- Should CMV –ve platelets not be available at any time, it is acceptable to use unscreened leucodepleted red cells or platelets. This is because CMV is carried predominantly in leucocytes.
- For allograft recipients, additional preventive measures are taken against CMV reactivation (📖 see CMV prophylaxis and treatment, p.440).

Indications for RBC and platelet transfusions

Identical to those for patients undergoing intensive chemotherapy (📖 see pp.670–766 & 768.

Management of ABO incompatibility

ABO incompatibility between donor and recipient does not affect the long-term success of the transplant or the incidence of graft failure or GvHD. However, major ABO incompatibility transfusion reactions will occur unless specific steps are taken to manipulate the graft where donor and recipient are ABO mismatched. Furthermore, additional care must be given post-transplant in providing appropriate ABO matched products.

ABO mismatched definitions

- *Major* ABO mismatch. This is where the recipient has anti-A or anti-B antibody to donor ABO antigens e.g. group O recipients with group A donor.
- *Minor* ABO mismatch. This is where the donor has antibodies to recipient ABO antigens e.g. group A recipient with group O donor.

Management of major ABO mismatch

Manipulation of donor marrow/stem cells: red cells are removed in the transplant laboratory by starch sedimentation or Ficoll centrifugation, prior to infusion of the graft.

Choice of red cell and platelet supportive transfusions

- Transfuse packed group O red cells only for all major mismatch donor–recipient pairs.
- The choice of platelet group is less critical and may be affected by availability. 1st, 2nd, and 3rd choice groups for platelet transfusions are shown in the table below.

Management of minor ABO mismatch

Manipulation of donor stem cells: prior to infusion, the product will have been plasma reduced in the transplant laboratory by centrifugation to remove antibody that could be passively transferred. Delayed immune haemolysis, which may be severe and intravascular, can occur after minor ABO mismatch due to active production of antibody by engrafting donor lymphocytes. Maximum haemolysis occurs 9–16d post-transplant.

Choice of red cell and platelet transfusions

- Always transfuse packed O red cells, i.e. the same as in major ABO mismatch.
- Platelet transfusions 1st, 2nd, and 3rd choice group is shown in the Table 9.8.

Table 9.8 Choice of ABO group of blood/platelets in ABO mismatch BMT

			Platelets		
Donor	**Recipient**	**Red cells**	**1st choice**	**2nd choice**	**3rd choice**
Major ABO mismatch					
A	O	O	A	B	O
B	O	O	B	A	O
AB	O	O	A	B	O
A	B	O	B	A*	O*
B	A	O	A	B*	O*
AB	A	O	A	B*	O*
AB	B	O	B	A*	O*
Minor ABO mismatch					
O	A	O	A	B*	O*
O	B	O	B	A*	O*
O	AB	O	A*	B*	O*
A	AB	O	A*	B*	O*
B	AB	O	B*	A*	O*

(*Risk of haemolysis but do not withhold)

Rh (D) mismatch

Anti-D is not a naturally occurring antibody but may be induced by sensitization with D +ve cells through pregnancy or previous incompatible transfusion. Important to screen both recipient and donor serum for the presence of anti-D.

- When either donor or recipient serum contains anti-D, Rh D –ve blood products should always be given post-transplant. Note: in the situation where a Rh D +ve recipient receives a graft from a donor whose serum contains anti-D, immune haemolysis may occur despite plasma reduction of the donor marrow due to active production of donor lymphocyte derived anti-D. Cannot be prevented but is rarely severe.
- Provided neither donor nor recipient have anti-D in the serum, specific pre-transplant manipulation of the product is only required in the situation of Rh D +ve donor going into Rh D –ve recipient where red cell depletion is required pre-transplant.
- It will occasionally be necessary to give Rh D +ve platelet support when Rh D –ve is preferable simply due to lack of abundant availability of Rh D –ve platelet products.
- If Rh D +ve platelets have to be given, give anti-D 250IU SC immediately post-transfusion.

GvHD prophylaxis

In vitro T-cell depletion of graft or *in vivo* T-cell depletion with Campath®-1H or anti-thymocyte globulin (ATG) are successful in reducing both the incidence and severity of GvHD in graft recipients. The former is associated with an ↑ risk of relapse. Both are used in UD and haploidentical grafts where the risk of severe GvHD is ↑. The 'Seattle protocol' is most commonly used post graft infusion: consists of a combination of stat pulses of IV MTX with bd infusions of ciclosporin:

MTX (IV bolus) 15mg/m^2 on day +1, then 10mg/m^2 days +3, +6, and +11. Folinic acid rescue 15mg/m^2 IV tds may be given 24h after each MTX injection for 24h (rescue protocol designed to reduce mucositis).

Dosage reductions

- If renal/hepatic impairment ↓ MTX dose as shown in Table 9.9:

Table 9.9 Methotrexate dosage reductions

Creatinine (micromol/L)	**MTX dose (%)**
<145	100
146–165	50
166–180	25
>180	omit dose
Bilirubin (micromol/L)	**MTX dose (%)**
<35	100
36–50	50
51–85	25
>85	omit dose

Side effects

Although reduced by folinic acid rescue, mucositis may remain severe and require IV diamorphine.

Ciclosporin administration

Powerful immunosuppressant with profound effects on T-cell suppressor function. Available for IV and oral use.

IV regimen

Commence on day −1 at 1.5mg/kg IV bd as IVI in 100mL 0.9% saline/2h. If flushing, nausea, or pronounced tremor, slow infusion rate 4–6h/dose. Following loading, on day +3 onwards, adjust ciclosporin dosage based on plasma ciclosporin A level together with renal and hepatic function.

Oral regimen

Switch IV → oral when patient can tolerate oral medication and is eating (usually day +10 to +20). Dosage on conversion is ~1.5–2.0 × IV dose (still bd).

Monitoring ciclosporin levels

- Ciclosporin is toxic and renal impairment is the most frequent dose limiting toxicity.
- Ciclosporin A levels should be monitored at least twice weekly.

- Never take blood for ciclosporin A levels from the central catheter through which ciclosporin has been given as ciclosporin adheres to plastic and falsely high levels will be obtained. One lumen should be marked for ciclosporin administration and another lumen marked for blood levels testing.
- 12h pre-dose trough whole blood levels are measured.

Instruct patient to delay the morning dose of ciclosporin until after the blood level has been taken. The optimum blood ciclosporin level is not known. Target range: 100–300ng/mL. Aim towards the top of the therapeutic range in the early post-transplant period and lower part of the range at other times. In practice, the dose is often limited by a rise in serum creatinine. If serum creatinine >130micromol/L—adjust dose. Do not give ciclosporin if serum creatinine >180micromol/L.

Dosage adjustment

Ciclosporin has a very long $t\frac{1}{2}$, so dosage adjustment similar to warfarin adjustment.

- To ↓ ciclosporin level omit 1–2 doses and make a 25–50% reduction in ongoing maintenance dose, recheck levels at 48h.
- To ↑ levels, give 1 additional dose, increase maintenance dose by 25–50%, recheck level in 48h.
- Monitor renal function and LFTs daily. Check serum calcium and magnesium twice weekly.

Ciclosporin toxicity

- Nephrotoxicity (📖 see Monitoring ciclosporin levels, p.420). Worse with concurrent use of aminoglycosides, vancomycin, and amphotericin.
- Hypertension—often associated with fluid retention and potentiated by steroids. Treat initially with diuretic to baseline weight and then nifedipine if persists. Sub-lingual nifedipine useful where emergency reduction of blood pressure is required.
- Neurological syndromes, esp. grand mal seizures (usually if untreated hypertension/fluid retention).
- Anorexia, nausea, vomiting, tremor (almost always occurs—if severe suggests overdosage).
- Hirsutism and gum hypertrophy with prolonged usage.
- Hepatotoxicity—less common than nephrotoxicity. Usually intrahepatic cholestatic picture on LFTs. Potentiated by concurrent drug administration e.g. macrolide antibiotics, norethisterone and the azole antifungals.
- Hypomagnesaemia commonly occurs. Potentiated by combination with amphotericin. Give 20mmol IVI if levels <0.5micromol/L or if symptoms develop.

Note: only one orally absorbed preparation of magnesium. For hypomagnesaemia persisting on ciclosporin post-discharge, consider magnesium glycerophosphate tablets qds.

Ciclosporin drug interactions

There are substantial and important drug interactions with ciclosporin (Table 9.10).

Table 9.10 Ciclosporin drug interactions

Drugs that ↑ ciclosporin A levels	Drugs that ↓ ciclosporin levels
Azole antifungals	Rifampicin → major effect
Digoxin	Phenytoin → major effect
Macrolide antibiotics, especially	Sulphonamides
Erythromycin	Carbamazepine
Imipenem/meropenem	
$Ca2^{+}$ channel blockers	
Oral contraceptives	

Drugs worsening ciclosporin nephrotoxicity

- Aminoglycosides.
- Amphotericin B.
- Ciprofloxacin.
- Cotrimoxazole.
- ACE inhibitors.

Note: This is not an exhaustive list. Check ciclosporin levels 48h after any drug addition or cessation.

Tacrolimus

- Calcineurin inhibitor that prevents early T-cell activation; mechanism of action, pharmacology, drug interactions, and toxicity similar to ciclosporin: renal impairment, neurotoxicity, and cardiomyopathy.
- Superior to ciclosporin in 3 randomized trials when used in combination with MTX as GvHD prophylaxis.
- Dosage: 0.03mg/kg/d by continuous IV infusion from day –2; taper 20% every 2 weeks from d180; monitor blood level and toxicities and modify dose accordingly; used with standard dose MTX or mini-MTX ($5mg/m^2$ IV days +1, +3, +6, and +11).

Mycophenolate mofetil (MMF)

- Recently added to the immuosuppressants used in prevention and treatment of GvHD; replaced MTX in trials of SCT using reduced intensity conditioning.
- MMF/CsA appears to have equivalent activity to CsA/MTX in control of acute GvHD with reduced mucositis and duration of neutropenia but a possible ↑ risk of viral infection, myelosuppression, and gut ulceration.

Acute GvHD

The major cause of early transplant-related mortality. Median incidence of clinically significant (grade II–IV) acute GvHD is ~40%. Risk factors for acute GvHD include: older recipients, older donors, ♂ recipient of ♀ SCT (↑ risk with previous donor pregnancies), matched unrelated donors, haploidentical sibling donor, PBSC graft (> BM > cord blood). Defined as GvHD occurring within 1st 100d post-transplant (usually starts between d7 and d28 post-transplant). Ranges from mild self-limiting condition to extensive disease and may be fatal. Characterized by fever, rash, abnormal LFTs, diarrhoea, suppression of engraftment and viral reactivation, particularly CMV.

Classified according to the Seattle system by a staging for each organ involved (skin, liver, gut) and overall clinical grading based on the organ staging (Table 9.11).

Skin—involved in >90% cases. May be mild and unremarkable maculopapular rash (esp. palms of hands and soles of feet, but can affect any part of the body). In more severe cases, erythroderma and extensive desquamation and exfoliation can occur.

Liver—typical pattern of LFT abnormalities is intrahepatic cholestasis with ↑ bilirubin and alkaline phosphatase (relative sparing of transaminases). *Note*: this picture often does not discriminate between other causes of post-transplant liver dysfunction (e.g. drugs, infection—particularly CMV and fungal).

Gut—may occasionally be only organ involved, with nausea, vomiting, diarrhoea. Stool appearance may be highly abnormal with mincemeat or redcurrant jelly stools or green coloration.

Diagnosis

- Perform skin biopsy—but do not delay treatment if strong clinical suspicion.
- Rectal biopsy may be helpful (to distinguish infective from pseudo-membranous colitis) but beware risk of bleeding and bacteraemia— perform only if it will alter management.
- Where GI symptoms are predominantly upper GI, gastroscopy with oesophageal, gastric, and duodenal biopsies may be helpful (e.g. to distinguish between CMV and fungal oesophagitis and gastritis). Liver biopsy is hazardous and should only be performed where other convincing diagnostic guides are not available. It should be performed only by the trans-jugular route by an experienced operator and covered appropriately with blood products.

Table 9.11 Consensus criteria for grading acute GvHD

Stage	Skin	Liver	Gut
1	Rash <25% body	Bilirubin 35–50micromol/L	Diarrhoea >0.5L/d or persistent nausea
2	Rash 25–50% body	Bilirubin 51–102micromol/L	Diarrhoea 1–1.5L/d
3	Rash >50% body	Bilirubin 103–255micromol/L	Diarrhoea >1.5L/d
4	Generalized erythroderma with bullae and desquamation	Bilirubin >255	Severe abdominal pain ± ileus
Overall clinical grading for the patient			
Grade			
I	Stage 1–2	None	None
II	Stage 3	***or*** Stage 1	***or*** Stage 1
III	–	Stage 2–3	***or*** Stage 2-4
IV	Stage 4	***or*** Stage 4	–

Treatment

General measures

Good nutrition and weight maintenance important. TPN may be necessary. IV antibiotics and antifungals often necessary in the absence of neutropenia and signs of infection may be masked by steroids. Continue ciclosporin during acute GvHD ensuring levels are not toxic.

Specific treatment

Should always be discussed with an experienced transplant haematologist. Now known that mild GvHD confers a GvL effect (📖 see Allogenic SCT, p.398) in the patient and mild forms of skin GvHD may require no treatment.

1st-line treatment

Methylprednisolone 2mg/kg/d IV is added to the ongoing ciclosporin regimen (if there is gut GvHD or diarrhoea administer ciclosporin IV) for 2 weeks then tapered slowly. In more severe cases 250–500mg/m^2 for 3d halving the dose thereafter every 48-–2h. Response to initial therapy has prognostic importance. 50–60% long-term survival in responders.

Side effects of methylprednisolone

- Gastritis/peptic ulceration—use proton pump inhibitors rather than H_2 blockers.
- Hyperglycaemia, particularly when TPN in use. May require insulin infusion.
- Hypertension may be potentiated by ciclosporin and by fluid retention—treat with diuretics and nifedipine.
- Insomnia and psychosis.

Supportive care

- Very important; includes GI rest, parenteral nutrition, replacement of enteral fluid loss, pain control and infection prophylaxis.

Failure of response to high dose methylprednisolone

Defined by:

- Progression after 3d.
- No change after 7d.
- Incomplete response after 14d.

Discuss with senior colleague. Outlook poor. Various empirical possibilities include tacrolimus, infusion of Campath® or ATG.

2nd-line treatment

Response to 2nd-line therapy ranges from 35–70% but 6–12-month survival is poor because of infectious complications or recurrence of GvHD. Long-term survival in not more than 25–35%. No systematic randomized studies. Options include:

- Tacrolimus + MMF.
- High dose methylprednisolone 5–20mg/kg.
- ATG or Campath®-1H.
- Extracorporeal photophoresis.
- TNF-blocking agent (infliximab).

Prognosis

Skin involvement is more likely to respond than liver or gut acute GvHD. Viral, bacterial, and mycotic infections are the most common cause of death in patients with severe acute GvHD. The outcome depends on:

- Overall grade of acute GvHD.
- Time of onset.
- Response to treatment.

Chronic GvHD

The 1° cause of late morbidity and mortality after an allograft. Occurs between 100–300d post-allogeneic transplant. Median incidence 30–45%. The major risk factor is previous acute GvHD. Other risk factors are increasing recipient age (children less frequently affected), ♀ donor to ♂ recipient, inadequate prophylaxis, busulfan conditioning, graft T-cell dose and DLI. There may not have been preceding acute GvHD or acute GvHD may have resolved prior to onset of chronic GvHD.

Diagnosis[1]

Diagnosis of cGvHD requires at least one *diagnostic* manifestation or at least one *distinctive* manifestation confirmed by the pertinent biopsy or test (📖 see Table 9.12).

Table 9.12 Signs & Symptoms of cGvHD

Organ/site	'Diagnostic'	'Distinctive'	Other	Both acute and chronic
Skin	Poikiloderma Lichen planus-like features	Depigmentation		Erythema, Maculopopular rash, prutitis
Nails		Dystrophy		
Scalp		Alopecia		
Mouth	Lichen planus	Xerostomia		Mucositis
Eyes		Kerato-conjunctivitis sicca	Photophobia, blepharitis	
Genitalia	Lichen planus			
GI tract	Strictues of oesophagus		Exocrine pancreatic insufficiency	Anorexia weight loss
Liver				Bilirubin or alk phos >2× ULN
Lung	Bronchiolitis obliterans			
Muscles, fascia, joints	Fasciitis, joint contractures	Myositis	Cramps arthralgias	
Haemopoietic and immune			Thrombocytopenia eosinophilia, Lymphopenia	
Other			Ascites, pericardial or pleural effusion	

From Apperley *et al.* EBMT Handbook Haemopoietic stem cell transplantation, EBMT, Paris, 2008. Reproduced with permission

Conventionally subdivided into limited or extensive chronic GvHD. Major clinical features are debility, weight loss with malabsorption, sclerodermatous reaction due to excessive collagen deposition, severe immunosuppression, and features of autoimmune disease.

Limited chronic GvHD—clinical features

- Localized skin involvement <50% total surface.
- Hepatic dysfunction—portal lesions but lacking necrosis, aggressive hepatitis, or cirrhosis.
- Other localized involvement of eyes, salivary glands, and mouth.

Extensive chronic GvHD—clinical features

- Generalized skin involvement >50% of surface—may include sclerodermatous changes and ulceration.
- Abnormal liver function—histology shows centrilobular changes, chronic aggressive hepatitis, bridging necrosis, or cirrhosis.
- Liver dysfunction ± localized skin GvHD with involvement of eyes, salivary glands, or oral mucosa on labial biopsy.
- Involvement of any other major organ system.
- See Table 9.13 for classification criteria.

Table 9.13 Criteria for classification of chronic GvHD

Classification	Criteria
Subclinical	Histological evidence on screening biopsies without clinical signs or symptoms.
Limited	Localized skin or single organ involvement not requiring systemic therapy.
Extensive low risk	Platelet count $>100 \times 10^9$/L and extensive skin disease or other organ involvement requiring systemic therapy.
Extensive high risk	Platelet count $<100 \times 10^9$/L and extensive skin disease or other organ involvement requiring systemic therapy.

The NIH Working Group[1] has proposed a new global staging which involves both the number of organs or sites involved and the severity of cGvHD within each organ: score 0 = no symptoms; score 1 = mild symptoms; score 2 = moderate symptoms; score 3 = severe symptoms. Mild cGvHD = only 1 or 2 organs (except lung) with a maximum score of 1.

Moderate cGvHD = at least 1 organ with score 2, or ≥ 3 organs with score 1 (or lung score 1)

Severe cGvHD = score 3 in any organ (or score 2 in lung).

Prognostic factors

Thrombocytopenia is an adverse prognostic factor for survival from diagnosis of chronic GvHD. Other factors associated with poor outcome are progressive onset, lichenoid skin rash, elevated bilirubin, poor performance status, alternative donor, and sex mismatched donor. A prognostic model for chronic GvHD survival has been proposed using 3 independent risk factors for shortened survival: thrombocytopenia $< 100 \times 10^9$/l, progressive type onset and extensive skin involvement (>50%)[2].

Treatment

Discuss with a senior member of transplant team. Limited chronic GvHD is much easier to treat than extensive chronic GvHD. Localized mucosal or skin involvement often responds to topical steroids, azathioprine, ciclosporin, and tacrolimus.

General measures

- Adequate nutrition, vitamin/calorie supplements may be required and severe cases may require TPN.
- Pneumococcal prophylaxis must be continued lifelong. (infection with *S. pneumoniae* and *H. influenzae* common)
- Restart conventional prophylactic antifungal (fluconazole or itraconazole), antiviral (aciclovir), and antibacterial agents.
- CMV surveillance is critical (reactivation is more common).
- *P. jirovecii* prophylaxis must be commenced with cotrimoxazole or nebulized pentamidine and continued for 6 months after immunosuppressive therapy.
- Ursodeoxycholic acid may be given for cholestasis in patients with hepatic chronic GvHD.
- Artificial tears for patients with ocular involvement.
- Skin hydration/emollients to lubricate skin; avoid perfume and sun-exposure.
- Regular dental care for patients with oropharyngeal involvement as caries are ↑.
- Bisphosphonates for patients on long-term steroids.
- Psychological support may be required to adjust to chronic disability.

Specific treatment

- Commonest protocol used is the Seattle regimen of prednisolone and ciclosporin A on alternate days; typically: begin daily prednisolone 1mg/kg/d with ciclosporin A 10mg/kg/d divided bd.
- If disease stable or improved after 2 weeks taper prednisolone by 25% per week to target dose of 1mg/kg every other day to minimize side effects.
- After successful completion of steroid taper, reduce ciclosporin A by 25% per week to alternate day dosage of 10mg/kg/d divided bd.
- If resolved completely at 9 months, slowly wean patient from both medications with dose reductions every 2 weeks.
- Incomplete responses should be re-evaluated after 3 months more therapy; if fail to respond or progress then salvage therapy required.
- If no response or progression add in azathioprine 1.5mg/kg/d initially (monitor FBC, renal, and liver function).
- Severe refractory cases may respond to thalidomide, tacrolimus, hydroxychloroquine, or MMF (all of which may at least have a steroid sparing effect) or experimental measures such as extracorporeal PUVA therapy or ATG.

Prognosis

In a retrospective series only 10–30% of patients with extensive chronic GvHD became long-term survivors. Prompt introduction of effective immunosuppressive therapy has improved the outcome for these patients.

1. Filipovich AH et al (2005) National Institute of Health consensus development project on criteria for clinical trials in chronic graft versus host disease: I Diagnosis and staging Working Group report. Biol Blood Marrow Transplant II: 945–56

2. Akpek, G. et al. (2003). Performance of a new clinical grading system for chronic graft-versus-host disease: a multicventre study. *Blood*, **102**, 802–9.

Veno-occlusive disease (*syn.* sinusoidal obstruction syndrome)

Presents clinically early post-transplant (usually within the first 14d). Pathophysiology poorly understood, probably due to damage to hepatic sinusoidal endothelial cells leading to venous occlusion and liver failure. A procoagulant state develops with low antithrombin and protein C levels, consumption of FVII, and ↑ levels of plasminogen activator inhibitor-1 (PAI-1). Multi-organ failure and death may follow.

Risk factors for severe VOD include: intensive conditioning regimens, pre-transplant hepatitis, and second transplants. VOD is characterized by a triad of hepatomegaly, jaundice and ascites. In addition there is fluid retention and weight gain as a result of this. Commoner in allografts than autografts.

Diagnosis is largely clinical but may be supported by typical findings on Doppler ultrasound study of hepatic arterial and venous flows, or by elevated plasminogen activator inhibitor (PAI-1) levels. However, the only definitive diagnostic investigation is trans-jugular liver biopsy, the risks of which must be weighed against the importance of the information obtained.

Differential diagnosis

- Acute GvHD
- Sepsis with renal failure
- Cholestasis due to medication or TPN
- Haemolysis
- CCF

Table 9.14 Criteria for diagnosis of VOD (SOS)

	McDonald (Seattle) *2 out of 3*	**Jones (Baltimore)** *hyperbilirubinaemia plus 2 out of 3*
Hepatomegaly or right upper quadrant pain	+	+
Weight gain (>2% from pre-transplant baseline)	+	+
Hyperbilirubinaemia (>2mg/dL or 34microμmol/L)	+	+
Ascites	-	+

* Adapted from reference 1, with permission of Macmillan Publishers Ltd., copyright 2003

Risk assessment

Table 9.15 Scoring system for VOD**

Clinical feature	Score
Progressive and persisting ↑ in bilirubin • Serum bilirubin ≥34 but <75micromol/L ***or*** • Serum bilirubin ≥75micromol/L	 1 2
Persisting hepatomegaly (>2cm from baseline)	1
Ascites	1
Persisting weight gain (from baseline) • ≥5% but <15% ***or*** • ≥15%	 1 2
Raised PT or need to transfuse platelets regularly	1
Risk factors (1 or more present) • Age <6 months or • Raised ALT pre-SCT	1
Associated organ system failure * (excluding liver failure) • Each system failure • Maximum	 1 2
Maximum total score	10
Calculate total score on daily basis: • Score of 4 suggests early or impending VOD • Score of 5–7 suggests moderate VOD and specific treatment is recommended • Score of 8–10 indicates severe VOD and a poor prognosis	

*Respiratory failure needing ventilation, circulatory failure needing inotropes, renal failure needing dialysis or need for abdominal paracentesis.

*Adapted from reference 2, with permission of Macmillan Publishers Ltd., copyright 2003

Treatment

- Supportive treatment: careful fluid and electrolyte balance; diuretics, analgesics, platelet transfusion and correction of deranged coagulation.
- Defibrotide: 5–60mg/kg/d × 2–3 weeks achieved complete resolution of severe VOD in 10–40% with 30–50% survival at d100; binds to vascular endothelium and stimulates fibrinolysis by increasing endogenous tPA function and decreasing PAI-1 activity; no significant toxicity.
- Antithrombotic and thrombolytic agents: recombinant tissue plasminogen activator (r-tPA) ± heparin was treatment of choice until recently; risk of fatal haemorrhage.
- Antithrombin concentrate: aim to maintain levels >120%.

Prognosis

Patients with mild VOD have no apparent adverse effects and generally respond to treatment with analgesics and diuretics and have a good prognosis. Patients with moderate VOD require specific treatment for symptomatic hepatic failure. Severe VOD is associated with severe effects from hepatocellular failure and patients require specific treatment but may fail to respond, progress to multi-organ failure, require ITU support and have a mortality >90%.

Prophylaxis

Ursodeoxycholic acid and/or heparin are widely used but a trial of defibrotide plus continuous low-dose heparin for 3 weeks from the day before SCT suggests this is an effective prophylactic regimen.

1. Abinun, M. and Cavet, J. (2007). Gastrointestinal, respiratory and renal/urogenital complications of HSCT. In *Practical Haemopoietic Stem Cell Transplantation.* (Cant AJ, *et al.* (eds.) Blackwell Publishing, Oxford, pp.126–32.

2. Bajwa, R.P.S. *et al.* (2003). Recombinant tissue plasminogen activator for treatment of hepatic veno-occlusive disease following bone marrow transplantation in children: effectiveness of a scoring system for initiating treatment. *Bone Marrow Transplant,* **31**, 591–7.

Invasive fungal infections and antifungal therapy

Invasive fungal infections are an important cause of morbidity and mortality after allogeneic SCT with a frequency of 10–25% and mortality of >70%.

Pathogenesis

- Majority of infections are due to *Candida* species and *Aspergillus* species though infections due to other opportunistic fungi increasing (*Trichosporon* spp., *Fusarium* spp., *Bipolaris* spp., and *Zygomycetes* amongst others).
- Invasive *Candida* infections classified as candidaemia or acute disseminated candidiasis, and arise from invasion of bloodstream from infected mucosal surfaces or via central venous catheters; decreasing incidence due to introduction of fluconazole prophylaxis though increased *non-albicans* spp. (esp. *glabrata* and *krusei*).
- Invasive *Aspergillus* infections affect paranasal sinuses and lungs and arise from airborne exposure; increasing incidence, particularly late after transplantation.
- Risk factors: prolonged and profound neutropenia; use of corticosteroids.

Prophylaxis

- Prophylaxis: high efficiency (>90%) particulate air (HEPA) filtration or positive pressure ventilation; prophylaxis with fluconazole (400mg/day does not cover *Aspergillus* spp., *C glabrata,* or *C krusei*) or itraconazole (200–400mg/d; poor absorption from capsules; extremely unpalatable liquid preparation).

Management

- If a febrile neutropenic transplant patient is unresponsive to 2nd-line antibiotics after 48–96h and/or there is a suspicion of possible fungal infection (unwell; chest symptoms; peripheral nodules, halo sign or cavitation on CT chest, evidence of candidaemia), then antifungal therapy should be started.
- Empirical therapy should be initiated with an agent active against *Aspergillus* spp as this is the major risk in adult patients with neutropenic sepsis; although standard amphotericin B deoxycholate has been widely used for several decades, it demonstrates efficacy in only ~33% of patients and has a high incidence of side effects and renal toxicity.

Treatment of invasive aspergillosis

Liposomal amphotericin

- AmBisome® achieves responses in ~50% of patients with proven/probable invasive aspergillosis at a dose of 3mg/kg/day with 12-week survival of 72% in a large randomized trial. It is better tolerated than amphotericin B lipid complex (Abelcet®) and more effective and better tolerated than amphotericin B colloidal dispersion though no trials have undertaken direct comparisons.
- Commence either liposomal amphotericin (AmBisome®) at 3mg/kg/d or amphotericin B lipid complex (Abelcet®) at 2.5mg/kg (in practice round up or down to standard vial size to avoid wastage and minimize cost). Follow data sheet instructions carefully, observing for anaphylaxis.

The dosage should be increased to a maximum of 5mg/kg Abelcet® or 3–5mg/kg AmBisome® in patients who have either a confirmed mycological diagnosis or a fever that does not respond within 72h on the lower dose.

- Paracetamol 1g PO 30min prior to infusion plus chlorphenamine 10mg IV pre-medication is advised for Abelcet® (may also be required for AmBisome®). Pethidine 25–30mg IV stat may be given if a troublesome reaction occurs.
- 0.9% saline preload used with standard amphotericin B is not normally required unless renal or liver function deteriorate during treatment. Renal function should be checked on alternate days for the duration of the treatment. Serum Mg^{2+} and LFTs should be checked weekly.

Voriconazole

- A 2nd-generation triazole. 48% response rate. Shown to be superior to standard amphotericin B in antifungal efficacy, safety, and survival in a randomized trial and widespread treatment of choice for invasive aspergillosis due to more favourable toxicity profile.
- Dose 6mg/kg IV bd d1 then 4mg/kg IV bd maintenance converting to oral 200mg bd (may commence orally with 400mg bd loading dose on d1).
- IV voriconazole is contra-indicated in renal insufficiency. Side effects: visual disturbances, rash, elevated LFTs and with IV administration, flushing, fever, tachycardia, and dyspnoea.

Caspofungin

- An echinocandin which targets the fungal cell wall and is active against *Candida* and *Aspergillus* spp. Higher response rate demonstrated in comparison to amphotericin in treatment of invasive candidiasis.
- Loading dose of slow IV infusion of 70mg on d1 followed by maintenance dose of 50mg/d (lower maintenance in moderate liver insufficiency).
- It may also be used for treatment of invasive aspergillosis refractory to amphotericin preparations. Caution with concomitant ciclosporin: monitor LFTs; adjust tacrolimus dose. Side effects: phlebitis, fever, headache, rash, abdominal pain, nausea, diarrhoea.

Combination therapy

- A combination of voriconazole and caspofungin as salvage therapy after failure of amphotericin B provided a substantially improved 3-month survival in allogeneic SCT recipients compared with a historical control group receiving voriconazole monotherapy.

Total duration of treatment is difficult to determine. General principles are that therapy should continue for at least 2 weeks, until neutrophil recovery and until there are no signs of progression radiologically.

Recommendations of ECIL Working Group[1]

Treatment of Invasive Aspergillosis

1° therapy

Voriconazole was strongly recommended as 1st-line therapy for pulmonary aspergillosis in patients with acute leukaemia or after SCT by a Working Group at the European Conference on Infections in Leukaemia (ECIL). Liposomal amphotericin and amphotericin lipid complex were graded as alternatives when voriconazole is contra-indicated or unavailable.

Amphotericin colloidal dispersion and standard amphotericin B deoxycholate were not recommended. There were insufficient data in this setting to grade caspofungin, itraconazole and posaconazole.

Salvage therapy

No data are available for any agent in the context of voriconazole failure. Caspofungin and posaconazole were similarly graded. Liposomal amphotericin, amphotericin lipid complex, and itraconazole were graded on the basis of expert opinions. Voriconazole is an option for patients who did not receive it as 1st-line therapy. Combinations of caspofungin and voriconazole or caspofungin and liposomal amphotericin were scored as options.

Optimal duration of therapy

Therapy must be long enough to achieve complete response and to allow recovery from immunosuppression. No fixed duration can be proposed.

Note

As with all protocols check local policies since these may differ from those outlined in this handbook.

Treatment of invasive candidiasis

- Treatment is initiated on detection of *Candida* spp. on blood culture before species and susceptibility are identified.
- Liposomal amphotericin, caspofungin, or voriconazole generally used as the patient has generally been on fluconazole prophylaxis.
- Caspofungin is the drug of choice for the treatment of confirmed *C. glabrata* or *C. krusei* infections. Voriconazole is an alternative and a switch to oral voriconazole can be considered when a patient is stable and able to take oral medication.
- Removal of indwelling IV catheters is recommended in patients with candidaemia.
- Neutropenic patients should receive antifungal therapy for 14d after the last +ve blood culture and resolution of signs and symptoms.

Recommendations of BCSH Guidelines for invasive fungal infection[2]

- Empirical therapy for antibiotic resistant febrile neutropenia discouraged
- Antifungal therapy for possible invasive fungal infection should be justified through CT scans and mycological tests.
- Choice of emperical therapy should be between liposomal amphotericin (not in escalated doses and caspofungin to minimise toxicity
- Proven intestine fungal infection may be treated with liposomal amphotericium, invasive or voriconazole; voriconazole is recommended in intracerebral aspergillosis.

1. Herbrecht, R. *et al.* (2007). Treatment of invasive candida and invasive aspergillus infections in adult haematological patients. *European J Cancer*, **5**(Suppl), 49–59.

2. Prentice, AG. *et al.* (2008). BCSH Guidelines on the management of invasive fungal infections during therapy for haematological malignancy 🖫 http://www.bcshguidelines.com/pdf/IFI_therapy.pdf

CMV prophylaxis and treatment

All transplant recipients who are CMV seronegative should receive CMV –ve blood products. If supplies are available, this is recommended also for CMV seropositive recipients. Limits risk of CMV blood product transmission regardless of donor/recipient serological status. Reactivation of the patient's own latent virus is the main source of CMV disease in recipients of allogeneic SCT (80% of previously seropositive patients reactivate). CMV status in the donor is an important consideration in donor selection. CMV disease has been a major cause of death in allogeneic SCT recipients except where both donor and recipient are seronegative.

CMV surveillance

- All allograft patients and CMV sero-positive autograft recipients should receive CMV surveillance as active CMV infection may remain asymptomatic and does not always progress to disease.
- Progression to CMV disease is predicted by detection of CMV viraemia with high viral loads by quantitative PCR in buffy coat of EDTA peripheral blood.
- 5mL EDTA blood should be sent weekly on the above cohort of transplant patients from admission until d100. Screening of allograft recipients should continue until 1 year post-transplant although the frequency of testing may be reduced in the absence of appropriate symptoms. Urine and throat washings are not sent routinely for CMV detection.

CMV prophylaxis

Indicated in allograft patients when either donor or recipient are CMV seropositive. Not recommended when both donor and recipient are seronegative, nor for autograft recipients, even if seropositive.

Suggested protocol

- Aciclovir 800mg tds IV from day –5 to discharge, then 800mg tds PO for 3 months ***plus***
- IVIg 200mg/kg IV day –1, day +1,3 and then every 3 weeks until day +100.
- *Note*: The graft suppression of this dose of aciclovir may sometimes be dose limiting.

Treatment of CMV infection

A +ve CMV identification in buffy coat by surveillance should be treated even if the patient is asymptomatic:

- Ganciclovir: 5 mg/kg IV bd for 14d minimum then continue maintenance dose 5mg/kg/day IV daily (6mg/kg/day 5d weekly as outpatient).
- Stop aciclovir when ganciclovir commenced.
- Side effects: myelosuppressive, may be abrogated by G-CSF, nephrotoxic
- Renal function must be monitored and dose reductions implemented according to the BNF.
- Abnormal LFTs may occur.
- Fever, rashes, and headaches.
- Alternative—foscarnet 90 mg/kg IV bd for 14d minimum.
- Administer through a central line as IVI over 2h (may be given as a peripheral IVI but should be given concurrently with a fast running litre

of 0.9% saline). Side effects: nephrotoxic and hepatotoxic (follow *BNF* dosage adjustments).

Treatment plan

On a 1st episode of CMV antigenaemia, start with ganciclovir. Failure to become CMV antigen –ve by the end of the 2-week course would lead to immediate progression to foscarnet. Valganciclovir, the oral pro-drug of ganciclovir is an alternative which is useful for patients who have been discharged.

CMV-related disease

May cause PUO, pneumonitis, oesophagitis, gastritis, hepatitis, retinitis, delayed engraftment, and myelosuppression. Where CMV antigenaemia accompanied by symptoms or signs of CMV disease high titre anti-CMV Ig 200mg/kg/d IV should be administered on d1, 3, 5, and 7 of antiviral therapy with ganciclovir or foscarnet. Broncho-alveolar lavage (BAL) should be performed to establish the presence of CMV locally in the lung.

Post-transplant vaccination programme

General

The subject of revaccination post-transplant remains a contentious topic. The general principles are that live vaccination is forbidden, probably for the lifetime of the patient. Secondly, antibody and T-cell responses to vaccination in the 1st year following transplantation are suboptimal. In allogeneic SCT recipients, immune reconstitution continues beyond 1 and up to 2 years post-transplant. These general considerations have been used to suggest the following policy.

Allogeneic transplants

No immunizations should be given in the presence of acute or chronic GvHD. In the absence of these conditions, proceed as follows:

At 12 months post-matched sibling donor SCT (18 months after others)

- Diphtheria tetanus toxoid and acellular pertussis 1° course (3 doses at monthly intervals).
- 1° course of inactivated polio vaccine (3 doses at monthly intervals).
- Conjugated 7-valent pneumococcal vaccine (2 doses at 8-week interval).
- Conjugated *Haemophilus influenzae* B (3 doses at monthly intervals).
- Conjugated meningococcal C (2 doses at monthly intervals).
- Influenza vaccine (and annually thereafter).

The vaccinations should be staggered with only diphtheria and tetanus being administered concurrently. It would be reasonable to leave a gap of several days between each vaccination. Not only may this enhance antibody responses but it will easily identify the cause if there are any reactions.

At 18 months post-matched sibling donor SCT (24 months after others)

- MMR.

At 2 years post-matched sibling donor SCT (30 months after others)

- HiB and conjugated meningococcal C vaccine.

At 25 months post-matched sibling donor SCT (31 months after others)

- MMR and conjugated 7-valent pneumococcal vaccine.

At 30 months post-matched sibling donor SCT (3 years after others)

- Polysaccharide pneumococcal vaccine.

Autologous SCT for lymphoma or myeloma—1 year post-transplant

- Tetanus booster.
- Inactivated polio vaccine booster.
- Pneumovax II (repeated every 6 years).
- *Haemophilus influenzae* B.
- Meningococcal C.
- Influenza vaccine (repeated annually).

Foreign travel

All transplant recipients should take medical advice from their transplant team before travelling abroad.

- Typhoid, cholera, hepatitis A/B, and meningococcal vaccines are safe.
- Yellow fever and Japanese B encephalitis are not safe.
- Remember malaria prophylaxis.

Avoid live vaccines. e.g.:

- Yellow fever
- BCG.
- Oral polio.
- Oral typhoid.

Post-transplant complications

- Bacterial and fungal infections.
- Pneumonitis.
- CMV reactivation.
- VOD—📖 see Veno-occlusive disease, p.432.

Allografts only

- Acute GvHD (📖 see Acute GvHD, p.424).
- Chronic GvHD (📖 see Chronic GvHD, p.428).

Longer term effects:

- Endocrine: hypothyroidism may occur post-transplant. Check TFTs at 3-monthly intervals → 1 year.
- Respiratory: check lung function tests at 6 months and 1 year if TBI has been given.
- Skin: advise about sun protection (following TBI avoid the sun). If exposure is unavoidable, total sun block factor 15 or higher is essential for at least 1 year.
- Fertility: most patients will be infertile after transplant (almost invariably if TBI given). Since this cannot be absolutely guaranteed, contraceptive precautions should be taken until the confirmatory tests have been performed.
  - ♂: check sperm counts at 3 and 6 months post-transplant. Zero motile sperm on both samples confirms infertility.
  - ♀: check FSH, LH, and oestradiol at 3 months. FSH and LH levels should be high and oestradiol levels low if no ovulation is occurring.
- Menopause: women may have an early menopause due to the treatment and may experience symptoms such as hot flushes, dry skin, dryness of the vagina, and loss of libido. Most women should have hormone replacement therapy (Prempak C 1.25 initially starting as soon as early menopause is confirmed) and counselled about HRT problems.
- Cataracts: patients who have had TBI are at risk of developing cataracts. Refer for ophthalmological assessment at 1 year post BMT.
- Immunizations at 12–30 months post-transplant (📖 see Post-transplant vaccination programme, p.442).

Treatment of relapse post-allogeneic SCT

Recurrence of leukaemia, myeloma, or lymphoma after an allogeneic SCT may be treated by DLI, a 2nd transplant (in those patients with a durable 1st response who are fit enough to withstand the rigours of a 2nd allograft) or conventional dose or palliative treatment.

DLI

- May be used in CML, AML, ALL, NHL, HL, and myeloma.
- DLI can promote full donor chimerism in patients with mixed chimerism or residual tumour after reduced intensity non-myeloablative conditioning.
- Patient should discontinue ciclosporin and steroid therapy at least 2 weeks before DLI and chemotherapy at least 24h before DLI.
- Donor lymphocytes are collected by leucapheresis; a typical collection of 150mL contains ~50×10^8 T lymphocytes.
- Escalating doses are generally used to limit GvHD e.g. 1st dose 10^7 donor lymphocytes followed 12 weeks later if no response by 5×10^7 cells, then if no response 12 weeks later 10^8 cells then $>10^8$ cells 12 weeks later if no response; lower initial doses and increments are utilized in UD SCT.
- Where possible e.g. CML, AML molecular monitoring may be under-taken and DLI may be utilized for molecular relapse with molecular monitoring of response.
- The main adverse effect of DLI is acute or chronic GvHD especially if administered early after SCT. The incidence of these complications has been reduced by the adoption of an escalating dose regimen but increased with UD SCT.

Discharge and follow-up

Criteria for discharge

Blood counts should ideally be: Hb >10.0g/dL (but may require transfusion), neutrophils >1.0 × 10^9/L, platelets >25 × 10^9/L, and patients should be able to maintain a fluid intake of 2–3L/d, tolerating diet and oral medications particularly in allografts on ciclosporin. Should be apyrexial and no longer losing weight.

Counsel patients

- Possible need for blood/platelets.
- Adherence to neutropenic diet.
- Check temperature bd and report immediately if febrile.
- Fatigue post-transplant in irradiated patients due to the late TBI effect usually 6–10 weeks post transplant.
- Risk of HZV (explain the early symptoms).
- To continue with mouth care.
- To report any new symptoms.

Blood tests—initially twice weekly

- FBC, reticulocytes, and blood film.
- Biochemistry including LFTs.
- Ciclosporin A levels pre-dose (EDTA sample)—allografts only.

Initially once a week

- Magnesium.
- CRP.
- Coagulation screen.
- CMV screening: allografts and seropositive autograft recipients only.
- Stool culture: allografts only unless relevant symptoms.

Drugs

- Ciclosporin capsules—allografts only.
- Aciclovir prophylaxis against HZV 400mg qds PO for minimum of 3 months in non-TBI patients and 6 months in TBI autografts and all allografts. Allografts may be on 800mg tds if aciclovir chosen for CMV prophylaxis. Consider low dose 200mg bd maintenance until 1–2 years post-transplant.
- Penicillin V 250mg bd PO should be given to all patients. Erythromycin 250mg od PO if penicillin allergic.
- Ciprofloxacin 250mg bd PO if neutrophils <1.0 × 10^9/L.
- Co-trimoxazole 480mg bd PO Monday, Wednesday, Friday for 1 year minimum and until CD4 count >500. Co-trimoxazole should be started when neutrophils >1.5 × 10^9/L and platelets >60 × 10^9/L. Until then, use nebulized pentamidine 300mg every 3 weeks.
- Itraconazole—allografts only.
- Nystatin mouth care.
- Folic acid 5mg bd until full engraftment.
- Multivitamins 1 daily may be advisable while gaining weight.
- Antiemetics PRN.

Follow-up

- Monitor closely for first 100 days (twice weekly for CMV monitoring in first 2 months) for engraftment, transfusion requirements, GvHD, CMV, opportunistic infection, side effects of therapy, chimerism, psychosocial needs and relapse.
- Review 4–8 weekly for first year after 100 days if uncomplicated.
- Review intervals may be extended after first year if uncomplicated.

Chapter 10

Haemostasis and thrombosis

Assessing haemostasis

Haemostatic capacity is assessed by:

- History.
- Examination.
- Laboratory investigations.

Haemophilia

Describes a tendency to bleeding and may be heritable (often congenital) or acquired. Acquired haemophilia due to anticoagulant drugs is very common in the UK as 1 in 100 of the population is receiving oral anticoagulant therapy with warfarin.

Thrombophilia

Describes a tendency to thrombosis and may be heritable (but usually late onset in adult) or acquired. Acquired thrombophilia is common in hospitalized patients by virtue of immobility, surgery, and multiple medical illness (VTE including DVT and PE,).

The haemostatic system maintains the integrity of the vascular tree through a complex network of cellular, ligand-receptor, and enzymatic interactions. It is essential that blood remains fluid within the circulation but clots at sites of vascular injury. This is achieved by the equilibrium between:

- Procoagulant and anticoagulant systems.
- Fibrinolytic and antifibrinolytic systems.

In response to endothelial damage there is rapid thrombin generation and antifibrinolysis at the site of injury. At adjacent areas of healthy intact endothelium there is enhanced natural anticoagulant activity and fibrinolytic activity to limit the clot to the site of injury and thus prevent thrombosis (a blood clot within the lumen of a blood vessel). Regulation of the haemostatic network in such a way results in localized clot formation with minimal loss of vascular patency. Pathological disruption of the network results in thrombosis or bleeding, or both; the most extreme example of haemostatic pathology is a complete breakdown as occurs in disseminated intravascular coagulation (DIC).

The coagulation system

The initiation of coagulation is triggered by tissue factor, a cell membrane protein which binds activated factor VII (factor VIIa). Although there is a small fraction of circulating factor VII in the activated state it has little or no enzymatic activity until it is bound to tissue factor.

Once bound to tissue factor, factor VIIa activates factor IX and factor X (to IXa and Xa respectively) leading to thrombin generation and clot formation (📖 Fig. 10.1).

Thrombin converts soluble fibrinogen into insoluble fibrin monomers which spontaneously polymerize to form the fibrin mesh that is then stabilized and crosslinked by activated factor XIII (factor XIIIa).

1. Baglin, T. (2005). The measurement and application of thrombin generation. *Brit J Haem*, **130**, 653–61.

2. Hoffman, M. and Monroe, D.M. (2001). A cell-based model of hemostasis. *Thromb Haemostasis*, **85**, 958–65.

3. Monroe, D. M. and M. Hoffman (2006). What does it take to make the perfect clot? *Arteriosclerosis Thrombosis and Vascular Biology*, **26**, 41–8.

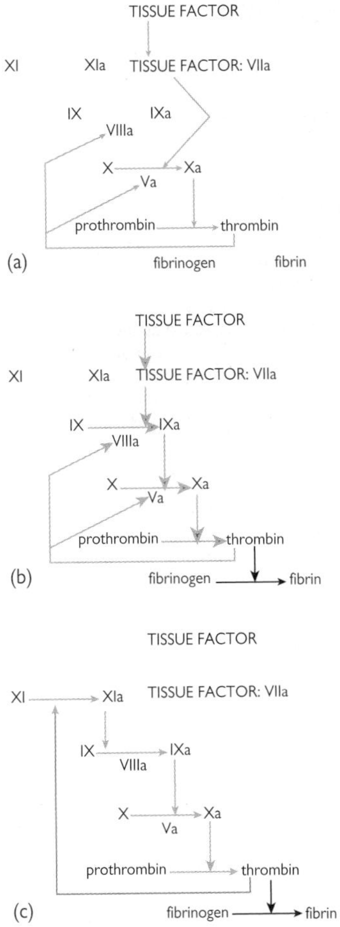

Fig. 10.1 Thrombin generating mechanism.
The thrombin explosion occurs in 3 phases, the first (Fig.10.1a: initiation) in which TF:VIIa generates small amounts of thrombin which enhances platelet activation (in conjunction with exposed subendothelial collagen at the site of vascular injury) and V and VIII to their active forms. The activation of Va and VIIIa opens the factor IX-dependent pathway to thrombin generation (Fig. 10.1b: amplification) and increasing concentrations of thrombin then lead to back activation of factor XI (Fig. 10.1c: propagation). The activated forms of factors V and VIII are non-enzymatic cofactors which assemble and orientate the enzymes (IXa and Xa) on the negatively charged surface of activated platelets.

Laboratory tests

- Prothrombin time (PT).
- Activated partial thromboplastin time (APTT).
- Fibrinogen (Fgn) level.
- Thrombin time (TT).
- Reptilase time (RT).
- Factor assays.
- Mixing studies.
- Thromboelastography (TEG).
- Tests of fibrinolysis.

Coagulation tests are typically performed on plasma that has been separated from a blood sample by centrifugation. Thrombin generation takes place on phospholipid surfaces (provided by platelets normally) and so an artificial lipid preparation is added as the platelets are removed by the centrifugation. Most routine clotting tests use the time taken for a clot to appear as the endpoint of the assay. Blood is usually taken into tubes containing citrate, which chelates Ca^{2+} and thereby prevents clotting. Blood is centrifuged and the plasma is removed and recalcified during the clotting assay.

PT

The PT is the time in seconds for a blood sample to clot after recalcification and addition of thromboplastin (a preparation of tissue factor which is the protein that activates factor VII). The normal PT is about 11–14sec, depending on the type of thromboplastin used.

The PT is prolonged by:

- Oral anticoagulant therapy (typically warfarin).
- Vitamin K deficiency.
- Liver disease.
- DIC.
- Factor VII deficiency.

APTT

The APTT is the time taken in seconds for a citrated blood sample to clot after recalcification and addition of a contact factor activator, such as kaolin.

The normal APTT is about 32–38sec, depending on the type of contact factor activator used.

The APTT is prolonged by:

- Unfractionated heparin (LMWH has minimal effect at therapeutic levels).
- Oral anticoagulant therapy (mildly, the PT is much more sensitive).
- Vitamin K deficiency (mildly, the PT is much more sensitive).
- Liver disease (mildly, the PT is much more sensitive).
- DIC.
- Dilutional coagulopathy (massive blood transfusion).
- Severe and moderate deficiencies of factors VIII, IX, or XI.
- Antiphospholipid antibodies (known as lupus anticoagulant activity).
- Contact factor deficiency (including factor XII and prekallikrein).

Fgn level

Fgn levels are low in:

- DIC.
- Dilutional coagulopathy (massive blood transfusion).
- Advanced liver disease.
- Following thrombolytic therapy.
- Congenital hypofibrinogenaemia (very rare).
- Acquired dysfibrinogenaemias.

TT

The TT (thrombin time) is the time in seconds for a citrated blood sample to clot after addition of thrombin.

The TT is prolonged by:

- Unfractionated heparin.
- Hypofibrinogenaemia (📖 see p.476 for low Fgn levels)
- Fibrin degradation products (high levels may occur in DIC and after thrombolysis).

RT

The RT(reptilase time) is a snake venom-based test. It is prolonged by low Fgn levels but not by heparin and so comparison of the TT and RT is useful for determining if a prolonged APTT is due to heparin; (long TT with ↔ RT = heparin)

Factor assays

Individual factor assays are useful in patients with a bleeding history and are guided by PT and APTT results. The cascade model of coagulation (Fig. 10.2) is no longer considered to represent the physiological process involved in coagulation. The cascade model was derived from observation of results using the PT and APTT assays which are not 'physiological' tests. Therefore, whilst the cascade model may not be 'physiologically true' it is still a useful framework for interpreting PT and APTT results. For example, in a patient with a bleeding history with a ↔ PT and a long APTT (not due to heparin or a lupus anticoagulant) there may be deficiency of factor VIII, IX, or XI.

Mixing studies

If the PT or APTT are prolonged then mixing with ↔ plasma and repeating the test will indicate if the prolongation is likely due to a factor deficiency (the mix corrects the abnormality) or an inhibitor such as heparin or a specific factor inhibitor (the mix does not correct the abnormality).

Thromboelastography

This test measures the physical strength of a clot as it forms. Its role in clinical practice is limited. It is often used as a near-patient testing device during surgical procedures with potentially massive blood loss (such as liver transplantation) when it is used to guide transfusion therapy. It is useful for identifying severe hyperfibrinolysis, as occurs during liver transplantation—an indication for using the antiplasmin drug aprotonin (unlicensed so its use is currently restricted).

Tests of fibrinolysis

These tests are not performed routinely. Defects of fibrinolysis have not been linked with a predisposition to thrombosis and bleeding disorders due to defective regulation of fibrinolysis being exceptionally rare. The fibrinolytic system may have a 1° role in clearing clot as part of wound healing rather than in the immediate haemostatic response to injury. Nevertheless pharmacological doses of fibrinolytic activators (e.g. recombinant tissue factor activator) have a very useful clinical role in rapidly lysing newly formed clot—'clot-busting drugs'.

Practical application of coagulation tests

Clotting tests are indicated in patients with a personal or family history of bleeding. They are not generally indicated as routine pre-operative screening tests as they have very low sensitivity and specificity for surgical bleeding in unselected patients. Preoperative assessment of bleeding risk is better determined by identification of a personal or family bleeding history, which should then be investigated accordingly.

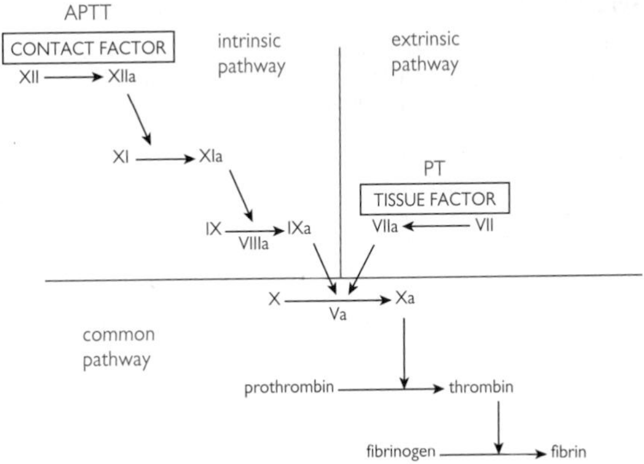

Fig. 10.2 Cascade model of coagulation.
The concept of the cascade model involves an extrinsic pathway (triggered by tissue factor and measured by the PT) and an intrinsic pathway (triggered by contact factor activation and measured by the APTT) joining in a common pathway (measured by both PT and APTT). The utility of this concept involves comparing the results of the PT and APTT to determine where there is a deficiency in the cascade, e.g. a ↔ PT with a prolonged APTT indicates a defect in the intrinsic pathway before it joins the common pathway, e.g. a deficiency of factor VIII.

Platelets

↔ platelet survival 7–10d. Platelets are activated by multiple agonists through numerous intracellular second-messenger pathways. The activation pathways converge on activation of the fibrinogen receptor, glycoprotein IIb-IIIa (integrin $\alpha_{IIb}\beta_3$), such that an induced conformational change results in fibrinogen/fibrin binding (📖 see Fig. 10.3).

As a result of occupation of the Fgn receptor (GPIIb-IIIa) 'outside-in signalling' consolidates the platelet activation process by upregulating second-messenger pathways and hence providing a +ve feedback loop. In addition to adhesion and aggregation at sites of vascular injury a major role of platelets in coagulation is the provision of an anionic phospholipid surface required for assembly of the coagulation factor enzymes and cofactors required for thrombin generation.

Following vascular injury platelets adhere to subendothelial collagen via the von Willebrand factor (vWF) ligand. Platelets then aggregate to form a platelet mass at the site of injury.

Laboratory tests

Blood collection needs to be with a non-traumatic venepuncture, rapid transport to the lab with storage at room temperature, and testing within a limited time.

- Platelet count and platelet size
- Blood film for platelet morphology
- Platelet function at high shear rate (PFA-100)
- Platelet function at low shear rate (platelet aggregation)
- Platelet granules and nucleotide quantification
- Bleeding time is no longer recommended as a routine test.[1]

Platelet count

- Normal range 150–450 × 10^9/L.
- Beware pseudothrombocytopenia—due to platelet clumping typically in EDTA (1% of blood counts)—check film for clumps and if suspicious repeat count on citrated or heparinized sample.
- Adequate function is maintained until platelet count <80 × 10^9/L.
- With platelet count <20 × 10^9/L there is often easy bruising and petechial haemorrhages and more serious bleeding can occur.
- The degree of bleeding is influenced by the cause of the thrombocytopenia—more bleeding with marrow failure syndromes (aplastic anaemia and post-chemotherapy)—less bleeding with peripheral platelet destruction, as in immune thrombocytopenic purpura (ITP).

1. Harrison, P. (2005). Platelet function analysis. *Blood Rev*, **19**, 111–23.

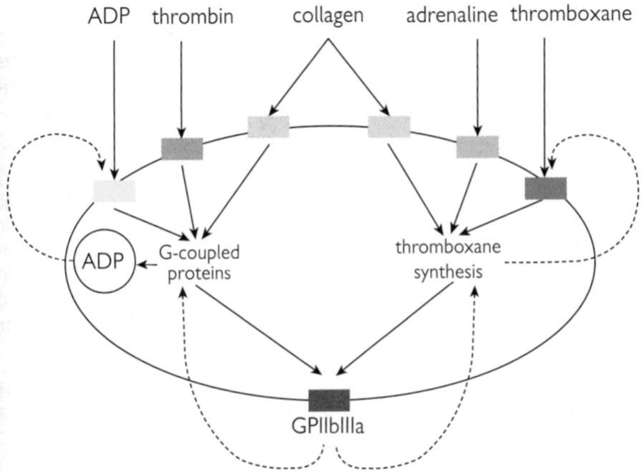

Fig. 10.3 Mechanisms of platelet activation.
Platelets are activated by multiple agonists through numerous intracellular second-messenger pathways. The activation pathways converge on activation of the fibrinogen receptor, glycoprotein IIb-IIIa, such that an induced conformational change results in fibrinogen/fibrin binding. Platelet activation is completed by occupation of the fibrinogen receptor resulting in 'outside-in signalling' and upregulation of second-messenger pathways.

Platelet size

Large platelets are often biochemically more active; high mean platelet volume (MPV >10fL) is associated with less bleeding in patients with severe thrombocytopenia, acquired BM disorders are a less likely cause of thrombocytopenia the higher the MPV (especially MPV >10fL).

Reticulated platelets can be counted by some new blood count analysers and may prove to be useful in assessing thrombocytopenia (often reported as 'immature platelet fraction' (IPF).

Altered platelet size is seen in inherited platelet disorders

- High MPV (>10fL) in May–Hegglin anomaly, gray platelet syndrome.
- Low MPV (<7fL) in Wiskott–Aldrich syndrome (WAS), X-linked thrombocytopenia.

Morphology

Pseudothrombocytopenia may be due to *in vitro* platelet clumping and clumps may be visible in blood film. Platelet morphology may be abnormal and white cells may contain inclusions in some inherited thrombocytopenias, e.g. May–Hegglin anomaly.

Platelet function at high shear rate (PFA-100)

Automated technique that measures the ability of platelets to occlude an aperture at high shear rate. Minimal sample manipulation. Test performed on citrated blood sample within 4h of sample collection. Abnormal in vWD and platelet function defects.

Platelet function at low shear rate (platelet aggregation)

Performed on platelet-rich plasma prepared by slow centrifugation of citrated blood sample. Performed within 4h of sample collection. Poor correlation with bleeding tendency except in specific congenital disorders with severe platelet function abnormality, e.g. Glanzmann's thrombasthenia (GT), Bernard–Soulier syndrome (BSS).

- Agonists used for aggregation studies include ADP, collagen, arachidonic acid, adrenaline (epinephrine).
- Response to ristocetin is an agglutination response dependent on induced conformational change of platelet membrane proteins e.g. glycoprotein Ib-IX-V, promoting interaction with vWF.
- Ristocetin-induced platelet agglutination (RIPA) is carried out at high (1.2mg/mL) and low ristocetin concentrations (0.5mg/dL). +ve RIPA at 0.5mg/dl is an abnormal result and is observed in type 2B vWD and with very high vWF levels, e.g. pregnancy.

Platelet granules and nucleotides

Platelet storage pool disorders (SPD) are characterized by absent platelet α or δ granules. α granule proteins include β-thromboglobulin (β-TG) and platelet factor 4 (PF4) which can be measured by ELISA—deficient in α-granule storage pool defects. Nucleotides (ADP/ATP) can be measured by a variety of techniques including HPLC and are deficient in dense granule δ-storage pool disorders. These are beyond the scope of the routine laboratory.

Clinical utility of platelet function tests

Main role is in diagnosis of inherited platelet functional defects. In acquired platelet dysfunction 2° to drugs (aspirin, clopidogrel), and disorders such as renal and hepatic disease, DIC, platelet function is rarely tested as the clinical utility is not established in this setting, i.e. no established correlation between test results and bleeding tendency. Therefore, platelet function testing is generally restricted for the investigation of possible congenital bleeding disorders.

Drugs impair platelet function

Many drugs impair platelet function e.g. aspirin, clopidogrel, dipyridamole, glycoprotein IIb/IIIa inhibitors such as abciximab, NSAIDs, alcohol. Many other drugs have subtle effects on platelet function that are rarely of clinical importance. Drug-induced thrombocytopenia is a more common and clinically important drug effect.

Bleeding

Major issues to be determined

- Is haemostatic capacity reduced or is there a non-haematological cause for bleeding?
- If haemostatic capacity is reduced is it due to a heritable defect with late clinical onset or is it the result of a newly acquired defect?
- If newly acquired is it due to an anticoagulant drug?
- If not due to reduced haemostatic capacity then what are the likely circumstances that resulted in abnormal bleeding?

Causes of bleeding

Surgery, trauma, non-accidental injury, coagulation disorders (including anticoagulant drugs), platelet dysfunction (including drug induced, e.g. aspirin), vascular disorders.

Clinical features

Is there a lifelong bleeding history, has the patient been previously challenged by surgery or dental extraction, is this an isolated symptom. Type of bleeding problem that led to presentation e.g. mucocutaneous, easy bruising, spontaneous, post-traumatic. Duration and time of onset. Menstrual history is important—menorrhagia has a low +ve predictive value for a bleeding disorder but absence of menorrhagia has a high –ve predictive value. Absence of obstetric bleeding does not exclude a bleeding disorder as haemostatic capacity increases significantly in pregnancy.

- ***Systemic enquiry:*** do symptoms suggest a systemic disorder, BM failure, infection, liver disease, renal disease?
- ***Past medical history***: previous episode, previous known disorder e.g. ITP, exposure to trauma, surgery, dental extraction, or pregnancies?
- ***Family history***: similar bleeding tendency in other family members? Pattern of inheritance—autosomal dominant, sex-linked?
- ***Drugs***: thrombocytopenia (📖 p.484), platelet dysfunction (📖 p.498), cause not always obvious—aspirin, warfarin? Drug reaction—allergic purpura.
- ***Physical examination***: signs of systemic disease—anaemia, lymphadenopathy ± hepato-splenomegaly? Assess bleeding site—check palate and fundi. Check size e.g. petechiae (pinhead); purpura (larger = 1cm); bruises (ecchymoses) =1cm— measure them. Joints—swelling or other signs of chronic arthritis, joint destruction, or muscle contractures from previous bleeds?
- ***Vascular lesions***: purpura e.g. allergic purpura, Henoch–Schönlein pupura (📖 p.500), senile purpura, steroid-related, hypergammaglobulinaemic purpura, hereditary haemorrhagic telangiectasia (HHT)—capillary dilatations which blanche on pressure, vasculitic lesions, autoimmune disorders, hyper-sensitivity reactions.
- ***Pre-operative history***: is an important aspect of identifying clinically significant bleeding risk. If abnormal bleeding does occur during operation then exclude surgical bleeding and take blood for testing. Results may not be reliable in immediate post-operative period due to effect of blood products and stress response of surgery (high vWF,

factor VIIIC and Fgn). Full investigation several weeks after surgery is recommended.

- ***The most common cause*** of an acquired bleeding disorder is anticoagulant therapy (📖 see p.490).

Antiplatelet drugs

Individual response to anti-platelet therapy is extremely variable and even aspirin or clopidogrel will produce a significant bleeding tendency in some patients.

Treatment: stop antiplatelet therapy. Platelet transfusion for acute severe bleeding.

Anticoagulants

Approximately 1 in 100 of the population of some countries are now receiving long-term oral anticoagulant therapy and overanticoagulation—often due to intercurrent illness and antibiotic use—is probably responsible for the majority of life-threatening bleeds due to antithrombotic therapy.

Surgical bleeding

Essential to examine the drug and infusion charts and check that the dose of any drug that may affect haemostasis is correct. Determine if the site of surgery is the only site of bleeding. If this is the case, e.g. there is no bleeding from venepuncture sites or an endotracheal tube and there is no history of previous abnormal bleeding, then depending on the results of coagulation tests it is important to keep the possibility of anatomical surgical bleeding as a likely possibility. In some cases of severe bleeding the patient may have to return to theatre to look for a bleeding point.

Critically ill patients

Many potential acquired disorders of haemostasis in critically ill patients. A coagulopathy due to vitamin K deficiency occurs within a few days in critically ill patients with no oral intake.

Treatment: IV vitamin K should be used routinely to prevent bleeding. Many critically ill patients develop disseminated intravascular coagulation.

Disseminated intravascular coagulation (DIC)

(📖 see p.488.) Major manifestations of DIC are end-organ damage due to microvascular thrombosis but the most readily apparent clinical manifestation is often bleeding due to the consumptive coagulopathy. DIC is a clinical diagnosis supported by the results of laboratory investigations.

Treatment: most important aspect of treatment is treating the underlying cause, e.g. sepsis or obstetric emergency such as placental abruption. FFP and platelet concentrates are used to treat bleeding or prevent haemorrhage associated with planned invasive procedures.

Massive transfusion

Dilutional coagulopathy resulting in deficiency of clotting factors and platelets will cause abnormal bleeding in patients receiving large amounts of plasma expanders and RBCs even in the absence of DIC.

Treatment: give replacement therapy with FFP and platelet concentrates guided by repeated measurement of the PT, APTT, and platelet count.

Thrombocytopenia

Many drugs result in a reversible idiosyncratic thrombocytopenia. In mos cases drug-induced thrombocytopenia is mild and does not cause bleedin Notable exceptions are quinine and gold-induced thrombocytopeni which are severe. Evaluation of drug history and cessation of possibl implicated drugs is essential in patients with acquired bleeding who ar found to be thrombocytopenic. Cytotoxic drugs produce a dose-depen dent suppression of BM platelet production and thrombocytopeni bleeding is common in oncology practice. BM suppression and BM failur syndromes, such as aplastic anaemia and myelodysplasia, often result i production of dysfunctional platelets and the bleeding tendency is signifi cantly greater than in patients with thrombocytopenia and an uncompro mised marrow, such as occurs in ITP.

Acquired inhibitors

Rare and most often autoantibodies. Platelet autoantibodies result i shortened platelet survival and thrombocytopenia (ITP). The bleedin manifestations of ITP (Immune Thrombocytopenic Purpura) are variabl and often mild, as compared with thrombocytopenia associated with inad equate platelet production (see p.484). Treatment-immunosuppressio Rarely, an autoantibody to a specific clotting factor, such as factor VI produces a severe acquired bleeding disorder.

Treatment: consult haematologist.

Bleeding: laboratory investigations

- FBC (platelet count).
- Blood film examination.
- PT, APTT.
- ESR.
- Biochemistry—creatinine, LFTs, and immunoglobulins.
- Factor assays and platelet function tests depending on type of bleeding.

When PT or APTT abnormal investigate accordingly (📖 p.452). Testing strategy depends on history as ↔ PT and APTT do not exclude moderate factor deficiency sufficient to cause abnormal bleeding tendency. LMWH, vWD, platelet abnormality, or very rare factor deficiency such as factor XIII. vWD often missed because PT and APTT and platelet count are ↔. If history suggestive of vWD then plasma level of vWF must be measured. The bleeding time is not a reliable test and is rarely performed. Fill blood sample tube to the mark to ensure correct anticoagulant concentration. Repeat test if result abnormal. Check patient not on anticoagulants. Family studies should be considered dependent on history.

Further investigations

- Check blood film for red cell fragments, platelet morphology, TT and RT (if abnormal APTT checking for heparin effect), Fgn, fibrin degradation products—XDPs/D-dimer.
- Vitamin K deficiency: give vitamin K and repeat 24h later, consider checking II, VII, IX, or X level (vitamin K-dependent) and comparing with factor XI or V (not vitamin K-dependent).
- Liver disease: check LFTs; will not correct to ↔ with vitamin K but may improve due to associated vitamin K deficiency.
- Isolated factor deficiency: assay as indicated by PT/APTT results.
- Inhibitor: lupus anticoagulant tests, check anticardiolipin antibodies, other factor-specific assays.
- Heparin: abnormal APTT (↑ APTT ratio), PT ↔ if heparin with APTT ratio <2.5. Prolonged TT with ↔ RT indicates heparin effect.
- Warfarin: PT prolongation > than APTT, low vitamin K dependent factors.
- vWD: diagnosis of vWD requires measurement of vWF level and function.

Bleeding: therapeutic products

FFP

Dose is 10–20mL/kg. Solvent-detergent virally-inactivated FFP is now produced and is used for rare bleeding disorders and patients with TTP who will require repeated exposure to FFP. Methylene blue-treated single donor unit FFP is also available as a virally-inactivated product.

Platelet transfusion

Typically used for thrombocytopenic bleeding, rarely required for abnormality of platelet function.

Desmopressin

A vasopressin analogue that increases the plasma levels of FVIII and vWF (mainly by release from stores) and directly activates platelets. Desmopressin is usually given subcutaneously or intravenously but the SC route reduces the severity of side effects of headache, flushing, and tachycardia. Tachyphylaxis (a progressively diminished response) can occur. Water retention and hyponatraemia may complicate therapy and for this reason it should not be used in very young children. Fluid intake should not exceed 1L in the 24h following treatment and with repeated doses the serum sodium should be monitored. Desmopressin will also shorten the bleeding time in patients with renal or liver failure.

Tranexamic acid

Inhibits the binding of plasminogen and t-PA to fibrin and effectively blocks conversion of plasminogen to plasmin—fibrinolysis is thus retarded. Used for menorrhagia, after prostatic surgery. Tranexamic acid may also reduce bleeding after ocular trauma and in vWD and FVIII deficiency after dental extraction where it is normally used in combination with desmopressin or clotting factor concentrate. May be of value in thrombocytopenia (idiopathic or following cytotoxic chemotherapy) reducing requirement for platelet transfusion. Contraindicated in patients with haematuria as it will prevent clot lysis in the urinary tract and can result in clot colic.

Aprotonin

Naturally-occurring inhibitor of plasmin and other proteolytic enzymes which has been used to limit bleeding following open heart surgery with extracorporeal circulation or liver transplantation. Currently unlicensed for this indication.

Clotting factor concentrates

Bleeding due to deficiency of specific coagulation factors is treated by either elevating the deficient factor—e.g. treatment of mild FVIII deficiency with desmopressin—or replacement of the missing factor. Recombinant factor VIII and IX are now available in some countries for routine use in patients with congenital deficiencies. For patients with rare coagulation factor deficiencies or multiple acquired deficiencies, as occurs with liver disease, massive blood loss with dilutional coagulopathy or DIC, replacement therapy still requires donor-derived FFP.

Recombinant VIIa and FEIBA

Products used to treat patients with inhibitory antibodies to factor VIII or IX. Recombinant factor VIIa also used for factor VII deficiency and Glanzmanns Thrombasthenia. It is also used in life-threatening haemorrhage after blood component transfusions.

1. British Committee for Standards in Haematology (2003). Guidelines for the use of platelet transfusions. *Brit J Haematol*, **122,** 10–23.

2. O'Shaughnessy, D.F. *et al.* (2004). Guidelines for the use of fresh-frozen plasma, cryoprecipitate and cryosupernatant. *Brit J Haematol*, **126**, 11–28.

von Willebrand disease (vWD)

Commonest heritable bleeding disorder. Autosomal inheritance. Low vWF level or reduced vWF function, affects both sexes but presents more frequently in ♀ because of menorrhagia. Incidence of 1 per few hundred.

Pathophysiology

vWF, produced in endothelial cells and megakaryocytes, is a protein of 250kDa molecular weight. Initial dimerization and subsequent removal of propeptide allows polymerization and secretion of large multimers. The higher molecular weight (HMW) multimers, up to 20×10^6Da, are particularly haemostatically active. vWF has two main functions:

- Its 1° haemostatic function is to act as a ligand for platelet adhesion and when this activity is reduced bleeding tendency increases.
- It has a 2° function as a carrier protein for factor VIII protecting it from degradation. In most patients with vWD the associated mild reduction in factor VIII level is not the cause of the haemostatic defect.

Many cases of heritable/congenital vWD are currently thought to be caused by genetic mutations at the vWF locus but some may be due to defects in other genes which affect vWF levels (epigenetic factors such as ABO blood group). Increasingly, vWF is considered a continuous variable with low levels associated with an ↑ bleeding tendency.

vWD is classified into 3 main types (Table 10.1)

- Type 1—quantitative deficiency of vWF (75% of cases).
- Type 2—qualitative deficiency of vWF (20% of cases).
- Type 3—complete deficiency of vWF (rare).

Clinical features

Presentation varies markedly but typically a mild-to-moderate bleeding tendency. Symptoms may be intermittent possibly related to fluctuating vWF levels. It may be necessary to test on repeated occasions to establish that vWF levels may be abnormally low on occasion.

- Bleeding type—mucocutaneous, easy bruising, nose bleeds, prolonged bleeding from cuts, dental extractions, trauma, surgery, and menorrhagia. Haemarthroses do not typically occur (except in type 3).
- Patients often present in 2nd or 3rd decade after prolonged bleeding after dental extraction or surgery.
- Type 2B causes thrombocytopenia.

Laboratory diagnosis

vWF is an acute phase protein—increasing with stress, oestrogens, pregnancy, malignancy, thyrotoxicosis. vWF levels are dependent on ABO blood group being lower in group O than non-O.

- Because vWF is the carrier protein for FVIII protecting it from proteolysis there is a 2° deficiency of FVIII associated with vWF deficiency, but it is a low vWF level that is primarily responsible for bleeding in most patients.
- vWF level and function typically mildly or moderately reduced.

Table 10.1 Classification of vWD

Type	VIII	vWF Ag	vWF activity	RIPA low dose	HMW multimer
1	↔/↓	↓	↓	↓/↔	↔
2A	↔/↓	↔/↓	↓	↓/↔	↓
2M	↔/↓	↔/↓	↓	↓/↔	↔
2B	↔/↓	↔/↓	↓	↑	↓
2N	↓	↔	↔	↔	↔
3	↓↓	↓↓	↓↓	↓↓	Usually undetectable

- FVIII may be ↔, or low in some patients. Factor VIII is seldom low enough to cause the joint bleeds seen in haemophilia except in type 3 which is a severe bleeding disorder.
- In type 1 vWD the PT, APTT, and platelet count are often ↔ (a 50% reduction in vWF is sufficient to reduce platelet adhesion and cause bleeding but the associated 50% reduction in FVIII is not sufficient to prolong the APTT).
- Bleeding time is often ↔ and is no longer used as a routine test. It has been largely replaced by automated in vitro platelet function analysis at high shear rate (PFA-100). PFA-100 has good sensitivity for vWD.
- When mild, the condition may be difficult to diagnose as many of the tests are ↔, including the VIII and variably the vWF level. Repeat testing is necessary. Family testing is useful.
- vWF activity measured as ristocetin cofactor activity (vWF:Rco) or collagen binding activity (vWF:CB), which is measured in plasma and is not the same as RIPA (📖 see p.458) which is the ability of ristocetin to agglutinate platelet rich plasma.
- Type 2 often diagnosed when vWF level is low and vWF:Rco/vWF:Ag ratio <0.7.
- The main subtypes of type 2 are 2A and 2M—in 2A there is a qualitative defect with absent HMW multimers and in 2M there is a qualitative defect but with HMW multimers present.
- RIPA is ristocetin-induced platelet agglutination performed on a patient's platelet rich plasma. Only use of RIPA test is for detection of type 2B when RIPA is ↑ due to high affinity variant vWF which produces thrombocytopenia and reduced circulating level of vWF
- Type 2N is rare autosomal recessive variant in which the FVIII:C carrier function of vWF is reduced. May be misdiagnosed as haemophilia A but clue is that ♀ are affected as well as ♂ and autosomal recessive inheritance.
- Majority of patients will have type 1 disease which rarely causes life-threatening bleeds; may have little impact on quality of life/life expectancy.

- Management with vWF rich FVIII concentrates as for severe haemophilia should enable patients with severe vWD to have good QoL.

Treatment

- Mainstay of treatment is desmopressin. Avoid aspirin and NSAIDs. Mild bleeding symptoms—easy bruising, bleeding from cuts may settle with local pressure. Tranexamic acid is a useful antifibrinolytic drug (15mg/kg oral tds), e.g. for dental extraction in conjunction with desmopressin.
- Vaccination against HBV and HAV recommended for all patients.
- Inhibitors infrequent—usually type 3 disease.

Moderate disease and minor surgery

- Desmopressin (0.3mcg/kg SC or by slow IV injection/infusion). Fewer side effects with SC route.
- Most responders have type 1 vWD but may work in some type 2 patients. ***Avoid in type 2B*** (may reduce platelets).

Major surgery, bleeding symptoms, or severe disease

- If desmopressin insufficient use vWF rich factor FVIII concentrate (intermediate purity VIII concentrate) e.g. Alphanate®, BPL 8Y®, Haemate P®.
- A high purity vWF concentrate (Wilfactin®) avoids extremely high FVIII levels when repeated dosing is required, e.g. surgery in type 3 patient.
- Monitor treatment with vWF:Rco or vWF:Ag assay.
- Bleeding time or PFA-100 (📖 see p.458) may not correct despite good clinical response. Treat post-op for 7–10d.

Pregnancy

FVIII and vWF ↑ in pregnancy so rarely presents a problem for type 1. Post-partum vWF ↓ so watch out for PPH in moderate/severely affected women. Give desmopressin or vWF concentrate to maintain levels >0.30u/mL if clinical problem. In Type 2B abnormal HMW multimers can cause platelet aggregation and thrombocytopenia in pregnancy. ***Avoid tranexamic acid in pregnancy/type 2B as there may be risk of thrombosis.***

Menorrhagia

May be major problem. Tranexamic acid for first 3 days of the menstrual period can reduce blood loss by 50%. Combined oral contraceptive pill is useful. Levonorgestrel (hormone impregnated) coil very effective in some patients.

Blood group O-associated low vWF levels

Major modifier of plasma vWF concentration is ABO blood group with vWF levels ranging from 0.35 to 1.50U/mL in group O and 0.50–>2.00U/mL in non-O. Many people with vWF levels of 0.35–0.50U/mL do not bleed but minor bleeding in the general population is common which may be due to lowish vWF levels in some people.

Distinguishing vWD from low-↔ vWF levels can be difficult. Some clinicians restrict diagnosis of vWD to patients with levels <0.30U/mL or a known mutation in the vWF gene and label other patients with bleeding history and vWF level between 0.30–0.50U/mL as 'low-vWF-related bleeding tendency'.

1. Laffan, M. *et al.* (2004). The diagnosis of von Willebrand disease: a guideline from the UK Haemophilia Centre Doctors' Organization. *Haemophilia*, **10**(3), 199–217.

2. Pasi, K.J. *et al.* (2004). Management of von Willebrand disease: a guideline from the UK Haemophilia Centre Doctors' Organization. *Haemophilia*, **10**(3), 218–31.

3. Sadler, J.E. (2003). Von Willebrand disease type 1: a diagnosis in search of a disease. *Blood*, **101**(6), 2089–93.

Haemophilia A and B

Congenital bleeding disorders with low levels of factor VIII (haemophilia A, classical haemophilia) or IX (haemophilia B, Christmas disease). Sex-linked inheritance. ♂ typically affected, ♀ carriers are rarely symptomatic.

Clinical presentation

Haemophilia A and B are clinically indistinguishable. Symptoms depend on the factor level. Bleeds into muscles, spontaneous bleeding into arms, legs, iliopsoas, or any site—may lead to nerve compression, compartment syndrome, muscle contractures—look for these. Haematuria is common (1 or 2 episodes per patient per decade), retroperitoneal and CNS bleeds are life threatening.

Chronic arthropathy

Repeated joint bleeds preventable but older patients often have arthropathy. Blood is highly irritant to synovium and cause synovial hypertrophy with hyperaemia and a tendency to rebleed. Rapid degenerative arthritis with features both of OA (mechanical pain—intermittent, worse on movement) and RA (inflammatory pain—constant but variable, morning stiffness, worse after rest) affecting predominantly hips, knees, and elbows.

Pseudotumours

Progressive cystic enlargement of an encapsulated haematoma. Due to recurrent subperiosteal bleeding and reactive new bone formation leading to destruction of bone, usually long bones in adults. Muscles also affected—iliopsoas.

Pathophysiology

Factor VIII activated by thrombin, and factor IX activated by the TF/factor VIIa complex, together activate factor X, leading to thrombin generation and conversion of soluble Fgn to insoluble fibrin. Haemophilia A and B are disorders characterized by inability to generate cell surface-associated factor Xa. ⅓ of haemophilia B patients have dysfunctional molecule (type II defect).

Genetic abnormalities

Include inversions within intron 22 of factor VIII gene in 50%, point mutations and deletions. Gross gene alterations common in haemophilia A but infrequent in haemophilia B. This may account for low frequency of inhibitors in haemophilia B.

Carrier detection and antenatal diagnosis now possible in many cases by direct gene mutation detection. Affected family member useful for identifying gene mutation. Linkage analysis no longer recommended as 1st-line method.

Epidemiology

- Haemophilia A occurs in 1:10,000, in ⅓ cases no family history as mutation is new. May present in neonatal period in previously unaffected family with prolonged bleeding from the cord or cephalhaematoma. May be erroneously diagnosed as 'non-accidental injury'.

- Haemophilia B occurs in 1:50,000 (i.e. 5 × less frequent than haemophilia A); no striking racial distribution.

Table 10.2

Severe disease (plasma level <0.01U/mL)	Usually presents in the first years of life with easy bruising and bleeding out of proportion to injury
Moderate disease (0.01–0.05U/mL factor level)	Intermediate and variable severity
Mild disease (>0.05U/mL)	May only present after trauma/surgery in later life
General features	Haemarthrosis; spontaneous bleeding into joints (knees>elbows>ankles>hips>wrists) produce local tingling, pain; later—swelling, limitation of movement, warmth, redness, severe pain

Diagnosis

Assess duration, type of bleeding, exposure to previous trauma/surgery and family history. Look for bruising, petechial haemorrhages, early signs of joint damage. Exclude acquired bleeding disorders.

Laboratory tests

PT ↔, APTT prolonged depending on degree of deficiency (*note*: a normal APTT does not exclude mild disease). Assay FVIII first, then FIX. Exclude vWD.

Radiology

Acute bleed—US or CT scan if in doubt. In established disease—chronic synovitis, arthropathy, and other pathological changes seen.

Complications

Factor VIII inhibitors

- Suggested by ↑ frequency of bleeding and/or reduced response to concentrates; occurs in 15–25% haemophilia A patients following treatment, usually after 5–20 treatment episodes (IX inhibitors are uncommon; <2%). Familial tendency, inhibitors occurring more often in patients with deletions or mutations within factor VIII gene. The antibody acts against part of the amino-terminal component of the A2 domain or the carboxyterminal part of the C2 domain of the VIII molecule. Inhibitor is detected by inhibitor screen and quantified by Bethesda assay.
- In 50% of patients inhibitors are transient and low titre (<5BU/mL) being noted incidentally on review.
- In 50%, however, a permanent high-titre inhibitor develops (>5BU/mL) and is a major complication.

Diagnosis

- Prolonged APTT with failure to correct with ↔ plasma.
- Inhibitor screen—APTT of mix of patient plasma and ↔ plasma compared immediately after mixing and after 2h incubation at 37°C.
- Inhibitor assay—factor assays performed on serial dilutions of patient's plasma in ↔ plasma after 2h incubation (Bethesda assay)—inhibitor titre (BU/mL) calculated from dilution that produces 50% reduction of ↔ factor VIII level.

Treatment

Requires a 'FVIII bypassing agent' for treatment of acute bleeds (rVIIa or FEIBA) and desensitization by immuntolerance with FVIII for high titre inhibitors. Various immune tolerance regimens have been tried—successful in up to 80% of patients but may take up to 2 years to eliminate inhibitor Treatment programme requires supervision in comprehensive care centre or similar expert centre with regular pharmacokinetic studies.

Example of immuntolerance programme:

- *Phase 1:* wait until FVIII titre <10BU/mL treating acute bleeds with bypassing agent.
- *Phase 2:* commence 100U/kg FVIII od or bd until inhibitor undetectable in Bethesda assay.
- *Phase 3:* perform half-life (t½) study 4–6-weekly after 3d wash out when inhibitor undetectable. When t½ >6h switch to 50U/kg 3 × weekly and continue to monitor t½.
- *Phase 4:* When t½ >6h for 3 months reduce to standard prophylaxis 25U/kg 3 × weekly.

Asymptomatic patients with low titre inhibitor—observation may be al that is necessary as the inhibitor may disappear.

Transmission of HBV, HCV, and HIV

Not a risk with recombinant products. Viral inactivation procedures fo plasma-derived products in mid 1980s limited transmission.

Treatment

General regular medical and haemophilia review and lifelong support are essential. At presentation establish:

- Factor level.
- Inhibitor screen.
- Mutation (useful for subsequent carrier detection and/or antenatal diagnosis and some predictive value for risk of inhibitor development).
- FBC—exclude anaemia due to bleeds including iron deficiency.
- Blood group.
- Liver function.
- Base-line viral status (HIV, HCV including genotype and HCV RNA level, HBV, HAV).
- Early treatment of bleeding episodes is essential. Prophylaxis is preferable to demand treatment for many patients with severe haemophilia. Prophylaxis started in 1st year or 2 of life can prevent most if not all joint damage and almost eliminate significant bleeding. Portacath may be required to deliver prophylaxis. Factor concentrate needs to be

administered every 2 or 3d. If not on prophylaxis, home demand treatment is preferable to hospital demand treatment.
- Regularly check inhibitor status, LFTs, FBC.
- Avoid aspirin, anti-platelet drugs, and IM injections.
- Vaccinate against HBV and HAV if not immune.

HIV management
Requires specialist involvement. Prophylaxis against infections and retroviral inhibition have significantly improved prognosis.

HCV management
Requires specialist involvement. HCV infected most haemophiliacs treated with pooled human factor concentrates before 1985. Approximately 20% have chronic liver disease. HCV genotyping and RNA detection by PCR is used to identify patients at higher risk of progressive liver disease. Liver biopsy if required is not contraindicated as factor levels are readily normalized with replacement therapy—need for biopsy has diminished as genotyping and RNA detection has become more informative. Combined antiviral therapy superior to IFN alone.

Variant CJD
No evidence as yet of transmission of vCJD by pooled human blood products.

Haemophilia A-specific treatment
- Minor bleeds may stop without factor concentrate therapy.
- Desmopressin for minor surgery and bleeds that fail to settle (0.3mcg/kg SC or slow IVI/20min)—may also be given by nasal spray. 30min later take blood sample to check response (if required)—plasma level ↑ 3–4-fold. Reduced response with repeated exposure sometimes observed.
- Tranexamic acid (15mg/kg tds oral)—useful for cuts or dental extraction. ***Do not use when haematuria***.
- Cryoprecipitate no longer recommended.
- Severe disease—factor VIII concentrate therapy necessary.
- Products—recombinant products are treatment of choice. 2nd generation recombinants do not contain any human material in product. Human donor-derived products are now subjected to multiple viral inactivation steps lyophilization (dry heat), pasteurization (wet-heat), solvent-detergent, nanofiltration)—good record of viral safety. High and intermediate purity human donor-derived products available for patients not receiving recombinant therapy. No particular advantage for high purity over intermediate except possibly useful in patients with allergic reactions to intermediate purity. Factor concentrate not available for majority of patients world-wide.
- Principle of treatment—raise factor VIII to haemostatic level (0.15–0.25U/mL for minor bleeds, 0.25–0.50U/mL for moderate bleeds, >0.50U/mL for severe bleeds, >0.40U/mL minor ops, >0.50U/mL for major surgery with achievement of 1.00U/mL for major surgery and life-threatening bleeds). ***Formula***: 1U/kg body weight raises plasma concentration by about 0.02U/mL (2U/dL). t½ 6–12h. Spontaneous

bleeds usually settle with single treatment if treated early. In major surgery replacement therapy required for up to 10d.
- Do not give IM injections when factor is low.

Haemophilia B-specific treatment

- General approach as for haemophilia A. Desmopressin typically of no value.
- Products—recombinant factor IX treatment of choice. If not recombinant then high purity factor IX preferable to intermediate (intermediate known as prothrombin complex concentrate) as high risk of thrombosis with intermediate purity product. ***Formula***: 1U/kg body wt raises plasma concentration by 0.01U/mL (1U/dL). t½ 12–24h.

Special considerations

Antenatal diagnosis

Carrier detection ideally by genetic mutation analysis. Phenotypic detection by FVIII:vWF ratios is unreliable. Antenatal diagnosis in carriers ideally performed by chorionic villus sampling (CVS) with mutation analysis at 10–12 weeks' gestation if termination preferred—rarer nowadays because of improved treatment and prognosis. Issue is complex and counselling testing should be at comprehensive care centre or similar expert centre.

Home treatment

Home treatment has transformed QoL of patients. Parents, the local GP the boy himself from age 6–7 years onwards can be trained to give IV factor concentrates at home. Treatment usually starts in 1st year or 2 of life and Port-A-Cath® may be needed until age 4 years or more.

Prophylaxis

E.g. 3 × weekly injections of concentrate (average dose 15–25U/kg) given at home.

Multidisciplinary support required

Physiotherapy plays key role in preservation of muscle and joint function in patients with haemarthroses. Combined clinics with orthopaedic surgeons, dental surgeons, hepatologists, paediatricians, HIV physicians, and geneticists are required to give comprehensive care.

1. Key, N.S. and Negrier C. (2007). Coagulation factor concentrates: past, present, and future. *Lancet*, **370**, 439–48.

Rare congenital coagulation disorders

Clotting factor deficiencies

Deficiency of coagulation factors other than vWF, FVIII, and FIX is rare with a prevalence of 1–2 per million. Autosomal recessive inheritance, the deficiency either due to reduced level (type 1) or production of a variant protein (type 2). t½ of factors vary and will determine the frequency and ease of treatment.

Rare factor deficiencies rarely produce haemarthrosis, except factor XIII deficiency, and may only present at time of surgery. Many patients with inherited coagulation deficiencies will not bleed unless exposed to surgery or trauma, and may seldom require treatment. When bleeding arises or cover for surgery is needed, the aim is to achieve a plasma factor concentration at least as high as the minimal haemostatic value and make sure it does not drop below this until haemostasis is secure.

Factor concentrates should be considered when available, e.g. factor XI, factor XIII, recombinant VIIa for FVII deficiency. The use of recombinant factor VIIa is rising and it is increasingly used to treat a variety of factor deficiencies and severe platelet function disorders. FFP can be used, e.g. when appropriate concentrate not available, and virally-inactivated plasma should be used when available. FFP is a source of all coagulation factors but large volumes may be required and even with viral inactivation there is risk of disease transmission.

Specific conditions

Factor XI deficiency

Deficiency more common in certain ethnic groups such as Ashkenazi Jews. Clinically of variable severity, often mild—even low factor levels may not produce symptoms whilst significant bleeding can occur with mild deficiency.

- *Diagnosis:* ↔ PT, ↔ APTT unless factor XI <0.40U/mL. Therefore necessary to measure factor XI level to make diagnosis in many cases.
- *Treatment:* tranexamic acid and desmopressin for oral and dental surgery. Factor XI concentrate sometimes available. Otherwise, use virally-inactivated FFP.

Hypo/afibrinogenaemia

↔ range 2.0–4.0g/L. Produced by liver; acute phase protein, raised in inflammatory reactions, pregnancy, stress, etc. Converted to fibrin by the action of thrombin and is a key component of a clot. Abnormalities of Fgn are more often acquired than inherited. Inherited defects are usually quantitative and include heterozygous hypofibrinogenaemia or homozygous afibrinogenaemia.

Bleeding usually only in afibrinogenaemic patients, hypofibrinogenaemia usually asymptomatic. Bruising, bleeding usually after trauma or operations will depend on the concentration and are more severe when <0.5g/L. Afibrinogenaemia (Fgn <0.2g/L) is a moderate-to-severe disorder with spontaneous bleeding; umbilical stump bleeding common, cerebral and gastrointestinal haemorrhage and haemarthrosis less common. Epistaxis, menorrhagia and post partum bleeding common.

- *Diagnosis*: prolonged (unclottable in afibrinogenaemia) PT, APTT, and TT. Fgn level measured by Clauss assay. Acquired hypofibrinogenaemia needs to be excluded (DIC, liver disease) and family studies are necessary.
- *Treatment*: Fgn has a long t½ (3–5d), severe deficiency managed by repeated (twice weekly) prophylactic injections with Fgn concentrates, FFP or cryoprecipitate. Fgn levels should be raised to 0.5–1.0g/L to achieve haemostasis.

Dysfibrinogenaemia

Qualitative defects of Fgn—the dysfibrinogenaemias—are inherited as incomplete autosomal dominant traits with >200 reported Fgn variants. Defective fibrin polymerization or fibrinopeptide release may occur. Most patients are heterozygous and asymptomatic, bleeding symptoms are not typical and usual clinical manifestation if any is arterial and/or venous thrombosis with some variants (although very rare at ~1 per million of population, <1% of patients with venous thrombosis). More likely to present with pregnancy-associated thrombosis.

- *Diagnosis*: possible prolongation of PT and APTT with variable abnormalities of TT and RT and Fgn-dependent platelet function may be defective. Diagnosis usually by demonstrating normal immunological Fgn concentrations with reduced functional activity in patient with a prolonged TT.

Factor VII deficiency

Vitamin K-dependent factor playing a pivotal role in initiating coagulation but low level required. The t½ is short (4–6h). In severe deficiency (<0.05U/mL), bleeding symptoms (similar to haemophilia) are not common but spontaneous intracerebral haemorrhage at a young age has been reported.

- *Diagnosis*: prolonged PT with ↔ APTT. Assay factor VII to assess severity.
- *Treatment*: recombinant VIIa (20mcg/kg) if available. Repeated doses required. Very short t½ makes management difficult, requiring repeated doses. If using FFP, give initial IV injection (10–15mL/kg) and check response with subsequent monitoring and repeat infusion.

Factor XIII (fibrin stabilizing factor) deficiency

Characteristically produces delayed post-operative bleeding (6–24h later). Neonatal umbilical stump bleeding more common than with other deficiencies. High risk of cerebral haemorrhage.

- *Diagnosis*: PT and APTT both normal so diagnosis will be missed unless specifically looked for. Screening tests are insensitive (clot solubility test with thrombin and acetic acid recommended if performed). Factor XIII antigen (α-subunit) level can be measured by ELISA.
- *Treatment*: very low levels required for haemostasis; t½ is very long. Severe deficiency should be treated with once-monthly prophylactic replacement with factor XIII concentrate.

Other deficiencies

Factor II, V, X deficiencies very rare. Bleeding less severe with factor V deficiency than with factor X or prothrombin deficiency. Consider consanguinity with rare autosomal recessive bleeding disorders.

Multiple defects

Rare familial coagulation factor deficiencies described; often involves factor VIII and another factor, e.g. combined FV and FVIII deficiency. Other combinations seen.

1. Bolton-Maggs, P.H. *et al.* (2004). The rare coagulation disorders–review with guidelines for management from the United Kingdom Haemophilia Centre Doctors' Organisation. *Haemophilia*, **10**, 593–628.

Congenital thrombocytopenias

Family history useful but –ve family history does not exclude inherited abnormality, usually autosomal recessive.

Non-inherited neonatal thrombocytopenia

Infection in the neonate: relatively common cause of neonatal thrombocytopenia. Also as a result of maternal toxoplasma, CMV, rubella when neonatal thrombocytopenia resolves over several months.

Maternal ITP: autoantibody crosses placenta and destroys fetal platelets, however severe thrombocytopenia rare and bleeding exceptional (unlike in NAIT *see below*). Recovery within 1–3 weeks.

Drugs: drugs taken by mother can cause thrombocytopenia, neonatal thrombocytopenia usually resolves rapidly without any haemorrhage

Neonatal alloimmune thrombocytopenia (NAIT): similar mechanism to rhesus haemolytic disease of the new born (HDN) but IgG antibody is to platelet antigen, usually in Pl-A1-+ve fetus of Pl-A1-–ve mother. Associated with severe bleeding including intracranial haemorrhage which may occur before delivery. Requires urgent diagnosis and transfusion of selected antigen-–ve platelets. Recovery may take several weeks.

Marrow infiltration: congenital leukaemia very rare.

Inherited neonatal thrombocytopenia

Very rare. Platelet size and presence or absence of other clinical features help to classify.

↓ ***platelet size***: WAS, X-linked, eczema, susceptibility to infection, death at early age from bleeding, infection or lymphoma.

↔ ***platelet size***: amegakaryocytic thrombocytopenia including TAR Syndrome (thrombocytopenia with absent radius). Schulman-Upshaw Syndrome—neonatal TTP

↑ ***platelet size***: commonest inherited thrombocytopenias, Mediterranean thrombocytopenias (asymptomatic), May–Hegglin anomaly (Dohle bodies in granulocytes, mild neutropenia, major haemorrhage rare, presence of other clinical features such as deafness, cataracts, nephritis identifies variants, all due to mutations of *MYH9* gene) BSS (associated with functional defect, 📖 see p.480), grey platelet syndrome (reduced α-granules), type 2B vWD (📖 see p.466) and pseudo-vWD (platelet type vWD due to mutation in platelet membrane GPIb-IX).

Congenital platelet function defects

Rare. Acquired platelet dysfunction is much more likely to be a cause of bleeding or easy bruising.

2 main hereditary qualitative defects are found:

- Defective platelet membrane glycoproteins (GPs)—GT(Glanzmann thrombasthenia), abnormal GPIIb/IIIa in which there is severe bleeding, and absent aggregation response to all agonists except ↔ agglutination with ristocetin, BSS(Bernard-Soulier syndrome), abnormal GPIb-IX-V complex, receptor for vWF, defective adhesion, variable bleeding can be severe, absent response to ristocetin.
- Abnormalities of platelet granules—storage pool disease (SPD)—α-granules (grey platelet syndrome), δ-granules (May–Hegglin anomaly, Hermansky–Pudlak syndrome, Chediak–Higashi syndrome, TAR syndrome).

Laboratory

- Platelet count.
- Platelet size.
- Blood film (examine granulocytes as well as platelets).
- PFA-100.
- Platelet aggregation.
- Flow cytometry for detection of platelet membrane glycoproteins.

Treatment

- Avoid antiplatelet drugs.
- Use pressure to control bleeding from minor cuts.
- Desmopressin.
- Tranexamic acid (15–25mg/kg body weight) 8-hrly for 7–10d for minor surgery and dental work.
- Platelet transfusions are effective in major surgery and severe bleeding but alloimmunization may occur causing platelet refractoriness.
- Recombinant VIIa considered for severe defects, e.g. GT.
- Splenectomy has been used in WAS.
- Allogeneic BMT has been performed (GT and WAS).

Congenital vascular disorders

Hereditary haemorrhagic telangiectasia (Osler–Weber–Rendu (OWR) syndrome)

Autosomal dominant, multiple mucocutaneous and skin telangiectasia which bleed easily. Recurrent epistaxis, menorrhagia, and GI bleeds causing Fe deficiency. Presentation may not be until later life. Development of pulmonary and cerebral AV malformations. Pulmonary AVMs may enlarge in pregnancy. Diagnosis by recognition of typical telangiectases and family history. Beware, another cause of bleeding may co-exist in a OWR patient.

Laboratory

- FBC and film may show Fe-deficient picture, i.e. microcytic, hypochromic anaemia, ↓ MCV, raised platelets, ↓ serum ferritin.
- Angiography of mesenteric circulation when recurrent bleeding.
- ENT examination.
- CT scan to identify pulmonary AV malformations or desaturation on exercise.

Treatment

- Fe supplementation if Fe deficient.
- Tranexamic acid if menorrhagia.
- Antibiotics for surgical/dental procedures as risk of cerebral abscess due to bacteraemia and shunting in lungs.
- Consider interventional procedure e.g. embolization (if angiography +ve).
- Oestrogen may reduce frequency of bleeding episodes.

Giant cavernous haemangioma

Venous malformation, may cause DIC-like features due to activation of coagulation system within haemangioma, spontaneous regression may occur.

Haemorrhagic disease of the newborn

- Caused by deficiency of the vitamin K dependent factors.
- Poor vitamin K transfer across placenta.
- Significant cause of bleeding in the neonatal period unless prevented by vitamin K.
- Three forms described—early, classic, and late.

Early

Due to maternal ingestion of drugs that interfere with vitamin K metabolism—warfarin, phenytoin, barbiturates, rifampicin. Presents in 1st day of life. Umbilical cord and skin bleeding, post circumcision bleeding, ICH is rare. Prevented by maternal administration of vitamin K.

Classic

Presents at 2–5d of birth, almost exclusively a disease of breast-fed babies, often full term and healthy, incidence 0.5/1000 deliveries. Human milk has less vitamin K than cows' and formula milk, reduced gut flora and synthesis of vitamin K2 may contribute, immaturity of the liver and impaired production of vitamin K-dependent factors may also be contributory.

- Bruising.
- Bleeding from venepuncture sites.
- GI bleeding.
- ICH.

Late

Presents at 2–12 weeks but can occur up to 6 months of age. Can present in breast-fed infants who did not receive vitamin K, may occur with chronic diarrhoea but cholestatic liver disease is often present—biliary atresia, cystic fibrosis, α-1 antitrypsin deficiency. ICH common.

Diagnosis—laboratory findings

- ↑ PT and APTT—may be markedly ↑↑.
- ↔ TT, Fgn, D-dimer/FDPs (*cf.* DIC).
- Factor assay (II, VII, IX, X) if in doubt.
- Correction of coagulation abnormality in 72h with parenteral vitamin K confirms diagnosis.

Differential diagnosis

Exclude other causes of bleeding in the neonatal period e.g. DIC, thrombocytopenia (platelets are ↔ in haemorrhagic disease of the newborn), haemophilia.

Radiology

Scan for ICH/internal bleeding as required.

Treatment

Prevention is indicated e.g. 1mg IM vitamin K_1 at birth (or multiple oral doses but not as effective as IM.

- Treatment should not be delayed when diagnosis suspected—1mg SC or IV vitamin K_1 (will correct PT and APTT to ↔ for age within 72h).

- If significant bleeding give PCC (factor concentrate of II, VII, IX, X) or FFP 15mL/kg.
- Previous concerns of a causal link between parenteral vitamin K administration to the neonate and childhood cancer have been shown to be unfounded.

Thrombocytopenia (acquired)

📖 see also Congenital thrombocytopenias, p.479 and beware pseudo-thrombocytopenia (p.456). Thrombocytopenia defined as platelet count <150 × 10^9/L.

May be due to:

- ↓ bone marrow production.
- Short platelet survival—↑ consumption, destruction, or sequestration (or combination).
- Dilution.

Platelet counts >100 × 10^9/L are not usually associated with bleeding. Purpura, easy bruising, and prolonged post-traumatic bleeding are increasingly common as the platelet count falls <50 × 10^9/L. Although there is no platelet count at which a patient definitely will or will not experience spontaneous bleeding, the risk is greater in patients with a platelet count <20 × 10^9/L and increases further in those with a count <10 × 10^9/L.

↓ bone marrow production of platelets

- ***Marrow failure***: aplastic anaemia (📖 see p.98).
- ***Marrow infiltration***: leukaemias, myelodysplasia, myeloma, myelofi-brosis, lymphoma, metastatic carcinoma.
- ***Marrow suppression***: redictable—cytotoxic drugs, radiotherapy. Idiosyncratic response—e.g. chloramphenicol.
- ***Megaloblastic anaemia*** (📖 see p.46).
- ***Amegakaryocytic***: ethanol, drugs (phenylbutazone, co-trimoxazole; penicillamine), chemicals, viral infection (e.g. HIV, parvovirus).
- ***Hereditary non-congenital***: Fanconi syndrome (📖 see p.590).

Short platelet survival

Consumption

- DIC (📖 see p.488).
- TTP/HUS (📖 see p.534).
- HITT (📖 see p.538).
- Haemangioma (Kasabach–Merritt syndrome).
- Congenital/acquired heart disease.
- Cardiopulmonary bypass.

Destruction

- Immune:
  - 1°: immune thrombocytopenic purpura.
  - 2° ITP: other autoimmune states (SLE, CLL, lymphoma)—drug-induced (heparin—also HITT (📖 p.538), gold, quinidine, quinine, penicillins, cimetidine, digoxin, vancomycin).
  - Infection (HIV, other viruses, malaria).
  - PTP (📖 see p.486).

Sequestration

- Hypersplenism (📖 see p.486).

Dilution

- Gestational thrombocytopenia.
- Massive transfusion (see p.504).
- Exchange transfusion.

Clinical assessment

- ***History***: drugs, symptoms of viral illness.
- ***Examination***: signs of infection, lymphadenopathy, hepatosplenomegaly.
- ***Investigations***: FBC, is thrombocytopenia isolated or not? MPV—acquired BM disorders are a less likely cause of thrombocytopenia the higher the MPV (especially MPV >10fL).
- ***Blood film***: platelet clumps (pseudothrombocytopenia), RBC
- fragmentation (DIC, TTP, HUS), white cells (atypical lymphocytes/ blasts).
- ***Others***: ANA, dsDNA, DAT, monospot, HIV serology, creatinine, LFTs.
- ***BM examination***: if clearly not due to short platelet survival.

1. British Committee for Standards in Haematology (2003). Guidelines for the investigation and management of idiopathic thrombocytopenic purpura in adults, children and in pregnancy. *Brit J Haematol*, **120,** 574–96.

Specific thrombocytopenic syndromes

ITP

2° thrombocytopenia (SLE and LPDs esp. low grade NHL and CLL) may present with isolated thrombocytopenia and underlying disorder may only be discovered on further investigation. Often refractory to therapy. Those with LPDs will require treatment of underlying condition.

ITP in pregnancy

Fetal thrombocytopenia may occur due to placental transfer of IgG anti-platelet antibodies in a pregnant woman with ITP but rare. Risk of ICH in fetus during delivery is very low, but may occur in the fetus of pregnancies in women with previously diagnosed ITP. No good predictor for fetal thrombocytopenia. Treatment with prednisolone, or IVIg should be administered to the mother with thrombocytopenia severe enough to constitute a haemorrhagic risk to her. Avoid splenectomy—high rate of fetal loss. Severe maternal haemorrhage at delivery is rare but may require platelet transfusion, IVIg and possibly splenectomy. Special antenatal treatment of the fetus is unnecessary but avoid prolonged and complicated labour. Ensure paediatric support at delivery and check neonatal platelet count—monitor for several days (delayed thrombocytopenia). IVIg, prednisolone or exchange transfusion may be required.

Differential diagnosis—gestational thrombocytopenia (common), pre-eclampsia, all other causes of thrombocytopenia.

Gestational thrombocytopenia

Benign thrombocytopenia (platelets >80 × 10^9/L) occurs in 5% of pregnancies. No treatment is indicated. Neonatal count ↔.

Neonatal alloimmune thrombocytopenia

(📖 see p.582)

Post-transfusion purpura

Rare but life-threatening. Causes severe haemorrhage due to thrombocytopenia 1 week after transfusion of blood or blood products. Thrombocytopenia may persist for several days. Occurs most commonly in platelet antigen HPA-1a –ve recipient (2% of population) of red cell or platelet transfusion from HPA-1a +ve donor. Patient usually previously sensitized by pregnancy.

Hypersplenism

Thrombocytopenia primarily due to platelet pooling in enlarged spleen. If haemorrhagic complications, consider splenectomy if the underlying cause is unknown or if treatment of underlying disorder has been ineffective.

Drug-induced thrombocytopenia

Many drugs cause idiosyncratic thrombocytopenia, largely through ↑ destruction—usually immune mechanism—patient may have been using the drug for several weeks/months, thrombocytopenia may be severe (<20 × 10^9/L) e.g. with gold or quinine. Drugs—heparin, quinine, quinidine, gold, sulphonamides, trimethoprim, penicillins, cephalosporins, cimetidine, ranitidine, diazepam, sodium valproate, phenacetin, rifampicin, thiazides, (furosemide), chlorpropamide, tolbutamide, digoxin, methyldopa, vancomycin, and teicoplanin. If drug-induced thrombocytopenia suspected, discontinue the suspected drug. If the patient is bleeding platelet transfusion should be administered. IVIg may be helpful. Thrombocytopenia usually resolves quickly but may persist for a prolonged period notably that due to gold which may be permanent. Implicated drugs should be avoided by that patient in future.

Disseminated intravascular coagulation (DIC)

A syndrome which complicates a range of illnesses. Characterized by systemic activation of coagulation resulting in the generation of fibrin clots that cause organ failure and consumption of platelets and coagulation factors resulting in bleeding.

Conditions associated with DIC

- Sepsis and severe infection.
- Trauma.
- Organ necrosis e.g. pancreatitis.
- Malignancy—solid tumours and leukaemia.
- Obstetric—amniotic fluid embolism, placental abruption, pre-eclampsia.
- Vascular abnormalities—large haemangiomas, aortic aneurysm.
- Severe liver failure.
- Toxic—snake bites, recreational drugs including 'Ecstasy'.
- Immunological challenges—ABO transfusion incompatibility, transplant rejection.

These conditions induce systemic activation of coagulation either by activating cytokines as part of a systemic inflammatory response or by causing exposure to procoagulant components, ↑ tissue factor expression, suboptimal function of natural anticoagulant systems, dysregulation of fibrinolysis and ↑ anionic phospholipid availability.

Diagnosis

No single laboratory test that can establish or rule out the diagnosis of DIC—therefore assess the whole clinical picture, taking into account the clinical condition of the patient, the diagnosis, and all available laboratory results.

Laboratory tests need to both keep pace with the rapidly changing condition of the patient.

- Thrombocytopenia.
- ↑ fibrin degradation products (inc. D-dimer).
- ↑ PT.
- ↑ aPTT.
- ↓ Fgn.

Platelet count is a sensitive (*but not specific*) marker of DIC and thrombocytopenia is a feature in up to 98% cases, with platelet count $<50 \times 10^9$/L in ~50% patients.

A scoring system aids diagnosis of overt DIC

Risk assessment—does the patient have an underlying disorder known to be associated with overt DIC?

If yes: proceed.
If no: do not use scoring algorithm.

- Platelet count (>100 = 0; <100 = 1; <50 = 2).
- Elevated FDPs e.g. D-dimer (no increase = 0; moderate increase = 2; strong increase = 3).

- Prolonged PT (<3 sec = 0; >3 but <6 sec = 1; >6 sec = 2).
- Fgn level (> 1g/L =0; < 1g/L = 1).

Calculate score:
- ≥5 compatible with overt DIC (repeat score daily).
- <5 suggestive for non-overt DIC (repeat next 1–2d).

Treatment
- Rapid treatment of the underlying disorder. In many cases the DIC will spontaneously resolve when the underlying disorder is treated, e.g. antibiotics and/or surgical drainage in patients with DIC due to severe infection and sepsis.
- Supportive treatment to minimize or correct coagulation abnormalities may be required.
- Transfusion of platelets or plasma (components) should not primarily be based on laboratory results but should in general be reserved for patients with bleeding.
- In patients with bleeding or at high risk of bleeding (e.g. postoperative patients or patients due to undergo an invasive procedure) and a platelet count of <50 × 10^9/L transfusion of platelets should be considered.
- In non-bleeding patients a platelet threshold for transfusion is 10–20 × 10^9/L. In patients at high risk of bleeding platelets may be transfused at higher levels e.g. 50 × 10^9/L.
- In bleeding patients with a prolonged PT and APTT administration of FFP should be considered.
- If transfusion of FFP is not possible in patients with bleeding who are fluid overloaded, consider using factor concentrates such as PCC (prothrombin complex concentrate)—this will only partially correct clotting abnormalities because they contain only selected factors. In DIC there is a global deficiency of coagulation factors.

1. Levi, M. (2004). Current understanding of disseminated intravascular coagulation. *Brit J Haematol* **124**, 567–76.

Anticoagulant drug therapy

Anticoagulant therapy not routinely indicated. Consider using therapeutic dose LMWH in patients with thrombotic complications e.g. large vessel arterial or venous thromboembolism, severe purpura fulminans associated with skin ischemia or skin infarction.

In critically ill, non-bleeding patients with DIC, prophylaxis for venous thromboembolism with prophylactic dose LMWH is recommended.

- Consider treating patients with severe sepsis and DIC with recombinant human activated protein C (rhAPC, continuous infusion, 24mcg/kg for 4d). Patients at high risk of bleeding should not be given rAPC and a platelet count of $<50 \times 10^9$/L is a relative contraindication. rAPC should be discontinued shortly before interventions (t½ ≈20 min) and may be resumed a few hours later, dependent on the clinical situation.
- Antithrombin concentrate not recommended.

Antifibrinolytic agents not routinely indicated. If 1° hyperfibrinolytic state (e.g. acute promyelocytic leukaemia) and bleeding then tranexamic acid can be considered.

Liver disease

Most coagulation factors, including the vitamin K-dependent factors, are made exclusively in the liver. Any damage to the liver may cause rapid reduction levels and resultant coagulopathy due to their short t½. Associated thrombocytopenia is common in established liver disease (30% of patients have count 70–100 × 10^9/L) and platelet function is reduced, increasing the risk of bleeding.

Pathophysiology

Haemostasis is a balance between procoagulant and anticoagulant mechanisms. Because of its central role in the production of these factors, haemostasis is often disturbed in liver disease. Clotting tests become abnormal and are useful monitors of liver function, especially PT. Low grade DIC may be present. Fibrinolysis may be ↑ in chronic liver disease (*cf.* during liver transplantation when it is ↑ causing bleeding). Dysfibrinogenaemia due to ↑ sialic acid content of the Fgn molecule is described. In obstructive jaundice, impaired bile flow leads to malabsorption of vitamin K, a fat soluble vitamin. A degree of intrahepatic obstruction 2° to hepatocyte swelling and fibrosis may also have this effect. Administration of IV vitamin K may partially correct clotting abnormalities. Thrombocytopenia may be due to portal hypertension, splenic pooling, alcohol, viral infection, drugs, or DIC. Altered platelet function with a prolonged bleeding time may occur.

Clinical features

Many patients with established hepatic dysfunction will have abnormal PT and thrombocytopenia but may be asymptomatic. Bleeding becomes a problem when other complications arise such as oesophageal varices, thrombocytopenia, surgery, liver biopsy, and infection.

Types of bleeding

- Ecchymoses.
- GI bleeding.
- Varicella bleeding.
- Epistaxis.
- Oozing from venepuncture sites and operative sites.

Laboratory

- Vitamin K deficiency—↑ PT > APTT.
- ↓ Fgn with advanced liver disease.
- ↑ TT due to ↓ Fgn, DIC with ↑ FDPs, dysfibrinogenaemia.
- Thrombocytopenia.

Treatment

- IV or SC vitamin K, 10mg daily × 3d.
- FFP (correction of clotting factor deficiency with partial correction of PT and APTT).
- Cryoprecipitate (for hypofibrinogenaemia)
- PCC (prothrombin complex concentrate).
- Platelets (if bleeding or high risk and very low count, e.g. <10 × 10^9/L).
- Desmopressin (improves platelet function).
- Red cell transfusion for anaemia.

- Stop NSAIDS, heparin flushes, and other drugs that may interfere with haemostasis.

Asymptomatic patients do not require treatment other than that directed at the underlying condition. Give vitamin K 10mg IV for 3d to exclude and correct vitamin K deficiency. Complete correction of the PT confirms this diagnosis—partial correction indicates combined hepatocellular dysfunction and vitamin K deficiency.

Liver biopsy

Aim for INR <1.4 and platelet count >70 × 10^9/L. Check on day of biopsy. Give FFP 10–15mL/kg. Check INR and repeat FFP dose until PT is satisfactory—not always achieved. Consider PCC (no longer contraindicated, previous concerns of DIC and/or thrombosis but low clinical risk). Platelet transfusion >70 × 10^9/L.

Active bleeding

Blood transfusion, vitamin K, FFP, platelets as for liver biopsy with monitoring and further therapy as required, may need repeating 6–12-hourly, surgical intervention for oesophageal bleeding (Sengstaken tube, sclerotherapy, desmopressin, TIPS). DIC is a feature of fulminant liver failure and after liver surgery and transplantation. Control underlying condition, support with platelet/FFP as required. Consider aprotonin or rVIIa for uncontrollable bleeding.

Renal disease

Uraemic bleeding

Bleeding common due to platelet dysfunction in patients with uraemia due to chronic renal failure correlating with the severity of the uraemia—exacerbated by anaemia. vWF levels ↔ but vWF function may be impaired. Abnormal bleeding time and abnormal platelet aggregation previously documented in studies but of little or no value in routine practice in individual patients. Bleeding time does not predict risk of haemorrhage and is not indicated. PFA-100 requires evaluation as a predictor of risk of bleeding in this situation.

Treatment

- Intensive dialysis.
- Maintain haemoglobin >10g/dL with transfusion/EPO.
- Desmopressin (0.3mcg/kg SC or slow IV injection, *beware hyponatraemia*).
- Cryoprecipitate (mechanism unknown, may be affect due to HMW vWF content, effect may last up to 36h, not always clinically effective).
- Conjugated oestrogens (oral Premarin 10–50mg/d or daily IV Emopremarin® 0.6mg/kg).

Often mucocutaneous bleeding but can be ICH and pericardial haemorrhage.

Acquired anticoagulants and inhibitors

The development of inhibitors against coagulation factors is uncommon other than antiphospholipid antibodies (📖 see Antiphospholipid Syndrome p.530). Factor VIII antibodies, either spontaneous or in treated haemophiliacs, are a major clinical problem. Acquired vWS may be due to antibodies (seen particularly in paraproteinaemias) or consumption when high platelet turnover (MPDs particularly essential thrombocythaemia). Inhibitors to other clotting factors and heparin-like inhibitors are very rare.

Factor VIII inhibitors

Alloantibodies

Occur in 15–25% haemophilia A patients following treatment, usually after 5–20 treatment episodes in severely affected patients (FVIII<0.01U/mL) (📖 see Haemophilia A complications, p,470). FIX inhibitors in haemophilia B patients are rare.

Autoantibodies

Spontaneous development of FVIII inhibitors in non-haemophiliacs is reported in 1 per million population. Antibody is usually IgG, occasionally IgM or IgA and will neutralize the functional VIII protein or result in ↑ clearance or both. Acquired FVIII inhibitors develop in the elderly, during pregnancy, in association with autoimmune and malignant disease, various skin disorders (psoriasis, pemphigus, erythema multiforme) infections, and drug therapy (penicillin, aminoglycosides, phenothiazines). Symptoms include bleeding (post-operatively this can be major), easy bruising. Haemarthrosis is unusual. Mortality is significant, as many as 25% patients with persisting VIII inhibitors will die from bleeding.

Diagnosis

- Prolonged APTT with failure to correct with ↔ plasma.
- Low plasma FVIII level.
- Inhibitor screen and inhibitor assay as for detection of FVIII inhibitor in patient with congenital haemophilia A (📖 see p.472), however assay is not quantitative in patients with acquired FVIII inhibitors and poor correlation between titre and bleeding.
- Differential diagnosis of spontaneous inhibitors—need to exclude non-specific inhibitors e.g. myeloma paraproteins which bind non-specifically to coagulation plasma proteins. Ensure sample not contaminated with heparin.

1. Collins, P.W. (2007). Treatment of acquired hemophilia A. *J Thromb Haemostasis*, **5**, 893–900.

Treatment of spontaneous FVIII inhibitor

- Prednisolone (1mg/kg/d)—may take weeks to work.
- Cyclophosphamide can be used or added to prednisolone initially or if no response after 6 weeks.
- Increasingly rituximab (375mg/m^2 weekly × 4 weeks) used with good response rate. Treat active bleeding with 'FVIII bypassing agent' (rVIIa or FEIBA).
- In past porcine FVIII was available and if no cross-reactivity porcine VIII treatment was often effective. A recombinant product is under development.
- Mild bleeding may respond to local pressure, tranexamic acid, or desmopressin.

Acquired vWS

Rare disorder presenting in later life, has a variable bleeding pattern similar to the inherited condition. An associated monoclonal gammopathy/LPD is common but the condition may be autoimmune or idiopathic. Bleeding symptoms vary from mild to major e.g. massive GI haemorrhage requiring frequent blood transfusion.

Diagnosis

- ↔ PT.
- ↑ APTT.
- ↓ VIIIC.
- ↓ vWF:Ag and vWF:Rco, in vitro evidence of the vWF inhibitor not always demonstrable.
- Paraprotein, often IgG.

Treatment

- High dose immunoglobulin (1g/kg/d × 2d) is often effective when IgG paraprotein, not effective when IgM. Regular treatment may be required, e.g. monthly.
- Bleeding treated with desmopressin, high purity vWF concentrate (Wilfactin®), vWF containing factor VIII concentrate (e.g. Alphanate®).
- Platelet transfusions may help if refractory major bleeding.

Other coagulation inhibitors

Inhibitors, spontaneous or post-treatment, are reported against most other coagulation factors (V, IX, and prothrombin, XI, VII, and X)—all very rare. Factor V antibodies may arise in congenitally deficient patients following treatment or spontaneously following antibiotics, infection, blood transfusion. Post-operative autoantibodies may develop as a result of exposure to haemostatic agents contaminated with bovine factor V, e.g. fibrin glue. Most are low titre and transient. Treat with FFP and platelets (a source of factor V).

Heparin-like inhibitors are reported in patients with malignant disease, following chemotherapy and may cause bleeding. Protamine sulphate neutralisation *in vitro* and *in vivo* is a feature of this inhibitor.

Diagnosis

- Screening tests (PT, APTT, TT) will give abnormal results depending on the factor involved, with failure to correct with ↔ plasma.
- Defining the specific factor requires factor assays.
- Exclude acquired deficiencies e.g. factor X deficiency in amyloidosis.
- Treatment for actively bleeding patients since acquired inhibitors may not give rise to symptoms.
- 1st-line treatment is often FFP but large volumes may be required and efficacy may be limited.
- Some specific concentrates are available.
- Recombinant VIIa can be considered in many cases.
- Treatment of the underlying condition may cause the inhibitor to disappear.

Acquired disorders of platelet function

Drugs associated with platelet dysfunction

- Aspirin, clopidogrel, dipyridamole, epoprosterol, IIb/IIIa antagonists.
- NSAIDs.
- β-lactam antibiotics: penicillins and cephalosporins.
- 'Antiplatelet agents': epoprostenol, dipyridamole.
- Heparin.
- Plasma expanders: dextran, hydroxyethyl starch.
- Other drugs: antihistamines, local anaesthetics, β-blockers.
- Food additives: fish oil.

Easy bruising, epistaxis, haematomas, haemorrhage after surgery especially in patients with a pre-existing bleeding tendency. NSAIDs cause reversible inhibition of cyclooxygenase. Effect on bleeding and platelet aggregation is brief (only as long as circulating drug present—up to 24h after ingestion) and less likely to cause clinical bleeding in patients without a prior bleeding disorder. β-lactam antibiotics affect platelet function by lipophilic attachment to cell membrane in dose-dependent manner—only after sustained high dosage though effect may last 7–10d. A diet rich in fish oils (omega-3 fatty acids) can cause mild prolongation of bleeding time but rarely bleeding. Ethanol has direct inhibitory effect on platelet function.

Aspirin should be avoided in patients with bleeding tendency. A patient on aspirin should discontinue the drug at least a week prior to a surgical procedure. Desmopressin or platelet transfusion may be used when bleeding due to aspirin-induced platelet function defect. In most cases discontinuation of drug is sufficient.

Systemic conditions which affect platelet function

- Renal failure.
- Liver failure.
- Glycogen storage disorders types Ia and Ib.
- Cardiopulmonary bypass surgery—abnormal platelet function and thrombocytopenia are frequently seen in patients subjected to cardiopulmonary bypass surgery. Impaired aggregation studies in vitro occur in proportion to duration of the bypass procedure. Possibly due to platelet activation and fragmentation in the extracorporeal loop. Desmopressin and platelet transfusion used in patients with bleeding.
- DIC.
- Valvular heart disease, renal allograft rejection, cavernous haemangioma.

Paraproteinaemias and antiplatelet antibodies

- Myeloma and Waldenström's macroglobulinaemia—haemorrhage is more commonly due to thrombocytopenia or hyperviscosity. Plasmapheresis to remove circulating protein may be tried.
- Autoimmune disorders (but thrombocytopenia usually more important).

Haematological conditions with production of abnormal platelets

- Chronic MPDs—especially essential thrombocythaemia—acquired vWS may also be contributory due to depletion of HMW vWF. ↑ whole blood viscosity in patients with polycythaemia causes bleeding.
- Myelodysplasia—abnormal morphology with ↓ granules, acquired storage pool defects.
- Leukaemia.

Henoch–Schönlein purpura

Immune complex disease characterized by a leucocytoclastic vasculitis. Purpura is not due to thrombocytopenia or impaired platelet function. Predominantly affects children aged 2–8 years. Clear preponderance in the winter. Commonly presents 1–3 weeks after upper respiratory tract illness. Various infections, toxins, physical trauma, possibly insect bites, and allergies have all been postulated as triggers of the disease but no clear causation established. May also occur with malignancy.

Clinical features

- Rapid onset usual.
- Classically a palpable purpuric rash over buttocks/legs (extensor surfaces).
- Urticarial plaques and haemorrhagic bullae seen, often symmetrical.
- Abdominal pain due to mesenteric vasculitis.
- Arthritis, particularly knees and ankles.
- Renal involvement—haematuria ± proteinuria, may lead to either acute or chronic renal failure.

Diagnosis

- Presence of typical findings above and exclusion of other causes.
- FBC and film ↔.
- Platelet numbers and function are ↔. ESR raised.
- Other markers of autoimmune disorders may be present.

Treatment and prognosis

- Spontaneous resolution within a month is commonest outcome in children.
- Long-term sequelae more common in adults e.g. chronic renal failure.
- Steroids may be of benefit particularly if joint pains are troublesome.

Peri-operative bleeding and massive blood loss

70–90% of abnormal intraoperative or postoperative bleeding is 'surgical (e.g. bleeding vessel due to failed ligature cautery) rather than haemostatic failure.

Distinguishing surgical bleeding and haemostatic failure

Features suggesting surgical bleeding

- Bleeding from a single site with other potential sites not bleeding.
- Sudden onset of massive and/or rapid bleeding.
- Bright red or pulsatile bleeding from an identifiable source.

Features suggesting haemostatic failure

- Multiple simultaneous bleeding sites—surgical incisions, vascular access sites, mucosal membranes, skin, haematuria.
- Slow persistent ooze of blood from a non identifiable source.
- Delayed haemorrhage following initial haemostasis.

Investigation

- Review drug chart—anticoagulants, antiplatelet drugs, NSAIDs.
- Were preoperative tests ↔ (PT, APTT, platelets if done, LFTs U&Es)?
- Take fresh samples for:
  - Platelet count.
  - PT and APTT (Fgn if either abnormal).
  - D-dimer if clinical suspicion of DIC and PT, APTT, and platelet count consistent with diagnosis (📖 see p.488).
- If liver transplantation consider hyperfibrinolysis—thromboelastography useful.
- Obtain history again from patient or relative regarding personal or family history of bleeding.
- Is patient septic—DIC?
- Does patient have multiorgan failure—DIC?
- Was surgery or anaesthesia prolonged—acidosis, hypothermia?
- Was patient transfused—dilutional coagulopathy?
- Estimate bleeding rate for later comparison.

Treatment

- Maintain tissue perfusion and oxygenation—fluid volume replacement and red cell transfusion if anaemic—aim to maintain Hb >8g/dL.
- Correct acidosis and hypothermia by restoring perfusion—use blood warmer if necessary for blood products.
- Explore surgical site when possible and when surgical bleeding suggested by clinical and laboratory findings.
- Correction of coagulopathy (PT and APTT ratios <1.5 × ↔) with FFP, platelet transfusion, and cryoprecipitate when necessary.
- Empirical administration of desmopressin.
- Empirical administration of antifibrinolytic drugs—tranexamic acid, aprotonin.

- In life-threatening cases not responding to treatment consider rVIIa use after consultation with haematologist. Ensure Fgn >1g/dL, platelets $> 50 \times 10^9$/L, PT and APTT corrected as far as possible with FFP.

1. Stainsby, D. *et al.* (2006). Guidelines on the management of massive blood loss. *Brit J Haematol*, **135**, 634–41.

Massive blood loss

- Total blood volume replaced within 24h, *or*
- 50% blood loss within 3h, *or*
- Blood loss at a rate of 150mL/min.

Treatment

- Maintain tissue perfusion and oxygenation.
- Correct surgical bleeding.
- Blood component therapy as for surgical bleeding—maintain Hb >8g/dL, platelets >75 × 10^9/L, PT and APTT ratios <1.5 × ↔, Fgn >1g/L.
- Contact key personnel—e.g. anaesthetist, blood bank.
- Consider use of VIIa.

Heparin

Heparin remains the most widely used parenteral antithrombotic.

- Naturally occurring glycosaminoglycan produced by the mast cells of most species. Pharmaceutical preparation is extracted from porcine (usually) or bovine mucosa.
- Heterogeneous mixture of straight chain anionic mucopolysaccharides spanning 20–100 monosaccharide units, alternating chains of uronic acid and glucosamine, sulphated to varying degrees.
- LMWH manufactured from unfractionated heparin (UFH) by chemical or enzymatic methods—no evidence that these differences in chemical structure affect biological function.
- The anticoagulant action of heparin is due to a combination of indirect anti-thrombin and anti-Xa activity.
- Elimination of heparin from the plasma appears to involve a combination of zero-order and 1st-order processes, the effect of which is that the plasma t½ alters disproportionately with dose, being 60min after 75U/kg and 150min after 400U/kg. LMWHs are less protein bound and have a predictable dose response profile. They also have a longer t½ than standard heparin preparations.
- Heparin is used when it is necessary to achieve immediate anticoagulation.
- Therapeutic dose UFH given either as a continuous IVI or by injection under the skin. Treatment is monitored by the APTT ratio, aiming to prolong the APTT to 2.0 × ↔ (range 1.5–2.5). ↔ starting dose is 15–20U/kg/h. The APTT should be measured within 6–12h of starting treatment and the dose of heparin adjusted accordingly. Thereafter, the APTT should be measured (preferably on a daily basis) and the dose of heparin adjusted each day. Unfractionated heparin is still used in some circumstances as the short duration of action can be advantageous when it is necessary to vary the intensity of anticoagulation over a short time period, e.g. in a high thrombosis risk patient undergoing surgery.
- Nowadays the heparin of choice for prevention and treatment of DVT and PE and unstable coronary disease is LMWH, given once daily SC injection without the need for monitoring or dose adjustment. Lower risk of HITT. Patients with acute VTE can be treated as outpatients.
- Osteoporosis may complicate long-term use. It is dose-related and is most frequently observed with use in pregnancy. The relative risk with LMWH is not yet established but appears less.
- Hypersensitivity reactions and skin necrosis (similar to that seen with warfarin) occur but are rare. Transient alopecia has been reported.

Bleeding due to heparin

- More common with impaired hepatic or renal function, with carcinoma and in patients >60 years of age .
- An APPT ratio >3.0 is associated with an ↑ risk of bleeding.

Treatment

- Effect of UFH is short and so reversal with protamine sulphate is seldom required, except after extracorporeal perfusion for heart surgery.
- Protamine sulphate, 1mg by slow IV neutralizes 80–100U of UFH.

- The dose given is usually estimated from the dose of heparin given and its expected t½.
- Protamine itself has some anticoagulant effect and overdosage must be avoided.
- The maximum dose must not exceed 50mg.
- Its clinical effectiveness in patients treated with LMWH is unknown.

. Baglin, T. *et al.* (2006). Guidelines on the use and monitoring of heparin. *Brit J Haematol*, **133**, 9–34.

Heparin induced thrombocytopenia/ with thrombosis (HIT/T)

HIT (📖 see Heparin-induced thrombocytopenia (HIT), p.538) with c without thrombosis (HIT/T) is due to an autoantibody against hepari complexed with PF4, causing platelet activation. It occurs most commonl with heparin derived from bovine lung. Thrombosis occurs in <1% c patients treated with LMWH but is associated with a mortality and lim amputation rate in excess of 30%.

Diagnosis

- Suspected in any patient in whom the platelet count falls by 50% or more after starting heparin.
- Usually occurs after ≥5d of heparin exposure (or sooner if the patient has previously been exposed to heparin).

Treatment

- When suspected all heparin (UFH and LMWH) stopped and an alternativ thrombin inhibitor, such as danaparoid or lepirudin should be given.
- Warfarin should not be started until adequate anticoagulation has bee achieved with one of these agents and the platelet count has returned to ↔.

Oral anticoagulant therapy (warfarin, VKAs)

Warfarin is a coumarin derivative that inhibits vitamin K epoxide reductase. Leads to intrahepatic depletion of the reduced form of vitamin K which is a necessary cofactor for the posttranslational modification of vitamin K-dependent proteins. Warfarin is the most widely used oral vitamin K antagonist. Rapidly accumulates in the liver with t½ >40h with a prolonged dose-dependent terminal phase of elimination with detectable warfarin levels 120h after a single dose. Average dose required to achieve an INR of 2.5 is between 3–5mg, although some patients require as little as 1mg and some as much as 30mg, or more. Warfarin is particularly effective for the prevention and treatment of venous thromboembolism and prevention of embolization in association with atrial fibrillation or prosthetic heart valves.

- Oral vitamin K antagonists (VKAs) take several days to produce an anticoagulant effect, hence the need for an immediate acting anticoagulant, such as a heparin, in the first few days of therapy if rapid anticoagulation is required.
- Response to warfarin, and other coumarins, varies within and between individuals and therefore the dose must be monitored regularly.
- Pharmacokinetics (absorption and metabolism) and pharmacodynamics (haemostatic effect) are influenced by vitamin K intake and absorption, by heritable functional polymorphisms affecting metabolism, by rates of synthesis, and clearance of coagulation proteins and by drugs.
- Anticoagulant therapy with oral VKAs is monitored by the international normalized ratio (INR). The INR is derived from the PT ratio and is a standardized method of reporting which permits comparability between laboratories. The ratio of the patient's PT is divided by the geometric mean ↔ PT (GMNPT) and the ratio is then raised to the power of the International Sensitivity Index (ISI) of the thromboplastin used to measure the PTs. Thus:

INR = (PT (patient) ÷ GMNPT)^{ISI}

> For example using a thromboplastin with an ISI of 1.2 and a GMNPT of 13.5sec a patient taking a daily maintenance dose of warfarin producing a PT of 27sec would have an INR of $(27 \div 13.5)^{1.2} = 2.3$.

For ***rapid induction of anticoagulation*** (e.g. treatment of VTE) commence loading dose (e.g. 5 or 10mg with daily or alternate day INR measurement and appropriate dose adjustment) (BCSH see p. 512) whilst treating with immediate acting anticoagulant, e.g. heparin. Daily maintenance dose is predicted by the INR on d4

For ***slow induction of anticoagulation*** (e.g. atrial fibrillation) a low dose can be started, e.g. 2mg of warfarin daily for 1 week and INR then measured—additional immediate acting anticoagulant not required. Daily dose of warfarin ↑ by 1mg each week, with weekly monitoring of the INR, and when the INR is >2.0 maintenance dose has been reached.

- Maintain as stable a level of anticoagulation as possible.
- Adopt the lowest effective target INR.
- Educate patients regarding risk, particularly that associated with additional drug use.

Bleeding due to oral VKA (warfarin)

Risk of bleeding greatest with:

- Age >65 years.
- A history of stroke.
- History of GI bleeding.
- Other medical illness, including renal failure and anaemia.

Warfarin embryopathy, central nervous system bleeding and fetal bleeding complicate administration of warfarin and other oral VKAs to pregnant women. Therefore:

- Warn women of childbearing age.
- Indicate need for early pregnancy test (within 6 weeks) and cessation of therapy with switch to heparin if +ve.

Acenocoumarol has a shorter t½ than warfarin. Indications, contraindications, and side effects are similar to warfarin. The dose required to produce the same intensity of anticoagulation as warfarin is about 50% of the warfarin dose.

Phenindione is an oral vitamin K antagonist that is not a coumarin derivative. It is an indanedione. It is more toxic than the coumarin derivatives and is associated with an ↑ risk of hypersensitivity reactions, including exfoliative dermatitis, renal and liver damage, and agranulocytosis. For this reason it is rarely used. It also produces taste disturbance and pink/orange urine. It is also teratogenic.

Management of overanticoagulation and/or bleeding due to oral VKA (warfarin)

- ***No bleeding, INR <8.0***: ↓ warfarin dose or stop warfarin and restart appropriate new dose when INR <5.0 (response to warfarin dose change is delayed so INR will continue to fall after restarting).
- ***No bleeding or minor bleeding, INR > 8.0:*** stop warfarin (restart when INR <5.0), consider oral vitamin K (0.5–2.5mg) especially if other risk factors for bleeding.
- ***Major bleeding***: stop warfarin, give factor concentrate (II, VII, IX, and X) or FFP, give 5–10mg IV vitamin K.

Perioperative management of oral anticoagulation

- Unless high risk of thromboembolism stop warfarin. Complete reversal of anticoagulation will require stopping 5d before surgery, for partial reversal 3d.
- Anticoagulation does not need to be stopped before dental surgery, including extraction. Safe to proceed as long as INR <4.0.
- Check INR pre-operatively.
- Short term risk of thromboembolism low in patients with mechanical prosthetic valves, mitral > aortic risk. When necessary to continue anticoagulation, e.g. metal mitral valve, bridge with heparin,

e.g. therapeutic dose LMWH starting 3d after stopping warfarin, omitting in 24h before surgery, continuing post-operatively until INR >2.0 in response to reintroduction of warfarin.

1. Baglin, T.P. *et al.* (2006). Guidelines on oral anticoagulation (warfarin): third edition—2005 update. *Brit J Haematol*, **132**, 277–85.

2. British Committee for Standards in Haematology (1998). Guidelines on oral anticoagulation: third edition. *Brit J Haematol*, **101**, 374–87.

Thrombosis

Thrombosis is defined as coagulation within the circulation. Thrombosis may occur in any part of the circulation including the heart, arteries, veins, and the microcirculation. The results of thrombosis are:

- Local obstruction of the circulation.
- Embolization of clot.
- Consumption of haemostatic factors (if thrombosis is extensive).

Venous thrombosis

DVT and PE are different clinical manifestations of a spectrum of disease termed collectively venous thromboembolism (VTE). Most patients presenting with PE have asymptomatic DVT and most patients presenting with symptoms of DVT alone have asymptomatic PE.

- Annual incidence of 1/1000 increasing with age.
- Case fatality rate range 1–5%.
- Post-thrombotic syndrome—characterized by chronic pain, swelling and sometimes ulceration of the skin of the leg occurs in up to ⅓ of patients. Can occur early or up to 10 years. Cumulative frequency 30% at 5 years.
- Chronic thromboembolic pulmonary hypertension develops in 2% of patients presenting with symptomatic PE. May require pulmonary artery endarterectomy.
- DVT usually starts in the calf but by the time symptoms develop 80% of patients have proximal DVT (popliteal vein and above).

Risk factors for VTE

📖 See VTE risk assessment and thromboprophylaxis, p.520.

DVT

Diagnosis

Investigation of suspected DVT is now frequently on combination of clinical assessment (pretest probability (PTP) score, Table 10.3) and result of D-dimer measurement. D-dimer is a fibrin degradation product. Test can be performed on plasma. Thrombosis results in high D-dimer (+ve result) ***but not specific,*** i.e. most patients with +ve D-dimer do not have thrombosis (infection, inflammation, malignancy, tissue trauma, pregnancy). Therefore, D-dimer cannot be used to diagnose DVT it can only be used to exclude it (depending on PPT probability score).

Table 10.3 Clinical probability (PTP) assessment (Well's score) score

Active cancer (treatment on-going or within previous 6 months or palliative)	1
Paralysis, plaster cast	1
Bed >3d or surgery within 4 weeks	1
Tenderness along veins	1
Entire leg swollen	1
Calf swollen >3 cm	1
Pitting oedema	1
Collateral veins	1
Alternative diagnosis likely	-2

Low: 0 or less; moderate: 1 or 2; high: 3 or more. 5%, 20% and 75% of patients with low, moderate or high pretest probability, respectively, have DVT.

D-dimer assay

Measurement of D-dimer can then be used to determine which patients require imaging (now usually compression ultrasound or CT angiography) and which patients do not.

- D-dimer should not be measured until after clinical score (pretest probability score).
- –ve D-dimer has a role in excluding VTE.
- D-dimer affected by heparin administration—potentially giving false –ve result.
- D-dimer may be false –ve if the patient has had symptoms for >2 weeks.
- D-dimer assay with appropriately high sensitivity must be used.[1]

Box 10.1

Low PTP + –ve D-dimer = DVT **excluded**
Moderate PTP + –ve D-dimer = US – if –ve DVT **excluded**
Moderate PTP + +ve D-dimer = US – if –ve repeat US in 1 week
High PTP = US

Radiology

Compression US is now preferred imaging technique. Inability to compres the vein lumen is the principle diagnostic criterion and other findings d not increase sensitivity. Sensitivity for proximal DVT of 97%. Advantag over conventional venography is the ability of US to identify alternativ diagnoses of leg pain and swelling. The 1st test will detect any proxima thrombosis, a calf vein thrombus may remain undetected but a repeat sca 1 week later will pick up clinically important calf DVT that has extende It is safe to withhold anticoagulant treatment from patients with clinicall suspected DVT who have –ve US and –ve D-dimer or –ve US and +ve D dimer and –ve repeat US 1 week later. If D-dimer not used it is safe to dis pense with the follow-up US with a –ve 1st US in patient with a low PTP.

Treatment

- Therapeutic dose LMWH for 3–5d (as outpatient for majority of patients but 🕮 see Contraindications to outpatient therapy, p.516).
- Loading dose of oral VKA when diagnosis confirmed, using loading nomogram with prediction of daily maintenance dose for target INR 2.5. Particular risk of overanticoagulation when elderly (>70 years), liver disease, alcohol abuse, body weight <50 kg, congestive heart failure.
- Oral anticoagulation for 3–6 months for first episode of VTE, longer if persistent risk factors (evidence of heritable thrombophilia not usually an indication of itself for prolonged anticoagulation).
- Compression stocking exerting pressure of at least 30mmHg at ankle (European Class 2, British Class 3 stocking). 50% reduction in post-thrombotic syndrome (PTS).
- Education of patient regarding risk avoidance and need for thromboprophylaxis at times of high risk.
- Testing for acquired thrombophilia as indicated. Antiphospholipid syndrome (APS, 🕮 see p.530), MPD including PNH.
- Review of family history with view to consideration of testing for heritable thrombophilia (🕮 see p.526) (may require completion of anticoagulant therapy for full assessment).

Contraindications to early/immediate outpatient treatment: co-existen serious medical pathology, severe acute venous obstruction (phlegmasi cerulean dolens), severe pain, active bleeding, or significant risk of bleedin renal impairment (creatinine in excess of 200micromol/L), liver diseas (PT >2sec beyond normal range), uncontrolled hypertension (diastoli >110mmHg, systolic >200mmHg), recent eye or CNS surgery (withi 1 month); recent haemorrhagic stroke (within 1 month), known hepari allergy or previous HIT/T, active peptic ulceration, thrombocytopeni (<100 × 10^9/L), suspected problems compliance.

Advantages of LMWH over UFH: once daily SC dose calculated fro patient weight, no monitoring of APTT required (platelet count at begin ning and on d3 or 4), low risk of HIT/T (🕮 see p.538), interpatient an intrapatient variability in UFH dosage requirement results in the APT being in the therapeutic range in only 50% of time.

PE

- PE carries a higher mortality than DVT. Whilst many patients will require hospital admission there is a subgroup of patients who present with peripheral PE (pleuritic chest pain and/or haemopytsis) who can safely be treated on an outpatient basis.
- Right heart strain and right ventricular muscle ischaemia causes release of troponin—sometimes used as prognostic indicator.

Diagnosis

All patients with possible PE should have clinical probability assessed.

Clinical probability (PPT)

Some assessment systems try and define PE as likely or unlikely but require complex scoring systems. A simple pragmatic approach is:

- Patient has clinical features compatible with PE—dyspnoea and/or tachypnoea with or without chest pain and/or haemoptysis (a).
- Absence of another diagnosis (b).
- Presence of a major risk factor (c).

Box 10.2

- **High probability** = (a) + (b) + (c) = CTPA.
- **Moderate probability** = (a) + (b) or (c) = CTPA or high sensitivity D-dimer, and CTPA only if D-dimer +ve.
- **Low probability** = (a) = D-dimer and CTPA if +ve.

D-dimer

Same considerations of assay as for DVT.

Radiology

- CT pulmonary angiography is now recommended imaging method for non-massive PE. V/Q scan if CTPA not available and CXR is ↔ and no significant pre-existing cardiopulmonary disease and non-diagnostic result is followed by further imaging.
- CTPA or echocardiography will reliable diagnose massive PE.
- Good quality normal CTPA excludes PE.

Treatment

- Thrombolysis is 1st-line treatment for massive PE—e.g. 10mg tPA over 2min followed by 90mg over 2h. May be started on clinical grounds if cardiac arrest imminent e.g. 50mg tPA IV bolus.
- Heparin should be started before imaging if moderate or high clinical probability.
- IV bolus of UFH recommended after thrombolysis for massive PE followed by LMWH.
- LMWH alone for non-massive PE.
- Oral VKA as for DVT when diagnosis confirmed—loading nomogram, target INR 2.5, 3–6 months duration for 1st episode of VTE.

Vena cava (VC) filters[2]

- VC filters are indicated to prevent PE in patients with VTE who have a contraindication to anticoagulation.
- Anticoagulation should be considered in patients with a VC filter when a temporary contraindication to anticoagulant therapy is no longer present.
- VC filters are not indicated in unselected patients with VTE who will receive conventional anticoagulant therapy.
- VC filter insertion may be considered in selected patients with recurrent PE despite therapeutic anticoagulation. Alternative treatment options
  such as long-term high-intensity oral anticoagulant therapy (INR target 3.5) or LMWH should be considered prior to VC filter placement, particularly in patients with thrombophilic disorders (e.g. antiphospholipid syndrome) or cancer.
- VC filter insertion may be considered in pregnant patients who have contraindications to anticoagulation or develop extensive VTE shortly before delivery (within 2 weeks). Retrievable filters should be considered.
- Free floating thrombus is not an indication for insertion of a VC filter.
- Thrombolysis is not an indication for filter insertion.
- VC filters should be considered in any pre-operative patient with recent VTE (within 1 month) in whom anticoagulation must be interrupted. Retrievable VC filters should be considered in this situation where a temporary contraindication to anticoagulation exists.

IV drug users—management of iliofemoral venous thrombosis in injecting drug users is problematic because of poor venous access, noncompliance with prescribed treatment, ongoing IV drug use, and co-existent sepsis. Treatment with antilation and LMWH results in a satisfactory clinical outcome.

Cancer—oral VKA therapy is inferior to therapeutic dose LMWH for treatment of VTE in patients with cancer. Therapeutic dose LMWH should be given for 4 weeks after which a 25% dose reduction can be made.

1. Keeling D. *et al.* (2006). on behalf of the Haemostasis and Thrombosis Task Force of the British Committee for Standards in Haematology. The management of heparin-induced thrombocytopenia. *Brit J Haematol*, **133**, 259–69.

2. Baglin, T.P. *et al.* (2006). Guidelines on use of vena cava filters. *Br J Haematol*, **134**, 590–5.

3. Keeling, D.M. *et al.* (2004). The diagnosis of deep vein thrombosis in symptomatic outpatients and the potential for clinical assessment and D-dimer assays to reduce the need for diagnostic imaging. *Brit J Haematol*, **124**, 15–25.

Risk assessment and thromboprophylaxis

Many studies have been performed to determine the incidence of DVT and PE in various groups of patients and to identify risk factors. The risk of VTE in a hospitalized patient depends not only on the reason for admission (procedural risk) but also on pre-existing patient-related factors (patient risk). Decision as to whether patient requires thromboprophylaxis depends on procedural and patient risks, and choice of prophylactic intervention depends also on procedural and patient bleeding risk.

Thrombosis risk factors

Procedural risk

- Major orthopaedic surgery to lower limb, e.g. hip or knee replacement.
- Abdominal or pelvic surgery lasting >30min under general anaesthetic.
- Major trauma is also a risk factor with hip fracture being associated with a very high risk of DVT.

Patient risk

- Age >40 years and particularly >60 years.
- Obesity—BMI >30kg/m^2 and particularly >35kg/m^2.
- Previous VTE.
- Known thrombophilia (a predisposing state which may be heritable).
- Malignancy.
- Heart failure.
- Respiratory disease.
- Severe infection.
- Oestrogen therapy and high dose progestogens.
- Pregnancy and the postpartum.
- Immobility.

Bleeding risk factors

Procedural risk

- Neurosurgery.
- Eye surgery.
- Other procedures with a high bleeding risk.

Patient risk

- Haemophilia and other bleeding disorders.
- Thrombocytopenia (platelets $<100 \times 10^9$/L).
- Recent cerebral haemorrhage (in previous month).
- Severe hypertension.
- Severe liver disease (↑ PT or oesophageal varices).
- Peptic ulcer.
- Endocarditis.

For each patient an assessment of risk should be undertaken on admission and reviewed periodically during hospitalization; depending on the degree of risk patients should receive advice and treatment to reduce risk. Patients should be mobilized early and low dose heparin (LMWH or UFH) and graded pressure stockings, or alternative mechanical devices, should be considered for patients at moderate-to-high risk.

Methods for prevention of VTE

Can be divided into mechanical and pharmacological methods:

Mechanical methods include:

- GCS.
- IPC.

The advantage of mechanical methods is the absence of an effect on coagulation so that there is no ↑ risk of bleeding. Disadvantages include cost (IPC), compliance (IPC and GCS), exacerbation of arterial insufficiency in patients with peripheral arterial disease, and possibly lower efficacy (GCS) than pharmacological methods.

Pharmacological methods include:

- LMWH.
- UFH.

The advantage of pharmacological methods is established efficacy and compliance, i.e. it is known when a dose is given. The disadvantage is bleeding due to an effect on coagulation and idiosyncratic drug reactions including heparin allergy, skin necrosis and HITT.

UFH at a dose of 5000U, 2 or 3 × daily by SC injection reduces the risk of DVT and PE by >50%. The risk of non-fatal haemorrhage is more than doubled but the absolute excess is small as most patients do not suffer any appreciable bleeding and there is no increase in life-threatening haemorrhage. The use of LMWH has the advantage of once daily injection, and a lower risk of bleeding relative to efficacy. It is at least as effective as standard heparin and probably more effective. The combination of graded pressure stocking plus heparin appears to be more effective than either alone. LMWH reduces the risk of DVT and PE in high risk medical patients by >50% when given at a high risk patient dose, e.g. (enoxaparin 40mg, dalteparin 5000U).

Suggested options for risk assessment and prophylaxis

Thromboprophylaxis in high risk medical patients

Risk assessment can be difficult and risk assessment methods are not fully validated.

- Age >60 years and likely hospitalization with immobility for >3d.
- **Or** age >60 years and a diagnosis of heart failure, respiratory disease, sepsis, or inflammatory disease.
- **Or** hospitalization with condition known to be associated with high risk of thrombosis, e.g. SLE with a lupus anticoagulant.
- Prophylaxis—if low bleeding risk LMWH at high risk dose (e.g. enoxaparin 40mg, dalteparin 5000U), if high bleeding risk graded pressure stockings.

Thromboprophylaxis in high risk non-orthopedic surgery

Risk assessment is easier.

- Abdominal or pelvic surgery lasting >30min under general anaesthetic.
- **Or** low risk procedure but 1 or more patient-related related risk factors.
- Prophylaxis—if low bleeding risk LMWH at standard risk dose (e.g. enoxaparin 20mg, dalteparin 2500U), if high bleeding risk appropriate mechanical intervention.

Thromboprophylaxis in high risk orthopaedic surgery

- Major orthopaedic surgery to lower limb, e.g. hip or knee replacement.
- ***Or*** hip fracture or major trauma.
- Prophylaxis—if low bleeding risk LMWH at high risk dose (e.g. enoxaparin 40mg, dalteparin 5000U), if high bleeding risk appropriate mechanical intervention.
- ***Or*** low risk procedure but one or more patient-related related risk factors.
- Prophylaxis—if low bleeding risk LMWH at standard or high risk dose depending on perceived risks of thrombosis and bleeding.

Example of VTE risk assessment

- Risk assessment is mandatory for all patients on admission to hospital. This example of a risk assessment model is not for use in pregnant women or children less than 18 years old.
- All patients should be assessed on admission and periodically during inpatient stay as risk may change. Reassessment after 48–72 hours is recommended and outcome and appropriate action must be recorded in the medical record.

Step one

- Review the patient-related factors shown on the assessment sheet against thrombosis risk, ticking each box that applies (more than one box can be ticked). Use the highest category of risk if more than one box is ticked (e.g. if both moderate and high risk are ticked, use guidance for high-risk patients).
- Any tick for thrombosis risk should prompt thromboprophylaxis. The choice of thromboprophylaxis will be determined by local policy but will likely utilize a combination of mechanical and pharmacological methods (📖 see Suggested options for risk assessment and prophylaxis, pp. 520–1).
- The risk factors identified are not exhaustive. Clinicians may consider additional risks in individual patients and offer thromboprophylaxis as appropriate.
- If the nurse or doctor completing this assessment is uncertain of risks e.g. duration of surgery, procedural bleeding risk, then medical staff should be consulted.

Step two

- Review the patient-related factors shown against bleeding risk and tick each box that applies (more than one box can be ticked).
- Any tick for bleeding risk should prompt medical staff review and to consider if bleeding risk is sufficient to preclude pharmacological intervention.

Step three

- If no boxes are ticked, then the patient is at low risk of VTE and no intervention is indicated.

Further reading

This topic draws on the VTE risk assessment guidance from the Department of Health, *Venous thromboembolism (VTE) risk assessemnt*, September, 2008.

Table 10.4 VTE risk assessment

Thrombosis risk	Patient-related	Procedure-related	Tick
HIGH	Age > 60 years Previous PE or DVT Active cancer Acute on chronic lung disease Acute on chronic inflammatory disease Chronic heart failure Lower limb paralysis (excluding acute stroke) Acute infectious disease e.g. pneumonia BMI > 30kg/m^2		
HIGH		Hip or knee replacement Hip fracture Other major orthopaedic surgery Surgical procedure lasting > 30min	
MODERATE		Plaster cast immobilization of lower limb	
LOW	None of above		
Bleeding risk	**Patient-related**	**Procedure-related**	**Tick**
	Haemophilia or other known bleeding disorder Known platelet count <100 Acute stroke in previous month (haemorrhagic or ischaemic) BP >200 systolic or 120 diastolic Severe liver disease (PT above normal or known varices) Severe renal disease Active bleeding Major bleeding risk, existing anticoagulant therapy or antiplatelet therapy		
		Neurosurgery, spinal surgery, eye surgery Other procedure with high bleeding risk LP / spinal / epidural in previous 4h	

Reproduced from Department of Health, *Venous thromboembolism (VTE) risk assessment*, September, 2008, with permission.

Heritable thrombophilia

Blood tests can be done after an episode of DVT or a PE to test for evidence of a genetic predisposition for heritable thrombophilia.

- Thrombophilia explains why some individuals suffer a blood clot.
- The risk of a recurrent blood clot is not significantly greater in most individuals with thrombophilia than it is in individuals without thrombophilia. Therefore, duration of treatment is not generally different in patients with and without laboratory evidence of thrombophilia.
- Treatment decisions are based on the circumstances that led to the thrombosis, e.g. whether or not the clot followed an operation and if there is a strong family history of DVT or PE.

The most common type of heritable predisposition to DVT and PE is a change in the genetic code known as a mutation. Some mutations are present in about 1 in 15 people. 2 common mutations, each present in 3.5% of the Caucasian UK population are:

- Factor V Leiden (FVL).
- *F2*G20210A, also known as the prothrombin gene mutation.

Less common mutations affect natural anticoagulants including antithrombin, protein C (PC), and protein S (PS) giving rise to low levels (type 1 defect) or impaired function (type 2 defects).

25% of unselected patients presenting with a 1st episode of VTE will have laboratory evidence of a heritable thrombophilic defect; 25–50% of patients with thrombosis and a +ve family history. The frequency of the commonly identified heritable major factors is shown in Table 10.5:

PC and PS deficiency

Many patients are asymptomatic and will never have a VTE. Clinically PC and PS deficiency are similar in terms of risk of thrombophlebitis and VTE. In neonates with severe PC deficiency (homozygous) purpura fulminans is life threatening. This is due to microvascular thrombosis (DIC). Skin necrosis may complicate warfarin therapy in patients with PC or S deficiency—less likely if slow loading regimen or when heparin used in combination with rapid loading.

Antithrombin (AT) deficiency

This was the first major familial defect described (1965). VTE thrombosis risk appears greater than PC/S deficiency particularly during pregnancy. Homozygous severe AT deficiency is probably incompatible with life.

Table 10.5 Heritable thrombophilic defects

Defect	Relative risk of VTE	Patients with 1st VTE	VTE with family history
FVL	2–4	15–20%	15–25%
F2G20210A	2–4	5%	5–10%
AT deficiency	10–20	1–2%	2–5%
PC deficiency	10	1–2%	2–5%
PS deficiency	5–10	3–6%	6–8%

FVL mutation/polymorphism

Coagulation system involves a complex network of interactions between clotting factors—the result of this interaction of clotting factors is the generation of enzymes (XIa, IXa, Xa, and thrombin—thrombin converts soluble Fgn → insoluble fibrin). These interactions take place on the surface of cells, e.g. on the surface of platelets, and require activated non-enzymatic cofactors—factors Va and VIIIa. Generation of thrombin is regulated by proteolysis of FVa by the activated form of PC (APC). APC inactivates membrane bound factor Va through proteolytic cleavage at 3 specific sites in the HC. >95% cases APC resistance due to factor V Leiden (mutation causes amino acid substitution glutamine to arginine at position 506). This reduces proteolysis promoting sustained thrombin generation.

- FVL is associated with an ↑ risk of a 1st episode of DVT.
- Risk of PE is not ↑ as much as DVT, if at all.
- Risk of recurrent VTE is no greater in carriers of FVL than in other patients with a history of VTE who are not carriers of FVL.
- Relative risk of DVT associated with COC is ↑ in carriers of FVL but this translates into an absolute risk of 15/10,000/year.
- Relative risk of DVT associated with HRT is ↑ in carriers of FVL but this translates into an absolute risk of 30/10,000/year.

Pregnancy

Risk of VTE estimated from personal and family history. Determines whether antenatal or postnatal prophylaxis is required.

Contraceptive pills

OCP-users have 4-fold VTE risk compared to non-users generally. The FVL mutation increase the risk a further 8-fold—the 30–35-fold ↑ risk in FVL +ve COC users compared to FVL −ve non-COC users translates into a low absolute risk, 📖 see Table 10.6.

These are overall risk estimates and some women with a strong family history of VTE may be at higher risk. Because thrombophilia is a polygenic disorder with significant environment–gene interaction a −ve thrombophilia result may give false reassurance of low risk.

Table 10.6 Annual VTE risk for FVL mutation and COC users

	Annual VTE risk per 10,000 women-years
FVL – COC –	0.5
FVL – COC +	1–2
FVL + COC –	2–4
FVL + COC +	15–20

Treatment

- Treatment as for any symptomatic VTE—heparin, warfarin thromboprophylaxis for high risk periods, e.g. surgery, pregnancy.
- AT deficiency—do not usually require higher heparin doses.
- Duration of anticoagulation following a 1st event will depend on the severity of the VTE and clinical risk factors for recurrence. Each patient needs to be individually assessed. Heritable thrombophilia is not an indication of itself for prolonged anticoagulation.
- Factor concentrates—AT and PC concentrates have been used in patients with heritable deficiency during surgical and pregnancy high risk periods but are not used routinely.
- PC concentrate should be used in fulminant neonatal thrombosis, including purpura fulminans, in severe homozygous deficiency.
- Thromboprophylaxis in pregnancy depends on family history and nature of thrombophilic defect if tested.

Case-finding and counselling

Identifying asymptomatic individuals by testing relatives of symptomatic patients (case-finding) is not routinely recommended for FVL and *F2*G20210A as the annual risk of VTE is marginally elevated above the general population. The risk is greater in asymptomatic relatives of affected patients with AT, PC, or PS deficiency but not high enough (<2% per year) to justify lifelong anticoagulant treatment. Therefore, high risk periods should be covered with thromboprophylaxis. It may be more sensible to offer thromboprophylaxis to all potentially affected relatives rather than to only those found to have a deficiency. VTE risk has been shown to be higher even in non-carriers of families illustrating the polygenic basis of VTE and the potential false reassurance of a –ve test result. Before embarking on a search for heritable thrombophilia it is essential that careful thought be given to any possible value for the patient and family. As a general rule young children should not be tested.

1. Greaves, M. and Baglin, T. (2000). Laboratory testing for heritable thrombophilia: impact on clinical management of thrombotic disease annotation. *Brit J Haematol*, **109**, 699–703.

Acquired thrombophilia

Antiphospholipid syndrome (APS)

Defined as the association between the persistent presence of circulating antiphospholipid antibodies, and a history of thrombosis ± pregnancy morbidity including fetal loss. Antiphospholipid antibodies are a group of antibodies that react with proteins associated with –vely charged phospholipids, e.g. β_2-glycoprotein 1 (β_2-GPI). Some patients have LA, some have ACL, and some have both. Strongest correlation with recurrent thrombosis is with +ve LA result. Diagnosis requires 1 or more clinical criteria and a +ve antiphospholipid antibody assay result.

Diagnostic criteria have been strictly defined:

Clinical, either:

- Thrombosis— 1 or more clinical episode of arterial, venous, or small vessel thrombosis, ***or***
- Pregnancy morbidity—either (i) unexplained fetal death after 10 weeks with normal fetal morphology, or (ii) 1 or more premature births before 34th week of gestation because of eclampsia or severe pre-eclampsia or placental insufficiency, or (iii) 3 or more unexplained consecutive spontaneous abortions before 10th week of gestation.

Laboratory, either:

- Lupus anticoagulant—on 2 or more occasions at least 12 weeks apart, ***or***
- Anticardiolipin antibody—on 2 or more occasions at least 12 weeks apart at moderate or high concentration.
- APTT may be prolonged and does not correct with ↔ plasma. ↔ result does not rule out the condition as different reagents have different sensitivity. PT usually ↔ unless hypoprothrombinaemia is present.
- LA tests include dilute Russell's viper venom time (DRVVT), Kaolin clotting time (KCT also known as Exner test), silica clot time (SCT). Principle of these tests is that prolonged clotting time is not observed when an excess of phospholipid is added (addition neutralizes the antibodies).
- Other features may be present which are not diagnostic criteria:
  - Thrombocytopenia, livedo reticularis, heart valve disease (usually without haemodynamic effects), myelopathy, migraine, visual disturbances.
  - Transient antiphospholipid antibodies are found after infection and may persist with hepatitis C or syphilis infection. Infection-related antibodies are not associated with thrombosis or obstetric problems.
  - Referred to as 2° APS when present in association with other autoimmune disorders, such as SLE, and 1° when there is no apparent underlying condition.

Lupus anticoagulant (LA)

The paradoxically named LA is arguably the most common clotting abnormality predisposing to thrombosis. It is an *in vitro* phenomenon and the term is a misnomer as it increases the risk of thrombosis not bleeding.

It is an IgG /IgM autoantibody which prolongs phospholipid dependent coagulation tests (hence the use of the term anticoagulant); bleeding is very rare despite the prolonged APTT. LA was first described in patients with SLE—hence the name. Other underlying disorders include the LPDs, HIV, other autoimmune disorders, and drugs (e.g. phenothiazines).

Thrombosis, the major defining feature, may be arterial (stroke, ocular occlusions, MI, limb thrombosis) or venous (DVT, PE, renal, hepatic, and portal veins). Fetal loss may be as high as 80% in women with APS. Catastrophic widespread intravascular thrombosis is reported (catastrophic APS).

Pathogenesis

The antibody specificity is to β_2-GPI, a phospholipid membrane-associated protein. Antibodies to prothrombin may also be present but rarely cause hypoprothrombinaemia and bleeding. Mechanism of thrombosis is not clear but may involve dimerization of β_2-GPI by antibodies on cell surfaces leading to cellular activation, e.g. platelet activation and tissue factor expression by monocytes and endothelial cells.

Treatment

Asymptomatic

Patients with +ve antibody assays without clinical manifestations require no specific action; the risk of thrombosis is estimated at <1% per patient-year.

Thromboembolic prophylaxis

Consider perioperative thromboprophylaxis.

APS

Acute thrombotic events should be treated as appropriate with heparin/warfarin. Long-term anticoagulation is considered by many clinicians as recurrence risk may be high. Target INR usually 2.5 e.g. PE but may be higher if history of arterial or cerebral small vessel thrombosis. Target INR 3.0 or 3.5.

Recurrent abortion

Subsequent pregnancies have been successfully achieved in women with APS with combined aspirin and heparin (UFH or LMWH) begun as soon as pregnancy is confirmed. Steroids are not indicated. Pregnancy in a woman with APS and a past history of thrombosis will require prophylactic anticoagulation with heparin (📖 see p.506).

Thrombophilia in pregnancy

Pregnancy is a hypercoagulable state with an ↑ risk of thrombosis throughout and up to 6 weeks post-partum. In addition to ↑ venous stasis 2° to abdominal pressure and reduced mobility, physiological prothrombotic changes—↑ Fgn, FVIII, vWF.

The risk of venous thromboembolic events (VTE) ↑ 10-fold in ↔ pregnancy—1/1000 deliveries, fatal PE 10/year in UK is the major cause of maternal death in pregnancy and the postpartum. Risk higher when the pregnancy is complicated (sepsis, prolonged bed rest, advanced maternal age, delivery by LSCS), previous VTE particularly in pregnancy, inherited/acquired thrombophilia.

Indications for anticoagulation in pregnancy

- Acute VTE presenting in pregnancy.
- Long-term anticoagulation for prosthetic heart valves/recurrent VTE.
- Previous VTE, particularly in pregnancy/post-partum.
- APS.
- Inherited thrombophilia ± a history of VTE.

There are no universally accepted protocols for the management of anti-coagulation in pregnancy. There are few controlled studies and much of the information relates to non-pregnant subjects. Both oral anticoagulants and heparin have advantages and disadvantages in pregnancy. LMWH is a significant advance in management. Warfarin crosses the placenta and is teratogenic in the 1st trimester. Exposure during weeks 6–12 can cause warfarin embryopathy with nasal hypoplasia, stippled epiphyses and other manifestations. Incidence ranges from <5% to 65% in reported series. Warfarin at any stage of pregnancy is associated with CNS abnormalities and ↑ risk of fetal haemorrhage *in utero* and at delivery.

Heparin (UFH and LMWH) does not cross the placenta and poses no teratogenic or haemorrhagic threat to the fetus. Maternal complications include haemorrhage (severe in <2%), thrombocytopenia (severe in <1%) and osteoporosis, usually asymptomatic and reversible but rare cause of vertebral fractures. LMWH may have fewer complications than UFH.

Treatment of VTE presenting in pregnancy

- Heparin 5–7d, either monitored IV UFH; aim for APTT ratio 1.5–2.5 or therapeutic SC LMWH based on body weight then monitored therapeutic dose SC LMWH, od or bd.
- Continue heparin until delivery; omit heparin during labour.
- Recommence heparin after delivery and start warfarin if desired.
- Continue treatment for at least 6 weeks post-partum, stop heparin once INR in therapeutic range.

Prophylaxis of thromboembolism in pregnancy

National guidelines should be consulted and patients treated in centres with special expertise.

Cardioversion

A target INR of 2.5 is recommended for 3 weeks before and 4 weeks after cardioversion to prevent thromboembolism. To minimize cardioversion cancellations due to low INRs on the day of the procedure a higher target INR, e.g. 3.0, can be used prior to the procedure.

Metal heart valve prostheses

The frequency of thromboembolism is lower with modern valves than 1st generation valves but oral anticoagulation is still required. For patients in whom valve type and location are known specific target INRs are recommended—otherwise a target INR of 3.0 is recommended for valves in the aortic position and 3.5 in the mitral position (Table 10.7).

Table 10.7 Target INRs for cardiac valves

Valve	Target INR
Bileaflet aortic	2.5
Tilting disk aortic	3.0
Bileaflet mitral	3.0
Tilting disk mitral	3.0
Caged ball or caged disk aortic or mitral	3.5

Peripheral arterial thrombosis and grafts

Antiplatelet drugs remain 1st-line intervention for 2° antithrombotic prophylaxis. If long-term anticoagulation is given to patients at high risk of femoral vein graft failure a target INR of 2.5 is recommended.

Paroxysmal nocturnal haemoglobinuria

Long-term anticoagulation with a target INR of 2.5 is recommended if large PNH clones (PNH granulocytes >50%) and a platelet count $>100 \times 10^9$/L. Anticoagulation can also be considered for patients with smaller clones and platelet counts $<100 \times 10^9$/L dependent on additional risk factors for thrombosis and bleeding.

1. Greaves, M. *et al.* (2000). Guidelines on the investigation and management of the antiphospholipid syndrome. *Brit J Haematol*, **109**, 704–15

2. Robertson, B. and Greaves M. (2006). Antiphospholipid syndrome: an evolving story. *Blood Rev*, **20**, 201–12.

Thrombotic thrombocytopenic purpura (TTP)

TTP is rare (4 per million). Early diagnosis and treatment is essential.

Clinical diagnosis—pentad of:

- Thrombocytopenia.
- Microangiopathic haemolytic anaemia.
- Fluctuating neurological signs.
- Renal impairment.
- Fever.

Often insidious onset. Neurological impairment has multiple manifestations including headache, bizarre behaviour, transient sensorimotor deficits (TIAs), seizure, and coma. Presence of coma at presentation is a poor prognostic indicator. Additional features may be present e.g. gastrointestinal ischaemia causing abdominal pain, myocardial ischaemia (📖 see Table 10.8).

Laboratory investigations

FBC and blood film, reticulocyte count, PT, APTT, Fgn and D-dimer, U&E, LFTs, lactate dehydrogenase, urinalysis, direct antiglobulin test.

Treatment

- Single-volume daily plasma exchange should be started within 24h of presentation.
- Plasma exchange using cryosupernatant may be more efficacious than FFP.
- Daily plasma exchange should continue for a minimum of 2d after complete remission.
- Steroid therapy should be given at a dose of at least 1mg/kg prednisolone; pulsed methylprednisolone 1g IV for 3d is often used.
- Low-dose aspirin 75mg daily should be commenced on platelet recovery (platelet count >50 × 10^9/L).
- For refractory disease, an alternative plasma product lacking HMW vWF
- Multimeric forms can be considered—cryosupernatant or SD plasma.
- Vincristine can be added—1mg every 3–4d.
- Malignancy and BMT-associated TTP are often refractory to plasma exchange.

Table 10.8 Clinical subtypes of TTP

Congenital		
Acquired	Acute idiopathic	No identifiable precipitant, low relapse rate
	Secondary	Drugs (oral contraceptive pill, ticlopidine, ciclosporin)
		Bone Marrow Transplantation
		SLE
		Malignancy
		Pregnancy
		Infection - HIV
Intermittent	Recurrent episodes	

1. Allford, S. L., *et al.* (2003). Guidelines on the diagnosis and management of the thrombotic microangiopathic haemolytic anaemias. *Brit J Haem* **120**, 556–73.

Haemolytic uraemic syndrome (HUS)

HUS is characterized by microangiopathic haemolytic anaemia, thrombocytopenia, and renal failure. There may be more extensive multiorgan disease (which may make distinction with TTP difficult). Epidemic form (D+) is associated with a prodromal illness often with bloody diarrhoea in contrast to the rare sporadic or atypical cases (D–) HUS. D+ seen increasingly following outbreaks of infection with verotoxin (VT)-producing organisms e.g. *E. coli* 0157:H7. After ingestion of contaminated food or water, the organisms bind to gut wall receptors and remain within the gut lumen. Toxin targets organs with specific globotriosyl ceramide (Gb) receptors, in particular glomerular microvascular endothelial cells.

Poor prognostic features:

- High neutrophil count.
- Severe thrombocytopenia uncommon.

Indicators of long-term renal disease are thrombocytopenia for >10d and proteinuria after 1 year.

Treatment

- D+ HUS: fluid and electrolyte balance and BP control.
- Dialysis.
- Anti-motility drugs and antibiotics not indicated.
- FFP and therapeutic plasma exchange not effective.

Heparin-induced thrombocytopenia (HIT)

HIT is caused by IgG antibody that recognizes multimolecular complexes of PF4 and heparin. PF4 is a 70-amino acid protein that self-associates to form tetramers of approximately 30kDa. HIT antibodies recognize a heparin-induced conformational change in the PF4 tetramer. The ability to induce the conformational change depends on the chain length and degree of sulphation of the glycosaminoglycan, which explains the differences in incidence of HIT observed with different heparins. PF4/heparin complexes bind to the platelet surface by binding to membrane Fc-receptors—this causes platelet activation.

- Incidence of HIT greater with bovine than with porcine heparin.
- Greater with UFH than with LMWH.
- All heparins used in the UK are of porcine origin.
- Frequency of HIT is greater in surgical than in medical patients.
- In orthopaedic patients given SC prophylactic heparin, the incidence is approximately 5% with UFH and 0.5% with LMWH.
- Risk is very low in obstetric patients given LMWH.
- Skin lesions occur at the site(s) of SC injection—range in appearance from indurated erythematous nodules or plaques to frank skin necrosis.
- If HIT develops the platelet count typically begins to fall 5–10d after starting heparin although in patients who have received heparin in the previous 3 months it can have a rapid onset because of pre-existing antibodies.
- Occasionally, the onset can occur after >10d of heparin exposure but it is rare after 15d.
- The platelet count normally falls by >50% and has a median nadir of 50×10^9/L but severe thrombocytopenia ($<15 \times 10^9$/L) is unusual.
- Half of the patients who develop HIT will have associated thrombosis.
- In patients without thrombosis (isolated HIT) there is a high risk of thrombosis if heparin is not stopped and an alternative anticoagulant (direct-thrombin inhibitor or danaparoid) given in therapeutic dose.

Diagnosis

Use pretest probability score to calculate likelihood of disease if HIT suspected (Table 10.9)

Treatment

High score:

- Heparin stopped and full-dose anticoagulation with a direct thrombin inhibitor, such as lepirudin or danaparoid commenced.
- Warfarin should not be used until the platelet count has recovered—the direct thrombin inhibitor must be continued until the INR is therapeutic (INR >2.0) for 2 consecutive days.
- Platelets should not be given for prevention of bleeding due to thrombocytopenia.

Intermediate score:

- Heparin stopped and prophylactic-dose anticoagulation with a non heparin parented anticoagulant.

Low score:

- Monitor platelet count.
- Consider stopping heparin and substituting prophylactic-dose anticoagulation with a direct thrombin inhibitor.

Table 10.9 Pretest probability score to calculate likelihood of disease if HIT suspected

Thrombocytopenia	0	Fall <30% or platelet count <10 × 10^9/L
	1	30–50% fall or platelet count 10–19 × 10^9/L
	2	>50% fall or platelet count 20–100 × 10^9/L
Timing of thrombocytopenia	0	<5d with no previous heparin exposure
	1	Possibly d5–10 but unclear, e.g. missing platelet counts
	2	D5–10 or less if previous heparin exposure
Thrombosis	0	None
	1	Progressive or recurrent thrombosis or skin lesions or suspected but unproven new thrombosis
	2	New thrombosis, skin necrosis, acute systemic reaction following heparin injection
Other cause of thrombocytopenia not evident	0	Definite other cause present
	1	Possible other cause evident
	2	No other cause evident

Score 0, 1, or 2 for each of 4 categories, maximum possible score = 8

1. Keeling, D. *et al.* (2006). The management of heparin-induced thrombocytopenia. *Brit J Haematol*, **133**, 259–69.

Chapter 11

Immunodeficiency

Congenital immunodeficiency syndromes

Incidence: rare, though as knowledge increases there is recognition of an increasing number of inherited defects in the complex human host defence system. The classical life-threatening disorders of specific immunity with major dysfunction or absence of T cells and/or B cells are all diseases that present in childhood, but milder variants may not be recognized until later life. 'Immunodeficiency' is a vague term that is generally taken to also encompass defects in opsonization and phagocytosis, so can be taken to include neutrophil and macrophage disorders of number, function, or both.

Classification of inherited immune deficiency syndromes

- Affecting T cells, B cells, and neutrophils.
- Affecting B and T cells.
- Affecting T cells.
- Affecting B cells.
- Affecting neutrophils.

Affecting T cells, B cells, and neutrophils

Reticular dysgenesis

An rare autosomal recessive or sometimes X-linked disorder where T cells, B cells, and granulocytes are absent. Such children present with serious infection at birth or shortly afterwards. They have no lymph nodes or tonsils, and the usual thymic shadow is absent. BM is hypoplastic, and there may also be thrombocytopenia and anaemia. It appears to be a pluripotential stem cell failure and carries a dire prognosis. The only curative therapy is BMT.

Affecting T cells and B cells (combined immunodeficiency disorders)

Severe combined immunodeficiency—SCID

A mixed group of disorders that all have grossly impaired T- and B-cell function leading to death normally within the first years of life. They can be broadly classified into 5 groups depending on their clinical and pathological characteristics. Reticular dysgenesis is generally considered to be a SCID variant, accounting for 3% of the total. Other types are:

- Adenosine deaminase deficiency (16%).
- T– B– SCID (27%).
- T– B+ SCID (44%).
- T+ B+ SCID (9%).

Adenosine deaminase deficiency

A recessively inherited enzyme deficiency. ADA is rate limiting in purine salvage metabolism and is essential for the synthesis of nucleotides in cells incapable of *de novo* purine synthesis—including lymphocytes. The gene for ADA is on chromosome 20q12–q13.11, and many mutations have been defined. Gene deletion leads to very low ADA activity and a profound T and B lymphopenia with early onset of clinical symptoms. Other tissues are involved, and there may be bony defects and neurologic disturbances.

A similar rare syndrome is seen with deficiency of the enzyme purine nucleoside phosphorylase. It is less severe and presents later.

Other forms of SCID

SCID with both T-cell and B-cell lymphopenia is a recessive disorder that also occurs without the enzyme deficiencies described above, but the commonest form of the disease is X-linked and shows a lack only of T cells. It appears to be due to a defect in the gene coding for the γ chain of the interleukin (IL)-2 receptor.

There are other rare SCID variants where T cells are present but dysfunctional, including MHC class II deficiency, where lymphocytes fail to express MHC class II molecules; and Omenn syndrome which presents in early infancy with the clinical features of acute widespread GvHD (skin rash, hepatosplenomegaly, diarrhoea, failure to thrive) coupled with persistent infections. Omenn syndrome is due to mutations in recombination activating genes 1 or 2 (*RAG1/2*) and is associated with absent B cells. In contrast to the more typical T-B-cell SCID defects, patients with Omenn syndrome have normal/elevated numbers of T and B cells. However, these cells lack the normal diverse T-cell repertoire, being oligoclonal in nature and having poor/absent proliferative capacity *in vitro* with no/low antibody responses to immunizations. The findings of activated T cells with ↑ production of IL-4, IL-5, and IL-10 at least in part may explain some of the clinical and laboratory manifestations of this syndrome. Recently a subtype of X-linked dyskeratosis congenita has also been recognized to present with SCID (T+ B– NK– phenotype).

Treatment of SCID

- Matched BMT is the treatment of choice for all varieties; a good outcome can be expected in >90%.
- No preconditioning needed for matched donors.
- Mismatched BMT results improving but donor marrow needs careful mature T-cell depletion and patients may need conditioning.
- ADA deficiency can be treated with regular enzyme replacement using a polyethylene glycol-linked ADA preparation.
- ADA deficiency has also been treated with gene replacement therapy, with so far only a transient effect, but the technique shows promise.
- X-linked SCID due to mutations in common γ-chain has been treated with gene replacement therapy in 19 patients with long-term efficacy.

Wiskott–Aldrich Syndrome

An X-linked congenital disorder with a triad of (i) eczema, (ii) thrombocytopenia with characteristically small platelets, and (iii) T- and B-cell dysfunction with susceptibility to infections, particularly otitis media and pneumonia. Due to a mutation in the gene encoding the Wiskott–Aldrich syndrome protein (WASP), important *inter alia* in regulating the cytoskeleton of haemopoietic cells.

- Presents in childhood.
- Tendency to immune cytopenias—compounding pre-existing thrombocytopenia and causing haemolytic anaemia.
- Herpes simplex, EBV, varicella, and CMV may be severe and life threatening.
- Greatly ↑ risk of lymphoid malignancy in adulthood for survivors.

- Splenectomy greatly ↑ risk of fatal infection.
- Need prophylactic antibiotics and immunoglobulin replacement therapy.
- BMT now treatment of choice; early in childhood if possible.

Ataxia telangiectasia

A recessive disorder with ↑ chromosome fragility and a single gene (*ATM*) defect on chromosome 11q22.3. This affects several systems. The first is neuromotor development with cerebellar ataxia appearing around 18 months of age and progressing to include dysarthria associated with degeneration of the Purkinje cells. Telangiectases appear between 2–8 years of age affecting the eyes, face, and ears. An immune deficiency is evident affecting both humoral and cellular immunity, though less severe than SCID. Affected children get:

- Sinopulmonary infections.
- Progressive failure of antibody production.
- Hypogammaglobulinaemia.
- CD4+ lymphopenia.
- Small thymus.
- ↑ incidence of lymphoid malignancies.

Affecting T cells

DiGeorge syndrome

Absence or hypoplasia of the thymus and parathyroid glands with aortic arch anomalies, contralateral cardiac abnormalities or other congenital heart defects. This congenital anomaly of the 3rd and 4th branchial arches usually presents with hypocalcaemic fits or problems with a heart defect. Total thymic aplasia occurs only in a minority, with severe immunodeficiency and a high risk of transfusion-transmitted GvHD. Most have some T-cell function, and relatively minor problems with impaired immunity for which treatment is supportive.

Affecting B cells

X-linked agammaglobulinaemia (Bruton tyrosine kinase deficiency)

Boys with this condition have mutations in the gene for Bruton tyrosine kinase (locus Xq22), resulting in a failure of B-cell development and lack of antibody production. Early infancy is not a problem because of maternally transmitted IgG, but by 2 years of age serious infections become apparent. These include bacterial invasion of the respiratory system, the GI tract, meninges, joints, and skin. Viruses, particularly coxsackie and echo viruses, are also a major threat.

- Absent or very low numbers of B cells.
- Absent or low levels of all immunoglobulins.
- Treatment is by regular antibody replacement with polyvalent IVIg.

Hyper IgM syndrome

An X-linked disorder with B-cell dysfunction due to defective T-cell CD40 ligand production and thus lack of signalling to B-cell CD40 receptors. B cells are normal, but receive no instructions to generate isotypes of Ig other than IgM. Low levels of IgG, IgA, and IgE result. There is also deficient function of some tissue macrophages and a tendency to develop *Pneumocystis jiroveci* (previously known as *Pneumocystis carinii*) pneumonia.

Treatment is with IVIg replacement therapy and cotrimoxazole prophylaxis.

IgA deficiency

A relatively benign and common disorder affecting 1:500 individuals. They may develop anti-IgA antibodies in serum which can cause urticarial and anaphylactic reactions to blood product infusions. No replacement therapy is needed.

Affecting neutrophils, monocytes and macrophages

Inherited disorders of neutrophil function mostly present in childhood and are described in the paediatric section on congenital neutropenia (📖 p.556). 1° functional disorders of monocytes and macrophages are also described in the paediatric section under histiocytic syndromes (📖 p.624).

Poorly characterized 1° immune deficiency syndromes.

There are a number of syndromes where susceptibility to certain types of infection is not associated with a clear pattern of inheritance and where the clinical picture is variable. Few are as severe as the specific syndromes referred to earlier in this section. They include *chronic mucocutaneous candidiasis*, where there is persistent superficial skin and mucous membrane fungal infection, and where there may be defective T-cell regulation or dendritic cell function. CMC is also associated with a wide variety of autoimmune phenomena, particularly thyroid and adrenal disease, and different patterns of inheritance are seen in different kindreds.

There is also a heterogeneous group of disorders collectively referred to as *common variable immunodeficiency*. Defined by the clinical susceptibility to infection and in the absence of any other apparent cause, this collectively named syndrome is usually a diagnosis of exclusion and presents in adult life. Low rather than absent levels of several isotypes of Ig are usual, and the condition is rarely life threatening.

Acquired immune deficiencies

Clinically important defects in lymphocyte numbers and/or function can be seen as a complication of a variety of acquired diseases. They can also be due to drugs, both those given deliberately to suppress an autoimmune process and those given primarily for other reasons. Similarly neutrophils can be reduced by a large number of acquired disorders and a long list of drugs and toxins. An acquired susceptibility to infection also arises in patients with absent or poorly functioning spleens.

Acquired hypogammaglobulinaemia

Causes

- Malignant LPDs including CLL and myeloma.
- Immunosuppressive therapy with e.g. azathioprine.
- Maintenance therapy for ALL.
- Nephrotic syndrome.

Clinical features

Bacterial infections—recurrent chest infections (may lead to bronchiectasis), sinus, skin, and urinary tract infections common. Fulminant viral infections, especially measles, varicella.

Treatment

- May improve with treatment of the underlying disease.
- IVIg should not be used routinely as prophylaxis.
- High titre specific antibody can be given for serious zoster/varicella infections if available; polyvalent for measles.
- Patients with severe hypogammaglobulinaemia and recurrent infections may be considered for IVIg replacement therapy every 4 weeks (400–600mg/kg).

Acquired T-lymphocyte abnormalities

Reduced numbers

- HIV infection (📖 see HIV infection and AIDS, p.548).
- High dose steroids.
- ALG.
- Purine analogues especially fludarabine and cladribine.
- Deoxycoformycin (adenosine deaminase inhibitor).
- After allogeneic STC.

Reduced function

LPDs, Hodgkin's disease, immunosuppressive agents e.g. cyclosporin and steroids, burns, uraemia.

Clinical features

↑ risk of viral, fungal, and atypical infections including HSV, HZV, CMV, EBV, *Candida*, *Aspergillus*, *Mycoplasma*, PCP, toxoplasmosis, TB, and atypical mycobacteria.

Treatment

Treat specific infection where possible. Consider prophylaxis against HZV, CMV, PCP, and *Candida* in high risk groups e.g. post-allogeneic stem cell transplant.

Combined B- and T-lymphocyte abnormalities

Causes

- Chronic lymphocytic leukaemia.
- Intensive chemotherapy.
- Extensive radiotherapy.
- Severe malnutrition.

Clinical features and treatment

📖 see Acquired T-lymphocyte abnormalities, p.546.

Neutrophil/macrophage abnormalities

Reduced numbers

📖 see Neutropenia, p.596.

Abnormal function

📖 see Myelodysplasia, p.620, Myeloproliferative disorders, p.620, Histiocytic syndromes, p.624.

Clinical features

Bacterial and fungal sepsis.

Treatment

Treat specific infections and consider prophylaxis.

Hyposplenism

Hyposplenism is an acquired immunodeficiency without lymphocyte or neutrophil abnormalities. It arises either following splenectomy, or due to functional deficiency as part of another disorder, especially sickle cell disease, inflammatory bowel disease, and following BMT. It gives rise to susceptibility to overwhelming infection with certain organisms due to lack of the spleen's function as a filter. These include:

- Streptococcus pneumoniae.
- *Neisseria menigitidis.*
- *Haemophilus influenzae* type B.
- Falciparum malaria.

The risk of hyposplenic infection is greatest in children in the first 6 years of life. It dwindles thereafter but the risk continues into adult life. All facing splenectomy should be vaccinated against HIB, pneumococcus, and meningococcus type B and all splenectomized children and young adults (and those with sickle cell disease) should take prophylactic penicillin 250mg bd (if allergic to penicillin use erythromycin).

HIV infection and AIDS

Infection with HIV-1 or HIV-2 produces a large number of haematological effects and can simulate a number of haematological conditions during both the latent pre-clinical phase and once clinical syndrome of AIDS has developed. HIV infection divided into 4 stages.

Stage 1: 1° infection

Entry of HIV-1 or HIV-2 through a mucosal surface after sexual contact, direct inoculation into the bloodstream by contaminated blood products, or IV drug abuse can be followed by a transient febrile illness up to 6 weeks later associated with oral ulceration, pharyngitis, and lymphadenopathy. Photophobia, meningism, myalgia, prostration, encephalopathy, and meningitis may also occur. FBC may show lymphopenia or lymphocytosis often with atypical lymphocytes, neutropenia, thrombocytopenia, or pancytopenia. Major differential diagnoses are acute viral meningitis and infectious mononucleosis. False +ve IM serology may occur. Specific IgM then IgG antibody to HIV appears 4–12 weeks after infection and routine tests for HIV may be –ve for up to 3 months. However, the virus is detectable in plasma and CSF from infected individuals during this period and the patient is highly infectious.

Stage 2: pre-clinical HIV infection

Although viral titres fall in the circulation at this time there is significant and persistent virus replication within lymph nodes and spleen. The clinically latent period may last 8–10 years and circulating CD4 T-cell count remains normal for most of this period. However, there is a delayed, gradual, but progressive fall in CD4 T lymphocytes in most patients, who may remain asymptomatic for a prolonged period despite modest lymphopenia. A number of minor skin problems such as seborrhoeic dermatitis are characteristic of the end of the latent phase.

A patient with latent HIV infection may have isolated thrombocytopenia on routine blood testing. This is due to an immune mechanism and may be confused with ITP as there is frequently ↑ platelet associated immunoglobulin.

Stage 3: clinical symptoms

Marked by onset of symptoms, rising titre of circulating virus, and decline in circulating CD4 T-cell count to $<0.5 \times 10^9$/L. Wide variation in individual patient's rate of progression at this stage. A number of minor opportunistic infections are common: oral/genital candida, herpes zoster, oral leucoplakia. Lethargy, PUO, and weight loss occur frequently. Deepening lymphopenia (CD4 $<0.2 \times 10^9$/L) invariably present when opportunistic infection occurs. Persistent generalized lymphadenopathy is a condition where lymphadenopathy >1cm at 2 or more extra-inguinal sites persists for >3 months. It is a prodrome to severe immunodeficiency, opportunistic infection and neoplasia.

Stage 4: AIDS

AIDS is now defined as the presence of a +ve HIV antibody test associated with a CD4 lymphocyte count $<0.2 \times 10^9$/L rather than by the development of a specific opportunistic infection or neoplastic complication. This final stage of HIV infection is associated with a marked reduction in CD4 T cells, severe life-threatening opportunistic infection, neoplasia, and neurological degeneration. Severity of these complications usually reflects the degree of immunodeficiency as measured by the CD4 T-cell count. However, there is evidence that prophylactic therapy reduces the incidence of complications and newer antiviral therapies slow the progression of this stage.

Haematological features of HIV infection

- Lymphopenia—CD4 lymphopenia may be masked by CD8 lymphocytosis in stage 2; improved by antiviral therapy.
- Neutropenia—marrow suppression by virus or therapy; splenic sequestration.
- Normochromic/normocytic anaemia due to suppression of marrow by virus or therapy. Microangiopathic haemolysis associated with TTP.
- Thrombocytopenia—suppression of marrow by virus or therapy or shortened survival due to immune destruction (may respond to antiviral therapy), infection, TTP, or splenic sequestration.
- BM suppression—direct HIV effect or complication of antiretroviral therapy, ganciclovir, trimethoprim, or amphotericin B therapy.
- BM infiltration—by NHL, Hodgkin's disease, granulomas due to *M. tuberculosis*, and atypical mycobacteria or disseminated fungal disease.

Complications of HIV infection

Opportunistic infections

Table 11.1 Complications of HIV infection

Fungal	*Pneumocystis jiroveci*	Pneumonia
	Candida albicans	Oro-oesophageal
	Aspergillus fumigatus	Pneumonia
	Histoplasma capsulatum	Meningo-encephalitis, pneumonia
Mycobacterial	*M. avium intracellulare*	Disseminated, intestinal
	M. tuberculosis	Pulmonary, intestinal
Parasitic	*Cryptosporidium*	Hepatobiliary, intestinal
	Isospora	Colon, hepatobiliary
	Toxoplasma gondii	Multiple abscesses: CNS ocular, lymphatic
Viral	Cytomegalovirus	Retinal, hepatic, intestinal, CNS
	Herpes zoster	Mucocutaneous
	Herpes simplex	Mucocutaneous
	JC virus	CNS
Bacterial	*Haemophilus influenzae*	Meningitis
	Streptococcus pneumoniae	Pneumonia, meningitis, septicaemia

Neoplasia

- AIDS-related Kaposi's sarcoma 20–30% of patients; multiple skin lesions; later lymph nodes, mucous membranes, and visceral organs. ?role of HHV8 (>95% +ve).
- NHL up to 10%; 65% diffuse large B-cell, 30% Burkitt-like; extranodal esp. small bowel and CNS; 1° effusion lymphomas; aggressive. ?role of EBV (100% +ve in 1° CNS NHL).
- Cervical carcinoma.
- Anal carcinoma.
- Hodgkin's disease; advanced stage, extranodal sites.

Direct effects of HIV infection

- BM suppression—dysplastic appearance; pancytopenia.
- Small bowel enteropathy—malabsorption syndrome.
- CNS—dementia, myelopathy, neuropathy.

Therapy of HIV infection

Table 11.2 Infection prophylaxis

Drugs	Activity against
Fluconazole/itraconazole	Oro-oesophageal candidiasis ± cryptococcal meningitis
Trimethoprim	*Pneumocystis jiroveci* ± ocular/ CNS toxoplasmosis
Dapsone/nebulized pentamidine	*Pneumocystis jiroveci*
Rifabutin/azithromycin/clarithromycin	*M. avium-intracellulare*
Aciclovir	HSV and HZV
?Ganciclovir	CMV

Antiviral therapy

- Nucleoside class of viral reverse transcriptase (RT) inhibitors have been widely used both as single agents and in combination: zidovudine (AZT), didanosine (ddl), zalcitabine (ddC), stavudine (d4T), lamivudine (3TC), and abacavir.
- Specific therapy is followed within hours by rapid clearance of virions from the circulation and subsequently by reappearance of circulating T cells and a rising count over several days. Viral resistance develops with time, especially to single agent treatment.
- Non-nucleoside class of reverse transcriptase inhibitors used in combination therapy: nevirapine and efavirenz.
- Protease inhibitors interfere with virus assembly and have dramatic effects on viral load: saquinavir, ritonavir, indinavir, amprenavir, nelfinavir.
- The most effective antiretroviral therapy uses a combination of 2 nucleoside RT inhibitors plus either a non-nucleoside RT inhibitor or 1 or 2 protease inhibitors and is currently recommended for all patients with stage 3 and 4 disease.

Table 11.3 Treatment of complications

Oro-oesophageal candidiasis	Systemic fluconazole or amphotericin then lifelong prophylaxis
Pneumocystis pneumonia	High dose co-trimoxazole or pentamidine then lifelong prophylaxis; pyrmethamine, dapsone, and leucovorin weekly
Tuberculosis	Multi-agent therapy (drug resistance common) ± lifelong isoniazid prophylaxis
Fungal pneumonia	Amphotericin B then lifelong prophylaxis
CMV pneumonitis/retinitis	Ganciclovir/foscarnet then lifelong prophylaxis
CNS toxoplasmosis	Pyrimethamine then lifelong prophylaxis; atovaquone (has *in vitro* activity against cysts of *Toxoplasma gondii* and has been used as salvage therapy for cerebral toxoplasmosis.
Cryptococcal meningitis	Amphotericin/fluconazole
AIDS-related Kaposi's sarcoma	Limited disease: local DXT, cryotherapy, intra-lesional vincristine, interferon-α; advanced disease: combination chemotherapy such as adriamycin, bleomycin, and vincristine (ABV), liposomal daunorubicin, paclitaxel
Non-Hodgkin's lymphoma	Poor prognosis; combination chemotherapy (often standard regimens at reduced dosage due to toxicity) 50% response, median survival <9 months; CNS lymphoma particularly poor prognosis; palliative dexamethasone DXT
2° prophylaxis	Sulfadiazine (2–4g daily in 4 divided doses) + pyrimethamine (25–50mg/d) is 1st choice for 2° prophylaxis. Folinic acid (10–25mg/d) is given concurrently

Chapter 12
Paediatric haematology

Blood counts in children

Blood counts in children are often different from adults, to varying degree at different ages. The differences are greatest during the neonatal period.

Red cells

The relatively hypoxic intrauterine environment means that the newbor is polycythaemic by adult standards, a phenomenon that self-correct during the first 3 months of life by which time the normal infant is anaemi relative to adults. Neonatal red cells are also macrocytic by adult stand-ards, a feature that also disappears during the first 6 months as HbA replaces HbF.

- Neonatal red cells show much greater variation in shape than those from adults, particularly in premature babies—alarming microscopists more used to adult blood films.
- Occasional nucleated red cells are normal in the first 24–48h of life.
- Fe lack is common around 12 months of age due to ↑ demand from ↑ red cell mass and (often) poor oral intake—cows' milk has virtually no Fe content. The MCV falls to what would be abnormally low levels for adults as a reflection of this.
- In healthy premature neonates all these red cell differences may be exaggerated, with a nadir Hb at 2–3 months of 8–9g/dL in those with birth weight 1–1.5kg.
- Children have slightly lower Hb than adults until puberty.

White cells

The most striking difference between children and adults is the high lymphocyte count in infants and young children. This means that the normal differential WBC in those <4 years shows more lymphocytes than neutrophils. Otherwise most of the changes in WCC seen in children are similar to those seen in adults and due to the same causes, with a few exceptions:

- Healthy term babies show a transiently raised neutrophil count in the first 24h after birth ($7–14 \times 10^9$/L) which returns to the normal (adult) range by 48h.
- Immature neutrophils (band cells and myelocytes) may comprise 5–10% of the total WBC in healthy neonates.
- Sick neonates with bacterial infections commonly show a paradoxical neutropenia, with or without an ↑ band cell count.
- Black children have lower neutrophil counts than other ethnic groups.
- Lymphocytoses with very high counts occur in children with specifici-nfections—notably pertussis.

Platelets

Platelet counts in children are essentially the same as adults as far as the lower limit is concerned, but there is greater volatility at the upper end and infants tend to produce high counts ($>500 \times 10^9$/L) as part of an acute phase reaction more frequently. There is a statistically significant fall in the upper limit (95th centile) from 4 years onwards from around 500 to reach 350–400 by the end of childhood.

Cord blood platelets are less reactive to aggregating agents *in vitro* and have other features of hypofunction compared with mature platelets.

Normal blood count values from birth to adulthood

📖 See Table 12.1.

Table 12.1 Normal blood count values from birth to adulthood[1]

Age	Hb (g/dL)	MCV (fL)	Neuts	Lymph	Platelets
Birth	14.9–23.7	100–125	2.7–14.4	2–7.3	150–450
2 weeks	13.4–19.8	88–110	1.5–5.4	2.8–9.1	170–500
2 months	9.4–13.0	84–98	0.7–4.8	3.3–10.3	210–650
6 months	10.0–13.0	73–84	1–6	3.3–11.5	210–560
1 year	10.1–13.0	70–82	1–8	3.4–10.5	200–550
2–6 years	11.5–13.8	72–87	1.5–8.5	1.8–8.4	210–490
6–12 years	11.1–14.7	76–90	1.5–8	1.5–5	170–450
Adult ♂	12.1–16.6	77–92	1.5–6	1.5–4.5	180–430
Adult ♀	12.1–15.1	77–94	1.5–6	1.5–4.5	180–430

Neuts, neutrophils; lymph, lymphocytes and platelets, all × 10^9/L

Other haematological variables in childhood

There are important differences in the concentration of various clotting factors during early infancy as described in Tables 21.3 and 21.4 (📖 p.810). Other laboratory investigations where children differ include:

- Reticulocyte counts low in the first 8 weeks of life as neonatal polycythaemia corrects itself.
- HbF comprises 75% of the total Hb at birth, 10% at 5 months, 2% at 1 year, and <1% thereafter.
- Some red cell enzymes (G6PD, PK, hexokinase) have greater activity (150–200% of adult values) in neonatal RBC.
- The lower limit of normal for serum ferritin at 1 year (12.5mg/L) is 50% of the LLN at 12 years (25mg/L).
- B_{12} and folate levels are around 2 × higher in infants and younger children than adults.

1. Lilleyman, J.S. *et al.* (eds.) (1999). *Pediatric Hematology*, 2e. Churchill Livingstone, London.

Red cell transfusion and blood component therapy—special considerations in neonates and children

Babies in Special Care Baby Units are now amongst the most intensively transfused of our hospital patients.

- To replace blood losses of investigative sampling.
- To alleviate anaemia of prematurity.

Note:

- Hb estimation alone is an inadequate assessment.
- Hb reduction with symptoms, e.g. failure to thrive, is needed to justify transfusion.
- Generally, neonatal Hb <10.5g/dL + symptoms—transfuse; if neonate requiring O_2 support, aim for Hb 13.0g/dL.

Source of blood

Directed donations from 'walking donors' (including donations from relatives) cannot be regarded as safe as microbiologically-screened volunteer donor blood—therefore not recommended.

Small volume transfusions

QUAD 'pedipacks' (SAGM blood) ensure that 4 transfusions possible from a single donor and so ↓ donor exposure in infant needing multiple transfusions.

Pre-transfusion testing

Maternal and neonatal samples should be taken and tested as follows:

Maternal samples

- ABO and Rh group.
- Antibody screen.

Infant samples

- ABO and Rh group.
- DAT.
- Antibody screen (if maternal sample unavailable).

Note: provided no atypical antibodies are present in maternal or infant serum and the DAT on the infant's cells is –ve, a conventional cross-match is unnecessary. Small volume replacement transfusions can be given repeatedly during the first 4 months of life without further serological testing. Transfusion centres may specifically designate a supply of low anti-A, B titre group O Rh (D) –ve blood for use in neonatal transfusions.

►After the first 4 months, compatibility testing should conform to requirements for adults.

Exchange transfusions

- To prevent kernicterus caused by rapidly rising bilirubin.
- Most commonly needed in haemolytic disease of the newborn.
- Plasma-reduced red cells (Hct 0.50–0.60).

- For small volume transfusions, age of red cells does not matter. For exchange transfusions within 5d of collection. ([K^+] levels rise in older blood).
- Transfusion should not take >5h/U due to risk of bacterial proliferation.
- Volumes of 5mL/kg/h usually safe.

Special hazards

- GvHD: in congenitally immunodeficient neonates immunocompetent donor T lymphocytes can cause GvHD—rare.
- Need to irradiate all blood products in these children. Also irradiate if 1st-degree relatives used as donors.
- CMV infection: particular risk in low birth weight babies, or immunocompromised children undergoing transplantation. CMV seronegative donations should be used. Alternatively use (modern) leucodepletion filter to reduce risk.
- Hypocalcaemia—rare now, due to change of additive.
- Citrate toxicity, also rare nowadays due to improvements in additive.
- Rebound hypoglycaemia, induced by high glucose levels of blood transfusion anticoagulants.
- Thrombocytopenia—dilution, DIC.
- Volume overload.
- Haemolytic transfusion reactions in necrotizing enterocolitis. Thought to be due to the 'T' antigen on baby's RBCs becoming exposed due to action of bacterial toxin entering the blood from diseased gut. Anti 'T' is present in almost all donor plasma.

Use of 4.5% albumin

Use controversial, but may be helpful after large volume paracentesis, as fluid replacement in therapeutic plasma exchange, or in nephrotic syndrome resistant to diuretics. There are better products for resuscitation and volume expansion. Should ***not*** be used in nutritional protein deficiency or chronic hypoalbuminaemia (e.g. cirrhosis or protein-losing enteropathy). Risk of infection transmission minimal but not zero.

Use of immunoglobulin

IV polyvalent immunoglobulin widely used as replacement therapy in immunodeficiencies, for Kawasaki disease to prevent the formation of coronary microaneurysms, and also as non-specific agent for reticuloendothelial blockade in immune cytopenias, chiefly (and usually unnecessarily) in childhood ITP. Can get immunoglobulin with particularly high titre against RSV, HZV, and hepatitis B. Usually this is for intramuscular use only and should not be given IV due to risk of complement activation. IVIg has transmitted hepatitis C in the past due to poor virus inactivation procedures, so should not be used in trivial conditions.

Use of FFP

Available in aliquots of 50mL. Must be ABO and Rh compatible. Infused via filter. Main indication—DIC. No need for CMV screening, or irradiation. Dose: 10–15mL/kg. Check PT and APTT. Repeat as necessary. May need cryoprecipitate also (📖 Massive blood transfusion, p.761; Cryoprecipitate, p.772), if evidence of ↓ Fgn (<1.0g/L). Both contain untreated plasma, so potential infection risk, though FFP should be virus-inactivated in future. For this reason methylene blue treated FFP now recommended for children <16 years.

Use of platelets

- Thrombocytopenia more hazardous in neonates, so prophylactic transfusion if count $<30 \times 10^9$/L.
- Reserve for children with marrow failure and counts $<10 \times 10^9$/L otherwise:
    - Only use in *immune* thrombocytopenia for life-threatening bleeding.
    - Then use massive 'swamping' dose to overwhelm antibody.
    - 1 dose (1 paediatric platelet concentrate) contained in ~50mL 'fresh' plasma, available either from apheresis or buffy coat derived.
    - Check increment 1h later if no clinical response.
    - Care with volume overload (give 10–20mL/kg).
    - Must be administered within 2h of receipt on ward.
    - Irradiate for immunosuppressed children.
    - Refractoriness can arise due to alloimmune antibodies.
    - For children < 16 years use platelets collected by apheresis from single donor.

Use of granulocytes

- Severely infected neonates may develop profound neutropenia.
- Usually respond to antibiotic therapy.
- Granulocyte transfusions very rarely given because of lack of effect, risk of CMV and toxoplasmosis, and respiratory distress syndrome.
- Blood products now routinely leucodepleted to reduce risk of CMV transmission.
- Granulocytes may be useful in patients with prolonged pancytopenia (e.g. in patients with aplastic anaemia or post-BMT) unresponsive to broad spectrum IV antibiotics.

Polycythaemia in newborn and childhood

As in adults, polycythaemia in children may be relative or absolute (📖 Polycythaemia vera, (PV) p.260). The condition is usually 2° nd most commonly seen as a clinical problem in neonates or older children with congenital cyanotic heart disease or high-affinity abnormal haemoglobins. 1° polycythaemia is very unusual in childhood; benign familial erythrocytosis is a very rare autosomal dominant self-limiting condition of unknown aetiology.

Pathophysiology

Polycythaemia is physiological in the neonatal period with ↑ Hct (range 42–60% in cord blood) persisting in the first few days of life. Pathological polycythaemia is defined in the neonate as Hct >65% (Hb >22.0g/dL), is uncommon (<5% of all births) and usually due to hypertransfusion or hypoxia.

Causes of polycythaemia in the newborn

- Relative (or 'pseudo'): dehydration, reduced plasma volume.
- Hypertransfusion: delayed cord clamping, maternofetal, twin to twin.
- Hypoxia: placental insufficiency, intrauterine growth retardation.
- Endocrine: congenital adrenal hyperplasia, thyrotoxicosis.
- Maternal disease; toxaemia of pregnancy, DM, heart disease, drugs e.g. propranolol
- Other miscellaneous conditions such as Down syndrome.

Clinical features

- Hyperviscosity may give rise to vomiting, poor feeding, hypotonia, hypoglycaemia, lethargy, irritability, and tremulousness.
- On examination— plethora, cyanosis, jaundice, hepatomegaly.
- Complications include intracranial haemorrhage, respiratory distress, cardiac failure, necrotizing enterocolitis, and neonatal thrombosis.

Diagnosis

- Clinical presentation may suggest the diagnosis e.g. anaemic twin.
- FBC (free-flowing venous sample) ↑ neonatal Hct >65%.
- Hypoglycaemia, hypocalcaemia, unconjugated hyperbilirubinaemia.
- Hb studies for excess HbA—?maternal haemorrhage.
- Radiology: CXR shows ↑ vascularity, infiltrates, cardiomegaly.

Management

- Supportive—IV fluids, close observation for complications.
- Exchange transfusion—partial with FFP/albumin to ↓ Hct<60%.

Neonatal anaemia

Intrauterine conditions require a state of polycythaemia. Congenita anaemia is present with cord blood Hb <14.0g/dL in term babies. In the healthy infant, Hb drops rapidly after birth (📖 Table 21.3, p.810) and by end of the neonatal period (4 weeks in a term baby), the mean Hb may be as low as 10.0g/dL. With ↑ RBC destruction, there is a concomitant ↑ in serum bilirubin. Thus complex changes occur in this period making distinction between physiology and pathology difficult.

Pathophysiology

In normal full-term babies, red cell production ↓ in the first 2–3 months of life. RBC survival shortens; reticulocytes and EPO production ↓; Fe folate and vitamin B_{12} stores are normal. Anaemia in the neonate may be due either to ***impaired production*** of RBCs or to ↑ ***destruction*** or ***loss*** (📖 Table 12.2).

Blood loss during delivery is common, in ~1% severe enough to produce anaemia. Infection is also a significant cause of anaemia; 1° haematologica disorders are rare. Anaemia in premature infant is almost invariably present induced and multifactorial. Jaundice arises in 90% healthy infants making interpretation of a raised bilirubin (📖 Hyperbilirubinaemia, p.578) a critica piece of the jigsaw when investigating an anaemic neonate.

Clinical features

History may make the diagnosis. Check events at time of delivery, past obstetrical history, maternal and family history. Non-specific symptoms—lethargy, reluctance to feed, failure to thrive—all may indicate anaemia Clinical features may be helpful in picking up inherited disorders such as Fanconi anaemia.

Laboratory tests

- FBC and reticulocytes.
- MCV and RBC morphology, bilirubin, and Kleihauer (on mother).
- Special tests may be necessary if cause not apparent (e.g. red cell enzyme defects, inherited BM failure syndromes).
- Glutathione peroxidase deficiency due to acquired selenium deficiency can present transiently with anaemia in neonates.
- Interpret as follows:
  - Reticulocyte count normally very low in first 6 weeks of life.
  - ↑ haemolysis, blood loss.
  - +ve Kleihauer suggests fetomaternal bleed (quantitate amount).
  - Bilirubin ↑ (unconjugated).
  - Check DAT: +ve in immune haemolytic anaemia (except ABO HDN).
  - –ve in other haemolytic anaemias, including ABO HDN).
  - Bilirubin ↑ (conjugated/mixed look for hepatobiliary obstruction/ dysfunction).
- Blood film
  - *Note*: ↑ polychromasia, occasional NRBC, poikilocytes and spherocytes d1–4 in healthy babies.

- RBC morphology may suggest congenital spherocytosis, other RBC membrane disorders or HDN.

- $\downarrow$ MCV—α thalassaemia syndromes.
- $\uparrow$ WBC—reactive, congenital leukaemia.
- Neutropenia—sepsis, marrow failure.

Table 12.2 Causes of neonatal anaemia

Impaired production	**$\uparrow$ destruction**	
Anaemia of prematurity	Overt or concealed haemorrhage; repeated	
Infection	venepuncture	
α thalassaemia	**Haemolytic anaemia**	
DBA	***Non-immune***	***Immune***
Fanconi anaemia	TORCH infection	Rh/ABOHDN
CDA	Congenital RBC abn.	Maternal autoimmune
	Drugs, MAHA	haemolytic anaemia

TORCH, toxoplasmosis, rubella, CMV, herpes simplex; DBA, Diamond–Blackfan anaemia; CDA, congenital dyserythropoietic anaemia; Rh/ABO HDN, rhesus/ABO haemolytic disease of the newborn; MAHA, microangiopathic haemolytic anaemia.

Anaemia of prematurity

Anaemia is an almost invariable finding in the premature infant. By week 3–4 of life the Hb may be as low as 7.0g/dL in untreated infants. In a study of very low birth weight infants (750–1499g) 75% required blood transfusion. A number of factors are causal.

Pathogenesis

- RBC production and survival are ↓.
- EPO production very low in the first few weeks.
- Iatrogenic from repeated blood sampling (depletes the RBC mass and Fe stores—by 4 weeks the premature baby may have had its total blood volume removed).

Clinical features

The ↑ oxygen needs and metabolic demand of the premature baby makes them less able to tolerate ↓ Hb. Over 50% infants <30 weeks' gestation develop tachycardia, tachypnoea, feeding difficulties and ↓ activity when anaemic. High HbF level and ↑ O_2 affinity exaggerates the hypoxia.

Treatment

- Delayed cord clamping ↑ Fe stores.
- Close control of blood sampling is important.
- Transfusion indications will vary in neonatal units—decide on clinical grounds, particularly if ventilated. The following are guidelines only:
  - Prems <2 week with Hb <14.0g/dL, Hct <40%.
  - Prems >2 week, Hb <11.0g/dL, Hct <32%.
- A rising reticulocyte count in some centres is used as a sign to withhold transfusion. Some studies have shown better weight gain in transfused infants (not confirmed by others).
- Fe supplementation (2mg/kg/d PO) after first 2 weeks and until Fe sufficient.
- EPO—controversial. It can be effective but its indiscriminate use is not encouraged. Large randomized trials have shown it to have an effect, but its expense makes cost effectiveness a concern and modern neonatal practice has already reduced the need for transfusion making it less necessary. Its best use is probably reserved for transfusion avoidance in infants weighing <1000g. A suitable regimen would be 200–250U/kg SC × 3/week between d3 and week 6.

Natural history

Despite the growing safety of blood and its ready availability and convenient packaging to reduce donor exposure, blood transfusion carries definite risks and is to be avoided. It is likely that in affluent societies the use of EPO will increase, despite its limited effect.

Haemolytic anaemia in the neonate

Normal red cell life span in term infants is <80 days, in pre-term infants <50 days. Red cell 'cull' in first month with jaundice is physiologic. Pathological haemolysis, when present, is most commonly due to iso-immune HDN 2° to fetomaternal blood group incompatibility in Caucasian populations. In other ethnic groups G6PD deficiency and congenital infection are major causes.

Pathophysiology

Physiological haemolysis occurs soon after birth and there is a marked drop in the Hb and RBC count in the first weeks of life. Neonatal RBCs are more susceptible to oxidative stress and there is altered RBC enzyme activity compared to adult RBC and reticulocytes. So pathological haemolysis occurs in the neonatal period more than at any other time.

Causes of haemolytic anaemia

Haemolysis may be due to intrinsic defects of the RBC, usually congenital or to acquired extracorpuscular factors which may be immune or non-immune.

Clinical features

Pathological jaundice may be clinically obvious at birth or within 24h (distinguishing it from the common physiological anaemia which occurs >48h after birth, 📖 Hyperbilirubinaemia, p.578).

- Anaemia may be severe depending on cause.
- Infections are common cause of hyperbilirubinaemia (📖 Hyperbilirubinaemia, p.578 with specific clinical findings. *In utero* infections (TORCH) do not usually cause severe jaundice *cf.* post-natal bacterial sepsis where jaundice may be striking and associated with MAHA.
- Splenomegaly at birth indicates a prenatal event; when noted later it may be 2° to splenic clearance of damaged RBC and is non-specific.
- Kernicterus is the major complication of neonatal hyperbilirubinaemia.
- Family history and drug history may be informative.

Laboratory diagnosis of haemolysis

- ↑ unconjugated bilirubin with anaemia is hallmark of haemolytic anaemia.
- ↑ reticulocytes (haptoglobins are unreliable in the newborn).
- Blood film—may show RBC abnormalities e.g. spherocytes, elliptocytes fragmented cells.
- DAT, if +ve indicates immune haemolysis; –ve does not rule this out— especially consider ABO HDN.
- Heinz body test—+ve in drug-induced haemolysis, G6PD deficiency and occasionally other enzyme disorders.
- Intravascular haemolysis—look for haemoglobinuria/haemoglobinaemia.

Congenital red cell defects

Pathophysiology

The neonate is uniquely disadvantaged when it comes to handling pathological haemolysis because of hepatic immaturity and altered enzyme activity. Thus congenital defects of the RBC commonly present in the newborn except for defects involving the β globin chain (e.g. SCD, β thalassaemia) which become clinically manifest several weeks after birth but can be diagnosed *in utero*, or in the neonatal period if suspected. HS is the commonest congenital haemolytic anaemia in Caucasian populations half present in the neonatal period. Worldwide, G6PD deficiency occurs in 3% population; neonatal presentation is common in Mediterranean and Canton peoples. α thalassaemia is incompatible with life causing hydrops fetalis (all 4 α globin genes deleted), or may present as HbH disease (3 of the 4 α globin genes deleted) with mild-to-moderate haemolysis in neonate.

Hereditary RBC defects in neonatal haemolytic anaemia

- Membrane defects:
  - Hereditary spherocytosis, hereditary elliptocytosis and variants e.g. stomatocytosis and pyropoikilocytosis (Afro-Americans).
- Haemoglobin defects:
  - αδβ thalassaemia.
  - Unstable haemoglobins (e.g. HbKöln, HbZurich).
- Enzyme defects:
  - Glycolytic pathway; pyruvate kinase and other enzyme deficiencies.
  - Hexose monophosphate shunt; G6PD deficiency, other enzymes.

Clinical features

Congenital haemolytic anaemia with mild or moderate unconjugated hyperbilirubinaemia. No gross excess of bile pigments in urine (old collective name for these diseases was 'acholuric jaundice'), ± hepatosplenomegaly. A +ve family history is common but not invariable.

Laboratory investigation

May be difficult to diagnose in neonate, especially if post-transfusion. Often have to wait until clinically stable some weeks/months later.

- Exclude acquired disorders, and immune lysis (DAT).
- RBC morphology is one key to diagnosis and further investigation, but spherocytes not specific for HS.
- Further tests for suspected:
  - Membrane defect (osmotic fragility, autohaemolysis, dye binding, membrane chemistry).
  - Hb defect; Hb electrophoresis, HbF, HbA_2 measurement.
  - Enzyme defect; Heinz body prep, screening tests for specific enzymes, G6PD, PK.
- Heinz body test +ve:
  - Drug or chemical induced in neonate without hereditary defect.
  - Enzyme deficiency: G6PD commonest but consider others.
  - Unstable Hb.
  - α thalassaemia.

Outcome

Given supportive management including transfusion if necessary, most problems due to congenital red cell defects other than haemoglobinopathies will improve during the first weeks and months of life as the infant matures.

Where the haemolysis is likely to be chronic folic supplementation should be commenced.

Acquired red cell defects

These may be either immune or non-immune. Main cause of the latter will be underlying infection either acquired *in utero* or in the days following delivery. Drug-induced haemolysis in the newborn is rare.

Pathophysiology

Neonatal RBCs have ↑ sensitivity to oxidative stress due to altered enzyme activity, and are more liable to be destroyed by altered physical conditions, mechanical factors, toxins and drugs than adult RBC. Infection acquired *in utero* post-natally is a common cause of mild-to-moderate haemolytic anaemia. The mechanism is multifactorial, and includes ↑ reticuloendothelial activity and microangiopathic damage. Drug-induced haemolysis and Heinz body formation is occasionally noted as a transient phenomenon in normal neonatal RBCs as a result of chemical or drug toxicity but is much more often seen when there is an underlying RBC defect such as G6PD deficiency.

Acquired RBC defects causing congenital haemolytic anaemia

- Infection:
  - Congenital TORCH infections also rare but serious are malaria (can cause stillbirth) and syphilis.
  - Post-natal, either viral or (more commonly) bacterial.
- Microangiopathy—2° to severe infections ± DIC, also Kasabach–Merritt syndrome (giant haemangioma with haemolysis and thrombocytopenia).
- Drug or chemically induced.
- Infantile pyknocytosis.
- (Rare) metabolic disease such as Wilson's disease, galactosaemia.

Clinical features

Congenital infections: all rare with adequate antenatal care. Most infants with herpes simplex will be symptomatic with DIC and hepatic dysfunction—haemolysis is not a major finding. Haemolytic anaemia is also mild in CMV and rubella infections but 50% infants with toxoplasmosis will be anaemic (may be severe).

Post-natal infections: viral, bacterial and protozoal (congenital malaria can be delayed for some days or weeks or it can be acquired early in life). Anaemia can be severe and associated with DIC.

MAHA 2° to toxic damage to the endothelium is rare in the neonate outside the context of DIC and sepsis, and is seen in burns and (classically) in the Kasabach–Merritt syndrome—a visible or covert giant haemangioma with haemolysis, RBC damage and profound thrombocytopenia.

Drugs/chemical exposure is more likely to cause Heinz body haemolysis in premature babies or those with G6PD deficiency. Incriminating agents include sulphonamides, chloramphenicol, mothballs, aniline dyes, maternal intake of diuretics, and, in the past, water-soluble vitamin K analogues. Vitamin E (a potent antioxidant) has a number of RBC stabilizing activities. Now rare due to dietary supplements, deficiency used to be seen occasionally in premature infants, following O_2 therapy and diets rich in polyunsaturated fatty acids. Clinical findings included haemolysis, pretibial oedema, and CNS signs. Acanthocytosis/pyknocytosis of the RBC is characteristic, and this may have been the main cause of infantile pyknocytosis.

Infantile pyknocytosis: indicates the diagnostic feature of this ncommon acquired disorder. Haemolysis with ↑ numbers (>6–50%) of pyknocytes (irregularly contracted RBCs with multiple projections) in the peripheral blood. Cause unknown, though may be associated with vitamin E deficiency. Anaemia may be severe and present at birth, and is most striking at ~3 weeks (Hb <5g/dL reported). Exchange transfusion occasionally required but the condition spontaneously remits by ~3 months. Its self-limiting nature and ill-understood pathology means that it may not be a distinct clinical entity.

Metabolic disorders—rare.

Laboratory investigation

Criteria set out above will establish the diagnosis of haemolytic anaemia. A +ve DAT points to an immune process—probably Rh/ABO disease. If non-immune, further tests to look for a congenital abnormality.

The diagnosis may be made by:

- Peripheral blood findings.
- Heinz body +ve—?chemical/drug-induced haemolysis.
- RBC enzyme screen to exclude G6PD or PK deficiency.
- Hb electrophoresis to exclude Hb defects.

Often no definitive cause is found and the HA will be presumed 2° to underlying systemic illness.

Management

1. General supportive measures for hyperbilirubinaemia (📖 Hyperbilirubinaemia, p.578).
2. Treatment of specific conditions
   - Haemolytic disease of the newborn—📖 HDN, p.574.
   - Neonatal infection as appropriate.
   - Exchange transfusion almost never needed.

Outlook

Prognosis is that of the underlying condition. Anaemia will usually respond as the underlying condition is brought under control.

Haemolytic disease of the newborn (HDN)

Arises when there is blood group incompatibility between mother and fetus. Maternal Abs produced against fetal RBC antigens cross the placenta and destroy fetal RBCs. Most commonly caused by the Rh (D) antigen, but maternal passive immunization with Rh (D) immunoglobulin (anti-D) introduced in the late 1960s transformed the outlook. Despite this, HDN due to anti-D and other red cell antibodies (e.g. anti-c anti-Kell) still remains an important cause of fetal morbidity.

Pathogenesis

Placental transfer of fetal cells → maternal circulation is maximal at delivery the condition does not usually present in the firstborn (*Note*: ABO incompatibility is an exception). Previous maternal transfusion, abortion, amniocentesis, chorionic villus sampling (CVS), or obstetric manipulations can cause antibody formation. Maternal IgG crosses placenta, reacts with Ag +ve fetal RBCs.

Rh HDN

Classically presents as jaundice in first 24h of life.

- ***Mild HDN:*** may go unnoticed and presents as persistent hyperbilirubinaemia or late anaemia weeks after birth.
- ***Severe HDN:*** may result in a macerated fetus, fresh stillbirth, or severely anaemic, grossly oedematous infant (hydrops fetalis) with hepato-splenomegaly 2° to compensatory extramedullary haemopoiesis in utero.
- ***Kernicterus:*** neurological damage 2° to bilirubin deposition in the brain, depends on a number of factors including the unconjugated bilirubin level, maturity of the baby, the use of interacting drugs.

Diagnosis

Rh HDN is the commonest cause of neonatal immune haemolysis; routine antenatal screening should identify most cases prior to delivery allowing appropriate action.

***In suspected case at delivery cord blood* is tested for:**

- ABO and Rh (D) group.
- Presence of antibody on fetal RBCs by DAT.
- Hb and blood film (spherocytes, ↑ polychromasia, NRBCs).
- Serum bilirubin (↑).

***Maternal blood* is tested for:**

- ABO and Rh (D) group.
- Serum antibodies against fetal cells (by indirect antiglobulin test, IAGT).
- Antibody titre.
- Kleihauer test—detects and quantitates fetal RBCs in maternal circulation.

Diagnostic findings include:

- DAT +ve haemolytic anaemia ± spherocytosis in the infant.
- Maternal anti-D, or other anti Rh antibody—the next most common to produce severe disease is anti-c.

ABO HDN

Theoretically should occur more frequently since ~1 in 4/5 babies and mothers are ABO incompatible. Usually occurs in group O mothers who may have high titres of naturally occurring IgG anti-A or B, and with a boost to this during pregnancy haemolysis can occur.

Clinical features

1st pregnancies are not exempt, but condition is usually mild. Presentation is later than with Rh HDN (2–4d, but may be weeks after birth).

Diagnosis

May be difficult—DAT commonly and puzzlingly –ve, but offending antibody can be eluted from infant RBC.

Antibody studies

Maternal high titre anti-A/B almost always in a group O mother cord-blood/infant's serum—an inappropriate antibody (e.g. anti-A in a group A baby).

Other blood group antibodies

Can occasionally produce severe HDN; anti-Kell in particular. Serological testing will establish diagnosis. Maternal autoimmune haemolytic anaemia may produce a similar picture to alloimmune HDN where the auto-antibody cross-reacts with the infant RBC. Usually the diagnosis will have been made antenatally. Severity in infant varies depending on maternal condition.

Management—prevention

Routine antenatal maternal ABO and Rh D grouping and antibody testing carried out at booking visit (~12–16 weeks).

- ***If antibody +ve*** repeat at intervals to check the antibody titre.
- ***If antibody –ve and Rh D –ve*** repeat at ~28 weeks' gestation. Establish if paternal red cells heterozygous, homozygous, or –ve for the specific Ag.

Anti-D prophylaxis

- 250IU IM during pregnancy to Rh D –ve women without antibodies to cover any intrauterine manoeuvre or miscarriage.
- After delivery, a standard dose of 500IU anti-D within 72h unless baby is known to be Rh (D) –ve.
- If Kleihauer test result shows a bleed of >4mL give further anti-D.

Treatment of affected fetus—before delivery

Treatment depends on past obstetric history, the nature and titre of the antibody, and paternal expression of the antigen. The fetal genotype can be established by CVS, fetal blood sampling, and PCR.

Examination of the amniotic fluid to assess the degree of hyperbilirubinaemia is indicated with a poor past history (exchange transfusion or stillbirth in previous baby) and high titre (1:8–1:64) of an antibody likely to cause severe HDN (e.g. anti-D, anti-c, or anti-Kell). The amniotic fluid bilirubin at optical density 450nm dictates treatment according to the Liley chart (📖 Fig. 12.1), which estimates the blood concentration.

Options include intrauterine transfusion (IUT) if fetus is not deemed mature enough for delivery (check lung maturity on phospholipid levels) or induction of labour if it is. Intensive maternal plasmapheresis may be useful to reduce antibody titre. Advances in management of very premature babies are such that nowadays IUT rarely performed.

After delivery

- Full paediatric support—metabolic, nutritional, and respiratory.
- If unconjugated hyperbilirubinaemia not a problem, treat anaemia (*Note*: cord blood Hb <14.0g/dL) by simple transfusion.
- Exchange transfusion with Rh (D) –ve and (if possible) group specific blood for:
  - A severely affected hydropic anaemic baby.
  - Hyperbilirubinaemia (bilirubin level at or near 340mmol/L (20mg/dL) or rapidly rising level e.g. >20mmol/h) in first few days of life.
  - Signs suggesting kernicterus—exchange transfusion may have to be repeated.
- Phototherapy to reduce the bilirubin level.
- Follow-up required—late anaemia can be severe particularly if exchange transfusion has not been carried out.

Outcome

With modern techniques, the outlook is good even for severely affected infants.

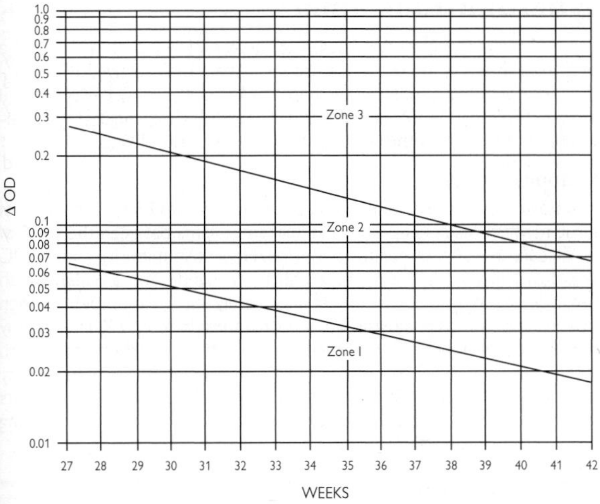

Fig. 12.1 Liley chart.

The amount of bilirubin can be quantitated by spectrophotometrically measuring absorbance at 450nm wavelength in a specimen of amniotic fluid that has been shielded from light. The results (delta 450) are plotted on a 'Liley' curve, which is divided into 3 zones.

A result in **Zone I** indicates mild or no disease. Fetuses in zone I are usually followed with amniocentesis every 3 weeks. A result in zone II indicates intermediate disease. Fetuses in low **Zone II** are usually followed by amniocentesis every 1–2 weeks. A result above the middle of Zone II may require transfusion or urgent delivery.

Hyperbilirubinaemia

Bilirubin results from the breakdown of haem, mostly Hb haem. It may be unconjugated, water insoluble, pre-hepatic (a mark of excessive RBC breakdown) or conjugated, soluble, post-hepatic (↑ in cholestasis). Unconjugated bilirubin ↑ in most neonates and is usually physiological; conjugated hyperbilirubinaemia, on the other hand, is almost always pathological.

Pathophysiology

Physiological jaundice is defined as a temporary inefficient excretion of bilirubin which results in jaundice in full-term infants between the d2–8 of life. Occurs in ~90% of healthy neonates. Hepatic immaturity and ↑ RBC breakdown overloads the neonate's ability to handle the bilirubin which is mainly unconjugated. The bilirubin is rarely >100micromol/L, though between 2–5d occasionally can be >200 in a term baby or 250 in a healthy pre-term. Levels much above this need investigation. Reaches a maximum by d3–6 and usually ↓ to normal by d10. In premature neonates it may take longer to settle. HDN due to blood group incompatibility accounts for ~10% cases of hyperbilirubinaemia and about 75% of those requiring exchange transfusion.

Causes

Table 12.3 Causes of hyperbilirubinaemia

Unconjugated	Conjugated
Physiological jaundice	Mechanical obstruction
Haemolytic anaemia	Bile duct abnormalities (e.g. atresia, cysts)
Haematoma	Hepatocellular disorders
Polycythaemia	Hepatitis
Biochemical defects	

Clinical features

- ►*Note: clinical jaundice in the first 24h of life is always pathological.*
- Presenting after this, the jaundice may/not be pathological—usually not. Inadequate food/fluid intake with dehydration can aggravate the physiological bilirubin. A higher concentration is acceptable for the full-term breast-fed baby (serum bilirubin 240micromol/L) than bottle-fed baby (190micromol/L).
- Jaundice in an active healthy infant is likely to be physiological.
- In a sick infant the underlying cause of the jaundice may be clinically evident—e.g. infection, anaemia, shock, asphyxia, haemorrhage (may be occult).
- Physical examination—hepatosplenomegaly is pathological.
- Maternal history (drugs, known condition) and family history may help.

Laboratory investigations

- FBC, reticulocyte count, and film—?haemolytic anaemia.
- Serum bilirubin—?conjugated or unconjugated:
  - Unconjugated hyperbilirubinaemia.
    —DAT, maternal and neonatal blood group serology.
    —Infection evaluation including TORCH.
    —Thyroid function.
    —Reducing substances.
  - Conjugated hyperbilirubinaemia.
    —Abdominal USS, bile pigments in stool, liver pathology.
- Further investigation as determined by results and clinical picture.

Management

- General—adequate hydration, nutrition, other supportive measures.
- Treat underlying cause—antibiotics, metabolic disturbances.
- Haemolytic anaemia—blood transfusion.
- Specific phototherapy (light source with wavelength between 400–500mm) effective in treating most causes of unconjugated hyper-bilirubinaemia. *Note*: contraindicated in conjugated hyperbilirubinaemia.
- Exchange transfusion—the indications are complex. Main indication is severe haemolytic anaemia and is used in full-term infants when the bilirubin is >340micromol/L and at a lower concentration in premature infants.
- Hyperbilirubinaemia due to mechanical obstruction may need surgery.

Outcome

In most infants hyperbilirubinaemia resolves by 2 weeks. When pathology has been excluded the commonest cause of prolonged hyperbilirubinaemia persisting beyond this period is breastfeeding. In 20% healthy breast-fed infants the bilirubin is still significantly ↑ at d21. Kernicterus is not a complication but the condition causes concern before it spontaneously remits.

Neonatal haemostasis

Neonates can develop bruising and/or purpura due to defects in platelets, coagulation factors, or both. Coagulation tests should be interpreted with caution because in the term infant the concentration of vitamin K-dependent proteins (II, VII, XI, and X together with protein C and protein S) are 50% of normal adult values, contact factors (XI, XII, PK, and HMWK) are 30–50% of adult concentrations, and all are lower in pre-terms. Factors VIII, V, and vWF are normal . Thrombin inhibitors antithrombin (AT, previously called antithrombin III) and HCII are ↓ but α2-M is ↑. Platelet count is the same as adults in both term and pre-term infants. There are technical problems in obtaining uncontaminated (heparin from catheters or IV lines) and adequate venous samples from neonates, causing *in vitro* inhibition or pre-test activation of clotting factors or dilution due to short sampling and thus excess anticoagulant. All can give spurious results.

Pathophysiology

Haemostatic and fibrinolytic system in neonates is immature. Sepsis, liver disease, necrotizing colitis and RDS can precipitate DIC easily. Thrombocytopenia can be caused by DIC and also immune mechanisms or marrow failure.

Clinical features

- Petechiae indicate problems with small vessels or platelets, bruises can be due to platelet deficiencies and/or coagulation disorders.
- Oozing from multiple venepunture sites in sick infants usually indicates generalized haemostatic failure and DIC.
- Haemorrhagic disease of the newborn due to functional vitamin K deficiency presents in 3 forms with bruising, purpura and GI bleeding in otherwise well babies; early (within 24h) usually due to maternal drugs such as warfarin; classical (days 2–5) in babies who have not been given adequate vitamin K prophylaxis and who have been breast fed; and late, a variant of the classical form (i.e. insufficient vitamin K, breast-fed) arising at 2–8 weeks and with a higher morbidity and ↑ incidence of ICH.
- Thrombosis usually catheter related, can be rarely associated with AT III deficiency or homozygous protein C and protein S deficiency (neonatal purpura fulminans—a life-threatening condition with wide-spread peripheral gangrene).
- Haemophilia and other coagulant deficiencies can cause large haematomas but rarely cause trouble in the neonatal period except factor XIII lack—typically presents with bleeding from the umbilical stump.
- In well babies, petechiae and bruises with thrombocytopenia suggests immune basis—antibody usually from mother (alloimmune or autoimmune). Rarely, infants under a month can develop endogenous ITP.
- Clear symptoms of thrombocytopenia with normal platelet count suggests major functional defect—Glanzmann's.
- Marrow failure due to infiltration, aplasia.

Table 12.4 Disorders causing bleeding in neonates

Inherited (rare)	Acquired (common)
• Haemophilia	• DIC (sepsis, necrotizing colitis, hypoxia, RDS)
• von Willebrand's disease (only type 3)	• Vitamin K deficiency
• Other inherited factor deficiencies	• Liver disease
• Inherited thrombotic disorders	• Acquired thrombotic disorders
• Glanzmann's thrombasthenia	• Neonatal alloimmune thrombocytopenia
• Inherited BM failure syndromes	• Maternally derived ITP • Endogenous ITP • Aplasia • Leukaemia

Neonatal alloimmune thrombocytopenia (NAIT)

Occurs when mothers form alloimmune antibodies against fetal platelet-specific antigens that their own platelets lack. These antibodies react with fetal platelets *in utero* causing thrombocytopenia which can be severe, and in some cases life threatening in late pregnancy and early life. A more serious condition with greater morbidity than thrombocytopenia due to maternal autoantibodies against platelets—i.e. where the mother has ITP.

Pathophysiology

In >90% cases the mother will be HPA-1a (old term = PLA1) –ve with anti-HPA-1a antibodies against the HPA-1a +ve fetus; only 2% population are HPA-1a –ve (i.e. homozygous HPA-1b). Incidence of NAIT is 1/1000 pregnancies and accounts for 10–20% cases of neonatal thrombocytopenia. Other antigens may be involved e.g. HPA-5 (Br) and HPA-3 (Bak) are the commonest.

Clinical features

- Commonly presents in first-born infant and recurs in 85–90%.
- Maternal platelet count normal with no past history of ITP.
- Bleeding manifestations in 10–20% evident within the first few days of life e.g. umbilical haemorrhage, petechiae, ecchymosis, internal haemorrhage, intracranial haemorrhage (ICH).
- Baby's platelet count ↑ to normal over the next 2–3 weeks as the antibody is cleared.
- Haemorrhage *in utero* with fatal ICH in ~1% cases.

📖 See Table 12.5 for laboratory diagnosis.

Management

Of bleeding neonate

Transfuse platelets –ve for Ag (usually HPA-1a –ve); use random donor platelets in an emergency. Maternal platelets (*irradiated*) are a good source. Repeat platelet transfusion PRN. IVIg as for ITP can be used in exceptional cases (response within days). Close observation (ICH is potentially lethal—screen using USS).

Of subsequent pregnancies

Cordocentesis *in utero* at ~24 weeks; take 1–3mL blood for platelet count and phenotype. If affected, treatment needs to be started immediately.

Options

1. *In utero* CMV –ve compatible platelet transfusions at 2–4-weekly intervals (depending on severity and history). Invasive and technically demanding. Keep platelet count >50 × 10^9/L (platelets ↓ rapidly so frequent follow-up mandatory).
2. Maternal administration of IVIg (1g/kg) weekly from ~24 weeks onwards: check fetal platelet count ~4 weeks later and again near term; response variable—around 75% respond—transfuse platelets if non-responsive. Check cord blood at birth and treat as necessary.

Outcome

With aggressive treatment the outcome is good, death in utero and ICH occur rarely. A history of a previous ICH correlates with severe thrombocytopenia in subsequent pregnancies.

Table 12.5 Laboratory diagnosis

Baby	Parents
• Severe thrombocytopenia platelets <20 × 10^9/L in 50%	• Mother's platelet count normal
• BM has megakaryocytes ++ (not usually necessary)	• Serology: • Mother's platelets usually HPA-1a –ve • Rarer Ab include anti-HPA-3 • HPA-5b, HPA-4 (Yuk/Pen) • Mother's serum contains anti-platelet antibody • (*Note*: antibody titre cannot predict degree of thrombocytopenia in fetus in subsequent pregnancies) • Father's platelets carry offending antigen

Congenital dyserythropoietic anaemias

A rare group of inherited lifelong anaemias with morphologically abnormal marrow erythroblasts and ineffective erythropoiesis. 3 clinically distinguishable types are recognized where inheritance may be recessive (types I and II) or dominant (type III), 📖 see Table 12.6. A number of families have been described that share some features but do not fit with the typical patterns.

Pathophysiology

Ineffective erythropoiesis (cell death within the BM); RBC survival in PB is not much reduced (III). Abnormal serological and haemolytic characteristics (type II CDA) and membrane abnormalities are described but as yet no defining shared defect in all cases of CDA.

Clinical features

- Age of presentation variable; but usually in older children (>10 years). Can rarely present as neonatal jaundice and anaemia.
- Anaemia—in type I, Hb 8.0–12.0g/dL; type II anaemia may be more severe, patient may be transfusion dependent. Type III (rare) anaemia is mild/moderate.
- Jaundice (2° to intramedullary RBC destruction).
- Gallstones.
- Splenomegaly common.

Laboratory diagnosis

- Peripheral blood—normocytic/macrocytic RBC with anisopoikilocytosis.
- WBC and platelets usually ↔; reticulocytes slightly ↑.
- BM appearance—striking, showing ↑ cellularity with excess abnormal erythroblasts.
- Type II shows +ve acidified serum test.
- ↑ serum ferritin due to ↑ Fe absorption; haemosiderosis can occur without transfusion dependence. Type III very occasionally Fe deficient due to intravascular haemolysis and haemosiderinuria.

Differential diagnosis

- CDA variants (CDA types IV to VII)—not all CDA falls neatly into 3 subtypes on BM findings, serology, or clinical features.
- PNH—acidified serum test is +ve with heterologous and autologous serum. In HEMPAS +ve with heterologous serum only.
- Other megaloblastic/dyserythropoietic anaemias—including vitamin B12 and folate deficiency.
- 1°/acquired sideroblastic anaemia.
- Erythroleukaemia (M6 AML).

Treatment

- Mostly unnecessary.
- Avoid blood transfusion if possible (Fe overload)—Fe chelation as necessary.
- Splenectomy not curative but may decrease transfusion requirements.
- Type I may respond to high dose IFN-α; not recommended as routine therapy.

Natural history

Severity of CDA varies considerably and many patients have good QoL with no therapy. Haemosiderosis is a long-term complication which may impact on survival.

Table 12.6 Types of congenital dyserythropoietic anaemias

Type	Bone marrow	Blood findings	Inheritance
I	Megaloblastic + intra-nuclear chromatin bridges	Macrocytic RBC	Recessive**
II (HEMPAS)*	Bi/multinuclearity with	Normocytic RBCs pluripolar mitosis. Lysis in acidified serum (not autologous serum)	Recessive
III	Giant erythroblasts with multinuclearity	Macrocytic	Dominant

*Hereditary erythroblast multinuclearity with +ve acidified serum test; commonest form, found in ~66% cases: **The *CDAN1* gene is mutated in majority of Type 1 patients

Congenital red cell aplasia

First desribed by Josephs in 1936 and subsequently by Diamond and Blackfan in 1938. Has come to be known as Diamond–Blackfan anaemia (DBA). Incidence now estimated to be 4–7/million live births.

Pathophysiology

DBA is a heterogeneous disorder with evidence for at least 3 genetic subtypes. Approximately 25% of DBA patients have a heterozygous mutation in the *RPS19* gene located on chromosome 19 (19q13.2). This gene has an ubiquitous expression profile and encodes a ribosomal protein. Its precise function is unknown but is predicted to have a role in ribosomal biogenesis. DBA therefore appears to be constitutional disorder arising from disruption of a key house keeping pathway. This is associated with pleotropic effects in many systems but the maximal impact is on erythropoiesis resulting in a deficiency of red cells.

Clinical features

- Usually presents in the 1st year of life: in 25% at birth and 90% <6 months of age. Rarely presents >1 year.
- Mildly affected individuals may rarely be detected as older children or adults during family studies.
- Associated physical anomalies in 50%; abnormal facies with abnormal eyes, webbed neck, malformed (including triphalangeal) thumbs, other skeletal abnormalities, short stature, congenital heart lesions, renal defects.
- Anaemia usually severe and child commonly transfusion dependent.
- Susceptibility to infection is not ↑.
- Hepatosplenomegaly absent.
- Family history is +ve in only 10–20% cases; most are sporadic.
- ↑ risk of AML in long survivors; ~5% in biggest series reported to date.

Laboratory diagnosis

- ↓ Hb, ↓ reticulocytes, ↑ MCV (> ↔ for age), WBC and platelets not ↓.
- Red cells—↔ morphology to red cell anisocytosis/macrocytosis, have ↑ i antigen positivity, ↑ ADA activity.
- ↑ HbF, ↑ EPO, ↑ serum Fe/ferritin.
- BM findings—usually absent erythroid precursors; other cell lines ↔.
- No evidence of parvovirus infection.
- Radiological investigation to define other congenital defects.
- Genetic diagnosis possible in 25% of DBA patients (*RPS19* gene).

Differential diagnosis

- TEC (📖 Transient erythroblastopenia of childhood, p.588; later presentation, transient, no other defects).
- Drugs, malnutrition, infection.
- Haemolytic anaemias in hypoplastic phase, with parvovirus B19, delayed recovery in HDN.
- Megaloblastic anaemia in aplastic phase.

Treatment

- Prednisolone 2mg/kg PO in divided doses, slowly ↓ over weeks; 70% respond well. Titrate to lowest dose to maintain Hb >7g/dL. Many achieve this on almost homeopathic doses despite true dependence. Around 10% need high dose maintenance and have trouble with side effects. 30% steroid resistant.
- Transfusion dependency usual in those who cannot be maintained on very low dose steroids. Need chelation to prevent Fe overload. Use CMV –ve leucocyte-depleted packed RBC.
- Splenectomy not helpful (unless hypersplenism).
- BM transplantation worth considering for transfusion dependents with suitable sibling donor; risk stratification as for severe thalassaemia (Fe overload). Complicated decision due to chance of spontaneous remission even after years of transfusion dependency.

Natural history

Spontaneous remission in 10–20% (even after several years). Median survival estimated at 30–40 years, though data patchy. Death due to haemosiderosis, complications of steroid therapy, or evolution of AML or aplastic anaemia. BMT may offer better outlook. DBA Registries are now prospectively gathering new data.

Acquired red cell aplasia

Isolated failure of erythropoiesis. Most commonly transient—either due to parvovirus B19 infection or transient erythroblastopenia of childhood (TEC). Acquired pure red cell aplasia (PRCA) seen in adults with or without thymoma and probably autoimmune in nature (📖 Aplastic anaemia, p.98) virtually unknown in childhood, though very occasionally seen in adolescents.

Parvovirus B19 infection

Clinical features

- Causes transient reticulocytopenia and (occasionally) neutropenia and thrombocytopenia in otherwise healthy individuals.
- In children with ↑ red cell turnover for any reason (compensated haemolysis, ineffective erythropoiesis) or those with reduced red cell production (marrow suppression or hypoplasia) can produce dramatic falls in Hb ('aplastic crisis').
- Can affect any age.
- Self-limiting as infection subsides following antibody response, 7–10d.
- In immunosuppressed children (e.g. chemotherapy, HIV) anaemia can occasionally become chronic with persisting viraemia.

Pathogenesis

Parvovirus shows tropism for red cells through the P antigen, and is cytotoxic for erythroid progenitor cells at the colony forming stage (CFU-E) *in vitro*.

Transient erythroblastopenia of childhood

Pathogenesis

Serum and cellular inhibitors of erythropoiesis and defective BM response to stimulating cytokines have been demonstrated. The condition may be idiopathic or associated with viral infection. It is uncommon but not excessively rare and there may be many subclinical cases where a blood count is not done.

Clinical features

- Boys and girls equally affected: age range 6 months–5 years; most commonly around 2 years.
- Typically a previously well young child presents with symptoms and signs of anaemia, sometimes but not invariably following an infection. Onset is insidious and the child becomes listless and pale—or just pale.
- Associated infections are usually viral (EBV, mumps), preceding the onset of TEC by some weeks.
- Fever is rare.
- Pallor may be striking.
- No lymphadenopathy or hepatosplenomegaly.
- No physical abnormalities.

Laboratory diagnosis

- Normocytic, normochromic anaemia which may be severe (Hb <5g/dL).

- Reticulocytes absent unless in early recovery phase; WBC and platelets usually normal .
- Blood film shows no abnormality other than anaemia.
- Biochemical profile normal.
- BM shows normocellular picture with absent erythroid precursors. normal Fe content.
- No karyotypic abnormalities.
- Exclude parvovirus infection (📖 Parovirus B19 infection, p.588).
- No other investigation is of diagnostic help.

Differential diagnosis

- Exclude acute blood loss and anaemia of chronic disease.
- Exclude common ALL.
- Diamond–Blackfan anaemia (📖 Congenital red cell aplasia, p.586). Usually presents within the first 6 months of life and other abnormalities (skeletal malformation, short stature, abnormal facies) are commonly present.
- Parvovirus infection (📖 Parovirus B19 infection, p.588)

Treatment

Blood transfusion should be avoided but may be necessary if symptomatic.

Natural history

Spontaneously remits (if not then diagnosis probably wrong) commonly within 4–8 weeks but may be up to 6 months. Relapse is rare. There are no long-term sequelae or associations.

Fanconi anaemia (FA)

First described by Fanconi in 1927, Fanconi anaemia (FA) is a clinically heterogeneous disorder usually presenting in childhood with the common feature being slowly progressive marrow failure affecting all 3 cell lines (RBC, WBC, and megakaryocytes) and manifest by peripheral blood pancytopenia and eventual marrow aplasia.

It is usually an autosomal recessive disorder with several different germ-line genetic mutations involving at least 12 genes (*FANCA* to *FANCM*), 11 of which have been identified and characterized, and all of which are on different chromosomes. One FA subtype (FAB) is X-linked. The products of the FA genes are components of the 'FA-BRCA pathway' important in the maintenance of genomic stability of the cell.

Pathophysiology of FA

FA affects all cells of the body and the cellular phenotype is characterized by ↑ chromosomal breakage, hypersensitivity to DNA cross-linking agents such as diepoxybutane (DEB) and mitomycin C (MMC), hypersensitivity to oxygen, ↑ apoptosis, and accelerated telomere shortening. The ↑ chromosomal fragility is characteristic and used as a diagnostic test. Apart from progressive marrow failure, 70% of FA patients show somatic abnormalities, chiefly involving the skeleton. 90% develop marrow failure and survivors show an ↑ risk of developing leukaemia, chiefly AML. Rarely, FA can present as AML. There is also an ↑ risk of liver tumours and squamous cell carcinomas.

Clinical features

- Autosomal recessive inheritance usually, rarely X-linked: in 10–20% the parents are related.
- Phenotypic expression of the disease varies widely, though often similar in any given kindred. Most commonly presents as insidious evolution of pancytopenia, presenting in mid-childhood with a median age of presentation of 9 years. Cell lines affected asynchronously; isolated thrombocytopenia may be first manifestation, lasting 2–3 years before other cytopenias occur.
- 10% present in adolescence or adult life, 4% present in early infancy (<1 year).
- Disorders of skin pigmentation common (60%)—café-au-lait spots, hypo- and hyperpigmentation.
- Short stature in 60%, microcephaly, and delayed development in >20%.
- Congenital abnormalities can affect almost any system—skeletal defects common, >50% in the upper limb especially thumb, spine, ribs.
- Characteristic facies described—elfin-like, with tapering jaw line.

Diagnosis

Laboratory findings

- Pancytopenia and hypoplastic marrow—patchy cellularity.
- BM may also show dyserythropoietic morphology.
- Anaemia varies in its severity and may be macrocytic (MCV 100–120fL).

- Excessive chromosomal breaks/rearrangements in culture of peripheral blood lymphocytes stressed with clastogens (DEB or MMC) is the defining abnormality, and can be used on fetal cell culture for antenatal diagnosis.
- Direct probing for mutations in the FA genes that have been identified and characterized permits molecular diagnosis in >95% of patients, but is complex, slow, and is not routinely available.
- Further investigation for systemic congenital abnormalities is indicated.

Differential diagnosis

- Acquired aplastic anaemia (📖 Aplastic anaemia, p.98)
- Other congenital or inherited childhood marrow failure syndromes—📖 see Rare congenital marrow failure syndromes, p.592.
- Bloom syndrome—clinically like FA with similar congenital defects, spontaneous chromosomal breaks, and a predisposition to leukaemia but without pancytopenia, or BM hypoplasia. Autosomal recessive. Characteristically have photosensitivity and telangiectatic facial erythema. Due to genetic mutations in the *RECQL3* helicase gene.

Treatment

General

- Supportive—blood transfusion with Fe chelation as required.
- Treatment of associated congenital anomalies where necessary.

Specific

- Combined therapy with steroids (moderate dosage alternate days) and androgens (oxymetholone 0.5–5mg/kg/d). Most patients respond to treatment but eventually become refractory.
- Haemopoietic growth factors may offer temporary relief from neutropenia and anaemia.
- BMT is potentially curative, but FA patients hypersensitive to conditioning agents cyclophosphamide and radiation. Using low doses, matched sibling grafts give 70% actuarial survival at 2 years; unrelated donor results less good but improving using fludarabine based protocols. Early survivors showed ↑ risk of tumours, especially head and neck.
- Much interest in gene therapy. Early trials have occurred, but no major therapeutic success. Theoretically should be possible to transduce patient stem cells from those with known mutations with the appropriate wild type FA gene, and for these stem cells to have a natural growth advantage over FA cells. So far responses have been disappointing and short-lived.

Outcome

Median survival of conventional treatment responders who do not undergo BMT is ~25 years. Non-responders have a median survival of ~12 years. Death most commonly due to marrow failure, but 10–20% will develop MDS or AML after a median period of observation of 13 years.

Rare congenital marrow failure syndromes

Amegakaryocytic thrombocytopenia (congenital amegakaryocytic thrombocytopenia—CAMT)

Presents in infancy (usually at birth or within 2 months) with profoundly ↓ platelets and associated physical signs (petechiae and bruising). Around 40% of affected children also have other congenital abnormalities—chiefly neurologic or cardiac. Developmental delay is common. The marrow completely lacks megakaryocytes and the disorder evolves to severe aplastic anaemia in around 50% of sufferers, usually in the first few years of life. Has none of the unstable DNA features of Fanconi anaemia (📖 see Fanconi anaemia, p.590). Also quite distinct from the syndrome of thrombocytopenia with absent radius (TAR syndrome) since it is a trilineage problem with a much greater mortality. Usually sporadic, but familial cases occur and disorder thought to be inherited. In a subgroup of CAMT patients mutations in the gene encoding for the thrombopoietin receptor (*c-mpl*) have been identified.

Outlook

Without BMT, mortality from bleeding, infection or (occasionally) progression to leukaemia near 100%.

Amegakaryocytic thrombocytopenia with absent radii (TAR syndrome)

- Usually diagnosed at birth because of lower arm deformity due to bilateral radial aplasia.
- No hyperpigmentation.
- Isolated thrombocytopenia with other cell lines ↔.
- BM lacks megakaryocytes; has adequate WBC/RBC precursors.
- No chromosomal breaks in cell culture.
- Autosomal recessive; no gene yet identified.
- Thrombopoietin ↑; platelets gradually increase as child grows.
- Bleeding problems greatest in infancy.
- Supportive therapy only needed.

Outlook

Usually good, with problems receding as childhood proceeds. Occasional patients continue to have problems with ↓ platelets. No ↑ malignancy.

Dyskeratosis congenita (DC)

- Inherited multi-system disorder including mucocutaneous and haemopoietic abnormalities.
- Clinical triad of skin pigmentation, leucoplakia of the mucous membranes, dystrophic nails and in 80% patients BM failure develops, usually in the 2nd decade.
- X-linked (due to mutations in *DKC1-Xq28*), autosomal dominant (heterozygous mutations in *TERC-3q26* and *TERT-5p15* genes) and autosomal recessive subtypes recognized. The DC genes identified to date have an important role in the maintenance of telomeres.

- Other congenital and immunological abnormalities described.
- Chromosome fragility on challenge with DEB or mitomycin C normal—important to distinguish DC from FA (see Fanconi anaemia, p.590).
- Despite this DC is a chromosome instability disorder due to defective telomere maintenance. Results of BMT for aplastic anaemia in DC patients poor, perhaps because of this.
- Anecdotal reports of good response to haemopoietic growth factors. Majority of patients also have a haemopoietic response to oxymetholone.

Outlook

10% develop cancers before the age of 40 years—mostly epithelial, but also MDS/AML. Life expectancy depends on development of aplasia or malignancy. 30% survive to middle age. Results of BMT improving with low-intensity fludarabine based protocols.

Kostmann's syndrome (congenital neutropenia)

- Autosomal recessive.
- Severe neutropenia with neutrophils $<0.2 \times 10^9$/L.
- Marrow shows maturation arrest at promyelocyte/myelocyte stage.
- High risk of severe infection in untreated state.
- Not due to germline mutation in G-CSF receptor gene, though abnormal receptor may be present in myeloid precursors. Some cases attributed to mutations in neutrophil elastase (*ELA2*)
- 90% will respond to pharmacological doses of G-CSF and continue to do so for years.
- Up to 10% develop AML/MDS—role of G-CSF not clear, but probably complication of disease revealed by longer survival.

Diagnosis

Distinguish from cyclical neutropenia (by observation); benign congenital neutropenia (by WBC), and reticular dysgenesis, a severe inherited immunodeficiency with congenital lack of all white cells, including lymphocytes.

Outlook

Good provided response to G-CSF satisfactory and maintained. Non-responders may need BMT.

Shwachman–Diamond syndrome

- Congenital exocrine pancreatic insufficiency; chronic diarrhoea, malabsorption and growth failure associated with neutropenia and skeletal abnormalities.
- BM failure – usually leads to neutropenia but can evolve to pancytopenia.
- BM morphology varies—may be dysplastic/hypo/aplastic.
- Autosomal recessive, majority of patients have mutations in the *SBDS* gene on 7q11.
- Psychomotor delay common.

Diagnosis

- Exclude cystic fibrosis (by normal sweat test).
- Exclude FA (by normal chromosome fragility).

- Pearson's syndrome clinically similar with severe pancreatic insufficiency but with anaemia rather than neutropenia and marrow shows ring sideroblasts and vacuolization of red and white cell precursors.
- Genetic diagnosis now possible in majority of patients.

Treatment

- Supportive with pancreatic enzymes, G-CSF and antibiotics.
- Greatly ↑ risk (up to 25%) of progression to MDS/leukaemia (AML > ALL).
- Limited experience with BMT for aplasia/leukaemia; may be ↑ risk of cardiotoxicity—ventricular fibrosis seen at autopsy in 2/5 patients who died post BMT.

Outlook

Depends on development of severe aplasia or leukaemia; long survivors few if so. Pancreatic insufficiency improves as childhood progresses.

Seckel's syndrome—bird-headed dwarfism

- Rare autosomal recessive disorder with (proportionate) very short stature and mental deficiency.
- Facial features fancifully described as bird-like.
- The *ATR* (ataxia-telenagiectasia and Rad3 related protein) gene is mutated in Seckel patients.
- Progression to aplastic anaemia common, clinically similar to FA (📖 see Fanconi anaemia, p.590) but chromosome fragility usually has different features to FA.

Infantile osteopetrosis

- Pancytopenia can arise in this autosomal recessive disorder where the marrow cavity is obliterated with cortical bone due to a functional deficiency of osteoclasts.
- It is a 1° marrow failure in the sense that there is no marrow, but is a failure of the microenvironment rather than haemopoietic stem cells.

Outlook

Poor due to cranial compression, and children usually die in early childhood unless successful allogeneic BMT can replace normal osteoclast function.

Neutropenia in childhood

Apart from 1° marrow failure due to aplastic anaemia, or other marrow failure syndromes (Aplastic anaemia, p.98), or marrow suppression due to antineoplastic, immunosuppressive, or antiviral chemotherapy, neutropenia can also arise as an immune phenomenon, a cytokine mediated problem or due to cyclic or non-cyclic disturbances of the homeostasis of neutrophil production.

Pathophysiology

- Commonest cause of a clinically important low neutrophil count in children ($<0.5 \times 10^9$/L) is myelosuppression due to drugs.
- 1° marrow stem cell failure failure either involving all cell lines or granulopoiesis alone is rare.
- Neutropenia can also be due to less serious inherited deficiencies of neutrophil production where neutropenia can be variable or cyclical and the problem seems to be one of production control rather than 1° stem cell failure.
- Probably due to cytokine disturbances, several microbial infections can cause paradoxical neutropenia, particularly in neonates but also in older children (Table 12.7).
- Autoimmune causes of neutropenia can arise in infancy or later in childhood.
- Isoimmune neutropenia in the newborn—due to maternal antineutrophil antibodies and analogous to HDN.

Homeostatic disorders

Cyclic neutropenia

Rare. Neutropenia arising every 21d lasting 3–6d. Counts may fall $<0.2 \times 10^9$/L. Associated with episodes of fever, malaise, mucous membrane ulcers, lymphadenopathy. Serious infection can arise and deaths. May improve after puberty. Usually +ve family history when problem encountered in childhood; due to mutations in neutrophil elastase (*ELA2*) gene. Treatment supportive with antibiotics. G-CSF may be useful.

Chronic benign neutropenia

More common. Persistent rather than cyclical, though often variable without clear periodicity. Neutrophil count usually $>0.5 \times 10^9$/L, so clinically mild or silent. May have autosomal dominant or autosomal recessive family history. Variable severity, often mild with few problems. To be distinguished from severe congenital neutropenia (Kostmann's syndrome, p.593) by milder clinical course and (usually) later presentation. Some of these patients will have mutations in *ELA2*. Therapy not usually necessary.

Table 12.7 Infections causing neutropenia

Viruses	Bacteria	Others
RSV	Tuberculosis	Rickettsiae
Malaria	Typhoid/paratyphoid	
Influenza	*E. coli* (neonates)	
Measles		
Varicella		
HIV		

Autoimmune neutropenia (AIN)

Infant form of isolated autoimmune neutropenia occurs within 1st year of life; demonstrable autoantibodies. Not familial; girls>boys. Self-limiting and usually relatively benign. Therapy supportive. Steroids not usually needed and can increase infection risk. IVIg has been used.

Older children may get

- Isolated AI neutropenia.
- Neutropenia as part of Evans' syndrome (📖 Immune thrombocytopenia, p.484).
- Neutropenia as part of multi-system AI disease—lupus erythematosus.
- Immune neutropenia following allogeneic BMT.
- Felty's syndrome (rheumatoid arthritis with splenomegaly and hypersplenic cytopenias may also be associated with neutrophil autoantibodies.
- All are potentially more serious and complicated than the infant form and may require immunosuppression as well as supportive therapy.

Isoimmune neutropenia of the newborn

- Maternal antibodies to fetal neutrophil antigens cross the placenta and give rise to neutropenia in the newborn child.
- Most commonly antibodies directed at neutrophil-specific antigens NA1 and NA2. (Maternal HLA antibodies do not cause trouble because antigens expressed on many tissues so quickly absorbed.)
- Estimated incidence up to 3% of newborns, so may be more common than generally appreciated; perhaps because usually clinically mild and neutropenia thought to be acquired due to drugs/infection.
- Condition resolves by 2 months as antibody disappears.
- Severely affected babies may show recurrent staphylococcal skin infections. Therapy supportive. Need for exchange transfusion very rare.
- Diagnosis based on serology.

Prognosis of neutropenia

Whatever the cause, severe neutropenia ($<0.2 \times 10^9$/L) is serious and incompatible with long survival if prolonged. It requires careful expert management.

Disorders of neutrophil function

Acquired

Mild defects arise in many clinical situations; following some infections associated with drugs (steroids, chemotherapy) and systemic disease (malnutrition, diabetes mellitus, rheumatoid arthritis, CRF, sickle cell anaemia)—here the underlying condition will dominate the clinical picture.

Congenital

Inherited defects rare but several important and disabling syndromes occur in children.

Pathophysiology

Neutrophils produced in BM are released into circulation where they survive for only a few hours. Fundamental role is to kill bacteria. Do this by moving to site of infection drawn there (chemotaxis) by interaction of bacteria with complement and Ig (opsonization) and engulf them (phagocytosis). Killing is accomplished by H_2O_2 generation, release of lysosomal enzymes, neutrophil degranulation (respiratory burst). Several enzyme systems are involved (MPO, cytochrome system, HMP shunt). In the neonate neutrophil function is defective (↓ chemotaxis, phagocytosis, motility) particularly if premature, jaundiced. Killing is normal.

Classification

Disorders of all aspects of neutrophil function are described and there is no consensus as to how best to classify them. All are rare. In several of the best described conditions multiple defects are present (Table 12.8).

Table 12.8 Classification

↓ Chemotaxis	↓ Opsonization	↓ Killing
Lazy leucocyte syndrome	Complement C_3 deficiency	Chronic granulomatous disease
Hyper IgE syndrome		MPO deficiency
Chediak–Higashi syndrome		
↓ Specific neutrophil granules		

Clinical features

All congenital syndromes are rare and diagnosis of the specific defect difficult. Few haematological/immunological labs are set up to perform the required range of tests. Specialist referral for diagnosis and treatment is indicated and may be able to alter the otherwise grim prognosis in many of these conditions.

Lazy leucocyte syndrome

Leucocyte adhesion deficiency (LAD) due to mutations in the gene encoding the β-subunit of the β_2-integrins (LAD1) or defective glycosylation of ligands on leucocytes recognized by selectin family (LAD2). Rare. Autosomal recessive. ↑ Recurrent infections often in oral cavity, delayed wound healing.

Lab findings: ↑ neutrophil count, ↔ BM, abnormal chemotaxis on Rebuck skin window test. The condition is relatively mild. Treatment is of specific infections with the need for prophylaxis in some patients.

Hyperimmunoglobulin E syndrome

Also known as Job's syndrome (Old Testament) because of recurrent staphylococcal abscesses. Autosomal recessive inheritance, associated with atopic dermatitis and other autoimmune phenomena. Bacterial/fungal infection, chronic dermatitis.

Lab findings: ↑ IgE, ↑ eosinophils.

Complement deficiency

Autosomal recessive inheritance of C_3 deficiency, homozygotes have severe recurrent bacterial infection, particularly encapsulated organisms.

Chronic granulomatous disease (CGD)

Though rare, commonest life-threatening inherited neutrophil functional defect. >1 disorder. Most are sex linked, boys affected 7 × more frequently than girls, but 3 autosomal mutations recognized. Presents in early life but also in adults; carriers asymptomatic. Multiple skin and visceral abscesses, systemic infection (pneumonia, osteitis etc.)—bacterial/fungal, lymphadenopathy, hepatosplenomegaly. Lab features: nitro blue tetrazolium (NBT) test (an index of defective respiratory burst) +ve. Specific mutational analysis now possible for earlier and prenatal diagnosis. Outlook better than it used to be. Improved by aggressive antibiotic policy and IFN-γ. BMT little used due to improving outlook with conservative/prophylactic treatment. Early results poor. Prospect of gene therapy attractive with some early progress.

Chediak–Higashi syndrome

Rare autosomal recessive disorder due to mutations in lysosomal trafficking regulator, *CHS1/LYST*, gene. Multiple defects. Partial oculocutaneous albinism, recurrent infection, lymphadenopathy, peripheral neuropathy and cerebellar ataxia. A fatal accelerated phase occurs in ~85%, usually in the 2nd decade, with lymphocytic infiltration of liver/spleen/nodes/BM, pancytopenia.

Lab findings

- ↓ Hb, ↓ neutrophil count, ↓ platelet count.
- Characteristic giant greenish grey refractile granules in neutrophils (also lymph inclusions).
- Treatment is supportive. High dose ascorbic acid may help some patients. Anecdotal reports of successful BMT.

Myeloperoxidase deficiency

Autosomal recessive. Commonest of neutrophil dysfunction conditions (1:2000) but also least serious. Often asymptomatic. Manifest in diabetics with recurrent infections—commonly *Candida albicans*. Good prognosis.

Lab findings

- ↑ neutrophil/monocyte peroxidase on histochemical analysis.
- Automated cell counters using MPO activity to count neutrophils may show spurious neutropenia.

Childhood immune (idiopathic) thrombocytopenic purpura (ITP)

ITP occurring in children differs from the adult form of the diseas (📖 Immune thrombocytopenia, p.484) in 2 ways—first, most cases are c abrupt onset and rapidly self-limiting, and secondly those that progress t chronicity have a lower morbidity and mortality.

Epidemiology

Incidence of ITP in children overall around 4–5 per 100,000 per yea 10–20% become chronic—i.e. last >6 months.

Pathophysiology

Thrombocytopenia mediated by antibodies opsonizing platelets that ar then destroyed by the reticuloendothelial system. Antibodies can be par of immune complexes non-specifically attached to platelet Fc receptor (as in typical acute childhood ITP) or true autoantibodies usually targete at glycoproteins IIb/IIIa and Ib (as found in up to 75% of chronic childhoo ITP and commonly in adults).

Clinical features

- Onset of bruising ± petechiae abrupt (80–90%) or insidious (10–20%).
- May have gingival and oral mucosal bleeding or epistaxis.
- Life threatening bleeding extremely rare.
- Child otherwise perfectly well.
- May have history of recent infection; specific (rubella, varicella) or nonspecific (URTI).
- Can follow vaccination.

Laboratory diagnosis

- Isolated thrombocytopenia; blood count otherwise normal.
- Marrow shows abundant megakaryocytes and is otherwise normal (not necessary to investigate unless clinical course or presenting features unusual).
- Platelet antibody studies difficult to perform and not necessary in most cases since they do not alter management.
- Exclude EBV infection (infectious mononucleosis).
- Exclude multisystem autoimmune disease (ACL, ANA, +ve DAT test—not necessary unless disease becomes chronic.
- Exclude underlying immunodeficiency syndrome (HIV, Wiskott–Aldrich).

Differential diagnosis

- Congenital or familial thrombocytopenias.
- Leukaemia or aplastic anaemia.
- Other rare thrombocytopenias (e.g. type IIB vWD).
- Multisystem autoimmune disease—Evans' syndrome (AIHA + immune thrombocytopenia), systemic lupus erythematosus.
- Immune thrombocytopenia associated with immunodeficiency due to other disease—HIV infection, Hodgkin's disease, Wiskott–Aldrich syndrome.

lanagement

lewly presenting

eldom require urgent therapy though this is frequently given, either olyvalent IVIg 0.8g/kg (single dose) or prednisolone 4mg/kg for 7d. Never istified in the absence of obvious bleeding since neither therapy without isk. Simple observation for spontaneous recovery should be preferred.

hronic

lo therapy is needed based on platelet count alone. Absence of symptoms nd signs is sufficient. Excessive restriction of activities is seldom justified. Open access to expert help and advice provides reassurance to families nd teachers. If therapy required to control symptoms (recurrent nose-leeds, menorrhagia) try local measures or hormonal control. Regular VIg or steroids seldom effective and may produce more problems than ntreated disease. For the most difficult cases (very rare) splenectomy till worth considering, though post-splenectomy mortality may be greater han that of untreated ITP. Newer therapies include danazol and rituximab, hough experience still anecdotal and long-term risks not yet evaluated.

ife-threatening haemorrhage or other emergency

Risk of life-threatening haemorrhage very small (<1/1000 in 1st week after iagnosis) though is a function of a platelet count <10–20 x 10^9/L and the ime exposed to this. Risk consequently rises in rare children with chronic nremitting severe disease for >1–2 years for whom more adventurous herapy (splenectomy, rituximab) can be contemplated, though risk still mall and those of treatment may be higher. If a large intracranial (ICH) or other catastrophic bleed occurs, this can be dealt with by simultaneous nassive platelet transfusion, IVIg, IV methylprednisolone and (if the diagnosis is beyond doubt) emergency splenectomy. Mortality of major ICH ess than 50% given active therapy.

Outlook

Most children with ITP recover irrespective of therapy, usually within weeks or occasionally within months. Even 75% of those whose problem persists for >6 months eventually spontaneously remit, sometimes several years later. It is very rare for children to carry ITP into adult life and beyond, and the occasional individuals who do are unlikely to be much troubled by it or to develop autoimmune disease of other systems.

1. Guidelines for the investigation and management of idiopathic thrombocytopenic purpura in adults, children and in pregnancy (2003). *Br J Haematol*, **120**, 574–96.

Haemolytic uraemic syndrome (HUS)

Characterized by a triad of *microangiopathic haemolytic anaemia (MAHA)*, *renal failure*, and *thrombocytopenia*. More common in children than adults and of 2 types; the more common epidemic form and the less common sporadic form closely related to thrombotic thrombocytopenic purpura (TTP)—a disease primarily of adults that also rarely occurs in children. TTP has the same triad of signs with two others—fever and neurologic disturbances (📖 Thrombotic thrombocytopenic purpura, p.534)

Pathogenesis

HUS usually occurs in outbreaks and in 90% is due to *Escherichia coli* 0157 and other verocytotoxin-producing *E. coli*. Food sources of the infection include uncooked/undercooked meats, hamburgers, and poor food hygiene. The verocytotoxin causes endothelial damage, particularly of the renal endothelium, leading to the formation of fibrin-rich microthrombi and MAHA. Familial haemolytic uraemic syndrome (5–10% of cases) have a deficiency or dysfunction of complement factor H, which results in excessive C3 activation.

Clinical features

- Young children (<4 years) are especially prone to the disease.
- Acute onset with a history of abdominal pain and bloody diarrhoea.
- Onset of ↓ urine output heralding renal failure occurs days later.
- In ~10% onset is non-epidemic and insidious—can be associated with chemotherapy/TBI.
- Other symptoms: anaemia (may be severe), jaundice, bruising, bleeding.
- Absence of fever and neurologic signs distinguish it from TTP.

Laboratory findings

- MAHA may be severe.
- Film shows fragmented RBCs/schistocytes/spherocytes.
- Thrombocytopenia.
- Coagulation tests: PT/APTT—usually ↔; Fgn and F/XDPs also ↔; reduced large vWF multimers.
- Proteinuria and haematuria.
- Biochemical evidence of renal failure.
- Stool culture may be +ve for *E. coli*.

Differential diagnosis

- TTP (📖 Thrombotic thrombocytopenic purpura, p.534).
- Other causes of MAHA and renal failure.

Complications

- ARF → CRF rare but more likely in older children and those with sporadic insidious onset HUS.
- Microvascular thrombosis and infarction of other organs.

Treatment

- Renal failure—fluid restriction, correct electrolyte imbalance.
- If anuria persists >24h—dialysis as necessary.
- Blood transfusion for anaemia.

- Platelet transfusion rarely needed—may ↑ thrombotic risk.
- Severe persistent disease may require plasmapheresis as for TTP (📖 Thrombotic thrombocytopenic purpura, p.534).
- Specific treatment: none of proven value. In familial form replacement of factor H with FFP may be helpful.

Outcome

Epidemic HUS has a good prognosis, patients usually recover and it rarely recurs. CRF does occur occasionally. Insidious onset HUS has a poorer prognosis. Overall mortality ~5%.

Childhood cancer and malignant blood disorders

Epidemiology

In Europe 1 child in 600 develops cancer before the age of 15. Annual incidence 1:10,000; ~1200 new cases/year in UK. Pattern of childhood cancers is very different from that seen in adults: carcinomas are rarely seen. Overall, childhood cancer is slightly more common in boys than girls.

- ***Leukaemias*** account for about 35% of the total: 80% are some type of ALL, 15% some type of AML. 5% CMLs, (adult and juvenile types) or myelodysplastic syndromes. CLL does not occur in children.
- ***Brain tumours*** are commonest solid malignancies, 25% of the total. Different tumour types from adults; commonest medulloblastoma in posterior fossa.
- ***Embryonal tumours*** 15%, seen almost exclusively in children. Include neuroblastoma, nephroblastoma (Wilms' tumour), rhabdomyosarcoma, hepatoblastoma.
- ***Bone tumours*** 5% osteosarcoma, Ewing's sarcoma.
- ***Lymphomas*** 9%—NHL and Hodgkin's disease. NHL in children closely related biologically to ALL; low grade disease very rare.
- Remainder of cases are mainly germ cell and primitive neuroectodermal tumours (PNETs), including retinoblastomas.

Aetiology

- Childhood cancer generally represents aberrant growth and development. Defective repair and renewal may also be important in some cancers.
- Growths arising in infancy are mostly congenital and the genetic mutations concerned arise *in utero*. Causes of such mutations and those arising later in childhood largely unknown.
- Although isolated cases are attributable to high dose radiation (e.g. thyroid cancer in Chernobyl survivors), there is no convincing link to levels of background radiation or electromagnetic fields.
- Population mixing studies have suggested that patterns of exposure to infection may contribute to some cases of ALL in the peak years of incidence (2–6 years).
- Childhood cancer rarely familial, but study of retinoblastoma (rare tumour that is commonly familial) has led to better understanding of tumour suppressor genes; germline mutation in 1 allele of RB gene in affected families only gives rise to tumours in cells where there is an acquired mutation in the other, healthy, wild type allele (the 'two hit' hypothesis).
- Cancer arising in older children may still be due to intrauterine event as concordance studies in identical twins with ALL have shown identical genetic mutations in malignant cells some years after birth. This suggests twin → twin transfer of potentially malignant clone through shared circulation.

Haematological effects of non-haemic tumours (for leukaemias, lymphomas, and MDS see appropriate sections)

- Marrow infiltration may be evident at the time of presentation (most commonly neuroblastoma, less commonly Ewing's sarcoma, rhabdomyosarcoma).
- Associated with anaemia, occasionally other cytopenias. Blood count hardly ever ↔ if marrow involved.
- Peripheral blood may show leucoerythroblastic picture, but not as commonly in adult cancers metastasizing to BM.
- Non-haemic tumours appear on cytomorphology as poorly differentiated fragile blast cells, often in sheets or clumps (unlike leukaemic blasts).
- Marrow infiltration may arise as a late event in terminally progressive disease in other tumours, including CNS malignancies, PNETS, and germ cell tumours.

Investigations in suspected childhood cancer

Haematology

- FBC and film. Leukaemia usually reflected in the blood count: ↑ or ↓ WBC, ± thrombocytopenia and anaemia. Blasts often present. In a small percentage, blood count entirely ↔. With other malignancies there may be signs of marrow infiltration, anaemia, or no abnormalities at all.
- BM aspirate and trephine if blood count abnormal. In children generally done under GA. Bilateral samples needed in the staging of neuroblastoma.

Biochemistry

- Full biochemical profile.
- Urinary catecholamines for neuroblastoma (easy test to do in unexplained bone pain).
- Tumour markers: α-FP, βHCG, in hepatoblastoma or germ cell tumours.

Radiology

- CXR for mediastinal mass (mandatory pre-anaesthetic).
- Abdominal USS.
- CT/MRI scan of 1° lesion. CT chest/abdomen may be required for staging. In young children sedation/general anaesthetic usually needed for CT/MRI scans.

Histology

Solid tumours need adequate biopsy material for diagnosis taken under general anaesthetic.

Genetics

Fresh tumour material from all childhood cancers should be sent for cytogenetic and molecular genetic studies. Information from these is increasingly being used in risk-stratifying therapy and in predicting outcome.

Specialist centres for treatment and investigation

Children with suspected malignancy should be referred to a specialist centre for investigation and initial treatment. Thereafter, shared care may be carried out nearer to home at a local hospital. Most children across the country receive treatment as part of a national trial or protocol. This is co-ordinated by the United Kingdom Children's Cancer Study Group and similar groups in other countries, and the success of such trials and studies is one of the reasons for the improved outlook for childhood cancer. Overall long-term survival is ~60%.

Late effects

It is estimated that soon 1:1000 adults will be survivors of childhood cancer. Long term follow-up clinics are needed to monitor growth, fertility, side effects from drugs (e.g. cardiotoxicity), and psychological well-being. There is an ↑ risk of further malignancy developing which varies according to both the 1° diagnosis and treatment used.

Childhood lymphoblastic leukaemia

Lymphoblastic leukaemia ('acute' is superfluous, but disease widely known as ALL) is a group of clonal malignancies all arising in developing lymphocytes. There is more overlap with lymphomas than in adults. Commonest malignant disease in childhood (35% of all cancers). Incidence 4–5/100,000 children per year with a peak incidence between 2–6 years of age.

Aetiology

Many cases thought to be due to antenatal mutations in developing B-cell clones; majority of cases B-cell derived, occur between 2–6 years, and may be abnormal response to infection where exposure to pathogens delayed or precipitated by population mixing. Evidence implicating background ionizing or electromagnetic radiation now discredited. Cause of T-ALL unknown.

Pathophysiology

- ~80% childhood ALLs arise in developing B lymphocytes; ~20% in developing T cells. Acquired genetic mutations found in the various subtypes are growing in number as the molecular biology of leukaemia unravels.
- In early B cells commonest mutation is a fusion between the *TEL* gene at 12p13 and the *AML1* gene at 21q22—arises in 20% overall; other common mutations are t(1;19)(q23;p13.3)—8% overall, t(9;22)(q34;q11.2) *BCR-ABL* (Ph chromosome); 5% overall.
- ~30% have 'high hyperdiploidy' (>50 chromosomes per cell) with or without translocations; 7% show hypodiploidy.
- Infants (<18 months) frequently have a mutation of the *MLL* gene on chromosome 11 involving a range of fusion partners; most commonly AF4 on chromosome 4.
- These changes mark biologically different types of precursor B-derived ALL in terms of clinical features and response to treatment.
- 1–2% of ALLs have features of mature B cells and a mutation where the *MYC* gene is translocated adjacent to the Ig heavy chain locus—t(8;14). Also called Burkitt-type as the cell biology is similar to that of Burkitt's lymphoma.
- T-ALL shows greater genetic diversity than B-derived disease but 12 recurring cytogenetic abnormalities now defined and under study. Clinical importance yet to be defined.
- ALL also classified by immunophenotyping using antibody cell markers for various differentiation antigens designated clusters of differentiation (CD), numbered according to their order of discovery. Immunophenotypes so defined include early pre-B (60%), pre-B (20%), transitional pre-B (1%), B-ALL (1%) and T-ALL (18%).

Clinical features

- Commonly presents insidiously in 3 ways, separately or combined.
- Signs of marrow failure—often anaemia predominates, with extreme pallor and listlessness (60%); also bruising/petechiae (40%).

- Hepatosplenomegaly and lymphadenopathy ('lymphomatous' features) 10–20%.
- Bone pain mimicking irritable hip(s) or juvenile rheumatoid 10–20%.

Laboratory features

- Usually pancytopenia with circulating blast cells indicates diagnosis.
- Confirmed by BM examination and classified by immunophenotyping and cytogenetic/molecular genetic analysis. Classification based on expression profiling might become available in the future.
- In sick children with very high blast cell counts classification studies can be carried out on peripheral blood, but marrow always preferred.
- Peripheral blood count may show cytopenias without obvious blasts (aleukaemic picture) when differential diagnosis is aplastic anaemia.
- Kidney/liver function usually normal, but ALLs with high blast counts and rapid cell turnover may have tumour-lysis organ dysfunction before therapy (urate nephropathy with ↑ urea, creatinine, and ↓ urine output).

Treatment of newly diagnosed disease

- All modern protocols have common elements of remission induction (RI), consolidation/intensification (C/I), CNS directed treatment, and continuing (maintenance) therapy with or without delayed intensification (DI).
- RI drugs include dexamethasone, vincristine, and asparaginase.
- C/I and DI drugs include anthracyclines, cytarabine, cyclophosphamide asparaginase, and thioguanine.
- CNS therapy is intrathecal cytarabine and MTX (radiotherapy now reserved for those with active CNS infiltration only).
- Maintenance therapy is a 2–3 year schedule of daily thiopurine (6-mercaptopurine) and weekly oral methotrexate.
- ALL is the only human malignancy that requires such a drawn-out chemotherapy module, immunosuppressive rather than antineoplastic.
- B-ALL is an exception; it does not respond to conventional ALL therapy, does not need maintenance and is treated on a 6 month intensive lymphoma schedule (📖 Childhood lymphomas, p.612).
- Treatment is usually risk-directed based on biological features of the disease with more intensive schedules reserved for those with adverse prognostic factors (📖 see Prognostic factors, p.610).
- BMT rarely used as 1st-line therapy.

Outlook

98% overall will remit on modern therapy, 75–80% overall will become long-term disease-free survivors—figures vary according to prognostic factors (📖 *see* Prognostic factors, p.610). >90% long-term survivors in low risk disease.

Treatment of relapse

- Some 20–25% of children will relapse; either on treatment or after its completion.
- Outlook depends on length of 1st remission; very bleak if relapse on treatment.

- Salvage therapy more successful if relapse >2 years off therapy.
- Relapsed T-ALL more difficult to treat successfully than other types.
- Treatment includes intensive chemotherapy with the addition of podophyllins, anthracycline analogues, and fludarabine.
- BMT reserved for those who show slow-to-clear residual disease by PCR amplification of unique disease-specific Ig or TCR gene rearrangements, those who relapse on treatment and those with relapsed T-ALL.

Prognostic factors

- Several features of ALL predict response to current standard therapies and are used to stratify treatment. Infants <1 year have a poor outlook, and older children >10 years do less well than those 1–10 years.
- High presenting WBC ($>100 \times 10^9$/L) in boys marks high risk, as do some genetic features (*MLL* gene rearrangements, *BCR-ABL* fusion genes, hypodiploidy).
- All children with T-ALL, and all with slow disease clearance during the 1st few days of therapy, are excluded from being classified as low risk.
- Low risk B-precursor ALL is that which shows none of these features.
- Minimal residual disease (MRD) monitoring by molecular methods is being incorporated into clinical trials to assist prognostic stratification.

Late effects of therapy

With ↑ long survivors, late effects of therapy are becoming more important. Most morbidity seen after TBI given for BMT.

Problems include:

- Growth failure due to CNS damage from radiation.
- Intellectual deficit due to CNS damage from radiation.
- Precocious puberty (girls>boys) after cranial radiation.
- Infertility (boys>girls) not dependent on radiation.
- Obesity (girls>boys) not dependent on radiation.
- 7–10-fold ↑ risk of brain tumours not dependent on radiation.

Childhood lymphomas

Lymphomas account for around 8–10% of all childhood cancers (this equates to around 1 per 100,000 children per year). Around 30–35% are Hodgkin's disease, the rest NHL.

Hodgkin's disease

Clinical features

Uncommon <5 years; incidence increases during the early teenage years. The disease is biologically the same as that of adults and the histological classification is identical (📖 see Hodgkins lymphoma ((HL, Hodgkin's disease), p.206 for more details), though mixed cellularity disease may be more common in the young. Staging is also similar to adults (📖 Table 5.8, p.210), but overall children and adolescents have a greater proportion of low-stage disease (I and II). Stage IV accounts for <10% of childhood cases.

Treatment and outcome

Treatment is so successful that most efforts are currently directed at reducing toxicity and late effects. Radiotherapy for stage I disease is being attenuated, and some therapists have abandoned it as 1st-line treatment and rely on chemotherapy alone. Chemotherapy regimens in turn are evolving (to avoid or minimize alkylating agents and their effect on fertility and anthracyclines with their potential for cardiotoxicity), but at present the traditional drugs are still being used with or without involved field radiotherapy, particularly in stage III or IV disease.

The outlook for even stage IV disease is good, given the best current regimen of chemotherapy and involved field radiotherapy, and over 80% should achieve long term EFS.

NHL

Childhood NHL are a heterogeneous group of tumours quite different from those seen in adults. Virtually all are disseminated, high-grade diffuse malignancies of immature B or T lymphocytes, and many are closely related to subtypes of ALL that occur in this age group.

Classification of NHL has always been confusing, but the Revised European American Lymphoma system is currently preferred. This maps disease in children into 6 categories:

1. Burkitt's lymphoma, Burkitt-like lymphoma, high grade B-cell disease

Different manifestations of biologically very closely related diseases and pathologically indistinguishable from B-ALL. ~45% of the total. Characteristic 'starry sky' histological pattern and deeply basophilic blasts on Romanowsky stains with prominent vacuoles (FAB L3 features). Associated with chromosomal translocation involving *MYC* locus on chromosome 8 and Ig heavy chain gene on 14 (or less commonly with a κ or γ light chain gene on 2 or 22) with resultant dysregulation of *MYC* gene transcription; the *MYC* product functions as a transcription factor.

2. Precursor B lymphoblastic lymphoma

Indistinguishable pathologically from common ALL. ~5% of the total. Commonly presents as a solitary SC swelling, typically on the scalp.

3. Precursor T lymphoblastic lymphoma

ndistinguishable pathologically from T-ALL. ~20% of the total. 66% have nediastinal involvement. Marrow involvement common in advanced lisease; so may be classified as T-ALL rather than stage IV NHL.

4. Diffuse large B-cell lymphoma

ncluding 1° sclerosing mediastinal form; no leukaemic counterpart, ccounts for ~3–4% of the total. Chiefly abdominal. Occasionally mediasinal. Has some features of Burkitt's but no *MYC* gene mutation.

. Peripheral T-cell lymphoma unspecified

Jo leukaemic counterpart. Skin involvement. Retrospective review shows nost so classified to be type 6 (large cell anaplastic, see category 6). 'oorly defined entity hardly ever seen in children.

. Large cell anaplastic, T, or null cell type

Jo leukaemic counterpart. More frequently recognized, and complex bioogical features gradually becoming better understood. ~15% of the total. Jsed to be diagnosed as peripheral T-cell lymphomas or 'malignant histioytosis'. Biological hallmarks are Ki-1 (CD30)+, also t(2;5).

\round 9% childhood NHLs defy classification and <1% adult type folcular lymphomas will occasionally arise in older children.

St Jude staging system for childhood NHL

\ staging system for childhood NHL has been developed (Table 12.9), hough therapy is increasingly being directed more by the biology of the lisease rather than its anatomical distribution or extent. Staging affects rognosis only within given tumour type.

Table 12.9 St Jude staging system for childhood NHL

Stage I	Single tumour (extranodal or single nodal anatomic area), excluding mediastinum or abdomen
Stage II	Single extranodal tumour with regional node involvement = 2 nodal areas on the same side of the diaphragm
	2 single extranodal tumours ± regional node involvement on same side of the diaphragm
	Primary GIT tumour, usually ileocaecal, ± involvement of associated mesenteric nodes
Stage III	2 extranodal tumours on opposite sides of the diaphragm = 2 nodal areas above and below the diaphragm
	Presence of 1° intrathoracic tumour (mediastinal, pleural or thymic)
	Presence of extensive 1° intra-abdominal disease
	Presence of paraspinal or epidural tumours, regardless of other sites
Stage IV	Any of the above with initial CNS and/or BM involvement

Treatment

- ***Burkitt's lymphoma/B-ALL***: short 6-month course of pulsed intensive high dose therapy (vincristine, steroids, MTX, cyclophosphamide, anthracyclines, and etoposide) including CNS treatment. No maintenanc treatment needed.
- ***B precursor lymphoblastic***: if isolated to one site, 6-month programme of ALL-type therapy may suffice, else treat as common ALL with extended maintenance (📖 Lymphoblastic leukaemia, p.608).
- ***T precursor lymphoblastic***: treated as T-ALL (📖 see Specific treatment, p.608).
- ***Diffuse large B-cell lymphoma***: treated as Burkitt's lymphoma (📖 p.196).
- ***Large cell anaplastic Ki-1+***: skin, CNS and mediastinal involvement anc splenomegaly are adverse features. Best therapy undefined but usually treated with short intensive Burkitt-like regimens. EFS is around ~75% (high risk cases ~60%).

General points on therapy/outlook

- Surgery usually indicated for the complete resection of a localized abdominal 1° tumour when possible.
- Low-dose involved field radiotherapy indicated for airway or spinal cord compression. Mediastinal irradiation for persistent local disease.
- Given best current therapy, the outlook for most patients is good with around 80% EFS for childhood lymphomas overall.

Childhood acute myeloid leukaemia (AML)

AML in children accounts for ~15% of all malignant blood disorders, with around 80–90 new cases arising in the UK each year. Unlike ALL, the disease is classified on morphological grounds using the FAB classification (Table 12.10), as is AML in adults (📖 see Table 4.1, p.122). The frequency of the different subtypes differs in children, however. M6 AML is very rare whereas M7 (megakaryocyte derived AML) is more common—especially in children with Down syndrome.

Table 12.10 Proportion of children with *de novo* AML by FAB type

	M0	M1	M2	M3	M4	M5	M6	M7
% of total	2	18	29	8	16	17	2	8

Pathophysiology

AML is a clonal neoplasm arising from developing blood cells affecting all haemopoietic cell lines, most commonly granulocyte or monocyte precursors but also occasionally involving immature erythroblasts or megakaryocytes. Apart from 1°, *de novo* disease for which no cause can be identified, some cases of AML are due to chemotherapy given for other diseases (2° AML), and some arise in children with predisposing syndromes where the risk is greatly ↑ and where specific subtypes of AML may develop.

- 2° AML caused by topoisomerase II inhibitors (e.g. etoposide) has a latency of 1–3 years and is of FAB type M4/M5 with a characteristic *MLL* gene mutation.
- 2° AML caused by alkylating agents (e.g. cyclophosphamide) has a latency of 4–6 years, a myelodysplastic phase, and loss or deletions of chromosomes 5, 7, or both.
- Down syndrome children are 20 × more likely to develop leukaemia than normal children; infants are more likely to develop M7 AML, older Down children develop ALL.
- Other conditions predisposing to AML in children are Fanconi anaemia and Bloom's syndrome (📖 Fanconi anaemia, p.590), dyskeratosis congenita, Kostmann's syndrome and Shwachman–Diamond syndrome (📖 Rare congenital marrow failure syndromes, p.592), Diamond– Blackfan anaemia (📖 Congenital red cell aplasia, p.586), and neurofibromatosis.

Apart from the specific changes in 2° AMLs, clonal chromosome abnormalities are found in blasts from ~90% of those with *de novo* disease. 2/3 of these are non-random, and many are associated with characteristic clinical and biological features.

Table 12.11 Commonest genetic mutations in childhood AML

Abnormality	Involved genes	FAB type	Frequency	Clinical features
t(8;21)	*ETO; AML1*	M2	10–15%	Extramedullary chloromas Good outlook
t(15;17)	*PML; RARA*	M3	5–10%	Coagulopathy Responds to retinoids
Inv16(p13q32)	*MYH11; CBFB*	M4eo	7–10%	Extramedullary deposits Good outlook
t(9;11)	*AF9; MLL*	M4/M5	7–10%	Infants, CNS disease Poor outlook
t(1;22)	*N/K*	M7	2–3%	2° myelofibrosis Down syndrome

Laboratory features

- Peripheral blood shows a variety of abnormalities—usually pancytopenia with circulating blasts.
- WBC seldom >50 × 10^9/L though can occasionally be very high with symptoms of leucostasis—deafness, confusion, and impaired consciousness.
- BM usually shows heavy overgrowth of blasts with different morphology depending on FAB type. Auer rods (abnormal elongated 1° granules seen on Romanowsky stains in cytoplasm of malignant myeloblasts) are diagnostic of AML and are not found in health. Seen in all types of AML except M6 and M7, most common in M1/2/3, particularly M3.
- Cytochemistry may help; non-specific esterase +ve in M4/M5 AML, not other types and myeloperoxidase positivity can help distinguish between poorly differentiated AML and ALL. M7 AML may develop extensive marrow fibrosis making aspiration difficult; trephine histology needed.
- Genetic abnormalities common in blast cells (📖 see Table 12.11).
- Immunophenotyping less important than in ALL, though essential for immediate diagnosis of M7 AML which has no distinguishing morphological or cytochemical features. CD antigens expressed vary according to FAB type; CD33 strongly +ve in all, CD13 in M2/3; CD4 in M4/M5 and CD41/61 in M7. M6 disease expresses glycophorin A.

Clinical features

Children with advanced AML are commonly sicker than those with ALL. They can present with bleeding, haemostatic failure, and/or septicaemia as manifestations of marrow failure and profound neutropenia. Extramedullary chloromas (solid deposits of malignant cells) arise in around 10% of cases They may precede marrow failure (or even detectable marrow infiltration). They can arise internally around the spine or spinal cord, causing pressure symptoms and mimicking non-haemic solid tumours. They are more common in AML with t(8;21). Peri-orbital chloromas are also not unusual in infants with M4/M5 AML.

Treatment and outlook

Outcome of therapy for childhood AML has shown a dramatic improvement over the last 15 years. From a dismal outlook in the 1970s through around 30% EFS in the 1980s we have now achieved >50% EFS at the turn of the 21st century. This has been due to increasingly intensive chemotherapy and parallel improvements in supportive treatment for the secondary marrow failure it produces.

The principle of treatment is to ablate marrow with chemotherapy to the point that endogenous recovery occurs within 4–6 weeks and to repeat the process with different drug combinations 4 or 5 times, giving a total treatment time of around 6 months. Results using this approach have improved for children in the best risk groups to the point where allogeneic BMT is no longer considered the consolidation treatment of choice even if a matched donor is available.

- Drugs used in remission induction include daunorubicin, etoposide, cytarabine, and mitoxantrone (mitozantrone).
- Drugs used in post induction and consolidation treatment include amsacrine, high-dose cytarabine, L-asparaginase, etoposide and mitoxantrone (mitozantrone).
- Good risk patients are those with t(8;21), t(15;17) and inv(16)—together accounting for around 20–25% overall; standard risk patients are those without good risk genetic changes but that respond well and remit after 1 course of chemotherapy (65% overall), and poor risk are those without good genetics who have residual disease at the start of course 2 of treatment (around 10% of the total).
- Long-term EFS for good risk children is around 75–80%, for standard risk around 60–65%, and for poor risk around 15%.
- Allogeneic BMT as consolidation therapy of 1st remission is reserved for children in standard and poor risk groups. It is also used as a salvage strategy for good risk patients who relapse.
- The role of autologous stem cell rescue following myeloablative conditioning in children with AML has not been established.
- The need for skilled supportive therapy confines AML therapy to specialist units.

Childhood myelodysplastic syndromes and chronic leukaemias

Myelodysplastic syndromes of childhood present a different spectrum of disease from that seen in adults. All are rare. The FAB classification of adult MDS (📖 Table 6.1, p.225) has been translated to paediatric disease, but sits uncomfortably and is of limited use clinically or in understanding the complex biology of this diverse group of clonal disorders of marrow function. The proportion that map to the various adult categories is shown in Table 12.12.

- Many children with MDS have a monocytosis which results in their being classified as CMML, also the clinical features and outlook for childhood CMML are quite different.
- RARS is virtually never seen in children.

Table 12.12 Paediatric modification of WHO classification of myelodysplastic disorders

Category	Diseases
Myelodysplastic/ myeloproliferative disease	Juvenile myelomonocytic leukaemia (JMML)
Down syndrome disease	Transient abnormal myelopoiesis Myeloid leukaemia of DS
Myelodysplastic syndrome	Refractory cytopenia (blood blasts <2%, marrow blasts <5%)
	Refractory anaemia with excess blasts (blood blasts <19%, marrow blasts 5–19%)
	Refractory anaemia with excess blasts in transformation (blood or marrow blasts 20–29%)

Individual disorders

Refractory anaemia

Children with a clonal genetic marker in the marrow who present with refractory anaemia usually progress to RAEB and AML. Those without such a marker probably do not have MDS but some other cause of erythropoietic failure.

RAEB and RAEB-t

Many of the RAEB syndromes in children arise in those with pre-existing disease like Down syndrome, trisomy 8, neurofibromatosis type 1, Fanconi anaemia, dyskeratosis congenita, Kostmann's syndrome, Diamond– Blackfan anaemia, and Shwachman–Diamond syndrome (📖 see Childhood acute myeloid leukaemia, p.616). All these diseases predispose to leukaemia, and RAEB is merely part of the evolution of AML. A substantial proportion of childhood MDS in the RA or RAEB category is also induced by previous chemotherapy as a prodrome to 2° AML. In other words all paediatric cases of RAEB/RAEB-t are best regarded as AML and treated as such if the diagnosis is not in any doubt.

- Down syndrome children have a particular predisposition to develop M7 (megakaryoblastic) AML in the first few years of life. This is commonly preceded by a RAEB prodrome where the marrow is hard to aspirate through 2° sclerosis. The decision when to start therapy is difficult, but the overall outlook is potentially good with EFS >50%.

Transient abnormal myelopoiesis (TAM)

Down children also have a predisposition to develop a transient blast cell overgrowth in infancy that looks like frank leukaemia with blasts in the peripheral blood. It is completely self-limiting within days or weeks and is not associated with marrow failure, arising alongside normal haemopoiesis. It is important that chemotherapy is withheld in what is regarded as a temporary stem cell instability. Rarely the problem can arise in non-Down children, where trisomy 21 is found in the BM only. TAM and M7 in Down syndrome patients has been recently shown to be associated with acquired mutations in *GATA-1*.

Juvenile chronic myelomonocytic leukaemia (JCMML)

Originally called juvenile chronic myeloid leukaemia to distinguish it from adult type chronic myeloid leukaemia (📖 ATCML, p.298), this pernicious disease still has a high mortality. It is now recognized to be a clonal disorder, with all marrow cell lines involved. It has several distinctive clinical and haematological features.

- Stigmata of fetal erythropoiesis; high HbF, ↑ red cell i antigen expression and carbonic anhydrase activity, ↑ MCV.
- Modest ↑ WBC; average 30–40 × 10^9/L, with evident monocytosis, blasts 5–10%, and occasionally a basophilia.
- Marrow appearances unremarkable; modest ↑ blasts.
- Thrombocytopenia; sometimes profound.
- Skin rashes; butterfly distribution on face.
- Increasing hepatosplenomegaly.
- Associated with neurofibromatosis type 1. May be present in >10% of cases.
- Poor outlook with progression associated with wasting, fever, infections, bleeding, and pulmonary infiltrations.

Monosomy 7 syndrome

Conventional cytogenetic analysis of the marrow in JCMML shows no abnormality in the classic syndrome, though there is a subvariety (or similar condition that may nevertheless be biologically distinct) where monosomy 7 is found. Whether this is a different disorder is not clear. Apart from the different genetics, monosomy 7 syndrome and JCMML have several features in common. However, monosomy 7 children may have:

- A longer prodrome with RA or RAEB and no monocytosis.
- They may respond to AML chemotherapy (JCMML responds poorly and seldom remits).
- They may remain stable for years without therapy.
- They respond better to BMT (JCMML achieve <40% EFS even with BMT).

Adult-type chronic myeloid (granulocytic) leukaemia (ATCML)

(📖 see Adult CML p.298.) More common than JCMML, though still rare ATCML arises in around 1 in 500,000 children per year (20 in whole of UK). Tends to affect older children (60% >6 years) though it has been reported in a 3-month-old infant.

- Associated with Ph chromosome and t(9;22) *BCR-ABL* fusion gene in all haemopoietic cells exactly as seen in adults.
- Natural history exactly the same as the disease in adults with chronic phase and eventual progression to accelerated acute phase.
- Only curative therapy is allogeneic BMT, but impressive remissions of so far unknown length are now being achieved with novel tyrosine kinase inhibitor imatinib (Glivec®). For patients who lack a compatible SCT donor this is becoming 1st-line therapy in place of IFNα or hydroxycarbamide

Histiocytic syndromes

Monocytes are formed in the marrow and move through the peripheral blood into the tissues where they become histiocytes, either in the mononuclear phagocytic system (MPS) or the dendritic cell system (DCS). MPS cells are antigen processing, are predominantly phagocytic and include many organ-specific cells such as Kupffer cells and pulmonary alveolar macrophages. DCS cells include tissue-based Langerhans cells (LC) which are antigen presenting. There is a variety of syndromes where histiocytes proliferate and malfunction and some of these carry a high mortality. A few are clonal neoplasms but most are produced by cytokine disturbances. In 1991 a new classification of histiocytic syndromes was set out as shown in Table 12.13.

Table 12.13 Histiocytic syndromes

Class I	*Disorders of dendritic cells* • Langerhans cell histiocytosis (LCH) (previously known as histiocytosis X)

Class II	*Disorders of macrophages*
	• Haemophagocytic syndromes
	• Haemophagocytic lymphohistiocytosis (HLH):
	  • 1° (genetic)
	  • 2° (to infection or malignant disease)
	• Sinus histiocytosis with massive lymphadenopathy
	• Histiocytic necrotising lymphadenitis

Class III	• Malignant histiocytic disorders:
	  • Malignant histiocytosis
	  • Monocytic leukaemias

Class I: Langerhans cell histiocytosis (LCH)

Cellular destructive tissue infiltration with LC. These are well differentiated large cells (15–25microm) with an indented nucleus and inconspicuous nucleolus; they are not phagocytic. Other reactive cells (granulocytes, eosinophils, macrophages) are often present. Diagnostic criteria of LC include the presence of Burbeck granules on electron microscopy and immunochemical positivity for CD1A. The aetiology of LCH remains unclear. Despite some evidence of clonality (not itself evidence of malignancy), no genetic mutations have been identified and the disorder is not regarded as a form of cancer.

Clinical features

LCH is primarily a disease of the very young with a peak incidence of 1–3 years. It can present in a variety of ways, from a small bone lesion heavily admixed with eosinophils (eosinophilic granuloma), through multiple lytic bone lesions, exophthalmos, and diabetes insipidus (Hand-Schuller–Christian disease) to multiple tissue infiltration involving skin liver, lung, bone, and BM (Letterer–Siwe disease). The eponymous terms are no longer used for what is now regarded as a common pathology and the overarching term LCH is preferred. This is staged on the basis of the number of organ systems showing infiltration, and virtually any can be involved. The skin rash of LCH is characteristically in skin folds and scaly with red/brown papules. It may be mistaken for nappy rash. Systemic symptoms including fever and weight loss arecommon in advanced disease. It can be staged as follows:

- *Stage A* Involvement of bones ± local nodes and adjacent soft tissue.
- *Stage B* Skin ± mucous membranes involvement, ± related nodes.
- *Stage C* Soft tissue involvement—not stage A, B or D.
- *Stage D* Multisystem disease with combinations of A, B, C.

Diagnosis

Based on tissue biopsy. Skeletal survey to define extent of disease; also bone scan, MRI. Urine osmolality studies for diabetes insipidus. BM aspirate and biopsy if anaemic or other cytopenias present.

Treatment

Local curettage of any isolated lesion, with or without intralesional steroids. Stable and symptomless disease can be simply observed for spontaneous resolution. Options for widespread disease include steroids and chemotherapy—rarely radiotherapy. Indications for chemotherapy include organ dysfunction and/or disease progression/recurrence. Drugs commonly used include steroids, vinblastine, or etoposide, singly or combined.

Outcome

Generally good, but widespread organ involvement with dysfunction and progression indicates a poor prognosis. Overall mortality 15–20%. Long term sequelae include pulmonary/liver fibrosis, diabetes insipidus, growth failure. Risk of malignant disease increased, chiefly leukaemias and lymphomas.

Class II: macrophage functional disorders—haemophagocytic syndromes

1°(genetic)

1° haemophagocytic lymphohistiocytosis (HLH) is an autosomal recessively inherited disease of infants and young children (>50% <1 year) also known as familial erythrophagocytic lymphohistiocytosis (FEL) due to the striking degree of marrow red cell phagocytosis. Genetic HLH is a heterogeneous disorder with at least 4 genetic subtypes (FHLH1-4). 3 genes (Perforin, *PRF1*, on 10q21; *Munc13-4* on 17q25; *Syntaxin 11* on 6q24) have been identified and account for ~50% of patients. Defects in these genes lead to cytokine dysregulation (high concentrations of IL-1 and 2, GM-CSF, and TNF) and 'activated' T cells and histiocytes prompting haemophagocytosis. CNS involvement is common. Laboratory investigation shows peripheral blood cytopenias, hypertrigliceridaemia, and hypofibrinogenaemia. Histopathology shows histiocyte/lymphocyte infiltration and haemophagocytosis in BM, nodes and spleen. Genetic testing possible in ~ 50%.

Treatment and outcome

The use of ALG and CSA in the 'HLH' protocol enables the disease to be brought under control. If this is followed by a SCT survival can be good. Otherwise the disease is usually rapidly fatal.

2°

- Clinical and laboratory picture is similar to 1° (genetic) HLH.
- Distinction between the 2 may be difficult.
- Affects more older patients, often immunocompromised.
- Commonly associated with underlying viral/bacterial infection when called infection-associated haemophagocytic syndrome (IAHS).
- Triggered by a wide variety of infections including (especially) EBV and malaria. Also associated with some malignancies (usually involving T cells) and lipid infusions.

Treatment and outcome

Good survival rates if underlying infection easily treatable. Otherwise has high mortality.

Class III: malignant histiocytosis

Monocyte-derived acute leukaemias account for 10% of AMLs arising in children. What used to be called 'malignant histiocytosis' with hepatosplenomegaly, fever, wasting, and pancytopenia and tissue infiltration with large monocytoid cells is now recognized as a lymphocyte-derived lymphoma (large cell anaplastic, CD30+, 📖 1° p.182). It is doubtful whether true histiocyte-derived malignancies other than AML occur in children.

Haematological effects of systemic disease in children

Non-haematological disease in children can produce a variety of haematological effects specific to the disease, to childhood, or both. Some of the more striking examples are listed here.

- *Wilson's disease:* genetic defect in copper metabolism that occasionally presents as a brisk non-immune haemolytic anaemia without specific features. More commonly presents with liver dysfunction, neurological symptoms, or renal disease.
- *Cyanotic congenital heart disease:* commonly associated with mild thrombocytopenia for ill-understood reasons.
- *Mast cell disease:* abnormal accumulations of mast cells in the skin or internal organs. Mast cell leukaemia does not occur in children. Commonest manifestation is urticaria pigmentosa in infants. Bullous or urticarial lesions eventually become infiltrated with mast cells. Marrow involvement rare. The cells produce histamine and cause itching. Condition resolves by adulthood.
- *Juvenile rheumatoid arthritis:* classically the anaemia of chronic inflammatory disease—a defective marrow response to anaemia in a variety of chronic inflammatory disorders primarily due to cytokine mediated inhibition of erythropoiesis rather than deficiency of EPO. True Fe deficiency also occurs due to NSAID therapy. Neutropenia may arise, either immune mediated or due to hypersplenism.
- *Systemic lupus erythematosus:* commonly associated with immune cytopenias (all cell lines) and anticardiolipin antibodies. May also produce marrow hypoplasia.
- *Epstein–Barr virus infection:* infects CD21 +ve B lymphocytes and other tissues including nasopharyngeal epithelium. 1° infection in the immunocompetent may be asymptomatic in the early years of childhood but in adolescence produces the syndrome of infectious mononucleosis ('glandular fever') associated with a striking atypical lymphocytosis. Occasionally there are associated self-limiting immune cytopenias—especially thrombocytopenia. The majority of adults harbour the latent virus in B cells. EBV in some cellular immune deficiency states (such as X-linked LPD also known as Purtilo's or Duncan's syndrome) can produce a fatal infection with uncontrolled lymphoproliferation and infection associated haemophagocytosis (📖 HLH, p.624).
- *Parvovirus B19 infection:* causes 'fifth disease' in infants and young children with the characteristic 'slapped cheek' rash on the face. More importantly shows trophism for marrow erythroblasts and causes temporary red cell hypoplasia. This causes very low Hb concentrations in children with chronic haemolysis (e.g. sickle cell disease). Persistent viraemia can arise in the immunosuppressed and can cause transfusion dependency.
- *TORCH infections:* a miscellaneous group of congenital infections—Toxoplasmosis, Rubella, Cytomegalovirus, Herpes simplex and syphilis. All can cause neonatal anaemia and thrombocytopenia.

- *Leishmaniasis:* the Mediterranean type of visceral leismaniasis primarily affects young children under 5 years. Infected sand flies transmit parasites that develop in macrophages and the child presents often several weeks or months later with fever and progressive pancytopenia and hepatosplenomegaly. Fatal if untreated but responds well to pentavalent antimony or amphotericin B.
- *Hookworms (ankylostoma):* are a common cause of Fe deficiency in tropical underdeveloped countries. Infestations may be heavy with each worm consuming up to 0.2mL blood per day.
- *Tapeworms:* a rare cause of vitamin B_{12} deficiency in societies that eat raw fish—Baltic states, Japan, and Scandinavia, due to infestation by *Diphyllobothrium latum*.
- *Kawasaki disease:* an acute multisystem disease of young children, presumed to be infective but no organism has so far been identified. Presents with conjunctivitis, rashes, reddening of the mucous membranes, hands and feet with desquamation and lymphadenopathy. Coronary artery aneurysms develop in ~20%; fatal in 3%. Haematological manifestations include anaemia (normochromic normocytic), neutrophilia, and a striking 2° thrombocytosis that may linger after the acute phase has passed. Treatment is with aspirin and high dose IVIg.

Nutritional disorders

Fe deficiency

Occurs in apparently healthy children (*cf.* adults where main cause is blood loss). Linked to rapid growth and poor intake the first 2 years of life and again at adolescence. Cows' milk is a poor source of iron. Cereals inhibit its absorption. Premature infants run out of Fe by 2 months of age.

Protein-calorie malnutrition

Covers adequate calories with protein lack (kwashiorkor) and simple calorie lack (marasmus)—or both. Chiefly in undeveloped countries, but also occasionally in vegan families, with gastrointestinal disease or other chronic illness. Concomitant Fe or folate deficiency may be present. Normochromic normocytic anaemia is usual.

Scurvy

Occasionally seen in infants due to poor intake with fruit juices being boiled. Pseudoparalysis due to painful legs. Petechial, periorbital, or sub-dural haemorrhages can arise. Bleeding tendency due to loss of vascular integrity with collagen deficiency.

Poisons

Lead poisoning

Inhibits haem synthesis and the activity of pyrimidine-5'-nucleotidase, causing hypochromic anaemia with basophilic stippling of red cells and ring sideroblasts in the BM. Also causes abdominal pain. Commonest in toddlers eating flakes of old lead-based paint.

Sodium chlorate

A common weedkiller, also a powerful oxidizing substance causing acute intravascular haemolysis and renal failure if ingested.

Nitrates, aniline dyes, nitrobenzene, and azo compounds

Can all cause methaemoglobinaemia. If >20% metHb formed, exchange transfusion may be needed.

Storage disorders

Gaucher's disease

Inherited (autosomal recessive) disorder resulting in deficiency of the enzyme glucocerebrosidase (β-glucosidase) Most common form has accumulated glycolipid in macrophages of spleen, liver, and BM. May be diagnosed at any time during life depending on severity. Some cases are not identified until adulthood. Rarer type 2 disease has severe progressive neurological deterioration from birth, usually fatal within 1 year due to glycolipid accumulation in the CNS. Diagnosis by assay of deficient enzyme, but characteristic (not diagnostic, 📖 see Marrow and blood cells in storage disorders, Gaucher cells evident in BM (laden macrophages with appearance of crumpled tissue paper).

Neimann–Pick (N-P) disease

Though rare, commonest cause of foamy macrophages in marrow of affected patients. Caused by the inherited deficiency of sphingomyelinase resulting in accumulation of sphingomyelin. 4 types of Niemann–Pick disease have been defined: type A (classic N-P disease) presents in the 1st year of life with developmental delay, neurodegeneration, and death within 3 years; type B with visceral rather than CNS involvement also presents in infancy and is also progressive and fatal but spares the CNS; type C presents later in childhood but then shows neurodegeneration with death in the 2nd or 3rd decade; and type D patients simply store sphingomyelin in viscera without ill health and live to adulthood.

Marrow and blood cells in storage disorders

The foamy macrophages seen in the marrow of N-P patients vary between types and are not in any way diagnostic or specific. Foamy macrophages are also seen in several other storage disorders and a variety of other clinical circumstances. Pseudo-Gaucher cells are seen in chronic granulocytic leukaemia, thalassaemia, and some atypical mycobacterial infections. Several storage disorders produce vacuolation of peripheral blood leucocytes, particularly lymphocytes, and this is also a non-specific finding. Diagnosis always rests on the appropriate enzyme assay.

Chapter 13

Haematological emergencies

Septic shock/neutropenic fever

►►One of the commonest haemato-oncological emergencies.

- May be defined as the presence of symptoms or signs of infection in a patient with an absolute neutrophil count of $<1.0 \times 10^9$/L. In practice, the neutrophil count is often $<0.1 \times 10^9$/L.
- Similar clinical picture also seen in neutrophil function disorders such as MDS despite ↔ neutrophil numbers.
- ***Beware***—can occur without pyrexia, especially patients on steroids.

Immediate action

►►Urgent clinical assessment.

- Follow ALS guidelines if cardiorespiratory arrest (rare).
- More commonly, clinical picture is more like cardiovascular shock ± respiratory embarrassment viz: tachycardia, hypotension, peripheral vasodilatation, and tachypnoea. Occurs with both Gram +ve (now more common with indwelling central catheters) and Gram –ve organisms (less common but more fulminant).
- Immediate rapid infusion of albumin 4.5% or Gelofusine® to restore BP.
- Insert central catheter if not in situ and monitor CVP.
- Start O_2 by face mask if pulse oximetry shows saturations <95% (common) and consider arterial blood gas measurement—care with platelet counts $<20 \times 10^9$/L—manual pressure over puncture site for 30min.
- Perform full septic screen (📖 see Guidelines for use of IV antibiotics, p.676).
- Give the first dose of 1st-line antibiotics immediately e.g ureidopenicillin and loading dose aminoglycoside (ceftazidime or ciprofloxacin if pre-existing renal impairment). Follow established protocols.
- If the event occurs while patient on 1st-line antibiotics, vancomycin/ciprofloxacin or vancomycin/meropenem are suitable alternatives.
- Commence full ITU-type monitoring chart.
- Monitor urine output with urinary catheter if necessary—if renal shutdown has already occurred, give single bolus of IV furosemide. If no response, start renal dose dopamine.
- If BP not restored with colloid despite ↑ CVP, consider inotropes.
- If O_2 saturations remain ↓ despite 60% O_2 delivered by rebreathing mask, consider ventilation.
- *Alert ITU giving details of current status.*

Subsequent actions

- Discuss with senior colleague.
- Amend antibiotics according to culture results or to suit likely source if cultures –ve (📖 see Treatment of neutropenic shock when source unknown, p.678 and Treatment of neutropenic shock when source known/suspected, p.680).
- Check aminoglycoside trough levels after loading dose and before 2nd dose as renal impairment may determine reducing or withholding next dose. Consider switch to non-nephrotoxic cover e.g ceftazidime/ciprofloxacin.

Continue antibiotics for 7–10d minimum and usually until neutrophil recovery.
If cultures show central line to be source of sepsis, remove immediately if patient not responding.

Transfusion reactions

Rapid temperature spike (>40°C) at start of transfusion indicates transfusi(should be ***stopped*** (suggests acute intravascular haemolysis).

If slow rising temperature (<40°C), providing patient not acutely unwe slow IVI. Fever often due to antibodies against WBCs (or to cytokines platelet packs).

►Immediate transfusion reaction

Intravascular haemolysis (→ haemoglobinaemia and haemoglobinuri Usually due to anti-A or anti-B antibodies (in ABO mismatched transfusio Symptoms occur in minutes/hours (Table 13.1).

If predominantly extravascular may only suffer chills/fever 1h after starti transfusion—commonly due to anti-D. Acute renal failure is *not* a featur

Mechanism

Complement (C3a, C4a, C5a) release into recipient plasma → smoo muscle contraction. May develop DIC (📖 see Disseminated intravascul coagulation, p.488, 642); oliguria (10% cases) due to profound hypotensio

Initial steps in management of acute transfusion reaction

- Stop blood transfusion immediately.
- Replace giving set, keep IV open with 0.9% saline.
- Check patient identity against donor unit.
- Insert urinary catheter and monitor urine output.
- Give fluids (IV colloids) to maintain urine output >1.5mL/kg/h.
- If urine output <1.5mL/kg/h insert CVP line and give fluid challenge.
- If urine output <1.5mL/kg/h and CVP adequate give furosemide 80–120 mg.
- If urine output still <1.5mL/kg/h consult senior medical staff for advice
- Contact Blood Transfusion Lab before sending back blood pack and fc advice on blood samples required for further investigation.

Complications

Overall mortality ~10%.

Table 13.1 Immediate transfusion reaction or bacterial contamination of blood

Symptoms	Signs
• Patient restless/agitated • Flushing • Anxiety • Chills • Nausea and vomiting • Pain at venepuncture site • Abdominal, flank or chest pain • Diarrhoea	• Fever • Hypotension • Oozing from wounds or venepuncture sites • Haemoglobinaemia • Haemoglobinuria

Immediate-type hypersensitivity reactions

May occur soon (30–90min) after transfusion of blood/component. Antiboc often unknown but in some cases is due to antibody directed against Ig (in recipients who have become sensitized).

- Mild reaction: urticaria, erythema, maculopapular rash, periorbital oedema.
- Severe reaction: bronchospasm.
- Hypotension.

Management

- Stop transfusion immediately.
- Change giving set.
- IV colloids to maintain BP/circulatory volume.
- Give
  - Epinephrine (adrenaline) 1:1000 1mL IM stat
  - Hydrocortisone 100mg IV stat
  - Chlorphenamine 10mg IV stat

Febrile transfusion reactions

Seen in 0.5–1.0% blood transfusions. Mainly due to anti-HLA antibodie in recipient serum or granulocyte-specific antibodies (e.g. sensitizatio during pregnancy or previous blood transfusion). Less common now th all blood is leucodepleted after donation.

Treatment

- Slow down rate of transfusion.
- Antipyretic.

Delayed transfusion reaction

Occurs in patients immunized through previous pregnancies or transfusion Antibody weak (so not detected at pretransfusion stage). 2° immun response occurs—antibody titre ↑.

Symptoms/signs

- Occur 7–10d after blood transfusion.
- Fever, anaemia, and jaundice.
- ± haemoglobinuria.

Management

- Check DAT and repeat compatibility tests.
- Transfuse patient with freshly cross-matched blood.

Bacterial contamination of blood products

Uncommon but potentially fatal adverse effect of blood transfusion affects red cells and blood products e.g. platelet concentrates). Implicated rganisms include Gram –ve bacteria, including *Pseudomonas, Yersinia,* and *'avobacterium.*

Features

Fever.
Skin flushing.
Rigors.
Abdominal pain.
DIC.
ARF.
Shock.
Cardiac arrest.

Management

As per *Immediate transfusion* reaction (📖 Transfusion reactions, p.636)
Stop transfusion.
Urgent resuscitation.
IV broad-spectrum antibiotics if bacterial contamination suspected.

Post-transfusion purpura

Profound thrombocytopenia occurring 5–10d after blood or platelet ransfusion. Usually due to high titre of anti-HPA-1a antibody in HPA-1a ve patient.

Features

Rare.
Multiparous ♀ most commonly (previous pregnancies or transfusions).
Caused by platelet-specific alloantibodies (usually anti-HPA-1a).
Platelets ↓↓ with associated bleeding/bruising—may be severe and even life threatening.

Management

IVIg if bleeding.
Plasma exchange worth considering.
If platelet transfusion needed, use random donor platelets (no evidence that HPA-1a superior).

Hypercalcaemia

Clinical symptoms

- General—weakness, lassitude, weight loss.
- Mental changes—impaired concentration, drowsiness, personality change and coma.
- GIT—anorexia, nausea, vomiting, abdominal pain (peptic ulceration an pancreatitis are rare complications).
- Genitourinary—polyuria, polydipsia.

Clinical effects

- Cardiovascular—↓ QT interval on ECG, cardiac arrhythmias and hypertension.
- Renal—dehydration, renal failure, and renal calculi.

Haematological causes

- Myeloma.
- High grade lymphoma.
- Adult T-cell leukaemia/lymphoma (ATLL).
- Acute lymphoblastic leukaemia.

Hypercalcaemia occurs in other clinical situations including metastat carcinoma of breast, prostate, and lung. Theories for occurrence in haema tological malignancy include ↑ bone resorption mediated by osteoclast under the influence of locally or systemically released cytokines such a PTH-related peptide, TGF, TNF-α, M-CSF, interleukins, and prostaglandin ↑ intestinal absorption of Ca^{2+} 2° to ↑ 1,25-hydroxycholecalciferol.

↔ range for plasma [Ca^{2+}] 2.12–2.65mmol/L. 40% of plasma Ca^{2+} is boun to albumin. Most laboratories measure the total plasma Ca^{2+} althoug only unbound Ca^{2+} is physiologically active. For accurate mea-surement c plasma or serum Ca^{2+} blood sampling should be taken from an uncuffe arm, i.e. without the use of a tourniquet. 📖 See Table 13.2.

Table 13.2 Correct for albumin

Albumin <40g/L	Corrected calcium = (Ca^{2+}) + 0.02 [40–(Albumin)]
Albumin >45g/L	Corrected calcium = (Ca^{2+}) – 0.02 [(Albumin)–45]

Management

►An emergency if Ca^{2+} >3.0mmol/L.

- Rehydrate with normal saline 4–6L/24h.
- Beware fluid overload—use loop diuretics and CVP monitoring if necessary.
- Stop thiazide diuretics and consider regular loop diuretics.
- Give bisphosphonates e.g. disodium pamidronate 60–90mg IV stat (📖 see Table 13.3) or zoledronic acid 4mg IV in 100mL N. saline over at least 15mins.
- Treat underlying malignancy.
- Consider dialysis if complicating factors (CCF, advanced renal failure).

- Other therapeutic options:
  - Calcitonin (salmon) 200IU 8-hourly.
  - Corticosteroids (e.g. prednisolone 60mg/d PO).
  - ↑ 25mcg/kg IV 3 weekly.
  - Plicamycin.

Table 13.3 Treatment of hypercalcaemia with disodium pamidronate

Serum Ca^{2+} (mmol/L)	Pamidronate (mg)
Up to 3.0	15–30
3.0–3.5	30–60
3.5–4.0	60–90
>4.0	90

Infuse slowly (📖 see *BNF*).
Response often takes 3–5d.

Hyperviscosity

Common haematological emergency. Defined as increase in whole blood viscosity as a result of an increase in either red cells, white cells, or plasma components, usually Ig.

Commonest situations arise as a result of:

- ↑ in red cell volume in PRV.
- High blast cell numbers in peripheral blood e.g. AML or ALL at presentation.
- Presence of monoclonal Ig e.g. Waldenström macroglobulinaemia (IgM).

Clinical features—polycythaemia (e.g. PRV)

Lethargy, itching, headaches, hypertension, plethora, arterial thromboses viz: MI, CVA, and visual loss (central retinal artery occlusion).

►*Emergency treatment*

Isovolaemic venesection. Remove 500mL blood volume from large bore vein (antecubital usually) with simultaneous replacement into another vein of 500mL 0.9% saline. Repeat daily until PCV <0.45.

Clinical features—high WBC (e.g. AML)

Dyspnoea and cough (pulmonary leucostasis); confusion, ↓ conscious level, isolated cranial nerve palsies (cerebral leucostasis), visual loss (retinal haemorrhage or CRVT).

►*Emergency treatment*

- Unless machine leucapheresis can be obtained immediately, venesect 500mL blood from large bore vein and replace isovolaemically with packed red cells if Hb <7.0g/dL—otherwise replace with 0.9% saline to avoid increasing whole blood viscosity.
- Arrange leucapheresis on cell separator machine. Use white cell interface program to apherese with replacement fluids depending on Hb as above. 2h is usually maximum tolerated.
- Initiate tumour lysis prophylactic protocol (📖 see Tumour lysis syndrome, p.684) in preparation for chemotherapy.
- Start chemotherapy as soon as criteria allow (high urine volume of pH>8 and allopurinol commenced). This is crucial as leucapheresis in this situation is only a holding manoeuvre while the patient is prepared for chemotherapy.
- Continue leucapheresis daily until leucostasis symptoms resolved or until WBC $<50 \times 10^9$/L.

Hypergammaglobulinaemia (e.g. Waldenström macroglobulinaemia)

Lethargy, headaches, memory loss, confusion, vertigo, visual disturbances from cerebral vessel sludging—rarely MI, CVA.

►*Emergency treatment*

- Unless immediate access to plasma exchange machine available, venesect 500mL blood from large bore vein with isovolaemic replacement with 0.9% saline unless Hb <7.0g/dL when use packed red cells.

- Arrange plasmapheresis on a cell separator machine using plasma exchange program (📖 see Plasma exchange (plasmapheresis), p.706). Replacement fluids on criteria as above. Aim for 1–1.5 blood volume exchange (usually 2.5–4.0L) starting at lower end of range initially. Repeat daily until symptoms resolved.
- Maintenance plasma exchanges at 3–6 weekly intervals may be sufficient treatment for some forms of Waldenström macroglobuli-naemia. However, if hyperviscosity due to IgA myeloma or occasionally IgG myeloma, chemotherapy will need to be initiated.

Note

Diseases in which the abnormal Ig shows activity at lower temperature e.g. cold antibodies associated with CHAD (📖 see Cold haemagglutin disease, p.96) require maintenance of plasmapheresis inlet and outlet venous lines and all infusional fluids at 37°C. Polyclonal ↑ in Ig (e.g. some forms of cryoglobulinaemia) can also rarely cause hyperviscosity symptoms. Management is as described for monoclonal immunoglobulins (📖 p.360).

Disseminated intravascular coagulation (DIC)

Pathological process characterized by generalized intravascular activation of the haemostatic mechanism producing widespread fibrin formation, resultant activation of fibrinolysis, and consumption of platelets/coagulation factors (esp I, II, V). Usually the result of serious underlying disease but may itself become life threatening (through haemorrhage or thrombosis). Mortality in severe DIC may exceed >80%. Haemorrhage usually the dominant feature and is the result of excessive fibrinolysis, depletion of coagulation factors and platelets, and inhibition of fibrin polymerization by FDPs. Wide range of disorders may precipitate DIC.

Pathophysiology—DIC may be initiated by:

- Exposure of blood to tissue factor (e.g. after trauma).
- Endothelial cell damage (e.g. by endotoxin or cytokines).
- Release of proteolytic enzymes into the blood (e.g. pancreas, snake venom).
- Infusion or release of activated clotting factors (factor IX concentrate).
- Massive thrombosis.
- Severe hypoxia and acidosis.

Causes of DIC

Tissue damage (release of tissue factor) e.g. trauma (esp brain or crush injury), thermal injury (burns, hyperthermia, hypothermia), surgery, shock, asphyxia/hypoxia, ischaemia/infarction, rhabdomyolysis, fat embolism.

Complications of pregnancy (release of tissue factor) e.g. amniotic fluid embolism, abruptio placentae, eclampsia and pre-eclampsia, retained dead fetus, uterine rupture, septic abortion, hydatidiform mole.

Neoplasia (release of tissue factor, TNF, proteases) e.g. solid tumours, leukaemias (esp. acute promyelocytic).

Infection (endotoxin release, endothelial cell damage) e.g. Gram –ve bacteria (e.g. meningococcus), Gram +ve bacteria (e.g. pneumococcus), anaerobes, *M. tuberculosis*, toxic shock syndrome, viruses (e.g. Lassa fever), protozoa (e.g. malaria), fungi (e.g. candidiasis), Rocky Mountain spotted fever.

Vascular disorders (abnormal endothelium, platelet activation) e.g. giant haemangioma (Kasabach–Merritt syndrome), vascular tumours, aortic aneurysm, vascular surgery, cardiac bypass surgery, malignant hypertension, pulmonary embolism, acute MI, stroke, subarachnoid haemorrhage.

Immunological (complement activation, release of tissue factor) anaphylaxis, acute haemolytic transfusion reaction, heparin-associated thrombocytopenia, renal allograft rejection, acute vasculitis, drug reactions (quinine).

Proteolytic activation of coagulation factors e.g. pancreatitis, snake venom, insect bites.

Neonatal disorders e.g. infection, aspiration syndromes, small-for-dates infant, respiratory distress syndrome, purpura fulminans.

Other disorders e.g. fulminant hepatic failure, cirrhosis, Reye's syndrome, acute fatty liver of pregnancy, ARDS, therapy with fibrinolytic agents, therapy with factor IX concentrates, massive transfusion, acute intravascular haemolysis familial ATIII deficiency, homozygous protein C or S deficiency.

Clinical features

Clinical features may be masked by those of the disorder which precipitated it and rarely is the cause of DIC obscure. DIC should be considered in the management of any seriously ill patient, 📖 see Table 13.4. The specific features of DIC are:

- Ecchymoses, petechiae, oozing from venepuncture sites, and post-op bleeding.
- Renal dysfunction, ARDS, cerebral dysfunction, and skin necrosis due to microthrombi.
- MAHA.

Table 13.4 Clinical features of DIC

Acute (uncompensated) DIC	Rapid and extensive activation of coagulation, fibrinolysis, or both, with depletion of procoagulant factors and inhibitors and significant haemorrhage.
Chronic (compensated) DIC	Slow consumption of factors with ↔ or ↑ levels; often asymptomatic or associated with thrombosis.

Laboratory features

The following investigations are useful in establishing the diagnosis of DIC though the extent to which any single test may be abnormal reflects the underlying cause of DIC.

- D-dimers—more specific and convenient than FDP titre (performed on plasma sample). Significant ↑ of D-dimers plus depletion of coagulation factors ± platelets is necessary for diagnosis of DIC.
- PT—less sensitive, usually ↑ in moderately severe DIC but may be ↔ in chronic DIC.
- APTT—less useful. May be normal or even <↔, particularly in chronic DIC.
- Fibrinogen (Fgn)—↓ or falling Fgn levels are characteristic of many causes of DIC in the presence of D-dimers. Greatest falls are seen with tissue factor release.
- Platelet count—↓ or falling platelet counts are characteristic of acute DIC, most notably in association with infective causes.
- Blood film may show evidence of fragmentation (schistocytes) though the absence of this finding does not exclude the diagnosis of DIC.
- Antithrombin levels are frequently ↓ in DIC and degree of reduction in plasma antithrombin and plasminogen may reflect severity.

- Factor assays rarely necessary or helpful. In severe DIC levels of most factors are reduced with the exception of FVIIIc and von Willebrand factor which may be ↑ due to release from endothelial cell storage sites.

Management of DIC

- 1Identify and, if possible, remove the precipitating cause.
- Supportive therapy as required (e.g. volume replacement for shock).
- Replacement therapy if bleeding: platelet transfusion if platelets $<50 \times 10^9$/L, cryoprecipitate to replace Fgn, and FFP to replace other factors (10U cryoprecipitate for every 3U FFP).
- Prophylactic platelet transfusion may be helpful if platelets $<20 \times 10^9$/L.
- Monitor response with platelet count, PT, Fgn, and D-dimers.
- Heparin (IVI 5–10IU/kg/h) for DIC associated with APML, carcinoma, skin necrosis, purpura fulminans, microthrombosis affecting skin, kidney, bowel, and large vessel thrombosis.
- ATIII concentrate in intractable shock or fulminant hepatic necrosis.
- Protein C concentrate in acquired purpura fulminans or severe neonatal DIC.

Overdosage of thrombolytic therapy

- Large doses of any thrombolytic agent (streptokinase, urokinase, TPA) will cause 1° fibrinolysis by proteolytic destruction of circulating Fgn and consumption of plasminogen and its major inhibitor α2-antiplasmin.
- Overdosage is associated with high risk of severe haemorrhage particularly at recent venepuncture sites or surgical wounds; intracranial haemorrhage occurs in 0.5–1% of patients treated with thrombolytic therapy.
- Superficial bleeding at venepuncture site may be managed with local pressure and the infusion continued.
- Bleeding at other sites or where pressure cannot be applied necessitates cessation of thrombolytic therapy (t½ <30min) and determination of the thrombin time (if used to monitor thrombolytic therapy) or Fgn level. If strongly indicated and bleeding minimal or stopped the infusion may be restarted at 50% the initial dose when the thrombin time has returned to the lower end of the therapeutic range (1.5 × baseline).

Treatment of serious bleeding after thrombolytic therapy

- Stop thrombolytic infusion immediately.
- Discontinue any simultaneous heparin infusion and any antiplatelet agents.
- Apply pressure to bleeding sites, ensure good venous access, and commence volume expansion.
- Check Fgn and APTT.
- Transfuse 10U cryoprecipitate.
- Monitor Fgn, repeat cryoprecipitate to maintain Fgn >1.0g/L.
- If still bleeding, transfuse 2–4U FFP.
- If bleeding time >9min, transfuse 10U platelets.
- If bleeding time <9min, commence tranexamic acid.

Heparin overdosage

The most serious complication of heparin overdosage is haemorrhage. The therapeutic range using the APTT is 1.5–2.5 × average ↔ control. The plasma t½ following IV administration is 1–2h. The t½ after SC administration is considerably longer.

Management guidelines—APTT > therapeutic range

See Table 13.5.

Table 13.5 Management guidelines

Without haemorrhage	***Continuous IV infusion*** Stop infusion, if markedly elevated, recheck after 0.5–1h; restart at lower dose when APTT in therapeutic range
	Intermittent SC heparin Reduce dose recheck 6h after administration
With haemorrhage	***Continuous IV infusion*** Stop infusion; if bleeding continues, administer protamine sulphate by slow IV injection (1mg neutralizes 100IU heparin, max. dose 40mg/injection)
	Intermittent SC heparin If protamine is required, administer 50% of calculated neutralization dose 1h after heparin administration and 25% after 2h

Heparin-induced thrombocytopenia (HIT)

Uncommon but sometimes life-threatening condition due to immun complex-mediated thrombocytopenia in patients treated with hepari Early recognition reduces morbidity and mortality.

Incidence

Estimated incidence 1–3% of patients receiving heparin for ≥1wee Occurs both with full dose regimens and 'minidose' regimens (5000IU bd or low doses used for 'flushing' IV lines. Less common with LMWH.

Pathogenesis

IgG antibodies formed in response to heparin therapy form immun complexes with heparin and PF4, bind to platelet Fc receptors, trigge aggregation and cause thrombocytopenia. Thrombin activation cause vascular thrombosis and microthrombi cause microvascular occlusion.

Clinical features

- HIT causes a fall in the platelet count ~8d (4–14d) after a patient's 1st exposure to heparin but may occur within 1–3d in a patient who has recently had prior exposure to heparin.
- Platelet count generally falls to ~60 × 10^9/L but may fall to <20 × 10^9/L
- Venous and arterial thromboses occur in up to 15%.
- Bleeding is rare.
- Microvascular occlusion may cause progressive gangrene extending proximally from the extremities and necessitating amputation. In patien with HITT (thrombocytopenia and thrombosis) limb amputation is required in ~10% and mortality approaches 20%.

HIT should be suspected in any patient on heparin in whom the platele count falls to <100 × 10^9/L or drops by ≥30–40% or develops a ne thromboembolic event 5–10d after ongoing heparin therapy.

►►Heparin should be discontinued immediately and confirmatory inves tigations undertaken.

Diagnostic test

ELISA using PF4 to detect antibodies to heparin-low molecular weig protein complex; may miss 5–10% of cases with antibodies to othe proteins and up to 50% false +ves after CABG.

Management

- Discontinue heparin (platelet count normally recovers in 2–5d).
- Substitute alternative anticoagulation where necessary and to prevent further thromboembolic events:
- Recombinant hirudin:
  - Thrombin inhibitor; anticoagulant effect lasts ~40min.
  - Slow IV bolus followed by IVI.
  - Dose determined by body weight and renal function (see product literature).

- Monitor 4h after IV bolus dose using APTT or ecarin clotting time (ECT); target range 1.5–2.5 mean ↔ APTT; reduce target to 1.5 if concomitant warfarin therapy and discontinue hirudin when INR ≥2.0.
- Adverse effects bleeding (esp. with warfarin), anaemia, haematoma, fever and abnormal LFTs.

Argatroban
- Thrombin inhibitor; t½ ~45min.
- Initiate IV infusion at dose of 2mcg/kg/min.
- Check APTT at 2h and adjust dose for APTT 1.5–3 baseline (max. 100sec).
- ↓ dose by 75% if hepatic insufficiency.
- Side effect—bleeding.

Danaparoid
- A heparinoid with low level cross-reactivity with HIT antibodies.
- IV bolus dose by weight (see product literature) followed by decremental infusion schedule and maintenance infusion.
- Monitor by factor Xa inhibition assay 4h after dose (target range 0.5–0.8U/mL).
- Prolonged t½ of 25h.
- Side effect—bleeding.

►► LMWHs frequently cross-react with HIT antibodies and are not recommended.

Warfarin overdosage

Haemorrhage is a potentially serious complication of anticoagulan therapy and may occur with an INR in the therapeutic range if there ar local predisposing factors e.g. peptic ulceration or recent surgery, or i NSAIDs are given concurrently.

Management guidelines

See Table 13.6.

Table 13.6 Management guidelines for warfarin overdose

INR	Action
>7.0	Without haemorrhage: stop warfarin and consider a single 5–10mg oral dose of vitamin K if high bleeding risk; review INR daily
4.5–7.0	Without haemorrhage: stop warfarin and review INR in 2d
>4.5	*With severe life-threatening haemorrhage:* give factor IX concentrate (50U/kg) or FFP (1L for an adult), consider a single 2–5mg IV dose of vitamin K
>4.5	*With less severe haemorrhage:* e.g. haematuria or epistaxis, withhold warfarin for =1d and consider a single 0.5–2mg IV dose of vitamin K
2.0–4.5	With haemorrhage: investigate the possibility of an underlying local cause; reduce warfarin dose if necessary; give FFP/factor IX concentrate only if haemorrhage is serious or life threatening

Vitamin K administration to patients on warfarin therapy

Effect of vitamin K is delayed several hours even with IV administratior Doses >2 mg cause unpredictable and prolonged resistance to oral anti coagulants and should be avoided in most circumstances where prolonge warfarin therapy is necessary. Particular care must be taken in patient with prosthetic cardiac valves who may require heparin therapy for severa weeks to achieve adequate anticoagulation if a large dose of vitamin K ha been administered.

Massive blood transfusion

Massive transfusion defined as replacement of >1 blood volume (5L) in less than 24h. Haemostatic failure may result from dilution or consumption of coagulation factors and platelets, DIC, systemic fibrinolysis, or acquired platelet dysfunction.

Pathophysiology

- *Dilution/consumption* e.g. replacement of intravascular volume with fluids lacking coagulation factors or platelets e.g. packed red cells and crystalloids.
- *DIC* may follow tissue damage, hypoxia, acidosis, sepsis or haemolytic transfusion reaction. Causes coagulopathy due to consumption of platelets and coagulation factors, fibrinolysis and circulating fibrin degradation products (📖 see Disseminated intravascular coagulation, p.488, 642).
- *Systemic fibrinolysis* particularly associated with liver disease; causes rapid lysis of thrombi at surgical sites and plasmin-induced fibrinogenolysis; may be assessed by the euglobulin lysis time.
- *Platelet dysfunction* may be due to circulating FDPs, exhausted platelets activated by intravascular trauma or effects of transfusion of stored platelets.

Investigations

- Baseline tests
  - Haematocrit.
  - Platelet count.
  - Fgn.
  - PT.
  - APTT ratio.
  - D-dimers.
- Frequent reassessment of tests to monitor effect of, and need for, further replacement therapy.

Management

📖 See Table 13.7.

Table 13.7 Management guidelines

Haematocrit	<0.30	Transfuse red cells
Platelet count	$<75 \times 10^9$/L	Transfuse platelets
Fgn	<1.0g/L	Transfuse cryoprecipitate
PT ± APTT ratio	>1.5 × control	Transfuse FFP

Red cell transfusion

- Full crossmatch takes 30–40min.
- Uncrossmatched group-specific blood can be available in 10min.

- Uncrossmatched group O Rh (D) –ve blood may be transfused in the emergency situation until group-specific blood can be made available; group O Rh (D) +ve red cells may be given to ♂ and older ♀ if necessary.

Platelet transfusion

- Usually available within 10–15min.
- Standard adult dose (6U equivalent) will raise platelet count by ~60×10^9/L in absence of dilution or consumption.
- As platelets do not carry Rh antigens, type incompatible platelets may be administered when necessary; Rh immune globulin should be administered when a Rh –ve patient has received Rh +ve platelets.
- 6U of platelets contain ~300mL plasma.

FFP

- Takes up to 30min to thaw; dose required ~10mL/kg.
- Use immediately for optimum replacement of coagulation factors.
- Each unit contains ~200–280mL plasma and 0.7–1.0IU/mL activity of each coagulation factor
- ABO group compatible FFP should be administered—no crossmatch is required.
- If large volumes infused, serum [Ca^{2+}] should be monitored to exclude hypocalcaemia due to citrate toxicity.

Cryoprecipitate

- Precipitate formed when FFP is thawed at 4°C; resuspended in 10–15mL plasma and refrozen at –18°C; takes up to 15min to thaw and pool.
- No grouping required.
- Contains 80–100IU FVIIIC, 100–250mg Fgn, 50–60mg fibronectin, and 40–70% of the original vWF.
- Should be used immediately for optimum replacement of Fgn and factor VIIIC.
- Infusion of 8–10 bags raises Fgn concentration by 0.6–1.0g/L in a 70kg patient.

Paraparesis/spinal collapse

May be due to tumour in the cord, spinal dura or meninges or by extension of a vertebral tumour into the spinal canal with compression of the cord or as a result of vertebral collapse.

Spinal cord compression from vertebral collapse in a haematological patient is most commonly due to myeloma (in up to 20% of patients) but may occur in a patient with HL (3–8%) or occasionally NHL. Spinal cord involvement by leukaemia is most common in AML, less so in ALL and CGL, and least common in CLL.

Onset of paraplegia may be preceded for days or weeks by paraesthesia but in some patients the onset of paraplegia may follow initial symptoms by only a few hours.

Symptoms suggestive of spinal cord compression require urgent assessment by CT or MRI and referral to a neurosurgical unit for assessment for surgical decompression. Where this is not possible early radiotherapy may provide symptomatic improvement. However, if treatment is delayed until paraparesis has developed, this often proves to be irreversible despite surgery and/or radiotherapy.

Leucostasis

Term is applied both to organ damage due to 'sludging' of leucocytes in the capillaries of a patient with high circulating blast count and to the lodging and growth of leukaemic blasts, usually in AML, in the vascular tree eroding the vessel wall and producing tumours and haemorrhage.

Features

- More common in AML and blast crisis of CML.
- Leucostatic tumours are associated with an exponential increase in blasts in the peripheral blood and, prior to the development of effective chemotherapy, haemorrhage from intracerebral tumours was not an uncommon cause of death.
- Pulmonary or cerebral leucostasis are serious complications which may occur in patients who present with a blast count $>50 \times 10^9$/L.
- Leucocyte thrombi may cause plugging of pulmonary or cerebral capillaries. Vascular rupture and tissue infiltration may occur.
- Less common manifestations are priapism and vascular insufficiency.
- Pulmonary leucostasis causes progressive dyspnoea of sudden onset associated with fever, tachypnoea, hypoxaemia, diffuse crepitations, and a diffuse interstitial infiltrate on CXR.
- Pulmonary haemorrhage and haemoptysis may occur. More common with monocytic leukaemias and the microgranular variant of acute promyelocytic leukaemia. Differentiation from bacterial or fungal pneumonia may be difficult.
- Cerebral leucostasis may cause a variety of neurological abnormalities.
- Anaemia may protect a patient with marked leucocytosis from the effects of ↑ whole blood viscosity. Transfusion of RBCs to correct anaemia prior to chemotherapy may initiate leucostasis.

Management

Urgent leucapheresis is required for a patient with marked leucostasis ($>200 \times 10^9$/L) or in any patient in whom leucostasis is suspected. Chemotherapy may be commenced concomitantly to further reduce the leucocyte count but may be associated with a high incidence of pulmonary and CNS haemorrhage.

Thrombotic thrombocytopenic purpura

Definition

Fulminant disease of unknown aetiology characterized by ↑ platele aggregation and occlusion of arterioles and capillaries of the microcircula tion. Considerable overlap in pathophysiology and clinical features with HUS—fundamental abnormality may be identical.

Incidence

Rare, ~1 in 500,000 per year. ♀:♂ = 2:1. HUS much commoner in children TTP commoner in adults—peak age incidence is 40 years, and 90% o cases <60 years old. There is some case clustering.

Clinical features

- Classical description is of a pentad of features:
  - 1. Microangiopathic haemolytic anaemia.
  - 2. Severe thrombocytopenia.
  - 3. Neurological involvement.
  - 4. Renal impairment.
  - 5. Fever.

In practice, few patients have the 'full monty'. 50–70% have renal abnormalities (*cf.* nearly all with HUS) and they are less severe. Neurological involvement is more prevalent in TTP than HUS. 40% of TTP patients have fever.

- *Haemolysis*—severe and intravascular causing jaundice.
- *Thrombocytopenia*—severe, mucosal haemorrhage likely and intracranial haemorrhage may be fatal.
- *Neurological*—from mild depression and confusion → visual defects, coma and status epilepticus.
- *Renal*—haematuria, proteinuria, oliguria and ↑ urea and creatinine. HUS>TTP.
- *Fever*—very variable, weakness and nausea common.
- Other disease features: serious venous thromboses at unusual sites (e.g. sagittal sinus—microthrombi in the brain seen on MRI scan). Abdominal pain severe enough to mimic an acute abdomen is sometimes seen due to mesenteric ischaemia. Diarrhoea is common, particularly bloody in HUS.

Diagnosis and investigations

- Made on the clinical features—exclude other diseases e.g. cerebral lupus, sepsis with DIC.
- FBC shows severe anaemia and thrombocytopenia.
- Blood film usually shows gross fragmentation of red cells, spherocytes, and nucleated red cells with polychromasia.
- Reticulocytes ↑↑.
- LDH ↑↑ (>1000IU/L).
- Clotting screen including Fgn and FDPs usually ↔ (*cf.* DIC).
- Serum haptoglobin low or absent.
- Urinary haemosiderin +ve.
- Unconjugated bilirubin ↑.

- DAT –ve.
- BM hypercellular.
- U&E show ↑ (HUS>TTP).
- Proteinuria and haematuria.
- Renal biopsy shows microthrombi.
- Stool culture for *E. coli* 0157 +ve in most cases of HUS in children, less often in adult TTP.
- MRI brain scan shows microthrombi and occasional intracranial haemorrhage.
- ► *Lumbar puncture—do not proceed with LP unless scans clear and there is suspicion of infective meningitis.*
- Look for evidence of viral infection. Association of syndrome with HIV, SLE, usage, and the 3rd trimester of pregnancy.

Treatment is a haematological emergency—seek expert help immediately

1. Unless antecubital venous access is excellent, insert a large bore central apheresis catheter (may need blood product support).
2. May need ITU level of care and ventilation.
3. Initiate plasmapheresis as soon as possible.
   Exchange 1–1.5 plasma volume daily until clinical improvement. May need 3–4L exchanges. Replacement fluid should be solely FFP. In the event of delayed access to cell separator facilities, start IV infusions of FFP making intravascular space with diuretics if necessary. Once response achieved, ↓ frequency of exchanges gradually. If no response obtained within 1 week, change FFP replacement to *cryosupernatant* (rationale: it lacks HMW multimers of vWF postulated in endothelial damage disease triggers).
4. Give RBC as necessary but reserve platelet transfusions for sever mucosal or intracranial bleeding as reports suggest they may worsen the disease.
5. Cover for infection with IV broad spectrum antibiotics including teicoplanin if necessary to preserve the apheresis catheter.
6. Start anticonvulsants if fitting.
7. Most would start high dose steroids (prednisolone 2mg/kg/d PO) with gastric protection although evidence is equivocal.
8. Aspirin/dipyridamole/heparin may be considered for non-responders.
9. Refractory patients (~10%) should be considered for IV vincristine.
10. Still refractory patients may achieve remission with splenectomy.
11. Response to treatment may be dramatic e.g. ventilated, comatose patient watching TV in the afternoon after plasma exchange in the morning!

Prognosis

- 90% respond to plasma exchange with FFP replacement.
- ~30% will relapse. Most respond again to further plasma exchange but leaves 15% who become chronic relapsers.
- Role of prophylaxis for chronic relapsers unclear. Intermittent FFP infusions or continuous low dose aspirin may help individual cases.

Sickle crisis

Management

►Early and effective treatment of crises essential (hospital).
►Rest patient and start IV fluids and O2 (patients often dehydrated through poor oral intake of fluid + excessive loss if fever).
►Start empirical antibiotic therapy (e.g. cephalosporin) if infection is suspected whilst culture results (blood, urine or sputum) are awaited.
►Analgesia usually required—e.g. IV opiates (diamorphine/morphine) especially when patients are first admitted to hospital. Switch later to oral medication after the initial crisis abates.
►Consider exchange blood transfusion (if neurological symptoms, stroke or visceral damage). Aim to ↓ HbS to <30%.
►Exchange transfusion if PaO_2 <60mm on air (►chest syndrome).
►α-adrenergic stimulators for priapism.
►Seek advice of senior haematology staff.
►Consider regular blood transfusion if crises frequent or anaemia is severe or patient has had CVA/abnormal brain scan.
►Top-up transfusion if Hb <4.5g/dL (hunt for cause).

Transfusion and splenectomy may be lifesaving in children with splenic sequestration.

Management of acute chest syndrome

- O_2 supplementation.
- Antibiotics (include cover for community-acquired organisms and atypicals).
- Monitor fluid balance aiming for euvolaemia.
- Implement pain management, avoid splinting and oversedation.
- Bronchodilator therapy.
- Red cell transfusion if respiratory compromise or clinical deterioration.

1. www.bcshguidelines.com/pdf/SICKLE.V4_0802.pdf

Chapter 14

Supportive care

Quality of life

In managing any disease problem a key objective is to improve the quality of a patient's survival as well as its duration. Part of the clinical decision-making process takes into account QoL in judging the most appropriate treatment. QoL is also evaluated as an outcome in clinical trials parallel to conventional measures such as survival.

Defining QoL precisely is not easy; it has been described as a measure of the difference at a particular time point between the hopes and expectations of the individual and that individual's present experiences. QoL is multifaceted and can only be assessed by the individual since it takes into account many aspects of that individual's life and their current perception of what, for them, is good QoL in their specific circumstances.

A clear distinction exists between performance scores (e.g. Karnofsky or WHO) which record functional status and assess independence; these are assessed by the physician according to pre-set criteria. They have erroneously been considered to be surrogate markers of QoL.

Patient QoL as assessed by the treating physician has been shown to be unreliable in an oncological setting.

There is no single determinant of good QoL. A number of qualities which go to make up QoL are capable of assessment; these include: *ability to carry on normal physical activities, ability to work, to engage in normal social activities, a sense of general well-being,* and a *perception of health.*

Several validated instruments now exist to measure QoL; these mainly involve questionnaires completed by the patient. They are simple to complete and involve 'yes' or 'no' answers to specific questions, answers on a linear analogue scale or the use of 4- or 7-point Likert scales.

Available QoL instruments include:

- Functional Living Index–Cancer (FLIC)[1]
- Functional Assessment of Cancer Therapy (FACT)[2]
- European Organisation for Research and Treatment in Cancer (EORTC) Quality of Life Questionnaire C-30 (QLQ C30)[3]

Data from validated QoL questionnaires are now accepted as a requirement and a clinical end point in many major clinical trials, especially in malignancies, particularly those where survival differences are minimal between contrasting therapy approaches. Where survivals are minimally affected it is then essential to focus on treatments which will offer the best QoL.

1. Schipper, H. *et al.* (1984). Measuring the quality of life of cancer patients: the Functional Living Index–Cancer: development and validation. *J Clin Oncol*, **2**, 472–83.
2. Cella, D.F. *et al.* (1993). The Functional Assessment of Cancer Therapy scale: development and validation of the general measure. *J Clin Oncol*, **11**, 570–9.
3. Aaronson, N.K. *et al.* (1993). The European Organization for Research and Treatment of Cancer QLQ-C30: a quality-of-life instrument for use in international clinical trials in oncology. *J Natl Cancer Inst*, **85**, 365–76.

Pain management

Pain is a clinical problem in diverse haematological disorders, notably in sickle cell disease, haemophilia, and myeloma. Acknowledgement of the need to manage pain effectively is an essential part of successful patient care and management in clinical haematology.

Pain may be local or generalized. More than one type of pain may be present and causes may be multifactorial. It is most important to listen to the patient and give them the chance to talk about their pain(s). Not only will this help determine an appropriate therapeutic strategy, the act of listening and allowing the patient to talk about their pains and associated anxieties is part of the pain management process.

Engaging the patient in 'measuring' their pain is often helpful; it enables specific goals to be set and provides a means to assess the effectiveness of the analgesic strategy. A variety of scales have been employed, with simple numerical values ('pain score out of ten') being the most common. These strategies must be tailored to the individual patient's comprehension—often young children are being assessed.

Basic to the control of pain is to manage and remove the pathological process causing pain, wherever this is possible. Analgesia must be part of an integrated care plan which takes this into account.

Analgesic requirements should be recorded regularly as these form a valuable 'semi-quantitative' end point of pain measurement. Reduction in requirements, for example, is an indicator that attempts to remove or control the underlying cause are succeeding.

Managing pain successfully involves patient and family/carer participation, a collaborative multidisciplinary approach in most categories of haematological disorder-related pain; medication should aim to provide continuous pain relief wherever possible with a minimum of drug related side effects. Anticipating pain with the use of regular medications rather than a 'prn' basis can be key to analgesic success. Treatment strategies are based on the WHO pain ladder, simple analgesics being used initially, in combination with opiates of ↑ strength if pain is not relieved.

Table 14.1 Analgesics

Simple non-opioid analgesics	Paracetamol: 1g 4–6-hourly, oral as tablets or liquid; suppositories available.
	No contraindication in liver disease; useful in mild-to-moderate pain.
Anti-inflammatory drugs	Ibuprofen 800mg or diclofenac 75–100mg bd as slow release formulations can be synergistic with other analgesics; combined formulations of diclofenac with misoprostol may reduce risks of gastric irritation bleeding, or used with gastric acid suppressants; useful in combination with paracetamol or weak opioids.
	Caution should be exercised in renal impairment (notably in myeloma).

Table 14.1 Analgesics (*continued*)

Weak opioids	Codeine 30–60mg usually combined with paracetamol 1g as co-codamol 30/500 tablets; usual dosage is 2 tablets 6-hourly or dihydrocodeine 30–60mg up to 4-hourly provide effective analgesia for moderate pain.
	Confusion, drowsiness may be associated with initial usage in some. Weak (and strong) opioids cause constipation; usually requires simple laxatives
Strong opioids	Morphine available as liquid or tablets commencing at 5–10mg and given 4-hourly is treatment of choice in severe pain.
	Once daily requirements are established patients can be 'converted' to 12-hourly slow release morphine preparations.
	Breakthrough pain can be treated with additional doses of 5–10mg morphine. Diamorphine preferred for parenteral usage. Highly soluble and suitable for use in a syringe driver for continuous administration or as a 4-hourly injection. Can be administered as a nasal spray in children. Accumulation can occur with renal impairment.
Alternatives to opioids	Tramadol may be given orally.
	Fentanyl given as slow release transdermal patches may be a valuable alternative to slow release morphine for moderate-to-severe chronic pain. It is also available in 'lollipop' form for rapid relief
	Oxycodone is a newer synthetic opiate which has been successfully employed as an alternative to morphine where analgesia is inadequate or adverse effects intolerable.

For chronic pain give analgesia PO regularly, wherever possible.

- Pain control is very specific to the individual patient, there is no 'correct' formula other than the combination of measures which alleviate the pain.
- The clinician should work 'upwards' or 'downwards' through the levels of available analgesics to achieve control.
- Constipation due to analgesics should be managed with aperients.
- Nausea or vomiting may occur in up to 50% patients with strong opiates; cyclizine 50mg 8-hourly, metoclopramide 10mg 8-hourly oraloperidol 1.5mg 12-hourly are available options to limit nausea orvomiting.
- Additional general measures include:
  - Radiotherapy for localized cancer pain and lytic lesions in myeloma.
  - Physical methods e.g. TENS or consideration of nerve root block.
  - Surgery, especially in myeloma where stabilizing fractures and pinning will relieve pain and allow mobility.

  - Encouraging/allowing patients to utilize 'alternative' approaches. including relaxation techniques, aromatherapy, hypnosis, etc.
- Additional drug therapy:
  - Antidepressants e.g. amitriptyline may help in neuropathic pain.
  - Anticonvulsants e.g. carbamazepine and gabapentin may be helpful in neuropathic pains especially in post-herpetic neuralgia.
  - Corticosteroids, particularly dexamethasone, to relieve leukaemic bone pain in late-stage disease.

Many hospitals also run specific pain clinics and have palliative care or pain control teams who can review inpatients and offer advice. The support and expertise available should be enlisted particularly for difficult problems with persistent localized pain e.g. post-herpetic neuralgia. For long-term painful conditions it is essential to work with medical and nursing colleagues in Primary Care and in Palliative Care so that the patient receives appropriate support in the community setting. Physiotherapy care can also be appropriate, particularly with chronic joint damage (for example in haemophilic arthropathy), and orthopaedic referral is often useful.

The severe acute pain in sickle crises often requires high and frequent doses of strong opiates. Health professionals unused to caring for patients with these conditions are sometimes cautious about use of such high doses and fear that patients may become addicted. Situations can arise whereby the patients are not receiving appropriate care because of such fears. These can be generally resolved by good communication and education. Psychological dependence on opiates is rare, and may be associated with difficult psychosocial circumstances which makes care for such patients challenging.

Psychological support

Many haematological disorders are long-term conditions; the specific diagnosis can be seen to 'label' the patient as different or ill and therefore will exert a profound influence on their life and that of their immediate family or carers. Patients (and their families) experience and demonstrate a number of reactions to their diagnosis, the clinical haematologist needs to have an awareness of this and respond accordingly.

Reactions to serious diagnosis include:

- Numbness.
- Denial.
- Anger.
- Guilt.
- Depression.
- Loneliness.

Ultimately most patients come to acceptance of their condition; carers/partners will also go through a similar range of reactions. The clinician needs to be aware of the way in which news of a diagnosis is likely to affect a patient and their family/carers and respond appropriately. In the first instance this will often involve the need to impart the diagnosis, what it means, and what needs to be done clinically. There is no 'right way' to impart bad or difficult news. It is very important to make and take time to tell the patient of the diagnosis. Wherever possible this should be done in a quiet, private setting. The presence of experienced nursing professionals is advised. Numbness at learning of a serious diagnosis often means that very little is taken in initially other than the diagnostic label. The various reactions listed above may subsequently emerge during the time the patient comes to accept the diagnosis, what it means, and what is to be done clinically. Literature can be very useful to convey disease information.

Within the haematological team there should be support available to the patient and family/carers which can provide them with practical information about the disease and its management. Simply knowing there is a sympathetic ear may be all that is required in the way of support; however, for some patients and families/carers more specialized support may be needed e.g. availability of formal counselling or access to psychological or psychiatric support.

Children may experience a variety of haematological diseases requiring admission to hospital. They will have ongoing needs as regards schooling and exams. Specialist professionals such as play therapists can help families through frightening and confusing experiences.

Use can be made of local or national patient support groups; knowledge of others in similar predicaments can help diffuse anger and loneliness. Support groups can also be a valuable resource in providing information and experience which patients and families/carers find helpful.

The most effective psychological support for haematological patients is to see them as individuals and not 'diseases'.

Chapter 15
Protocols and procedures

Note

Please check local protocols since these may differ to those outlined in this handbook.

Acute leukaemia—investigations

- FBC, blood film, reticulocytes, ESR.
- Serum B12, red cell folate, and ferritin.
- Blood group, antibody screen, and DAT.
- Coagulation screen, INR, APTT, fibrinogen, (and D-dimers if bleeding).
- BM aspirate for morphology, cytogenetics, immunophenotype (type peripheral blood if relevant) plus samples required by the MRC trials.
- BM trephine biopsy.

Biochemistry

- U&E, LFTs.
- Ca^{2+}, phosphate, random glucose.
- LDH.
- Serum and urine lysozyme (if M4 or M5 AML suspected).

Virology

- Hepatitis BsAg.
- Hepatitis A antibody.
- Hepatitis C antibody.
- HIV I and II antibody (counselling and consent required).
- CMV IgG and IgM.

Immunology

- Serum immunoglobulins.
- Autoantibody screen profile.
- HLA type—class 1 always in case HLA matched platelets are required, class 1 and 2 if allogeneic transplant indicated.

Bacteriology

- Baseline blood cultures.
- Throat swab.
- MSU.
- Stool for fungal culture.
- Nose swab for MRSA if transferred from another hospital/unit.

Cardiology

- ECG.
- Echocardiogram, only if in cardiac failure or infective endocarditis suspected or significant cardiac history.

Radiology

- CXR.

Other

- If any evidence of severe dental caries or gum disease refer patient for dental assessment before chemotherapy.
- Consider semen/embryo storage.

Platelet storage and administration

Storage

- Platelets should be stored at room temperature (20–22°C) in a platelet agitator until infused. Helps to retain function. Use before expiry date on pack.
- Platelet packs should be inspected before infusion—platelet packs that look visibly pink due to RBC contamination should not be used.
  - Occasionally fine fibrinoid strands may be seen in concentrates (give a slightly stringy or cloudy appearance). Such strands disperse with gentle massage and are safe to use.
  - Occasionally larger aggregates of platelets and/or white cell clumps are seen in the bags which do not disperse with gentle massage. Such bags are dangerous and should never be infused.

Dosage and timing

- A single dose of platelets is generally supplied as a single bag.
- Represents a standard transfusion dose although twice this amount may be required to cover insertions of central lines or minor surgery.
- Occasionally double doses may be required for patients becoming refractory.
- The frequency of platelet transfusion will be determined by clinical circumstances. In general, a patient who is well, afebrile, and with no evidence of new bruising or bleeding need only have a platelet count maintained above 10×10^9/L. May be achieved with platelets given as infrequently as every 2–4d with this interval being guided on daily platelet counts.
- Patients who are infected or bleeding have much greater platelet requirements—aim to keep the platelet count $>20 \times 10^9$/L. This will usually mean daily platelet infusions for the duration of this clinical episode.
- Platelet counts of $<10 \times 10^9$/L should always be avoided but within these constraints the fewer platelets transfused the better since this reduces the risk of alloimmunization to HLA and platelet antigens.
- Anyone with a persistent platelet count $<10 \times 10^9$/L should be started on tranexamic acid 1g qds PO or IV unless specific contraindications exist such as genitourinary tract bleeding.

Choice of blood group for platelet support

At diagnosis, all patients should have a blood group and CMV antibody status determined. Patients should receive platelets of their own blood group as far as possible. Due to fluctuations in supply, this is not always possible and the choice is less critical than for red cell transfusions as platelet ABO blood group antigen expression is weak and the recipient exposed only to donor plasma. 📖 See Table 15.1.

- Occasionally necessary to give Rh (D) +ve platelets to Rh (D) –ve patients. The Blood Bank should be informed as all future red cell transfusions must be Rh (D) –ve. Anti-D administration may be given to such patients routinely or may be reserved for women of child-bearing age (dose: 250IU (50mcg). Anti-D SC immediately after the transfusion

Table 15.1 Choice of blood group for platelet support

Patient's blood group	1st choice	2nd choice
O	O	A
A	A	O
B	B (if available)	A preferably or O
AB	A	O

Rh (D) +ve patients may receive Rh (D) +ve or Rh (D) –ve products.
Rh (D) –ve patients should receive Rh (D) –ve platelets.

Platelet transfusion support

📖 See Platelet transfusion, p.768.

Platelet reactions and refractoriness

Reactions to platelet transfusion are common and range from mild temperatures to rigors. The development of an urticarial rash is also frequently seen. When a transfusion reaction develops, the following steps should be taken:

- ► Stop the transfusion.
- ► Give 10mg chlorphenamine (chlorphenamine) IV and 1g of paracetamol PO.
- ► Cover future transfusions with chlorphenamine and paracetamol 30min pre-transfusion.
- Hydrocortisone 100mg IV stat may be (sparingly) used for refractory reactions
- Pethidine is a suitable alternative for severe reactions and is almost invariably effective. Give 25mg IV stat with repeat dose if necessary or set up an IVI of 25–50mg IV over 8h.
- The possibility of generation of HLA and platelet-specific antibodies should also be considered (📖 see Proceed as follows, p. 672).

Platelet refractoriness

Occasionally patients show little/no increment in the platelet count after platelet transfusions. This is called platelet refractoriness. May be due to physical or immunological mechanisms in the patient. The commonest physical mechanism is of platelet circulatory half-life reduction caused by concurrent sepsis or coagulopathy e.g. DIC. Immunological causes include induction of anti-HLA antibodies due to allosensitization from previous transfusions or generation of anti-platelet antibodies such as in ITP. Investigation should be considered if platelet transfusions fail to maintain a platelet count $>10 \times 10^9$/L at all times.

Proceed as follows

- Check FBC pre-platelet infusion, 1 and 12h post-infusion to assess the rate of platelet count decay. Failure to show a rise of platelet count by at least 10×10^9/L at 1h or any rise after 12h post-infusion merits further testing.
- Samples should be sent to a blood transfusion centre for HLA and platelet antibody screening (10mL EDTA samples and 20mL serum).
- The patient's own HLA type should be checked.
- If HLA or platelet antibodies are identified, the provision of HLA or platelet antigen matched platelet products may improve the platelet transfusion responsiveness.

Platelet refractoriness

More than two-thirds of patients receiving multiple transfusion with random platelets develop anti-HLA antibodies. Refractoriness defined as failure of 2 consecutive transfusions to give corrected increment of $>7.5 \times 10^9$/L 1h after platelet transfusion in absence of fever, infection, severe bleeding, splenomegaly, or DIC.

GvHD

Rare complication where there is engraftment of donor lymphocytes in platelet concentrate in severely immunocompromised patients. Filtration reduces risk.

Box 5.1 Calculating platelet increment $[(P_1–P_0)\ SA]/n$

P_0 = platelet count pre-transfusion ($\times 10^9$/L)
P_1 = platelet count post-transfusion ($\times 10^9$/L)
SA = surface area
n = number of units of platelets transfused

Corrected increment 60min after transfusion $>7.5 \times 10^9$/L indicates successful platelet transfusion (P_1–P_0).

1. Hows, J.M. and Brozovic, R. (1992). In *ABC of Transfusion* 2nd edn, Contreras, M., (ed). BMJ Publishing, London.

Prophylactic regimen for neutropenic patients

Infective risk is related to the severity and duration of neutropenia. Higher risk is associated with concurrent immunological defects e.g. hypogammaglobulinaemia in myeloma, T-cell defects e.g. HIV disease, additional immunosuppressive agents e.g. ciclosporin post-transplant, and older patients. Principal risk is from bacterial organisms but fungi and viruses, especially herpes (HSV, HZV) and CMV are also seen in prolonged neutropenia.

Typical protocols include:

- ***Isolation procedures***—strict handwashing by all patient contacts is the only isolation measure of universally proven benefit. Others include visitor restriction, gloves, aprons, gowns, masks, and full reverse barrier nursing. Isolation rooms with +ve pressure filtered air will reduce risk of fungal infection.
- ***Drinks***—avoid mains tap water/still mineral water (use boiled water or sparkling mineral water). Avoid unpasteurized milk and freshly squeezed fruit juice.
- ***Food***—avoid cream, ice-cream, soft, blue, or ripened cheeses, live yoghurt, raw eggs or derived foods e.g. mayonnaise and soufflés, cold chicken, meat paté, raw fish/shellfish, unpeeled fresh vegetables/salads, unpeeled fruit, uncooked herbs and spices, ground pepper (contains *Aspergillus* spores).
- ***General mouthcare***—antiseptic mouthwash e.g. Chlorhexidine gluconate 10mL 4-hourly swish and spit. If soreness develops, substitute benzydamine mouth-wash. For discrete oral ulcers, use topical triancinolone dental paste; for generalized ulceration use 0.9% saline mouthwash hourly, swish and spit. Chlorhexidine gluconate 1% gel should replace standard toothpastes. Oral antifungal prophylaxis should be nystatin susp. 1mL 4-hourly swish and spit or swallow, or amphotericin lozenges, 1 to suck slowly 4-hourly.
- ***Antibacterial prophylaxis***—aim to alter flora and prevent exogenous colonization. Principal agents: ciprofloxacin 250mg bd, or co-trimoxazole 480mg bd, or colistin 1.5MU tds and neomycin 500mg qds. All given PO starting 48h after antifungal prophylaxis.
- ***Antifungal prophylaxis***—a systemic imidazole compound is most routinely used e.g. fluconazole 100mg PO od. Itraconazole liquid 2.5mg/kg bd PO may offer additional protection against *Aspergillus*.
- ***Antiviral prophylaxis***—aciclovir is the most useful drug at preventing herpes reactivation. Dose is dependent on degree of immunosuppression and thus the likely organism to be encountered. 400mg bd will prevent HSV reactivation e.g. post-standard chemotherapy; 400mg qds may prevent HZV reactivation e.g. post-SCT; 800mg tds or more may prevent CMV reactivation post-allogeneic SCT.
- ***Additional prophylaxis for specials situations***—history of, or radiological evidence of, tuberculosis (TB). Consideration should be given to standard anti-TB prophylaxis e.g. isoniazid for 6 months particularly if prolonged neutropenia expected. Splenectomized patient—at extra

risk from encapsulated organisms particularly *Streptococcus pneumoniae, Haemophilus influenzae and Neisseria meningitidis*. Use penicillin V 500mg od PO or erythromycin 250 mg bd PO if penicillin allergic as prophylaxis switching to high dose amoxicillin/cefotaxime if febrile. Post-SCT (📖 see p. 445).

Guidelines for use of IV antibiotics in neutropenic patients

Urgent action required if neutropenic patient develops:

- Single fever spike >38°C.
- 2 fever spikes >37.5°C 1h apart.
- Symptoms or signs of sepsis even without fever.

Assessment

- Search for localizing symptoms or signs of infection.
- Full clinical examination noting BP, pulse, mouth, chest, perineum, line sites, skin. and fundi.
- O_2 saturation (pulse oximetry).
- FBC, U&E, creatinine, LFTs, CRP, PT, APTT, fibrinogen.
- Perform a septic screen:
  - 3 sets of blood cultures (10mL per bottle optimizes organism recovery) if central line present, take paired peripheral and central samples.
  - Single further blood culture set if non-response at 48–72h or condition changes.
- Swab relevant sites: wounds, central line exit site, throat.
- Sputum culture.
- MSSU.
- Faeces if symptomatic incl. *C. difficile* toxin.
- Viral serology if clinically relevant.
- CXR.
- Other imaging as relevant, consider sinus CT.
- Consider bronchoalveolar lavage if chest infiltrates present.
- Consider risk of invasive fungal infection: CT chest if high risk.

Empirical treatment

Start IV antibiotics to provide broad spectrum cover. Stop prophylactic ciprofloxacin. Follow local protocol if available.

1st line: Tazocin® 4.5g tds plus gentamicin 6mg/kg/day.

If patient has history of penicillin allergy use ceftazidime 2g tds instead of Tazocin®; if anaphylaxis with penicillin discuss with microbiologist.

If suspected line infection (exit site inflammation) add vancomycin 1g bd and consider line removal. Vancomycin dose should be split and administered through each lumen. May be locked in the line for 1h then flushed.

If there are signs of perianal sepsis, mucositis or intra-abdominal infection or if *C. difficile* is suspected add metronidazole 500mg tds IV.

- Patients on od gentamicin should have pre-dose level checked 24h after 1st dose then twice weekly if satisfactory.
- Patients on vancomycin should have predose levels checked immediately before 3rd or 4th dose (2nd if renal impairment) then twice weekly if satisfactory.

Reassess at 48–72h

If no response to antibiotics and –ve blood cultures:

- Add vancomycin 1g bd.
- If already on vancomycin, consider line removal.
- Consider risk of invasive fungal infection. CT chest if high risk.

Reassess after further 48–72h

If no response to antibiotics and –ve blood cultures:

If high risk for invasive fungal infection:

Stop antibiotics. Commence anti-fungal therapy (e.g. liposomal amphotericin 3mg/kg/day) plus ciprofloxacin 500mg bd PO/IV. Stop prophylactic fluconazole/itraconazole.

If low risk for invasive fungal infection:

Switch antibiotics to meropenem 1g tds plus gentamicin 6mg/kg/d.

Reassess after further 48h

- If no response to anti-fungal therapy, change ciprofloxacin to meropenem 1g tds plus gentamicin 6mg/kg/d.
- If not on anti-fungal therapy, consider switching to liposomal amphotericin 3mg/kg/ day plus ciprofloxacin 500mg bd PO/IV. Stop prophylactic fluconazole/itraconazole.

Duration of therapy

If temperature responds but cultures are –ve, continue anti-infective treatment until apyrexial for 72h or minimum 5d course. If still neutropenic restart prophylactic anti-infectives. Anti-fungal therapy should be continued until complete response and neutrophil regeneration; no fixed duration can be recommended; oral voriconazole or posaconazole can facilitate early discharge during this period.

+ve cultures

Antibiotic therapy may be changed on the basis of +ve cultures.

Treatment of neutropenic sepsis when source unknown

►► One of the commonest haemato-oncological emergencies.

- May be defined as the presence of symptoms or signs of infection in a patient with an absolute neutrophil count of $<1.0 \times 10^9$/L. In practice, the neutrophil count is often $<0.1 \times 10^9$/L.
- Similar clinical picture also seen in neutrophil function disorders such as MDS despite ↔ neutrophil numbers.
- *Beware*—can occur without pyrexia, especially patients on steroids.

Immediate action

►► Urgent clinical assessment.

- Follow ALS guidelines if cardiorespiratory arrest (rare).
- More commonly, clinical picture is more like cardiovascular shock ± respiratory embarrassment viz: tachycardia, hypotension, peripheral vasodilatation, and tachypnoea. Occurs with both Gram +ve (now more common with indwelling central catheters) and Gram –ve organisms (less common but more fulminant).
- Immediate rapid infusion of albumin 4.5% or Gelofusine® to restore BP.
- Insert central catheter if not *in situ* and monitor CVP.
- Start O_2 by face mask if pulse oximetry shows saturations <95% (common) and consider arterial blood gas measurement—care with platelet counts $<20 \times 10^9$/L—manual pressure over puncture site for 30min.
- Perform full septic screen (📖 see Guidelines for use of IV antibiotics in neutropenic patients, p. 676).
- Give the 1st dose of 1st-line antibiotics immediately e.g ureidopenicillin and loading dose aminoglycoside (ceftazidime or ciprofloxacin if pre-existing renal impairment). Follow established protocols.
- If the event occurs while patient on 1st-line antibiotics, vancomycin/ciprofloxacin or vancomycin/meropenem are suitable alternatives.
- Commence full ITU-type monitoring chart.
- Monitor urine output with urinary catheter if necessary—if renal shutdown has already occurred, give single bolus of IV furosemide. If no response, start renal dose dopamine.
- If BP not restored with colloid despite elevated CVP, consider inotropes.
- If O_2 saturations remain low despite 60% O_2 delivered by rebreathing mask, consider ventilation.
- *Alert ITU giving details of current status.*

Subsequent actions

- Discuss with senior colleague.
- Amend antibiotics according to culture results or to suit likely source if cultures –ve.
- Check aminoglycoside trough levels after loading dose and before 2nd dose as renal impairment may determine reducing or withholding next dose. Consider switch to non-nephrotoxic cover e.g. ceftazidime/ciprofloxacin.

- Continue antibiotics for 7–10d minimum and usually until neutrophil recovery.
- If cultures show central line to be source of sepsis, remove immediately if patient not responding.

Treatment of neutropenic sepsis when source known/suspected

Central indwelling catheters

Very common. Organisms usually *Staph. epidermidis* but can be other *Staph* spp. and even Gram –ve organisms. May be erythema/exudate around entry or exit sites of line, tenderness/erythema over SC tunnel or discomfort over line track. Blood cultures must be taken from each lumen and peripherally and labelled individually. Add vancomycin 1g bd IV if not in standard protocol. Split dose between all lumens unless cultures known to be +ve in one lumen only. Lock and leave in line for 1h, then flush through. If no response or clinical deterioration, remove line immediately.

Perianal or periodontal

Both are common sites of infection in neutropenic patients. Perianal lesions may become secondarily infected if skin abraded. Add metronidazole 500mg IV tds to standard therapy. Painful SC abscesses may form and may require surgical incision. Gum disease and localized tooth infections/abscesses are frequently seen. Add metronidazole to therapy as above, arrange OPG and dental review as surgical intervention may be required in non-responders. If possible, best delayed until neutrophil recovery in most cases—then do electively before next course of chemotherapy.

Atypical organisms

Risk group

- HIV infection, HCL, post-SCT.
- *Mycoplasma* and other atypicals are commonly found and usually community acquired (*except Legionella*)—typically occur shortly after return to hospital and in patients with chronic lung disease.

Treatment

Azithromycin (or clarithromycin if IV preparation needed) is now treatment of choice—well absorbed and fewer side effects than erythromycin. 5d rather than 3d course may be needed.

Pneumocystis jiroveci pneumonia

Risk group

Lymphoid malignancy long-term treatment esp. ALL, steroid usage, purine analogues e.g. fludarabine and cladribine.

Treatment

High dose cotrimoxazole IV initially—watch renal function and adjust dose to creatinine. Give short pulse of steroid 0.5mg/kg at start of treatment. At-risk patients should remain on long-term prophylaxis until chemo finished and absolute CD4 lymphocyte count >500 × 10^6/L. Use co-trimoxazole 480mg bd on Monday, Wednesday, and Friday only, provided neutrophil count maintained >1.0 × 10^9/L. Otherwise use nebulized pentamidine 300mg every 3 weeks with preceding nebulized salbutamol 2.5mg.

Fungal

Risk group

Prolonged, severe neutropenia, chronic steroid and antibiotic usage, GvHD. *Aspergillus* and other moulds increasingly common with intensive chemotherapy protocols and post-stem cell transplant esp. MUDs.

Treatment

- Liposomal amphotericin or voriconazole IV (📖 see Invasive fungal infections and antifungal therapy, p. 436).
- Once neutrophil recovery has occurred, maintenance may be with oral itraconazole liquid 2.5mg/kg bd or oral voriconazole 400mg bd × 24h then 200mg bd—may also be used for prophylaxis.

Viral—CMV

Risk group

Allogeneic SCT esp. UDs where donor or recipient is CMV +ve. Disease usually due to reactivation rather than *de novo* infection. Apart from pneumonitis, may cause graft suppression, gastritis, oesophagitis, weight loss, hepatitis, retinitis, haemorrhagic cystitis, and vertigo.

Treatment

Ganciclovir or foscarnet (📖 see CMV, p. 440) + IV immunoglobulin. Lack of response, switch to the other drug.

Viral—HSV/HZV

Risk group

Rare causes of lung disease. SCT recipients at greatest risk esp. UDs and intensively treated lymphoid malignancy.

Treatment

High dose IV aciclovir 5–10mg/kg tds IV for minimum 10d.

Viral—RSV

Risk group

Post-SCT recipients esp. UDs.

Treatment

Consider ribovarin therapy.

TB and atypical mycobacteria

Risk group

Prolonged T-cell immunosuppression e.g. chronic steroid or ciclosporin therapy, chronic GvHD, previous history and/or treatment for TB, HIV-related disease.

Treatment

Often difficult to diagnose—empirical treatment required with standard triple therapy.

Prophylaxis for patients treated with purine analogues

The purine analogues fludarabine and cladribine used in standard lymphoproliferative protocols induce neutropenia in all cases. Nadir ~14d post-treatment initiation and neutrophil counts may fall to zero for several days or even weeks. They are therefore associated with the usual neutropenic infections. In addition, purine analogues have a particular property of inhibition of CD4 helper lymphocyte subsets within weeks of initiation of therapy (nadir at 3 months) and may last for >1 year following cessation of therapy. This profound CD4 function inhibition predisposes to fungal infection, as well as a higher incidence of *H zoster* infection and *P. jiroveci*. ↓ lymphocyte function also predisposes to transfusion associated GvHD by passenger lymphocytes in donor blood transfusions.

The following preventive measures are recommended:

Recommended

- Irradiation of cellular blood products (2500cGy) from d1 of initiation of therapy and continue until 2 years post-treatment.
- *P. jiroveci* prophylaxis from start of therapy—usually cotrimoxazole 480mg bd Mondays, Wednesdays, and Fridays. In patients who are already severely neutropenic, cotrimoxazole may be substituted by pentamidine nebulizers 300mg 4-weekly with 2.5mg of salbutamol nebulizer pretreatment. *P. jiroveci* prophylaxis should continue for 3 months after the end of treatment.
- HZV prophylaxis—aciclovir 400mg qds is the minimum continuous dose required to prevent HZV reactivation. Most physicians will not wish to have patients continuously on this dosage throughout the treatment cycle and for a year post-treatment so suggest: counsel patients about the risk of shingles and advise to contact the hospital immediately if shingles suspected. Patients who have already had a zoster reactivation should be maintained continuously on aciclovir 400mg qds and continuation of the purine analogue reviewed.

Optional

- Anti-bacterial prophylaxis—consider use of ciprofloxacin 250mg bd PO from d7 → d21 of each course.
- Anti-fungal prophylaxis: patients with no history of fungal reactivation should perform nystatin suspension 1mL qds mouthcare from d7 → d21 of each course, taught symptoms of oral and genital thrush, and supplied with fluconazole 200mg to be taken daily for 7d in the event of thrush.
- Patients with previous history of suspected fungal infection with a mould-type organism e.g. *Aspergillus*—give itraconazole oral liquid 2.5mg/kg bd throughout treatment.

Tumour lysis syndrome (TLS)

Potentially life threatening metabolic derangement resulting from treatment-induced or spontaneous tumour necrosis causing renal, cardiac, or neurological complications. Usually occurs in rapidly proliferating, highly chemosensitive neoplasms with high tumour load: leukaemias with high WBC counts (ALL >50 × 10^9/L; AML >100 × 10^9/L; CML blast crisis >100 × 10^9/L; CLL >200 × 10^9/L; PLL or ATLL >100 × 10^9/L) and high grade NHL (particularly Burkitt lymphoma or high serum LDH). May occur before or up to 5d (usually 48–72h) after initiation of chemotherapy.

Pathophysiology and clinical features

Rapid lysis of large numbers of tumour cells releases intracellular ions and metabolites into the circulation causing numerous metabolic abnormalities to develop rapidly:

- *Hyperuricaemia* due to metabolism of nucleic acid purines; (solubility ↓ by high acidity); may cause arthralgia and renal colic.
- *Hyperkalaemia* due to rapid cell lysis; often earliest sign of TLS; aggravated by renal failure; may cause paraesthesiae, muscle weakness, and arrhythmias.
- *Hyperphosphataemia* due to rapid cell lysis,; precipitates calcium phosphate in tissues (insolubility exacerbated by overzealous alkalinization).
- *Hypocalcaemia* secondary to hyperphosphataemia; may cause paraesthesiae, tetany, carpo-pedal spasm, altered mental state, seizures, and arrhythmias.
- *Acute renal failure* predisposed by volume depletion and pre-existing dysfunction; due to uric acid nephropathy, acute nephrocalcinosis, and precipitation of xanthine; oliguria → volume overload and pulmonary oedema; uraemia causes malaise, lethargy, nausea, anorexia, pruritus, and pericarditis; may require dialysis; usually reversible with prompt therapy.

Principles of management

- Identify high-risk patients, initiate preventative measures prior to chemotherapy and monitor for clinical and laboratory features of TLS.
- Detect features of TLS promptly and initiate supportive therapy early.

Prevention and management

- Monitor weight bd, urine output, fluid balance, renal function, serum K^+, phosphate, Ca^{2+}, uric acid, and ECG daily for 72h after initiation of chemotherapy; monitor parameters at least 3 × daily in patients with TLS.
- Ensure aggresive IV hydration:
  - Aim for urine output >100mL/h (>3L/d) and total input >4L/d (3L/m^2/d) from 24–48h prior to chemotherapy and in high-risk patients, until 48–72h after completion of chemotherapy.
  - Furosemide (20mg IV) may be given cautiously to maintain adequate diuresis in well-hydrated patients; may be used to treat hyperkalaemia or fluid overload but may cause uric acid or Ca^{2+} deposition in dehydrated patients; no proven benefit in initial treatment of TLS.

- Prevent hyperuricaemia:
  - *Allopurinol*: xanthine oxidase inhibitor; 300–600mg/d PO for prophylaxis if renal function ↔ (100mg/d if creatine >100mmol/L) up to max. 500mg/m²/d for treatment of TLS; may be given IV if necessary (max. 600mg/d); side effects: rash, xanthine urolithiasis; reduce dose in renal impairment or mercaptopurine, 6-thioguanine or azathioprine therapy.
  - *Rasburicase*: recombinant urate oxidase; converts uric acid to water-soluble metabolites without increasing excretion of xanthine and other purine metabolites; very rapidly ↓ uric acid levels and simplifies management of high-risk patients; dose 200mcg/kgld IVI over 30min for 5–7d; recommended in BL, high count leukaemia and as rescue treatment in hyperuricaemia plus rapidly rising creatinine, oliguria, phosphate ≥2mmol/L or K^+ ≥5.5mmol/L; side effects: fever, nausea, vomiting; less common: haemolysis, allergic reactions or anaphylaxis; contraindicated in G-6-PD deficiency and pregnancy.
- Alkalinization of urine:
  - Not routine; administer $NaHCO_3$ PO (3g every 2h) or IV through central line (500mL 1.26% $NaHCO_3$ over 1h; 1L 5% dextrose over 4h; 500mL 0.9% NaCl over 1h, repeated 6-hourly) to ↑ urinary pH to 7.0 and maximize uric acid solubility.
  - Risk of more severe symptoms or hypocalcaemia and ↑ $CaPO_4$ precipitation in tubules. Requires close monitoring of urinary pH (test all urine passed), serum bicarbonate, and uric acid; withdraw IV sodium bicarbonate when serum bicarbonate >30mmol/L, urinary pH>7.5 or serum uric acid normalized.
- Control of electrolytes:
  - Hyperkalaemia: treat aggressively:

    —Restrict dietary K^+ intake and eliminate K^+ from IV fluids.

    —Use K^+ wasting diuretics with caution.

    —Measure arterial blood gases (correction more difficult if acidosis).

    —K^+ >5mmol/L, start Ca^{2+} resonium 15g PO qds and ↑ hydration; recheck K^+ after 2h.

    —K^+ >6mmol/L, check ECG; commence IVI of 50mL 50% dextrose with 20U actrapid insulin over 1h.

    —ECG changes or K^+ >6.5mmol/L, give 10mL Ca^{2+} gluconate 10% or $CaCl_2$ 10% IV cardioprotection.
  - Hyperphosphataemia:

    —Commence oral phosphate binding agent, e.g. aluminium hydroxide 20–100mL or 4–20 capsules daily or sevelamer 2.4–4.8g/d in divided doses; adjust dose according to serum phosphate.

    —Infuse 50mL 50% dextrose with 20 U actrapid insulin IV over 1h.
- Dialysis:
  - Seek renal and critical care consultations early if initial measures fail to control electrolyte abnormalities or renal failure. Dialysis indicated if persistent hyperkalaemia (>6mmol/L) or hyperphosphataemia (>3.33mmol/L) despite treatment, fluid overload, rising urea or creatinine (>880mmol/L), hyperuricaemia (>0.6mmol/L), or symptomatic hypocalcaemia.
  - HD achieves better phosphate and uric acid clearance than PD.

Management of chronic bone marrow failure

Introduction

Common haematological problem. Occurs as result of marrow infiltrated with disease e.g. MDS, or following chemotherapy or other causes of marrow aplasia. Extent of RBC, WBC, and platelet production failure varies greatly in individual clinical situations. Production failure may not affect all 3 cell lines equally.

Management

- Mainstay is supportive treatment with blood products and antibiotics.
- In patients who may be SCT candidates, give CMV–ve blood product until CMV-status known.
- Underlying disease should be treated where possible.

Red cell production failure

- Where anaemia is due solely to absence of RBC production, transfusion requirement should be ~1U packed red cells/week. Suitable protocol is 3U transfusion every 3 weeks as day case.
- If requirement is greater, investigate for bleeding and haemolysis.
- If requirement is chronic e.g. a young patient with MDS, consider giving desferrioxamine or deferasirox with long-term Fe chelation (📖 see Management, p.106).
- EPO may be tried where some red cell production capacity remains and transfusion needs to be avoided or minimized e.g. Jehovah's Witnesses.

White cell production failure

- Mainstay of treatment is with antibiotics.
- Prompt treatment of fever in neutropenic patient with combination IV antibiotics is lifesaving.
- Simple mouthcare with chlorhexidine gluconate or similar mouthwash, plus nystatin suspension orally reduces risk of bacterial and fungal colonization in oropharynx. Dietary modifications may also be helpful.
- Role of prophylactic antibiotics remains controversial as resistance generation is an increasing problem.
- Ciprofloxacin 250mg bd PO is probably the best single agent.
- Patients with recurring foci of infection may have prophylaxis targeted to their usual or most likely organisms.
- Patients with neutropenia and low Igs who have developed bronchiectasis may benefit from regular infusions of IVIg 200mg/kg every 4 weeks ± rotating antibiotic courses.
- WBC infusions are not generally useful except in rare situations—they are toxic and cause HLA sensitization. In prolonged neutropenic sepsis unresponsive to antibiotics, granulocyte infusions may be useful
- Haemopoietic growth factors should not be used routinely.
- Life-threatening infections despite IV antibiotics and anti-fungals can be considered for trial of G-CSF at 5mcg/kg/d SC.

Platelet production failure

- Where low platelets are due solely to absence of platelet production, transfusion requirement should be ~1–2 adult dose packs/week. Tranexamic acid 1g qds PO may reduce clinical bleeding episodes and transfusion requirement. Thrombopoietin (TPO) is a potent in vitro platelet growth and maturation factor but its clinical role remains to be defined.

Venepuncture

Blood samples are best taken from an antecubital vein using a 21G needle and a Vacutainer® system or syringe. If a large volume of blood is required a 21G butterfly may be inserted to facilitate changing the vacutainer sample bottle or the syringe.

A tourniquet should be gently applied to the upper arm and the antecubital fossa inspected and palpated for veins. In an obese individual antecubital veins may be more easily palpated than seen. The skin over the vein should be 'sterilized' (alcohol swab or Mediswab™) and allowed to dry. The needle should then be gently introduced along the line of the chosen vein at an angle of 45° to the skin surface. It may be helpful to attempt to penetrate the skin with the initial introduction of the needle and then slowly penetrate the vessel wall by continuing the forward movement of the needle. The tourniquet on the upper arm should be loosened once the needle has been inserted into the vein to reduce haemoconcentration. If a syringe is used the piston should be withdrawn slowly to prevent collapse of the vein. Once an adequate sample has been obtained, the tourniquet should be completely removed, a dry cotton wool ball applied gently above the site of venepuncture and gentle pressure ↑ as the needle is removed. Firm pressure should be directly applied to the venepuncture site for 3–5min to ensure haemostasis and prevent extravasation and bruising. A small adhesive plaster or if allergic, suitable light dressing, should be applied to the venepuncture site.

In patients in whom it is difficult to obtain a sample, the arm should be kept warm, a sphygmomanometer cuff inflated on the upper arm to the diastolic pressure, and the vein may be dilated by smacking the overlying skin. With patience it is rarely impossible to obtain a venous sample. In very obese individuals or those in whom iatrogenic thrombosis or sclerosis has occurred in the antecubital veins, the dorsal veins of the hand may be used for sampling, though a smaller gauge needle (23G) or butterfly is often necessary.

N. B. In children use a 23G butterfly after application of Emla® cream.

In patients with thrombocytopenia, apply firm pressure to the venepuncture site for a minimum of 3 min.

Do not use the swab to apply pressure as this will sting and slows down haemostasis.

Venesection

Aim of venesection or phlebotomy is the removal of blood for donation to the Blood Transfusion Service or as a therapeutic manoeuvre for a patient with haemochromatosis or PRV or for a patient who requires an exchange transfusion or to obtain blood for autologous transfusion during elective surgery. In patients with haemochromatosis or PRV the therapeutic effect of the venesection programme to date should be assessed on a FBC sample taken prior to venesection.

Procedure

- Patient or donor is best placed lying on a couch with the chosen arm placed comfortably on a supporting pillow.
- A large gauge needle attached to a collection pack containing anticoagulant is inserted in an antecubital vein or forearm vein after application of a sphygmomanometer cuff to the upper arm (inflated to diastolic pressure) and sterilization of the skin. It is widespread practice to infiltrate the skin over the chosen vein with local anaesthetic (1% lidocaine) prior to insertion of the large bore needle.
- Inflation of the sphygmomanometer cuff is maintained until the desired volume of blood is collected.
- The patient may assist the flow of blood by squeezing a soft ball or similar object in the hand of the arm from which the blood is drawn.
- Blood is allowed to drain into the collection pack until the desired volume has been obtained (usually 500mL).
- The volume collected may be monitored by suspension of the pack from a simple spring measuring device.
- The positioning of the collection pack below the patient's (or donor's) level facilitates blood flow into the bag.
- Once the desired volume has been collected the cuff is deflated, the line should be clamped and the needle removed and a dry cotton wool ball used to apply pressure to the venesection site.
- Direct firm pressure should be applied for 5min and the site inspected for haemostasis prior to application of a firm bandage.
- The patient should slowly adopt the erect posture and should remain seated for several minutes if symptoms of lightheadedness occur.
- Patients should not be permitted to drive after venesection.
- The collected blood from a therapeutic venesection should be disposed of by incineration.

Note: for patients with PPP/PRV isovolaemic venesection is recommended to minimize volume depletion whilst still reducing Hct.

Tunnelled central venous catheters

A tunnelled central venous catheter is required in all patients undergoing intensive cytotoxic chemotherapy and those undergoing BM or peripheral blood SCT. Also indicated for some patients on long-term regular transfusion programmes.

Catheter type

A double or triple lumen catheter preferred, and essential for patients undergoing transplantation procedures. Hickman catheters are available from Vygon UK and the Groshong lines (Bard) are available for use in all patients except those needing stem cell collections who will require apheresis catheters (Kimal).

Requirements

An x-ray screening room with facility for aseptic procedures or an operating theatre is required. A trained radiographer must be available for x-ray screening throughout the procedure. In addition a minimum of 2 staff are required for the safe execution of this procedure. 1 should be a member of medical staff (radiologist/surgeon/anaesthetist/haemato-oncologist) to insert the catheter and administer sedation and antibiotics and the other to generally assist. The 2nd person can be an IV trained nurse.

Patient assessment

Assess for fitness for sedation and the ability to lie flat. Plan position of central venous catheter in advance. The 1st choice is the right subclavian vein, followed by the left subclavian vein. Check FBC and clotting screen. Platelets should be available if platelet count is less than 50×10^9/L.

Patient preparation

The patient should be well hydrated (↓ CVP makes procedure difficult), and fasting for 6h prior to the procedure as sedative drugs will be administered. Good peripheral venous access must be established (with Venflon™) before commencing central venous cannulation, for the administration of sedative drugs and prophylactic antibiotics as well as for emergency venous access.

Technique

Follow manufacturer's instructions. Sequence of stages during insertion is as follows:

1. Cannulation of the central vein, placement of guide wire and creation of the upper central wound.
2. Creation of lower peripheral wound, formation of SC tunnel and threading of the catheter through SC tunnel with cuff buried.
3. Placement of the vessel dilator/sheath in the central vein over the guide wire.
4. Placement of the catheter into the sheath.
5. Careful removal of the sheath whilst retaining position of catheter.
6. Suturing of the upper and lower wounds with suture around the body of the catheter close to the exit site to hold the catheter in position.
7. Manipulate catheter so tip lies in SVC above right atrium. Patency must be confirmed by easy aspiration of blood, and the catheter flushed with heparinized saline. Check position with standard PA chest radiograph.

Sedation and analgesia

IV sedation is used if the patient is particularly anxious before or during the procedure.

Prophylactic antibiotics

- Teicoplanin 400mg is administered by peripheral vein immediately prior to central venous cannulation.
- 400mg teicoplanin is also administered into the central venous catheter immediately after the insertion procedure (200mg is locked into each lumen for 1h and then the catheter is flushed with heparinized saline).

Catheter aftercare

- Catheter may be used immediately after above procedures. All patients should be educated in the care of their indwelling tunnelled IV catheter. This may include self-flushing of the catheter. Catheter should be flushed after each use with saline and locked with heparinized saline. Flush twice weekly when not in use.
- Urokinase may be used if line blockage occurs, insert urokinase and leave for 4–12h and remove.
- Clindamycin roll-on lotion may be applied to the exit site to minimize local infections.
- Upper wound suture is removed 7d post-insertion.
- Lower exit site suture can be removed at 2 weeks post-insertion for most lines and 3 weeks for apheresis lines to ensure SC embedding of the cuff.

Bone marrow examination

BM is the key investigation in haematology. It may prove diagostic in the follow-up of abnormal peripheral blood findings. It is an important staging procedure in defining the extent of disease, especially LPDs. It is a helpful investigative procedure in unexplained anaemia, splenomegaly or selected cases of pyrexia of unknown origin (PUO). Preferred site for sampling → posterior iliac crest; aspirate and biopsy material can easily be obtained from this location. The anterior iliac crest is an alternative. The sternum is suitable only for marrow aspiration.

Marrow aspirate material provides information on:

- Cytology of nucleated cells.
- Qualitative and semi-qualitative analysis of haematopoiesis.
- Assessment of Fe stores.
- Smears for cytochemistry of atypical cells.

Suspensions of marrow cells in medium are suitable for:

- Chromosome (cytogenetic) analysis.
- Immunophenotype studies using monoclonal antibodies directed against cell surface antigens.
- Aliquots of marrow can be cryopreserved for future molecular analysis.
- Quantitative and qualitative haemopoietic progenitor cell assays.

Marrow trephine biopsy yields information on:

- Marrow cellularity.
- Identification/classification of abnormal cellular infiltrates.
- Immunohistochemistry on infiltrates.

Note: cytology of trephine imprints can be helpful, especially when aspirate yields a 'dry tap'. Trephine biopsy information complements that obtained at aspiration.

Contraindications

None, other than physical limitations e.g. pain or restricted mobility. Avoid sites of previous radiotherapy (inevitably grossly hypocellular and not representative).

Procedure

1. BM aspiration may be performed under local anaesthesia alone, but short acting IV benzodiazepines (e.g. midazolam) may be administered—with appropriate monitoring (pulse oximetry), O_2 administration and available resuscitation equipment—when trephine biopsy is performed. General anaesthesia rarely used (except in children).
2. Best position is with patient in L or R lateral position.
3. Skin and periosteum over the posterior iliac spine are infiltrated with local anaesthetic.
4. A small cutaneous incision is made, the aspirating needle is introduced through this and should penetrate the marrow cortex 3–10mm before removal of the trocar.
5. No more than 0.5–1mL marrow should be aspirated initially, and smears made promptly.

6. Further material can be aspirated and placed in EDTA or other anticoagulant media for other studies.
7. An Islam or Jamshidi needle is preferred for trephine biopsy.
8. The needle is advanced through the same puncture site to penetrate the cortex.
9. The trocar is removed and using firm hand pressure the needle is rotated clockwise and should be advanced as far as possible.
10. The needle is removed by gentle anti-clockwise rotation. In this manner an experienced operator should regularly obtain biopsy samples of 25–35mm in length.
11. Simple pressure dressings are sufficient aftercare and minor discomfort at the location may be dealt with by simple analgesia such as paracetamol.

Administration of chemotherapy

Cytotoxic chemotherapeutic drugs may cause serious harm if not prescribed, dispensed, and administered with great care. Drugs should be prescribed, dispensed, and administered by an experienced multidisciplinary team with shared clear information on:

- The fitness of the patient to receive chemotherapy (e.g. recent FBC for myelosuppressive agents, renal function studies for cisplatinum).
- Appropriate protocol and chemotherapeutic regimen for the patient.
- Prescribed drugs and individualized dosage for the patient's surface area (📖 see Body surface area nomogram, p. 804), taking note of cumulative maximum doses (e.g. anthracyclines).
- Appropriate supportive treatment required e.g. allopurinol, antiemetic prophylaxis, anti-infective prophylaxis, and hydration.

Chemotherapy for IV administration should be reformulated carefully in accordance with the manufacturer's instructions by an experienced pharmacist using a class B laminar airflow hood or isolator. Care should be taken to ensure that the drug is administered within the expiry time after it has been reformulated in the form chosen.

Many cytotoxic drugs are best administered as a slow IVI in dextrose or 0.9% saline over 30min–2h. Vesicants e.g. mitoxantrone, daunorubicin, adriamycin and should be administered as a slow IV 'push'. However this should only be administered through the side access port of a freely flowing infusion of 0.9% saline or dextrose and should never be injected directly into a peripheral vein. N.B. Following 2008 NPSA alert, vinca alkaloids must be administered as a short IV infusion to avoid the risk of inadvertent intrathecal administration.

If the patient does not have an indwelling IV catheter (Hickman line), a Teflon or silicone IV cannula of adequate bore (≤21G) should be inserted into a vein of sufficient diameter to permit a freely flowing 0.9% saline infusion to be commenced. Site chosen should be one where cannula can be easily inserted and observed, can be fastened securely and will not be subject to movement during drug administration. The veins of the forearm are the most suitable for this purpose followed by those on the dorsum of the hand. Antecubital fossae and other sites close to joints are best avoided. The risk of extravasation (📖 see Management of extravasation, p.700) is ↑ by the use of a cannula which has not been inserted recently and by the use of steel (butterfly) cannulae.

A slow 'push' injection should be administered carefully into the side access port on the IV line with continuous observation of the drip chamber ensure that the infusion is continuing to run during injection of the cytotoxic drug. The patient should be asked whether any untoward sensations are being experienced at the site of the infusion and the site should be carefully observed to ensure that no extravasation is occurring. Patency of the IV site should be verified regularly throughout the procedure. The saline or dextrose infusion should be continued for 30min after the chemotherapy administration has been completed before the cannula is removed.

The administration of potentially extravasable chemotherapy, site of cannulation, condition of the site and any symptoms associated with administration should be clearly documented in the patient's notes.

Prevention of extravasation

- Use a PIC line or central line for slow infusion of high-risk cytotoxics.
- Administer cytotoxics through a recently sited cannula located where it cannot be dislodged, e.g. the forearm rather than near joints.
- Administer vesicants by slow IV push into the side arm port of a fast-running IV infusion of compatible solution.
- Administer the most vesicant drug first.
- Assess a peripheral site continuously for signs of redness or swelling.
- Verify the patency of the IV site prior to vesicant infusion and regularly throughout. If in doubt, stop and investigate. Resite if not satisfactory.
- Ask the patient to report any sensations of pain or burning at the infusion site.
- Never hurry. Administer cytotoxics slowly to allow dilution and assessment of the site.

1. The National Extravasation Information Service Protocol for Management of Chemotherapy Extravasations. www.extravasation.org.uk/CEG.htm

Antiemetics for chemotherapy

Classification of antiemetics

Dopamine antagonist—block D_2 receptors in the chemoreceptor trigger zone (CTZ). Examples are metoclopramide and domperidone—both have additional effect on enhancing gastric emptying. Side effects with metoclopramide, include extrapyramidal reactions and occasionally oculogyric crisis (younger patients at most risk therefore use domperidone).

Phenothiazines—examples are prochlorperazine and cyclizine—particular benefit in opioid-induced nausea. Side effects include anticholinergic effects and drowsiness.

Benzodiazepine—lorazepam commonest used. Advantages are long t½ and additional anxiolytic effect. Side effects include drowsiness.

5HT3 antagonists—block $5HT_3$ receptors in the CTZ. Examples include ondansetron, granisetron and tropesitron. Side effects include headaches, bowel disturbance, and rashes.

Cannabinoids—nabilone is the major drug. Side effects include depersonalization experiences.

Steroids—examples are dexamethasone and prednisolone. Side effects include predisposition to fungal infection, hypertension, irritability and sleeplessness, gastric erosions and, with chronic use, diabetes and osteoporosis.

NK1 receptor antagonists—e.g. aprepitant, used in addition to dexamethasone and 5HT3 antagonist for highly emetic chemotherapy e.g. high dose cisplatin.

Emesis with chemotherapy

Categorized as anticipatory, early, or late.

Anticipatory—occurs days to hours in advance of chemotherapy. Psychogenic in origin, it occurs in patients with previous bad experiences of nausea and vomiting and almost unknown prior to first dose. May be largely prevented by ensuring a positive experience with first dose by use of prophylactic antiemetics.

Early—occurs <24h, sometimes within minutes of IV chemotherapy or within hours of oral chemotherapy. Generally responds best to antiemetics.

Late—occurs >24h after the end of a chemotherapy course—up to 7d. The most difficult form to treat—requires continuation of antiemetics throughout post-chemo period and even the newer agents such as the $5HT_3$ receptor antagonists are relatively ineffective.

Antiemetics—may be used singly or in combination and should be administered regularly, prophylactically and orally. Optimal control in the early phase is essential to prevent nausea and vomiting in the late phase. IV antiemetics are only required if patient is unable to take oral drugs. Choice of antiemetic is determined largely by patient preferences and degree of emetic potential of the chemotherapy regimen used, classed as high, moderately high, moderately low, and low.

Risk factors—female sex, age <30 years, history of sickness in pregnancy or with travel, prior chemotherapy-induced nausea/vomiting, anxiety, other factors: radiotherapy, other medications, metabolic disorders, constipation

GI obstruction. If ≥3 factors, consider additional antiemetic therapy from start of chemotherapy.

High emetic risk

Cisplatin ≥50mg/m^2, high dose cyclophosphamide >1.5g/m^2, carmustine >250mg/m^2, dacarbazine, chlormethine (mustine), TBI.

Moderately high emetic risk

Cisplatin <50mg/m^2, daunorubicin, doxorubicin ≥60mg/m^2, idarubicin, cytarabine ≥1g/m^2, ifosfamide, carboplatin, carmustine ≤250mg/m^2, lomustine.

Antiemesis of high and moderately high emetic risk

- *Early*—5HT$_3$ antagonist PO prior to each IV cytotoxic *plus* dexamethasone 20mg PO/IV on each day of chemotherapy *or* additional 2 days of 5HT$_3$ antagonist.
- *Late*—dexamethasone 4mg PO bd for 2–5d *plus* metoclopramide 10–20mg PO tds (*or* domperidone 20mg PO tds) for 3–4d then prn.
- *Second line*—add lorazepam 1mg PO/IV/SL up to 8hrly *or* levomepromazine 6.25–12.5mg PO in the evening *or* cyclizine 50mg PO tds *or* 150mg/d by SC infusion *plus* dexamethasone 4mg PO bd for up to 1 week.

Moderately low emetic risk

Doxorubicin <60mg/m^2, mitoxantrone, gemcitabine, etoposide, methotrexate (MTX) 50–250mg/m^2, oral cyclophosphamide, oral procarbazine.

Antiemesis of moderately low emetic risk

- *Early*—dexamethasone 8mg PO/IV prior to each day of chemotherapy *plus* metoclopramide 10–20mg PO tds (*or* domperidone 20mg PO tds).
- *Late*—metoclopramide 10–20mg PO qds/prn (*or* domperidone 20mg PO tds/prn) for 3–4d.
- *Second line*—5HT$_3$ antagonist PO prior to each day of chemotherapy *plus* dexamethasone 8mg PO prior to each day of chemotherapy with 4mg PO bd for 2 further days if necessary *plus* metoclopramide 10–20mg PO tds/prn (*or* domperidone 20mg PO tds/prn) for 3–4d.

Low emetic risk

Examples include oral chlorambucil, oral melphalan, oral busulfan, oral hydroxycarbamide, oral 6-mercaptopurine, vinca alkaloids, MTX<50mg/m^2, fludarabine, cladribine (2-CDA), bleomycin, asparaginase and most steroid-containing protocols.

Antiemesis of low emetic risk

- *Early and late*—no routine prophylaxis required *or* metoclopramide 10–20mg PO tds/prn (*or* domperidone 20mg PO tds/prn) for 3–4d.
- *Second line*—dexamethasone 8mg PO/IV prior to chemotherapy *plus* metoclopramide 10–20mg PO tds/prn (*or* domperidone 20mg PO tds/prn) for 3–4d.

1. www.aswcs.nhs.uk/pharmacy/ChemoHandbook/NetworkPolicies/ProtA21.pdf.
2. Gralla, R.J. *et al.* (1999). Recommendations for the use of anti-emetics: evidence-based clinical practice guidelines. *J Clin Oncol*, **17**, 2971–94.
3. Hesketh, P.J. (2008). Chemotherapy-induced nausea and vomiting. *N Engl J Med*, **358**, 2482–94.

Intrathecal chemotherapy

In the UK administration of intrathecal (IT) chemotherapy is controlled by strict national guidelines to prevent inappropriate administration of IT chemotherapy. These require all medical staff, nursing staff and pharmacists involved in the procedure to undergo training and annual refresher courses to remain eligible to administer IT chemotherapy, require strict compliance with grades of staff who may be involved in IT therapy, checking procedures, administration of IT therapy at separate times from IV chemotherapy and specify sites at which the procedure may be carried out.

Indications

- Given for both prophylaxis and treatment of CNS disease.
- May be used in addition to other CNS disease strategies such as high-dose IV MTX or cranial irradiation.
- CNS involvement is detected by presence of blasts on CSF cytospin and/or abnormalities on MRI or CT.
- The ONLY cytotoxic drugs used intrathecally are:
  - MTX.
  - Cytarabine (Ara-C).
  - Hydrocortisone.
  - All have strict upper dosage limits—follow the protocol.

►► Never use any other cytotoxic drugs for intrathecal injection—fatal consequences may ensue.

Common protocols

- CNS prophylaxis for ALL and high grade NHL:
  - MTX 10mg/m^2 (max. 12.5mg) 6 injections at weekly intervals.
- CNS prophylaxis for AML:
  - cytarabine 30mg/m^2 (max. 50mg), dosage schedule varies.
- CNS treatment for ALL:
  - Triple IT regimen viz:
    —MTX 15mg/m^2 (max. 12.5–15mg).
    —cytarabine 30mg/m^2 (max. 50mg).
    —hydrocortisone 15mg/m^2.

Usually given twice weekly until CSF clear of blasts then weekly to a maximum of 6 total courses. Consider using folinic acid rescue.

Technique

- Standard contraindications to lumbar puncture apply—alternatives will be needed in these situations. Cytotoxics should be made up freshly in smallest possible volume in a sterile pharmacy.
- Consider GA for children and IV sedation for adults.
- Use special LP 'blunt' needle or small gauge bevelled LP needle.
- Aim to remove the same volume of CSF as you are injecting intrathecally (may be several mL if giving triple chemotherapy).
- Take samples for CSF cytospin to determine blast cell concentration, microbiology for M/C/S, biochemistry for protein and glucose.
- Check syringe cytotoxic dose carefully with another person before connecting.

- Connect syringe and aspirate gently to confirm position in CSF. Inject slowly, drawing back at intervals to reconfirm position. Disconnect syringe and connect other syringes in turn if giving 'triple'.
- Follow standard post-LP precautions. Document procedure in notes. Repeated IT chemotherapy carries risk of CSF leakage and post-LP headache. Manometry pre-injection may help assess whether less CSF should be withdrawn pre-injection.
- A syndrome of MTX-induced neurotoxicity occurs in a few patients presenting with features of meningo-encephalitis. Aetiology is unknown. Treat with short pulse of high dose steroids.
- Do not give further IT MTX to these patients.

Management of extravasation

Inappropriate or accidental administration of chemotherapy into SC tissu rather than into the IV compartment causes pain, erythema, and inflam mation which may lead to sloughing of the skin and severe tissue necrosi Appropriate early treatment can prevent the most serious consequence of extravasation. All chemotherapy units should have a protocol wit which all staff administering chemotherapy are familiar and a regularl updated extravasation kit for the management of extravasation giving firs aid instructions and further directions.

The risk of tissue damage relates to the drug's ability to bind to DN to kill replicating cells, to cause tissue or vascular dilatation and its p osmolarity, concentration, volume and formulation components e. alcohol, polyethylene glycol.

Cytotoxic drugs are classified into 5 groups by their potential to caus serious necrosis when extravasated.

Group 1: neutrals
Asparaginase; bleomycin; cladribine; cyclophosphamide; cytarabin edroclomab; fludarabine; gemcitabine; ifosfamide; melphalan; pentostati rituximab; thiotepa; beta-interferons; aldesleukin (IL-2); trastuzumab.

Group 2: inflammitants
Etoposide phosphate; fluorouracil; MTX; raltitrexed.

Group 3: irritants (cause local inflammation, pain, and necrosis)
Carboplatin; etoposide; irinotecan; teniposide.

Group 4: exfoliants
Aclarubicin; cisplatin; liposomal daunorubicin; docetaxel; liposomal doxoru bicin; floxuridine; mitoxantrone; oxaliplatin; topotecan.

Group 5: vesicants
Amsacrine; carmustine; dacarbazine; dactinomycin; daunorubicin; doxoru bicin; epirubicin; idarubicin; mitomycin; chlormethine (mustine); paclitaxe streptozocin; treosulfan; vinblastine; vincristine; vindesine; vinorelbine.

Symptoms and signs

- Burning, stinging or pain at the injection site.
- Induration, swelling, venous discolouration/erythema at the site.
- No blood return from the cannula.
- Reduced flow rate.
- ↑ resistance to administration.

Pre-extravasation syndrome

- Severe phlebitis and/or local hypersensitivity.
- Local risk factors e.g. difficult cannulation and one patient symptom.
- Act promptly.
- Stop IV therapy immediately to prevent progression to extravasation.

Type I extravasation

- Bleb or blister with defined area of induration around site of extravasation.
- Often due to rapid IV bolus injection with excessive pressure.

ype II extravasation

Diffuse boggy tissue injury with dispersal into the intracellular space.
Associated with IV infusion or IV bolus into side arm port of infusion with dislodged cannula.

eneral treatment guidelines

Act promptly; for prevention.
Stop the infusion, disconnect the IV line but **do not remove the cannula**.
Mark the area of injury/extravasation around the cannula tip.
Seek the help of a more experienced individual if available.
Aspirate the site of extravasation to remove as much of the offending drug as possible through cannula with a fresh 10mL syringe; this may be facilitated with SC injection of 0.9% saline to dilute the drug or 1500U of hyaluronidase in 2mL water for injection.
Now remove the cannula.
Administer a further 100mg hydrocortisone locally by 6–8 × 0.1–0.2mL SC injections around the area of injury.
Administer 100mg hydrocortisone intravenously at another site if large-scale inflammation or flare has occurred.
Consult the management chart for specific treatments and/or the National Extravasation Information Service on 0121–554–3801 bleep 3007 or www.extravasation.org.uk
Treatment is then either:

- *'Spread & dilute'* using normal saline, hyaluronidase and warm, continuous compression & elevation of limb; or
- *'Localize & neutralize'* using specific antidote if available and intermittent cold compression.

Administer analgesia if required (indometacin 25mg tds).
Document site and extent of extravasation and treatment in case notes; photograph site if possible.
Complete a 'Green Card' to report the extravasation episode.
Instruct the patient on the correct care of the injury and the use of any ongoing treatment.
Monitor injured site twice daily for erythema, induration, blistering, or necrosis.
Photograph injured site weekly until healed.

The National Extravasation Information Service Protocol for Management of Chemotherapy xtravasations. www.extravasation.org.uk/CEG.htm

Specific procedures after extravasation of cytotoxics commonly used in haematology

Table 15.2 Specific procedures following extravasation[1]

Group & drugs	Aspirate & instill steroids	'Spread & dilute'	'Localize & neutralize'	Specific Management
1. Neutrals				
Asparaginase; Bleomycin; Cladribine; Cyclophosphamide; Cytarabine; Fludarabine; Gemcitabine; Ifosfamide; Melphalan; Pentostatin	Y	Y		Infiltrate with 1500 units hyaluronidase as 0.2mL SC injections over and around affected site; apply heat and compression
2. Inflammitants				
MTX	Y		Y	Apply topical hydrocortisone and cover area with ice pack for next 4h. If local reaction then settled, apply heat for next 24–48h. SC hyaluronidase may facilitate dispersion of large volume extravasations.
3. Irritants				
Etoposide	Y	Y		Apply topical hydrocortisone and cover area with ice pack.
4. Exfoliants				
Cisplatin	Y	If <24h	If >24h	Infiltrate site with 1–3mL 3% sodium thiosulphate, aspirate back then give 1500 units hyaluronidase, topical hydrocortisone and warm compression.
Mitoxantrone	Y		Y	Apply topical DMSO to site every 2h followed by hydrocortisone cream and a cold compress.

Table 15.2 Specific procedures following extravasation (*continued*)

Group & drugs	Aspirate & instill steroids	'Spread & dilute'	'Localize & neutralize'	Specific Management
5. Vesicants				
Amsacrine; Dacarbazine; Daunorubicin; Doxorubicin; Idarubicin	Y		Y	Apply topical DMSO to site every 2h followed by hydrocortisone cream and a cold compress. Avoid contact with good skin. If blistering occurs, stop and seek advice. Surgical excision sometimes required.
Carmustine	Y		Y	Infiltrate with 2.1% sodium bicarbonate; leave for 2 mins and aspirate off again; N.B. sodium bicarbonate is a vesicant.
Chlormethine (mustine)	Y		Y	Infiltrate site with 1–3mL 3% sodium thiosulphate, then introduce 100mg of hydrocortisone to site. Apply cold compress for 24h. Surgical excision may be required.
Vinblastine; Vincristine; Vindesine; Vinorelbine	Y	Y		Infiltrate area with 1500 units of hyaluronidase as 0.2mL SC injections over and around the affected area; apply heat and compression for 24h then apply topical non-steroidal anti-inflammatory cream to the area qds.

1. Adapted from The National Extravasation Information Service Protocol for Management of Chemotherapy Extravasations. Consult www.extravasation.org.uk/CEG.htm for further information or specific information on other drugs

Splenectomy

Splenectomy is an established procedure in management of selected haematological disorders. Removal of the spleen is usually required for 1 or more of the following reasons:

- Extreme enlargement.
- Hyperfunction.
- Autoimmune activity.
- Diagnostic and therapeutic purposes.

Indications include:

- LPDs—e.g. CLL, MZL, HCL. Reasons include massive organomegaly, occurrence of autoimmune complications and for diagnostic and/or therapeutic purposes.
- MPDs—commonly used in myelofibrosis to reduce transfusion requirements, abdominal discomfort from massive splenic enlargement, and may reduce constitutional symptoms e.g. weight loss and night sweats. Occasionally used in the management of CML.
- Autoimmune conditions—an accepted treatment in autoimmune thrombocytopenic purpura and autoimmune haemolytic anaemia following the failure of immunosuppression with corticosteroids and immunoglobulin (in the case of thrombocytopenic purpura). The procedure is not curative but may result in prolonged remissions and certainly will have steroid-sparing effect.
- Hereditary disorders—reduces red cell sequestration and transfusion requirements in homozygous β-thalassaemia. Recurrent, severe hereditary spherocytosis. Rare indications include pyruvate kinase deficiency and type 1 Gaucher's disease. Other circumstances where splenectomy may help include Felty's syndrome.
- Staging splenectomy is no longer a routine procedure for NHL or HL.

The clinician has to balance the risks and benefits of the procedure in an individual patient bearing in mind the long-term risk of post-splenectomy sepsis as well as immediate surgical factors. There are now established consensus guidelines for carrying out splenectomy.

Pre-operatively the need for the procedure is agreed with the patient and surgical team. At least 2 weeks pre-operatively immunization with pneumococcal and *Haemophilus* vaccine should be given. Meningococcal vaccine may be offered but this covers sub-types A and C only and does not give long-lasting immunity. Peri-operative thromboembolic risks should be considered (e.g. standard surgical risks and those posed by the rebound thrombocytosis after splenectomy). Low dose heparin may be appropriate peri-operatively followed by low dose aspirin (may require modification in thrombocytopenia or if platelet dysfunction). Before discharge, patients must be given a leaflet/card which they carry. Lifelong prophylaxis with penicillin V 500mg bd recommended or erythromycin 250mg bd if the patient is allergic to penicillin. The patient and his/her family must be advised to report urgently profound systemic symptoms, most promptly to their nearest local Emergency department.

Plasma exchange (plasmapheresis)

Plasmapheresis is the therapeutic removal of plasma from the peripheral blood usually carried out by a cell separator machine. The removed plasma is replaced isovolaemically usually by albumin/saline combinations depending on indication, plasma albumin level, and frequency of exchange. Blood products may also be given as part of replacement which is useful in patients with fluid intolerance e.g. on renal dialysis. The exception to this is TTP where the replacement fluid is always FFP or cryosupernatant. ~1–1.5 × plasma volume is exchanged in each procedure, i.e. 2.5–4L for average adult. Procedure takes 2–4h depending on volume to be exchanged and the line flow rates. Procedure may need to be repeated daily until response e.g. TTP, or until a total volume exchange has been achieved e.g. 10–15L over 2 weeks (e.g. Guillain–Barré syndrome), or monthly to control hyperviscosity (e.g. WM).

Indications—generally accepted in:

- Hyperviscosity syndromes.
- Guillain–Barré syndrome resistant to IVIg.
- Myasthenia gravis: peri-operatively for thymectomy, and refractory disease.
- Paraproteinaemic neuropathy.
- Goodpasture's syndrome.
- TTP.
- Post-transfusion purpura.
- Cold haemagglutinin disease.

Efficacy contentious but may be indicated in:

- Severe warm type AIHA.
- Lupus, Wegener's, and other vasculitides.
- Rheumatoid arthritis.
- Peripheral neuropathies other than paraproteinaemic neuropathy.
- Multiple sclerosis.
- Chronic inflammatory demyelinating polyradiculopathy.
- Eaton–Lambert syndrome.
- Renal transplant rejection.

Venous access

If exchange is to be performed via peripheral veins, one large antecubital vein is required sufficient to tolerate cannulation by a 16G butterfly needle as the drawing line (return line need only be 18G). If not possible, make arrangements for insertion of a central line prior to the planned exchanges inserting a double lumen renal dialysis type catheter of 16G or larger. Regular medication due immediately prior to exchange may be best deferred until immediately post-exchange particularly for drugs which are predominantly protein bound (📖 see Table 15.3).

Problems with apheresis

- General—patient anxiety, discomfort and boredom.
- Citrate toxicity—parasthesiae, tremors, tetany.
- Vascular and cardiac—poor venous access giving poor flow rates. Extravasation with haematoma at puncture sites, local vein

thrombosis—during and after procedure, sepsis at puncture sites, hypo/hypervolaemia, vasovagal attacks, arrhythmias.
- Metabolic and pharmacological—hypoalbuminaemia, hypoglycaemia, removal of drugs (plasma bound).
- *Allergic reactions*—including anaphylaxis.

Drugs >75% bound

f drugs in Table 15.3 are due immediately prior to exchange, delay administration until after procedure.

Table 15.3 Medication that must be administered after plasmapheresis

Beta blockers	**Antipsychotics**
Propranolol	Chlorpromazine
Timolol	Haloperidol
Penbutolol	Thioridazine
Ca^{2+} channel blockers	**Antifungal agents**
Diltiazem	Amphotericin B
Nifedipine	Ketoconazole
Verapamil	**Antihistamines**
Anti-arrhythmics	Chlorphenamine
Amiodarone	**Antimalarials**
Prepafenone	Mepacrine
Quinidine	Pyrimethamine
Digitoxin (digoxin is OK)	**Antibiotics**
Diuretics	Cloxacillin
Furosemide (frusemide)	Flucloxacillin
Metolazone	Penicillin V
Bendroflumethazide (bendrofluazide)	Sulphonamide
Diazoxide	Doxycycline
Antiepileptics	**Anti-TB**
Carbamazepine	Rifampicin
Phenytoin	**Anticoagulants**
Sodium valproate	Heparin
Hypolipidaemics	Warfarin
Clofibrate	**Thyroid drugs**
Gout drugs	Levothyroxine
Probenecid	Tri-iodothyronine
Sulfinpyrazone	Propylthiouracil
Analgesics	**Oestrogens and progestogens**
NSAIDs (all)	All
Aspirin	**Hypoglycaemics**
Co-proxamol	Tolbutamide
Benzodiazepines	Glipizide
All	Gliclazide
Antidepressants	Glibenclamide
All	Chlorpropamide
Antiepileptics	
Carbamazepine	
Phenytoin	
Sodium valproate	

Leucapheresis

Leucapheresis is the removal from the peripheral blood of white blood cells, usually leukaemic blasts, via a cell separation machine.

Procedure

Usually now a standard computer controlled program on modern machines e.g. Cobe Spectra™ or Fenwall CS™. May be performed manually in an emergency (📖 see Hyperviscosity, p. 640).

Indications

In patients with high WBC e.g. AML, CML, and with symptoms or signs of leucostasis, leucapheresis should be performed urgently. Leucostatic features are less common in lymphoid than in myeloid malignancies.

Leucostatic features

- Confusion.
- ↓ conscious level.
- Fits.
- Retinal haemorrhages.
- Papilloedema.
- Hypoxia and miliary shadowing on CXR.
- Bleeding and coronary ischaemia.

Should not be performed routinely just because of a high WBC. Leucostatic clinical features are the indication. Conversely, leucostasis may occur in some patients with AML without a very high blast count but these patients should be considered for leucapheresis.

Chemotherapy should be started as soon as possible after leucapheresis as WBC will 'rebound' quickly due to outpouring of cells from marrow. Leucapheresis may need to be repeated daily until chemotherapy has suppressed marrow.

Other indications

- Leucapheresis should be performed routinely at diagnosis of CML in patients <60 years for stem cell cryopreservation which can be used in the future as a stem cell rescue procedure.
- Leucapheresis may be used as an alternative to chemotherapy in low grade haematological malignancies in pregnancy.

Anticoagulation therapy—heparin

For acute thrombosis DVT/PE start with heparin and warfarin simultaneously. Essential to confirm diagnosis—but start treatment whilst awaiting results of investigations. When warfarin stable—stop heparin.

Heparin

Main advantage over oral anticoagulation is immediate anticoagulant effect and short t½. Two main products: *standard UFH*, a mixture of polysaccharide chains, mean MW 15,000, t½ 1.0–1.5h, and *LMWH*, fragments of UFH (mean MW 5000) with longer t½ (3–6h) and greater bioavailability. LMWH has significant advantages: 1 daily SC injection, no monitoring, no dose adjustment, low risk of HITT. Heparins act by potentiating coagulation inhibitor antithrombin resulting in antithrombin and anti-Xa activity. Both UFH and LMWH depend on renal clearance.

Therapeutic anticoagulation

LMWH—given SC once daily on basis of weight (see individual products for dosage). Usually continued for 4–7d until warfarin effect, INR>2.0.

Standard IV UFH—initial IV bolus 5000IU in 0.9% saline given over 30min (lower loading dose for small adult/child). Follow with 15–25IU/kg/h using a solution of 25,000IU heparin in 50mL 0.9% saline (= 500IU/mL) and a motorized pump, e.g. for 80kg adult dose is 80 × 25 = 2000IU/h. Monitor IVI with APTT ratio, aim for ratio of 1.5–2.5, check 6h after starting treatment. Adjust dose as shown in Table 15.4.

Check APTT ratio 10h after dose change; daily thereafter. Use fresh venous sample—do not take from line. Continue heparin until INR in therapeutic range for warfarin—takes ~5d; massive ileo-femoral thrombosis and severe PE may require 7–10d of heparin.

Contraindications

Caution if renal, hepatic impairment, recent surgery, known bleeding diathesis, severe hypertension.

Immediate complications of therapy

- Bleeding occurs even when APTT ratio within the therapeutic range but risk ↑ with ↑ APTT ratio. Treatment: stop heparin until APTT ratio <2.5. In life-threatening bleeding use protamine sulphate: 1mg/100IU of heparin given in preceding hour.
- Thrombocytopenia—mild ↓platelets common early in heparin therapy; not significant. Severe thrombocytopenia less common (HITT); occurs 6–10d after therapy begun; may be associated thrombosis. Stop heparin Give alternative antithrombin drug such as lepirudin or danaparoid. Do not start warfarin until thrombocytopenia resolved.

Prophylactic anticoagulation

LMWH now used in preference to UFH. LMWH given at low dose SC once daily. Recommended dose usually greater for orthopaedic surgery than general surgery. Continue until patient discharged and mobile.

- Moderate/high-risk patients—LMWH given 2h pre-op and once daily (📖 see *BNF* for dosage). UFH SC 5000IU 2h before surgery and bd until patient is mobile.
- Medical patients are also at risk of VTE and should be assessed for risk and considered for LMWH prophylaxis.

Conclusions

The ↑ convenience and proven efficacy means that for most clinical situations LMWH will now be preferred to UFH.

Table 15.4 Heparin infusion adjustment

APTR	>5.0	4.1–5.0	3.1–4.0	2.5–3.0	**TARGET (1.5–2.5)**	<1.2	1.5–2.5
DOSE	Stop* ↓500U/h	↓300U/h	↓100U/h	↓50U/h	**No change**	↑400U/h	↑200U/h

* Nil for 0.5–1.0h; check APTT ratio

Doses and dose adjustments (UFH) should follow local guidelines

1. Weitz, J.I. (1997). Low-molecular-weight heparins. *N Engl J Med*, **337**, 688–98.

Oral anticoagulation

Warfarin is the drug of choice; few side effects, well tolerated. A vitamin K antagonist, it takes ~72h to be effective; stable state takes 5–7d. t½ ~35h. Circulates mainly bound to albumin; free warfarin is active. Many drugs ↑ warfarin effect by displacing it from albumin. Monitored by PT using the international normalized ratio (INR).

Administration

Given daily. Usually given with heparin on d1. If massive thrombosis, delay warfarin for 2–3d. Standard adult regimen = 10mg/d for 2d. Load with caution using reduced dose if liver disease, interacting drugs, patient >80 years. Check INR <1.4 before loading. Check INR daily for 1st 4d[1] on d3 ~16h after 2nd dose, and adjust as follows.

Target INR usually 2.5 except for mechanical heart valves in mitral position when target is 3.0 or 3.5.

Complications

Haemorrhage. Easy bruising common within therapeutic range—is patient on aspirin? Rate of major bleeds ~2.7/100 treatment years, ↑ age ↑ INR. Rare side effects—alopecia, warfarin-induced skin necrosis, hypersensitivity, purple toe syndrome.

📖 See Warfarin overdose, p. 650 for details.

Asymptomatic patient

- ***INR >5.0***—stop warfarin and reduce dose by at least 25%. Check INR within 1 week.
- ***INR >8.0***—consider oral vitamin K 1–5mg.

Symptomatic patient

Moderate bleeding, INR 5.0–8.0, give vitamin K 1mg slowly IV. INR >8.0: give vitamin K 1mg and FFP or factor concentrate. Severe bleeding: vitamin K 5mg IV, and concentrate containing factors II, VII, IX, and X (e.g. beriplex). Observe in hospital. Vitamin K reverses over-anticoagulation in 24h. Look for causes of over-anticoagulation e.g. heart failure, alcohol, drugs.

1. Appendix II, Guidelines on oral anticoagulation: third edition, (1998). *Brit J Haematol*, **101**, 374–78)
2. Kearon, C. & Hirsh, J. (1997). Management of anticoagulation before and after elective surgery. *N Engl J Med*, **336**, 1506–1511.

Management of needlestick injuries

Every doctor dealing with high-risk patients is concerned to prevent exposure to blood and body fluids, particularly a needlestick injury. The UK DoH published guidance on post-exposure prophylaxis (PEP) for HIV in 1997 (tel. 0203 9724385 for copy). Your hospital/GP surgery should have a policy for the prevention and management of contamination incidents—check this out. Hospitals should have a 24h service providing advice and treatment.

Risk to health care workers

2 types of injury—*sharps injury* where intact skin is breached by sharp object contaminated with blood/blood-stained body fluids or unfixed tissue, and *contamination injury* where blood/blood-stained body fluid comes into contact with mucous membranes or non-intact skin. HBV and HIV are the 2 major concerns. All health care workers should be vaccinated against HBV. Risk of contracting HIV from percutaneous exposure to HIV-infected blood is ~0.3%. The amount of blood injected and a high viral load in the patient's blood ↑ the risk.

General guidelines

Prevention

All health care workers must adopt universal precautions when handling blood/blood stained fluids—wear gloves, avoid blood spillage, use decontamination procedures if spillage occurs, label high risk specimens, care with needles (do not resheath), disposal in burn bins, etc.

Immediate action in event of exposure

- Encourage bleeding and/or wash under running water.
- Contact Occupational Health/Emergency departments for help.
- Establish patient status re: blood-borne viruses.
- Take blood from patient/test for viruses (with consent).
- Take blood from needlestick victim and store. Check HBV immunity/later tests if necessary.

Treatment

- Decision to treat will be made by an experienced medical staff member. Treatment recommended for 'all health care workers exposed to high risk body fluids or tissues known to be, or strongly suspected to be, infected with HIV through percutaneous exposure, mucous membrane exposure or through exposure of broken skin'. Zidovudine alone given as soon as possible ↓ risk of seroconversion by 80% but failures are well described. Prophylaxis with triple therapy now recommended. Treat for 4 weeks as soon as possible with:
  - Zidovudine 200mg tds/250mg bd + lamivudine 150mg bd + indinavir 800mg tds. A 'starter pack' should be available in an accessible place at all times.
- Known exposure to hepatitis B:
  - No immunity—give HepB Ig 500mg IM; vaccinate immediately.
  - Known immunity with HepB Ab >100IU/L in past 2 years—no action.
  - Immunity—HepB Ab status not known—give booster dose.

Follow-up

Occupational Health Department appointment for advice re further management and tests. Counselling as required. 6 months after the incident a –ve test indicates infection has not occurred. Report incident to PHLS CDSC tel. 0208 2006868. In Scotland to SCIEH tel. 0141 9467120.

1. Beltrami, E.M. *et al.* (2000). Risk and management of blood-borne infection in healthcare workers. *Clin Microb Rev*, **13**, 385–407.

2. Cardo, D.M. *et al.* (1997). A case-control study of HIV seroconversion in health care workers after percutaneous exposure. Centers for Disease Control and Prevention Needlestick Surveillance Group. *N Engl J Med*, **337**, 1485–90.

3. Health Protection Agency (2006). *Eye of the needle: United Kingdom surveillance of significant exposures to bloodborne viruses in healthcare workers*. London: HPA

4. http://www.clinicalcareoptions.com/upload/hiv/guidelines/uk%/20pep.2004.pdf

Chemotherapy protocols: ABVD

Indication

HL.

Schedule: 28-day cycle (Table 15.5)

Table 15.5 ABVD

Days	Drug	Dose	Route
1 & 15	Doxorubicin	25mg/m^2	IV bolus
1 & 15	Bleomycin†	10,000IU/m^2	IVI in 500mL 0.9% saline
1 & 15	Vinblastine	6mg/m^2 IV (max l0mg)	IVI in 50mL 0.9%
1 & 15	Dacarbazine	375mg/m^2	IVI in 250mL 0.9% saline over at least 60min Saline over 5–10min

†Administer 100mg hydrocortisone IV before bleomycin when dexamethasone not used as an anti-emetic.

Administration

- Out-patient regimen.
- Consider sperm banking in ♂.
- Add allopurinol 300mg/d (100mg/d if creatinine clearance <20mL/min) for first 6 weeks.
- Antiemetic therapy for highly emetogenic regimens: at least a 5-HT$_3$ antagonist ± dexamethasone on 1st 2 days of each treatment.
- In patients with hepatic dysfunction, reduce doxorubicin & vinblastine to 50% dose for bilirubin 1.7–2.5 x ULN and reduce to 25% dose for bilirubin 2.5–4 x ULN.
- Proceed to next treatment if neutrophils >1.5 × 10^9/L and platelets >125 × 10^9/L; reduce doxorubicin & vinblastine to 50% dose if neutrophils 0.8–1.49 × 10^9/L or platelets 75–124 × 10^9/L; delay all drugs 1 week if neutrophils <0.8 × 10^9/L or platelets <75 × 10^9/L.
- Add G-CSF SC daily on days 5–11 and 20–26 of each cycle if 2 count related treatment delays or neutropenic septic episodes occur.
- Treat to complete remission + 2 cycles (maximum 8 cycles).

1. Canellos, G.P. *et al.* (1992). Chemotherapy of advanced Hodgkin's disease with MOPP, ABVD, or MOPP alternating with ABVD. *N Engl J Med*, **327**,1478–84.

BEACOPP & escalated BEACOPP

Indication

HL, advanced stage.

Schedule: 21-day cycle (Table 15.6)

Table 15.6 BEACOPP and escalated BEACOPP

Days	Drug	Standard dose	Escalated dose
1	Doxorubicin	25mg/m^2 IV bolus	35mg/m^2 IV bolus
1	Cyclophosphamide	650mg/m^2 IVI	1250mg/m^2 IVI
1–3	Etoposide †	100mg/m^2/d IVI	200mg/m^2/d IVI
1–7	Procarbazine	100mg/d PO	100mg/d PO
1–14	Prednisolone	40mg/m^2/d PO	40mg/m^2/d PO
8	Bleomycin‡	10,000iu/m^2 IVI	10,000IU/m^2 IVI
8	Vincristine	1.4mg/m^2 IVI in 50mL 0.9% saline (max 2mg)	1.4mg/m^2 IVI in 50mL 0.9% saline (max 2mg)
8 until neutrophils >1.0x10^9/L	G-CSF	Only if necessary	5mcg/kg/d filgrastim or 263mcg/d lenograstim SC

† Etoposide may be given orally at 200mg/m^2. ‡Administer 100mg hydrocortisone IV before bleomycin when dexamethasone not used as an anti-emetic.

Administration

- Out-patient regimen.
- Consider sperm banking in ♂.
- Add allopurinol 300mg/day (100mg/d if creatinine clearance <20mL/min) throughout first three treatment cycles.
- Antiemetic therapy for highly emetogenic regimens from d1–7.
- Infection prophylaxis with co-trimoxazole and aciclovir.
- Reduce bleomycin & etoposide doses to 75% for creatinine clearance 12–60mL/min & to 50% dose if <12mL/min.
- Reduce doxorubicin, etoposide & vincristine doses to 50% if bilirubin 1–2 x ULN, to 25% if 2–4 x ULN and omit if >4 x ULN.
- Withhold procarbazine if myelosuppression develops, restart at reduced dose after recovery.
- Discontinue procarbazine if paraesthesia, neuropathy, confusion, stomatitis or diarrhoea; restart at reduced dose after recovery
- Consider G-CSF support after first episode of febrile neutropenia or delay of treatment ≥1week
- Repeat treatment if neutrophils ≥1.5 × 10^9/L and platelets ≥100 × 10^9/L.
- Delay treatment if neutrophils <1.0 × 10^9/L or platelets <50 × 10^9/L until neutrophils ≥1.5 × 10^9/L or platelets ≥100 × 10^9/L.
- If it is considered essential to continue or delays of 2–3weeks fail to achieve adequate recovery:
  - 25% dose reduction if neutrophils ≥1.5 × 10^9/L and platelets 70–100 × 10^9/L.
  - 50% dose reduction if neutrophils 1–1.49 × 10^9/L and/or platelets 50–70 × 10^9/L.
- Administer every 3 weeks for 6–8 cycles; follow with 30 Gy radiotherapy to initial sites >5cm and 40 Gy to sites of residual disease.

1. Diehl, V. *et al.* (2003). Standard and increased-dose BEACOPP chemotherapy compared with COPP-ABVD for advanced Hodgkin's disease. *N Engl J Med*, **348**, 2386–95.

BEAM

Indications

Myeloablative conditioning regimen for autologous SCT in:

- Aggressive NHL with chemo-sensitive relapse or to consolidate remission in poor prognostic disease.
- HL: refractory or second remission.
- Indolent NHL refractory to second-line therapy.

Schedule (Table 15.7)

Table 15.7 BEAM

Days	Drug	Dose	Route
–7	Carmustine	300mg/m^2	IVI in 500mL 5% dextrose over 1h; avoid storage in PVC container for >24h
–6 to –3 (inclusive)	Cytarabine	200mg/m^2 bd	IVI in 100mL 0.9% saline over 30 min
–6 to –3 (inclusive)	Etoposide	200mg/m^2/d	IVI in 1L 0.9% saline over 2h
–2	Melphalan†	140mg/m^2	IVI in 250mL 0.9% saline within 60min of reconstitution
0	Thaw and reinfuse haematopoietic stem cells‡		

†Ensure excretion of melphalan by aggressive hydration (± furosemide).

‡Ensure stem cell dose ≥ 2.0 × 10^6/L CD34+ cells; do not re-infuse stem cells within 24h of melphalan infusion.

Administration

- In-patient regimen.
- Ensure adequate venous access by inserting a dual lumen tunnelled central venous catheter.
- Severe myelosuppression is expected (neutrophils <0.1 × 10^9/L and platelets <20 × 10^9/L).
- Add allopurinol 300mg (100mg if creatinine clearance <20mL/min) od for first week.
- Antiemetic therapy for highly emetogenic regimens.
- Give mouth care (nystatin and chlorhexidine M/W) and oral systemic antibacterial (e.g. ciprofloxacin) and antifungal prophylaxis (e.g. itraconazole) until neutrophil recovery ≥ 1.0 × 10^9/L—refer to local protocol for patients with severe neutropenia.
- Consider H_2 antagonist or PPI
- Consider starting G-CSF 5μg/kg/day on day +5 to shorten the duration of neutropenia.
- Consider aciclovir antiviral prophylaxis if previous history of HZV or HSV reactivation.
- Consider oral systemic *P. jirovecii* prophylaxis for 6 months after count recovery—refer to local protocol (generally co-trimoxazole 480mg bd tiw).
- Do not use BEAM if creatinine clearance is <40mL/min.

All patients must receive irradiated cellular blood components for at least 12 months post-SCT to prevent transfusion associated GvHD.

. Chopra, R. *et al.* (1993). The place of high-dose BEAM therapy and autologous bone marrow ransplantation in poor-risk Hodgkin's disease. A single-center eight-year study of 155 patients. *lood*, **81**, 1137–45.

. Mills, W. *et al.* (1995). BEAM chemotherapy and autologous bone marrow transplantation for atients with relapsed or refractory non-Hodgkin's lymphoma. J Clin Oncol, 13, 588–95.

CHOP 21 & CHOP 14

Indications

- Aggressive non-Hodgkin lymphoma.
- Low grade non-Hodgkin lymphoma resistant to first-line therapy.
- Rituximab may be added to either regimen (R-CHOP, see p.740) fo CD20+ NHL

Schedule: (Tables 15.8 and 15.9)

Table 15.8 CHOP 21 21-day cycle

Days	Drug	Dose	Route
1	Cyclophosphamide	750mg/m^2	IVI in 250mL 0.9% saline over 30min
1	Vincristine	1.4mg/m^2 (max. 2mg†)	IVI in 50mL 0.9% saline over 5–10min
1	Doxorubicin	50mg/m^2	IV bolus
1–5	Prednisolone	50mg/m^2/d (max 100mg)	PO in a.m. with food

† cap vincristine at 1mg for patients aged >70 years

Table 15.9 CHOP 14 14-day cycle

Days	Drug	Dose	Route
1	Cyclophosphamide	750mg/m^2	IVI in 250mL 0.9% saline over 30min
1	Vincristine	1.4mg/m^2 (max. 2mg†)	IVI in 50mL 0.9% saline over 5–10min
1	Doxorubicin	50mg/m^2	IV bolus
1–5	Prednisolone	50mg/m^2/d (max 100mg)	PO in a.m. with food
4–13	G-CSF filgrastim or lenograstim	5mcg/kg/d or 263mcg/d	SC

† cap vincristine at 1mg for patients aged >70 years

Administration

- Out-patient regimen.
- Consider sperm banking in ♂.
- Add allopurinol 300mg/d (100mg if creatinine clearance <20mL/min) throughout first treatment cycle.
- Antiemetic therapy for moderately emetogenic regimens.
- CNS chemoprophylaxis with intrathecal MTX should be administered for patients with aggressive NHL involving peripheral blood, testis, orbit, paranasal or paraspinal areas.
- With CHOP 14, consider oral systemic *P. jiroveci* prophylaxis —refer to local protocol (generally co-trimoxazole 480mg bd).

In patients with renal impairment, reduce cyclophosphamide dose to 75% for creatinine clearance 10–50mL/min and to 50% for clearance <10mL/min.
In patients with hepatic dysfunction, reduce doxorubicin dose by 50% for bilirubin 1.5–3× ULN and to 25% for bilirubin >3× ULN.
Repeat treatment when neutrophils ≥1.0 ×10^9/L and platelets ≥75 ×10^9/L; delay all drugs for 1 week if neutrophils <1.0 ×10^9/L or platelets <50 ×10^9/L; give 75% cyclophosphamide & doxorubicin doses if platelets 50–74 ×10^9/L and neutrophils ≥1.0 ×10^9/L.
Treat to complete remission + 2 cycles (max 8 cycles).
Mitoxantrone 10mg/m^2 may be substituted for doxorubicin (CNOP) in patients with previous cardiac disease.

. Fisher, R.I. *et al.* (1993). Comparison of a standard regimen (CHOP) with three intensive hemotherapy regimens for advanced non-Hodgkin's lymphoma. *N Engl J Med*, **328**, 1002–6. **1.**
. Pfreundshuh, M. *et al.* (2004). Two-weekly or 3-weekly CHOP chemotherapy with or without toposide for the treatment of elderly patients with aggressive lymphomas: results of the NHL-B2 rial of the DSHNHL. *Blood*, **104**, 634–41.

ChlVPP

Indication

HL in elderly patients unfit for ABVD or MOPP.

Schedule: 28-day cycle (Table 15.10)

Table 15.10 ChlVPP

Days	Drug	Dose	Route
1–14	Chlorambucil	6mg/m^2/d	PO
1 & 8	Vinblastine	6mg/m^2 (max 10mg)	IVI in 50mL 0.9% saline over 5–10min
1–14	Procarbazine	100mg/m^2/d (max 150mg)	PO
1–14	Prednisolone	40mg/m^2/d (max 60mg)	PO in a.m. with food

Administration

- Out-patient regimen.
- Less effective than ABVD; less toxic than MOPP.
- Consider sperm banking in ♂.
- Add allopurinol 300mg/d throughout first treatment cycle.
- Antiemetic therapy for moderately emetogenic regimens.
- Consider H_2-antagonist or PPI.
- Alcohol prohibited with procarbazine; avoid tyramine containing foods
- In patients with renal failure, consider dose reduction of procarbazine i creatinine >180micromol/L.
- In patients with hepatic dysfunction, reduce vinblastine dose to 50% if bilirubin 26–51 µmol/L or AST 60–180 IU/L; omit vinblastine if bilirubin >51µmol/L and AST/ALT >180 IU/L; consider dose reduct ion of chlorambucil in severe hepatic dysfunction.
- Repeat treatment cycle when WBC >3.5 × 10^9/L and platelets >100 × 10^9/L, otherwise delay 1 week.
- At day 8, if WBC ≥3.5 × 10^9/L and platelets >100 × 10^9/L, 100% doses; i WBC 3.1–3.49 × 10^9/L and platelets 81–99 × 10^9/L, give 50% vinblastine dose and 67% chlorambucil & procarbazine doses; if WBC 2.1–3.0 × 10^9/L or platelets 51–80 × 10^9/L, give 50% vinblastine & chlorambucil doses, stop procarbazine; if WBC <2.0 × 10^9/L or platelets <50 × 10^9/L, omit vinblastine and stop chlorambucil and procarbazine.
- Treat to complete remission + 2 cycles.

1. Dady, P.J. *et al.* (1982). Five years experience with ChlVPP: effective low-toxicity combination chemotherapy for Hodgkin's disease. *Br J Cancer*, **45**, 851–9.

CODOX-M/IVAC

Indication

Burkitt lymphoma or Burkitt-like lymphoma.

Schedule

Administer 2 alternating cycles of each regimen, i.e. A/B/A/B. Start each regimen as soon as possible after regeneration of neutrophils to >1.0 $\times10^9$/L and unsupported platelets to >75 $\times10^9$/L. In low risk patients (≥3 of normal LDH, WHO performance status 0–1, Stage I–II, ≤1 extra-nodal site), administer 3 cycles of CODOX-M only (Tables 15.11 and 15.12).

Table 15.11 Regimen A: CODOX-M

Days	Drug	Dose	Route
1	Cyclophosphamide	800mg/m^2	IVI in 500mL 0.9% saline over 30min
2–5		200mg/m^2/d	IVI in 250mL 0.9% saline over 15min × 4d
1 & 8	Vincristine	1.5mg/m^2 (max 2mg)	IV bolus
1	Doxorubicin	40mg/m^2	IVI in 50mL 0.9% Saline over 5–10min
1 & 3	Cytarabine [a]	70mg	IT injection
10	MTX [b]	300mg/m^2	IVI in 250mL 0.9% saline over 60min
		2700mg/m^2	IVI in 1L 0.9% saline over 23h
11	Calcium folinate [c]	15mg/m^2	IV 36 h after **start** of MTX; repeat 3hrly for 12 h then 15mg/m^2 IV/PO 6hrly until serum MTX level <5 $\times10^{-8}$ M.
13 until neutrophils >1.0 $\times10^9$/L	G-CSF (filgrastim or lenograstim)	5mcg/kg/d or 263mcg/d	SC
15	MTX[a]	12mg	Intrathecal injection
16	Calcium folinate[a]	15mg	PO 24h after IT MTX

[a] In patients with CNS involvement at diagnosis intensified CNS therapy is required during the first two cycles: cytarabine 70mg IT on days 1, 3 & 5; MTX 12.5mg IT on days 15 & 17; calcium folinate 15mg on days 16 & 18. [b] MTX should only be given if creatinine clearance >50ml/min/m^2. UK trials have used a lower dose of MTX than the original published regimen. Reduce MTX dose in patients aged >65 years (day 10: 100mg/m^2 IVI over 60min then 900mg/m^2 IVI over 23h). Alkalinise urine to pH ≥7 with 3L/m^2 IV fluids plus Na HCO_3 from 24h prior to start of MTX until serum MTX level <5 $\times10^{-8}$ M (i.e. until calcium folinate no longer required). Check serum MTX levels every 24h from 48h after start of MTX infusion. [c] If 48h serum MTX level >2 $\times10^{-6}$ M (2.0micromols/L) dose of calcium folinate should be doubled. Calcium folinate may be administered PO after 24h of IV administration if patient not vomiting.

Table 15.12 Regimen B: IVAC

Days	Drug	Dose	Route
1–5	Etoposide	60mg/m^2/d	IVI in 500mL 0.9% saline over 60min
1–5	Mesna [a]	300mg/m^2/d	IV bolus or IVI over 15min immediately before ifosfamide
		1500mg/m^2/d	IVI mixed with ifosfamide in 500mL 0.9% saline over 60min
		900mg/m^2/d	IVI in 500mL 0.9% saline over 12h
1–5	Ifosfamide [b]	1500mg/m^2/d	IVI over 60min mixed with Mesna in 500mL 0.9% saline
1 & 2	Cytarabine [c]	2g/m^2 every 12h (4 doses)	IVI in 1L 0.9% saline over 3h
5	MTX [d]	12mg	IT injection
6	Calcium folinate[d]	15mg	PO 24h after IT MTX
7 until neutrophils >1.0 x10^9/L	G-CSF (filgrastim or lenograstim)	5mcg/kg/d or 263mcg/d	SC

[a] In patients aged >65 years, reduce mesna doses to 200mg/m^2 IVI over 15min, 100mg/m^2 over 60min with Ifosfamide & 600mg/m^2 over 12h.[b] In patients aged >65 years, reduce Ifosfamide dose to 1000mg/m^2 IVI over 60 min.[c] Add Prednisolone 0.5% eye drops tds for 5–7 days during & after cytarabine. In patients aged >65 years, reduce cytarabine dose to 1g/m^2 IVI over 3h every 12 h (total 4 doses). [d] In patients with CNS involvement at diagnosis, intensified CNS therapy is required during the first two cycles: MTX 12.5mg IT on day 5; calcium folinate 15mg PO on day 6; cytarabine 70mg IT on days 7 & 9.

Administration

- Very intensive in-patient regimen; insert tunnelled central venous catheter if possible.
- Discuss risk of infertility and consider sperm storage.
- Check creatinine clearance before high dose MTX.
- High risk of tumour lysis syndrome; start IV hydration with ≥4.5 L/m^2/day with furosemide PRN. to maintain urine output ; add Na HCO_3 (start with 50mmol/L) if uric acid elevated and stop when uric acid normalizes, serum HCO_3 >30mmol/L or immediately prior to chemotherapy administration.
- Commence rasburicase (0.2mg/kg for 5–7 days) or allopurinol 10mg/kg/d in 2–3 divided doses x 3d then 5mg/kg/d x 14d.
- Infection prophylaxis with ciprofloxacin 250mg bd and nystatin mouthwash 1mL qds; fluconazole 100mg/day during CODOX-M; itraconazole 2.5mg/kg bd during IVAC .
- Prophylactic PPI, omeprazole 20mg od or equivalent.

- CODOX-M highly emetogenic on d1, use 5-HT_3 antagonist plus metoclopramide 10mg qds or domperidone 20mg qds for 2 days or cyclizine 50mg tds IV/ SC continuous infusion 150mg/d; IVAC days 1–5 very highly emetogenic, use 5-HT_3 antagonist plus dexamethasone 8mg bd plus metoclopramide or domperidone or cyclizine.

1. Magrath, I. *et al.* (1996). Adults and children with small non-cleaved-cell lymphoma have a similar excellent outcome when treated with the same chemotherapy regimen. *J Clin Oncol*, **14**, 925–34.
2. Lacasce, A. *et al.* (2004). Modified Magrath regimens for adults with Burkitt and Burkitt-like lymphomas: preserved efficacy with decreased toxicity. *Leuk Lymphoma*, **45**, 761–7.

CTD & CTDa

Indications

- Multiple myeloma.
- AL amyloid.
- Waldenström's macroglobulinaemia.

CTD schedule: 21-day cycle (Table 15.13)

Table 15.13 CTD

Days	Drug	Dose	Route
1, 8, 15	Cyclophosphamide	500mg/d	PO
1–21	Thalidomide	100mg/d for 3 weeks then 200mg/d	PO
1–4 & 12–15	Dexamethasone	40mg/d	PO

CTDa schedule: 28-day cycle (Table 15.14)

Table 15.14 CTDa

Days	Drug	Dose	Route
1, 8, 15, 22	Cyclophosphamide	500mg/d	PO
1–21	Thalidomide	50mg/d for 4 weeks increasing by 50mg/d every 4 weeks to 200mg/d	PO
1–4 & 15–18	Dexamethasone	20mg/d	PO

Administration

- Out-patient regimens; use CTDa in elderly patients with co-morbidities.
- Women of childbearing potential must have negative pregnancy test within 24h before starting thalidomide; repeat every 2–4 weeks while on thalidomide and 4 weeks after last dose.
- All patients should be enrolled in a pregnancy-prevention programme.
- Add allopurinol 300mg od PO (100mg if significant renal impairment) for first cycle.
- Add low dose aspirin (75mg/d) for patients at standard risk of thrombosis; add warfarin (target INR 2–3) or prophylactic dose LMW heparin (enoxaparin 40mg or equivalent) for patients with previous thrombosis or at higher risk (see p. 351).
- Antiemetic therapy for mildly emetogenic regimens.
- Commence H_2 antagonist or PPI.
- Consider regular laxative.
- Do not give cyclophosphamide if serum creatinine >300micromol/L after rehydration.
- Omit cyclophosphamide for 3 weeks if neutrophils $<1.0 \times 10^9$/L or platelets $<100 \times 10^9$/L. Reintroduce at 300mg or 400mg per dose.
- Consider G-CSF if treatment delays are prolonged or frequent
- Omit thalidomide for one cycle if grade 3/4 constipation, neuropathy, fatigue, sedation, rash, tremor, or oedema; reintroduce at 50mg/day.
- Treat with full dose warfarin or therapeutic doses of LMW heparin if thromboembolic event. Stop thalidomide and restart at 50mg/day escalating on the subsequent cycle to 100mg/day.
- Repeat for 4–6 cycles.

1. MRC Myeloma IX Trial Protocol (2004)

DHAP ± R

Indications

- Salvage chemotherapy for relapsed/refractory NHL and HL ± mobilization of peripheral blood stem cells.

Schedule: 21–28-day cycle depending on count recovery (Table 15.15)

Table 15.15 DHAP±R

Days	Drug	Dose	Route
−1	Rituximab	375mg/m^2	IVI in 500mL 0.9% saline over 3–5h
1–4	Dexamethasone	40mg/d	PO in the morning with food
1	Cisplatin	†100mg/m^2	IVI in 500mL 0.9% saline over 1h
2	Cytarabine	†2g/m^2 × 2	IVI in 1L 0.9% saline over 3h twice 12h apart

†cap surface area at 2m^2

Administration

- In-patient regimen.
- Ensure adequate venous access by inserting a dual lumen tunnelled central venous catheter.
- Severe myelosuppression (neutrophils <0.2 × 10^9/L and need for red cell and platelet transfusion support) should be expected.
- Allopurinol 300mg od PO (100mg if renal impairment) for first 2 cycles.
- For premedication and administration of rituximab 📖 see page 742.
- Consider aciclovir prophylaxis if previous history of HZV or HSV reactivation.
- Antiemetic therapy for highly emetogenic regimens.
- Aggressive pre- and post-hydration including potassium/magnesium supplementation is required with cisplatin.
- Prednisolone 0.5% eye-drops qds until 5d after completion of chemotherapy.
- Standard antimicrobial prophylaxis as dictated by local policy to cover duration of severe neutropenia.
- G-CSF 5–10mg/kg SC daily starting day +5 optional to shorten neutropenia and necessary to mobilize peripheral blood stem cells.
- Reduce cisplatin to 75% dose if creatinine clearance 45–60mL/min, 50% dose if creatinine clearance 30–45mL/min; do not give if creatinine clearance <30mL/min.
- Creatinine clearance should be assessed before each course of treatment.
- Cytarabine should be used with caution in severe renal impairment; consider reducing dose of cytarabine if hepatic impairment.
- Delay next cycle for 1 week if neutrophils <1.0 × 10^9/L or platelets <100 × 10^9/L.
- Patients with HL and those in whom stem cell collection is planned within 2 weeks must receive irradiated cellular blood components to prevent transfusion-associated GvHD.
- 2–6 cycles in total but usually consolidated with high dose therapy and autologous stem cell transplant in responding patients <65 years of age.

1. Velasquez, W.S. *et al.* (1988). Effective salvage therapy for lymphoma with cisplatin in combination with high dose Ara-C and dexamethasone (DHAP). *Blood*, **71**, 117–22.

EPOCH & DA-EPOCH ± R

Indications

- Treatment of refractory/relapsed aggressive NHL.
- Treatment of newly diagnosed aggressive NHL (DA-EPOCH)

Schedule: 21-day cycle (Table 15.16)

Table 15.16 EPOCH

Days	Drug	Dose	Route
–1	Rituximab	375mg/m^2	IVI in 500mL 0.9% saline over 3–5h
1–4	Etoposide	50mg/m^2/d	IV continuous infusion in 0.9% saline
1–4	Doxorubicin	10mg/m^2/d	IV continuous infusion in 0.9% saline
1–4	Vincristine	0.4mg/m^2/d	IV continuous infusion in 0.9% saline
1–5	Prednisolone	60mg/m^2/d	PO BID
5	Cyclophosphamide	750mg/m^2	IVI in 100mL 0.9% saline over 15min
6	G-CSF (filgrastim or lenograstim)	5mcg/kg/d or 263mcg/d	SC daily until neutrophils >0.5 × 10^9/L

Administration

- Outpatient continuous infusion regimen using portable pump.
- Ensure adequate venous access by inserting a tunnelled central venous catheter.
- Patients should have cardiac ejection fraction >40% but no cumulative doxorubicin limit is applied.
- Add allopurinol 300mg (100mg if creatinine clearance <20mL/min) od for first 2 cycles.
- For premedication and administration of rituximab see p. 742.
- Oral systemic *P. jiroveci* prophylaxis according to local protocol (generally co-trimoxazole 480mg bd three days per week) throughout treatment and for 8 weeks after completion.
- Antiemetic therapy for moderately emetogenic regimens.
- In EPOCH adjust cyclophosphamide dosage according to neutrophil count, reducing by 187mg/m^2 if nadir <0.5 × 10^9/L.
- In dose-adjusted or DA-EPOCH, increase doses of etoposide, doxorubicin and cyclophosphamide by 20% to achieve neutrophil nadir <0.5 × 10^9/L on 1 or 2 measurements biweekly.
- Delay next cycle may if neutrophils <1.0 × 10^9/L or platelets <100 × 10^9/L; give G-CSF until neutrophils >1.0 × 10^9/L.

Administer 2 additional cycles (minimum 6) beyond CR in patients with relapsed NHL, unless proceeding to stem cell transplantation.

1. Gutierrez, M. *et al.* (2000). Role of a doxorubicin-containing regimen in relapsed and resistant lymphomas: an 8-year follow-up study of EPOCH. *J Clin Oncol*, **18**, 3633–42.
2. Wilson, W.H. *et al.* (2002). Dose-adjusted EPOCH chemotherapy for untreated large B-cell lymphomas: a pharmacodynamic approach with high efficacy. *Blood*, **99**, 2685–93.
3. Wilson, W.H. *et al.* (2008). Phase II study of dose-adjusted EPOCH and rituximab in untreated diffuse large B-cell lymphoma with analysis of germinal center and post-germinal center biomarkers. *J Clin Oncol*, **26**, 2717–24.

ESHAP ± R

Indications

- Treatment of refractory/relapsed aggressive NHL and HL.
- Mobilization of peripheral blood stem cells for NHL and HL.

Schedule: 21–28-day cycle as soon as neutrophils >1.0 × 10^9/L and platelets (unsupported) >100 × 10^9/L (Table 15.17)

Table 15.17 ESHAP±R

Days	Drug	Dose	Route
–1	Rituximab	375mg/m^2	IVI in 500mL 0.9% saline over 3–5h
1	Cytarabine	2g/m^2	IVI in 500mL 0.9% saline over 2h
1–4	Etoposide	40–60mg/m^2/d	IVI in 250mL 0.9% saline over 60min
1–4	Cisplatin	25mg/m^2/d	IVI in 1L 0.9% saline over 24h
1–5	Methylprednisolone	500mg/d	IVI in 100mL 0.9% saline over 30min

Administration

- In-patient regimen.
- Ensure adequate venous access by inserting a dual lumen tunnelled central venous catheter.
- Severe myelosuppression (neutrophils <0.1 × 10^9/L and platelets <20 × 10^9/L) is expected.
- Add allopurinol 300mg (100mg if creatinine clearance <20mL/min) od for first 2 weeks.
- Administer rituximab after first dose of prednisolone on d1 before administering chemotherapy.
- For premedication and administration of rituximab 📖 see p. 742.
- Antiemetic therapy for highly emetogenic regimens.
- Aggressive pre- and post-hydration including potassium/magnesium supplementation required with cisplatin.
- Prednisolone 0.5% eye-drops qds until 5 days after completion of chemotherapy.
- Give mouth care (nystatin and chlorhexidine mouthwash) and oral systemic antibacterial and antifungal prophylaxis until neutrophil recovery ≥ 1.0 × 10^9/L.
- Consider H_2 antagonist or PPI.
- Consider starting G-CSF 5μg/kg/day on d7 either to shorten
- neutropenia or to facilitate peripheral blood stem cell collection around d16.
- Reduce cisplatin to 50% dose if creatinine clearance 40–60mL/min; do not give if creatinine clearance <40mL/min.
- Reduce cytarabine to 50% dose and omit etoposide if serum bilirubin >50micromol/L.
- Creatinine clearance should be assessed before each course of treatment

- Patients with HL and those in whom stem cell collection is planned within 2 weeks must receive irradiated cellular blood components to prevent transfusion-associated GvHD.
- 2–6 cycles in total but usually consolidated with high dose therapy and autologous stem cell transplant in responding patients <65 years of age.

1. Velasquez, W.S. *et al.* (1994). ESHAP – an effective chemotherapy regimen in refractory and relapsing lymphoma: a 4-year follow-up study. *J Clin Oncol*, **12**, 1169–76.

FC ± R

Indications
- CLL.
- Indolent lymphomas.
- Mantle cell lymphoma.

Schedule: 28-day cycle (Table 15.18)

Table 15.18 FC±R

Days	Drug	Dose	Route
1	Rituximab	375mg/m^2	IVI in 500mL 0.9% saline over 3–5h
1–3	Cyclophosphamide	250mg/m^2/d	IV bolus in 50mL 0.9% saline immediately prior to fludarabine
1–3	Fludarabine	25mg/m^2/d	IV bolus in 10mL 0.9% saline
Alternative oral schedule			
Days	**Drug**	**Dose**	**Route**
1	Rituximab	375mg/m^2	IVI in 500mL 0.9% saline over 3–5h
1–5	Cyclophosphamide	150mg/m^2/d†	PO
1–5	Fludarabine	24mg/m^2/d†	PO

†Appropriate rounding to the next available tablet size.

Administration
- Out-patient regimen.
- Check direct antiglobulin test (DAGT) pre-treatment; +ve DAGT is a relative contraindication to fludarabine therapy.
- Allopurinol 300mg od PO (100mg if significant renal impairment) for first 2 cycles.
- For premedication and administration of rituximab 📖 see p. 742.
- Oral systemic *P. jiroveci* prophylaxis according to local protocol (generally co-trimoxazole 480mg bd three days per week) throughout treatment and for 8 weeks after completion.
- Consider aciclovir prophylaxis if previous history of HZV or HSV reactivation.
- Antiemetic therapy for moderately emetogenic regimens.
- Reduce to 50% doses if renal impairment (creatinine clearance 30–60mL/min); do not give if creatinine clearance <30mL/min.
- Delay next cycle for 1 week if neutrophils $<1 \times 10^9$/L or platelets $<75 \times 10^9$/L.
- All cellular blood components should be irradiated for 1 year after therapy to prevent transfusion associated GvHD.
- Administer 6 cycles.

1. Hochster, H.S. *et al.* (2000). Phase I study of fludarabine plus cyclophosphamide in patients with previously untreated low-grade lymphoma: results and long term follow-up – a report from the Eastern Co-operative Oncology Group. *J Clin Oncol*, **18**, 987–94.
2. Keating, M.J. *et al.* (2005). Early results of a chemoimmunotherapy regimen of fludarabine, cyclophosphamide, and rituximab as initial therapy for chronic lymphocytic leukemia. *J Clin Oncol*, **23**, 4079–88.

FMD ± R (FND ± R)

Indications

- Follicular and other indolent NHL (beyond second line).
- Waldenström's macroglobulinaemia (beyond second line).
- Chronic lymphocytic leukaemia (beyond second line).

Schedule: 28-day cycle (Table 15.19)

Table 15.19 FMD ± R (FND ± R)

Days	Drug	Dose	Route
1	Rituximab	375mg/m^2	IVI in 500mL 0.9% saline over 3–5h
1–3	Fludarabine	25mg/m^2/d or 40mg/m^2/d	IV bolus in 10mL 0.9% saline or PO
1	Mitoxantrone	10mg/m^2	IV bolus in fast-running drip or infusion in 100mL 0.9% saline over 15min
1–5	Dexamethasone	20mg/d	PO/IV

Administration

- Out-patient regimen.
- Check DAGT pre-treatment and after each cycle; positive DAGT is a relative contraindication to fludarabine therapy.
- Allopurinol 300mg od PO (100mg if significant renal impairment) for first 2 cycles.
- Administer rituximab after first dose of dexamethasone on d1 before administering chemotherapy.
- For premedication and administration of rituximab 📖 see p. 742.
- Oral systemic *P. jiroveci* prophylaxis according to local protocol (generally cotrimoxazole 480mg bd three days per week) throughout treatment and for 8 weeks after completion.
- Consider aciclovir prophylaxis if previous history of VZV or HSV reactivation.
- Antiemetic therapy for moderately emetogenic regimens.
- Consider antagonist or PPI.
- Reduce fludarabine to 50% dose if renal impairment (creatinine clearance 30–60mL/min); do not give if creatinine clearance <30mL/min.
- Reduce mitoxantrone to 50% dose if serum bilirubin >1.5 upper limit normal and 25% if >3 upper limit normal.
- Delay next cycle for 1 week if neutrophils $<1.5 \times 10^9$/L or platelets $<100 \times 10^9$/L.
- All cellular blood components should be irradiated for 1 year after therapy to prevent transfusion associated GvHD.
- Repeat to maximum clinical response; usually 6 cycles.

1. McLaughlin P *et al* (1994) Phase I study of the combination of fludarabine, mitoxantrone and dexamethasone in low-grade lymphoma. *J Clin Oncol* **12**, 575–9.

Hyper-CVAD ± R / MA± R

Indications

- Mantle cell lymphoma.
- Burkitt lymphoma.

Schedule

► Administer 4 alternating cycles of each regimen, i.e. A/B/A/B/A/B/A/B (Table 15.20 and 15.21)

Table 15.20 Regimen A: (R-)Hyper-CVAD

Days	Drug	Dose	Route
1	Rituximab	375mg/m^2	IVI in 500mL 0.9% saline over 3-5h
2–4	Cyclophosphamide [a]	300mg/m^2	IVI in 500mL 0.9% saline over 2h 12hrly x 6 doses
2–5 & 12–15	Dexamethasone	40mg/day	IV/PO
5–6	Doxorubicin	25mg/m^2	IV continuous infusion in 0.9% saline
5 & 12	Vincristine [b]	1.4mg/m^2 (max 2mg)	IV bolus
7 until neutrophils >1.0 x10^9/L	G-CSF (Filgrastim or Lenograstim)	5µg/kg or 263µg	SC daily

[a] Begin Mesna 600mg/m^2/d by continuous infusion 1 hour before first dose of cyclophosphamide until 12h after final dose. [b] Administer day 5 vincristine 12h after last dose of cyclophosphamide.

Table 15.21 Regimen B: (R-)MA

Days	Drug	Dose	Route
1	Rituximab	375mg/m^2	IVI in 500mL 0.9% saline over 3-5h
2	Methotrexate (MTX)	200mg/m^2 then 800mg/m^2	IVI over 2h then IV continuous infusion over 22h
3	Calcium Folinate [a]	50mg then 15mg[a]	PO PO 6hrly x 8 doses
3–4	Cytarabine [b]	3g/m^2	IVI in 500mL 0.9% saline over 3h every 12h (total 4 doses)
4 until neutrophils >1.0 x10^9/L	G-CSF (Filgrastim or Lenograstim)	5µg/kg or 263µg	SC daily

[a] Adjust dose to MTX levels taken at 24h and 48h after completion of MTX [b] Add predinisolone 0.5% eye drops tds for 5–7 days during & after cytarabine. In patients aged >60 years or with creatinine >1.5mg/dL, reduce cytarabine dose to 1g/m^2 IVI over 3h every 12 h. [c] In patients with Burkitt lymphoma, add MTX 12mg IT on day 2 and cytarabine 100mg IT on days 7 with rituximab on days 1 & 11 of Hyper-CVAD and days 2 & 8 of MA during first 4 regimens only.

Administration

- Very intensive in-patient regimen; insert tunnelled central venous catheter if possible.
- Discuss risk of infertility and consider sperm storage.
- Allopurinol 300mg od PO (100mg if significant renal impairment) for first 2 cycles. Consider IV hydration and rasburicase in patients with bulky disease or Burkitt lymphoma.
- Administer rituximab after first dose of dexamethasone on d1 before administering chemotherapy.
- For premedication and administration of rituximab 📖 see p. 742.
- Oral systemic *P jiroveci* prophylaxis according to local protocol (generally co-trimoxazole 480mg bd three days per week) throughout treatment and for 4 weeks after completion; stop 1 day prior to MTX until neutrophils >1.0 $\times 10^9$/L.
- Commence bacterial infection prophylaxis with ciprofloxacin.
- Commence systemic oral antifungal prophylaxis, e.g. fluconazole.
- Consider aciclovir prophylaxis if previous history of HZV or HSV reactivation.
- Antiemetic therapy for highly emetogenic regimens.
- Reduce MTX dose in patients with pleural effusions or ascites (↓50%), grade 3/4 mucositis (↓25%) or renal impairment.
- In patients with renal impairment, reduce cytarabine dose by 1g/m^2 and MTX dose by 50% if creatinine 177–265 µmol/L and MTX dose by 75% if >265 µmol/L.
- In patients with hepatic dysfunction, reduce vincristine dose to 1mg if bilirubin ≥34micromol/L and doxorubicin dose by 25% if bilirubin ≥34, 50% ≥51 & 75% ≥68 micromol/L.
- Delay next cycle by 7d if neutrophils <1.0 $\times 10^9$/L or platelets <100 $\times 10^9$/L at d21; reduce cyclophosphamide by 20%, doxorubicin by 20%, MTX by 25% and cytarabine by 33% if same at d28.

1. Romaguera, J.E. *et al.* (2005). High rate of durable remissions after treatment of newly diagnosed aggressive mantle-cell lymphoma with rituximab plus hyper-CVAD alternating with rituximab plus high dose MTX and cytarabine. *J Clin Oncol*, **23**, 7013–23.

2. Thomas, D.A. *et al.* (2006). Chemoimmunotherapy with hyper-CVAD plus rituximab for the treatment of adult Burkitt and Burkitt-like lymphoma or acute lymphoblastic leukemia. Cancer, **106**, 1569–80.

ICE ± R

Indications

- Treatment of refractory/relapsed aggressive NHL and HL.
- Mobilization of peripheral blood stem cells for NHL and HL.

Schedule: 14-day cycle: 2 cycles for HL; 3 cycles for NHL (Table 15.22)

Table 15.22 ICE ± R

Days	Drug	Dose	Route
1	Rituximab [a]	375mg/m^2	IVI in 500mL 0.9% saline over 3-5h
1–3	Etoposide	100mg/m^2/d	IVI in 500mL-1L 0.9% saline over 30-60mins
2	Ifosfamide	5g/m^2	IV continuous infusion in 1L 0.9% saline over 24h
2	Mesna (mixed with Ifosfamide)	5g/m^2	IV continuous infusion over 24h
2	Carboplatin [b]	AUC 5 (capped at 800mg)	IVI in 250mL 0.9% saline over 1h
7–14	G-CSF [c] (filgrastim or lenograstim)	5mcg/kg/d or 263mcg/d	SC

[a] An initial dose of rituximab is administered 48h before initiation of cycle 1 (d2); patients completing 3 cycles receive 4 doses of rituximab. [b]Calculate creatinine clearance (Cl_{cr}) from 12h urine sample collected on day of admission; carboplatin dose based on Calvert formula: dose = 5 x [25 + Cl_{cr}]. [c] Double G-CSF dose on final cycle and continue until end of stem cell collection.

Administration

- Intensive in-patient regimen; insert tunnelled central venous catheter if possible.
- Discuss risk of infertility and consider sperm storage.
- Allopurinol 300mg od PO (100mg if significant renal impairment) for first 2 cycles.
- For premedication and administration of rituximab 📖 see p. 742.
- Commence bacterial infection prophylaxis with ciprofloxacin.
- Commence systemic oral antifungal prophylaxis, e.g. fluconazole.
- Consider aciclovir prophylaxis if previous history of HZV or HSV.
- Antiemetic therapy for highly emetogenic regimens.
- Delay next cycle if neutrophils <1.0 ×10^9/L or platelets <50 ×10^9/L at d15.
- Patients who achieve CR or PR with ICE ± R should proceed to autologous stem cell transplantation.

1. Moskowitz, C.H. *et al.* (2001). A 2-step comprehensive high-dose chemoradiotherapy second-line program for relapsed and refractory Hodgkin disease: analysis by intent to treat and development of a prognostic model. *Blood*, **97**, 616–23.

2. Kewalramani, T. *et al.* (2004). Rituximab and ICE as second-line therapy before autologous stem cell transplantation for relapsed or primary refractory diffuse large B-cell lymphoma. *Blood*, **103**, 3684–8.

MCP ± R

Indication

Indolent NHL.

Aggressive lymphoma where more intensive chemotherapy contraindicated.

Schedule: 28-day cycle (Table 15.23)

Table 15.23 MCP±R

Day	Drug	Dose	Route
1	Rituximab	$375mg/m^2$	IVI in 0.9% saline over 3–5h
3 & 4	Mitoxantrone	$8mg/m^2$	IV bolus or IVI over 30min in 100mL 0.9% saline
3–7	Chlorambucil	$9mg/m^2/d$	PO
3–7	Prednisolone	$25mg/m^2/d$	PO in a.m. with food

Administration

- Out-patient regimen.
- Add allopurinol 300mg/d (100mg/d if creatinine clearance <20mL/min) for first 2 cycles.
- Antiemetic therapy for moderately emetogenic regimens.
- Consider H_2-antagonist or PPI.
- An alternative MCP regimen with mitoxantrone $12mg/m^2$ by IVI on d1 and chlorambucil 10mg/d PO on days 1–10 with prednisolone 40mg/d PO on days 1–10 has been widely used in the UK.
- For premedication and administration of rituximab 📖 see p. 742.
- If neutrophils $<1.0 \times 10^9/L$ and/or platelets $<100 \times 10^9/L$, delay treatment for 1 week; if persistant, reduce mitoxantrone & chlorambucil dosage to 75%.
- Repeat to maximum clinical response (maximum 8 cycles).

1. Wöhrer, S. *et al.* (2005). Effective treatment of indolent non-Hodgkin's lymphomas with mitoxantrone, chlorambucil and prednisolone. *Onkologie* **28**,73–8.

2. Herold, M. *et al.* (2007). Rituximab added to first-line mitoxantrone, chlorambucil, and prednisolone chemotherapy followed by interferon maintenance prolongs survival in patients with advanced follicular lymphoma: an East German Study Group Hematology and Oncology Study. *J Clin Oncol*, **25**, 1986–92.

MINE

Indications

- Salvage treatment of refractory/relapsed Hodgkin lymphoma.
- Mobilisation of peripheral blood stem cells.

Schedule: 28-day cycle: 2–3 cycles followed by ASCT (Table 15.24)

Table 15.24 MINE

Days	Drug	Dose	Route
1 & 5	Mitoguazone	500mg/m^2	IVI in 500mL 0.9% saline over 1–3h
1–5	Ifosfamide	1.5g/m^2/d	IVI in 250mL 0.9% saline over 1h
1–5	Mesna (mixed with Ifosfamide)	1.5g/m^2/d	IVI over 1h
1 & 5	Vinorelbine	15mg/m^2	IVI in 50mL 0.9% saline over 30min
1–3	Etoposide	150mg/m^2/d	IVI in 500mL–1L 0.9% saline over 1–3h

Administration

- Intensive in-patient regimen; insert tunnelled central venous catheter if possible.
- Discuss risk of infertility and consider sperm storage.
- Allopurinol 300mg od PO (100mg if significant renal impairment) for first 2 cycles.
- Commence bacterial infection prophylaxis with ciprofloxacin.
- Commence systemic oral antifungal prophylaxis, e.g. fluconazole.
- Consider aciclovir prophylaxis if previous history of HZV or HSV reactivation.
- Antiemetic therapy for highly emetogenic regimen.
- Delay next cycle if neutrophils $<1.0 \times 10^9$/L or platelets $<100 \times 10^9$/L.
- Mobilize stem cells after MINE therapy by addition of G-CSF (5mcg/kg filgrastim or 263mcg lenograstim) from d6 until end of stem cell collection.
- Patients who achieve CR or PR with MINE should proceed to autologous stem cell transplantation.

1. Ferme, C. *et al*, (1995). The MINE regimen as intensive salvage chemotherapy for relapsed and refractory Hodgkin's disease. *Ann Onc*, **6**, 543–9.

Mini-BEAM ± R

Indications

- Salvage therapy of refractory/relapsed NHL and HL.
- Mobilization of peripheral blood stem cells.

Schedule (Table 15.25)

Table 15.25 Mini-BEAM±R

Days	Drug	Dose	Route
−1	Rituximab	375mg/m^2	IVI in 500mL 0.9% saline over 3–5h
1	Carmustine	60mg/m^2	IVI in 250mL 5% dextrose over 1h; avoid storage in PVC container for >24h
2–5	Cytarabine	100mg/m^2 bd	IVI in 100mL 0.9% saline over 30min
2–5	Etoposide	75mg/m^2	IVI in 500mL 0.9% saline over 1h
6	Melphalan†‡	30mg/m^2	IV bolus in 100mL 0.9% saline within 30min reconstitution

†Ensure adequate diuresis is achieved before administering melphalan.

‡ Ensure that melphalan is administered on a weekday; Mondays or Tuesdays provide optimal timing for stem cell collection.

Administration

- In-patient regimen.
- Ensure adequate venous access by inserting a dual lumen tunnelled central venous catheter.
- Severe myelosuppression (neutrophils <0.1 × 10^9/L and platelets <20 × 10^9/L) is expected.
- Add allopurinol 300mg (100mg if creatinine clearance <20mL/min) od for first 2 weeks.
- For premedication and administration of rituximab 📖 see p. 742.
- Antiemetic therapy for moderately emetogenic regimens
- Give mouth care (nystatin and chlorhexidine mouthwash) and oral systemic antibacterial and antifungal prophylaxis until neutrophil recovery ≥1.0 × 10^9/L.
- Consider H_2 antagonist or PPI.
- Consider starting G-CSF 5μg/kg/d on d9 either to shorten neutropenia or to facilitate peripheral blood stem cell collection around d18.
- Note: do not use mini-BEAM if creatinine clearance ≤40mL/min.
- Patients with HL and those in whom stem cell collection is planned within 2 weeks must receive irradiated cellular blood components to prevent transfusion-associated GvHD.
- A second course can be given when neutrophils >1.0 × 10^9/L and platelets (unsupported) >100 × 10^9/L; generally 4–6 weeks.
- Consolidate in responding patients with high dose therapy and autologous stem cell transplant.

1. Linch, D.C. *et al.* (1993). Dose intensification with autologous bone marrow transplantation in relapsed and resistant Hodgkin's disease: results of a BNLI randomized trial. *Lancet*, **341**, 1051–4.
2. Girouard, C. *et al.* (1997). Salvage chemotherapy with mini-BEAM for relapsed or refractory non-Hodgkin's lymphoma prior to autologous bone marrow transplantation. *Ann Oncol*, **8**, 675–80.

R-CHOP

Indication

- B-cell NHL
- Addition of rituximab approved in UK only for first line treatment of CD20+ diffuse large B cell lymphoma stage II, III or IV.

Schedule: 21-day cycle (Table 15.26)

Table 15.26 R-CHOP

Day	Drug	Dose	Route
1	Rituximab	375mg/m^2	IVI in 500mL 0.9% saline over 3–5h
1	Cyclophosophamide	750mg/m^2	IVI in 250mL 0.9% saline over 30mins
1	Vincristine	1.4mg/m^2 (max 2mg*)	IV bolus
1	Doxorubicin	50mg/m^2	IV bolus
1–5	Prednisolone	50mg/m^2/d (max 100mg)	PO in a.m. with food

* max 1mg for patients>70 years.

Administration

- Outpatient regimen.
- Consider sperm banking in ♂.
- Add allopurinol 300mg/d (100mg/d if creatinine clearance <20mL/min) throughout first 2 treatment cycles.
- Antiemetic therapy for moderately emetogenic regimen.
- CNS chemoprophylaxis with IT MTX should be administered for patients with aggressive NHL involving peripheral blood, testis, orbit, paranasal, or paraspinal areas.
- Administer rituximab after first dose of prednisolone on d1 before administering chemotherapy.
- For premedication and administration of rituximab 📖 see p. 742.
- In patients with renal impairment, reduce cyclophosphamide dose to 75% for creatinine clearance 10–50mL/min and to 50% for clearance <10mL/min.
- In patients with hepatic dysfunction, reduce doxorubicin dose by 50% for bilirubin 1.5–3x ULN and to 25% for bilirubin >3 x ULN.
- Repeat treatment when neutrophils ≥1.0 ×10^9/L & platelets ≥75 ×10^9/L; delay all drugs for 1 week if neutrophils <1.0 ×10^9/L or platelets <50 ×10^9/L; give 75% cyclophosphamide & doxorubicin doses if platelets 50–74 ×10^9/L and neutrophils ≥1.0 ×10^9/L.
- Treat to complete remission + 2 cycles, max 8 cycles.

1. Coiffier, B. *et al.* (2002). CHOP chemotherapy plus rituximab compared with CHOP alone in elderly patients with diffuse large-B-cell lymphoma. *N Engl J Med*, **346**, 235–42.

R-CVP & CVP

Indications

- Low grade NHL.
- R-CVP approved in UK for first line treatment of follicular lymphoma only.
- Advanced chronic lymphocytic leukaemia.

Schedule: 21-day cycle (Table 15.27)

Table 15.27 R-CVP & CVP

Day	Drug	Dose	Route
1	Rituximab	375mg/m^2	IVI in 500mL 0.9% saline over 3–5 h
1	Cyclophosphamide	750mg/m^2	IV bolus
1	Vincristine	1.4mg/m^2 (max. 2mg)*	IVI in 50mL 0.9% saline over 5–10min
1–5	Prednisolone	60mg/m^2/d (max. 100mg)	PO in a.m. with food

*consider maximum 1mg vincristine in patients >70

Administration

- Out-patient regimen.
- Consider sperm banking in ♂.
- Add allopurinol 300mg/d (100mg/d if creatinine clearance <20mL/min) throughout first 2 treatment cycles.
- Antiemetic therapy for moderately emetogenic regimens.
- Administer rituximab after first dose of prednisolone on d1 before administering chemotherapy.
- For premedication and administration of rituximab 📖 see p. 742.
- Repeat treatment when neutrophils >1.5 × 10^9/L & platelets ≥100 × 10^9/L; reduce cyclophosphamide to 75% dose if neutrophils 1.0–1.49 × 10^9/L & platelets ≥100 × 10^9/L and reduce to 50% dose if neutrophils 0.5–1.0 × 10^9/L &/or platelets 50–100 × 10^9/L; omit cyclophosphamide if neutrophils <0.5 × 10^9/L and/or platelets <50 × 10^9/L.
- Repeat to maximum clinical response; usually 6–8 cycles.

1. Marcus, R. *et al.* (2005). CVP chemotherapy plus rituximab compared with CVP as first-line treatment for advanced follicular lymphoma. *Blood*, **105**, 1417–23.

Rituximab

Indications

- CD20+ NHL and LPD; approved by NICE in UK only for follicular NHL (monotherapy, first line in R-CVP, maintenance in 2nd remission) and for diffuse large B-cell NHL as first-line in R-CHOP.

Monotherapy schedule for FL: single 28-day cycle (Table 15.28)

Table 15.28 Rituximab monotherapy

Days	Drug	Dose	Route
1, 8, 15, 22	Rituximab	375mg/m^2	IVI in 500mL 0.9% saline over 3-5h

Maintenance schedules for FL (Table 15.29)

Table 15.29 Rituximab maintenance

Months[a]	Drug	Dose	Route
2, 4, 6, 8	Rituximab	375mg/m^2	IVI in 500mL 0.9% saline over 3–5h

[a] Ghielmini, M. *et al.* (2005). Prolonged treatment with rituximab in patients with follicular lymphoma significantly increases event-free survival and response duration compared with the standard weekly x 4 schedule. *Blood*, **103**, 4416–23.

Months[b]	Drug	Dose	Route
3, 6, 9, 12, 15, 18, 21, 24	Rituximab	375mg/m^2	IVI in 500mL 0.9% saline over 3–5 h

[b] van Oers, M.H. *et al.* (2006). Rituximab maintenance improves clinical outcome of relapsed/resistant follicular non-Hodgkin lymphoma in patients both with and without rituximab during induction: results of a prospective randomized phase 3 intergroup trial. *Blood*, **108**, 3295–301.

Administration

- Premedication with paracetamol (1g) and chlorphenamine (10mg) should be administered before each rituximab infusion.
- In combination regimens rituximab may be given 1–2 days before chemotherapy if it is difficult to fit all infusions into a single day.
- Monitor closely for cytokine release syndrome: fever, chills, rigors within first 2 hours usually.
- Less common side effects include: flushing, angioedema, nausea, urticaria/rash, fatigue, headache, throat irritation, rhinitis, vomiting, tumour pain and features of tumour lysis syndrome, bronchospasm, hypotension.
- Interrupt rituximab infusion if severe dyspnoea, bronchospasm, or hypoxia.
- If lymphocyte count <20.0 × 10^9/L and if patient has previously tolerated rituximab with steroid-containing chemotherapy regimen,

Rituximab may be infused over 1.5h or if tolerated ≥2 prior doses within 3 months, may infuse over 1h.

- When lymphocyte count $\geq 20.0 \times 10^9$/L or bulky disease (>10cm), split dose and administer 100mg on day 1 and remainder on day 2.

1. McLaughlin, P. *et al.* (1998). Rituximab chimeric anti-CD20 monoclonal antibody therapy for relapsed indolent lymphoma: half of patients respond to a four-dose treatment program. *J Clin Oncol*, **16**, 2825–33.

2. Byrd, J.C. *et al.* (1999). Rituximab therapy in hematologic malignancy patients with circulating blood tumor cells: association with increased infusion-related side effects and rapid blood tumor clearance. *J Clin Oncol*, **17**, 791–5.

3. Sehn, L.H. *et al.* (2004). Rapid infusion rituximab in combination with steroid-containing chemotherapy can be given safely and substantially reduces resource utilization. *Blood*, **104**, 1407a.

4. Ghielmini, M. *et al.* (2005). Infusion speed escalation trial to give full-dose rituximab in one hour without steroids premedication. *Blood*, **106**, 2451a.

Stanford V

Indications

- HL, except stage IA or IIA without locally extensive disease (e.g. bulky mediastinal disease or ≥2 extranodal sites).

Schedule: 12 weeks of chemotherapy comprising 3 cycles of 28-days followed in 2–4 weeks by 36 Gy involved field radiotherapy in patients with disease >5cm or splenomegaly (Tables 15.30 and 15.31)

Table 15.30 Stanford V

Days	Drug	Dose	Route
1 & 15	Doxorubicin	$25mg/m^2$ [a]	IV bolus
1 & 15	Vinblastine [b]	$6mg/m^2$ [a]	IVI in 50mL 0.9% saline over 5–10min
1	Mechlorethamine (mustine)	$500mg/m^2$ [a]	IV bolus
1–28 [c]	Prednisolone	$40mg/m^2$ on alternate days [a]	PO in a.m. with food
8 & 22	Vincristine [d]	$1.4mg/m^2$ (max 2mg) [a]	IVI in 50mL 0.9% saline over 5–10min
8 & 22	Bleomycin [e]	$5000units/m^2$	IVI in 250mL 0.9% saline over 1h
15 & 16	Etoposide	$60mg/m^2/d$ [a]	IVI in 250mL 0.9% saline over 45min

[a]Cap surface area at $2m^2$ for calculating dose. [b]Reduce vinblastine dose to $4mg/m^2$ after second cycle for patients >50. [c]Taper prednisolone dose by 10mg every other day during weeks 10 – 12. [d]Reduce vincristine dose to $1mg/m^2$ after second cycle for patients >50. [e]Administer hydrocortisone 100mg IV before infusion of bleomycin unless dexamethasone used as anti-emesis therapy.

Table 15.31 Indications for involved field radiotherapy

Initial bulky disease: >33% of maximal trans-thoracic diameter on CXR
Initial individual or confluent nodal masses ≥5cm in diameter
Initial splenic disease: macroscopic nodules on CT when spleen not surgically removed; N.B. splenomegaly is not a criterion for splenic irradiation

Administration

- Intensive regimen.
- Discuss risk of infertility and consider sperm storage; child-bearing ♀ should commence oral contraceptive.
- Consider IV hydration for patients with bulk disease.
- Allopurinol 300mg od PO (100mg if creatinine clearance <20mL/min) for first 6 weeks.

- Anti-emetic therapy for highly emetogenic regimens with chlormethine (mustine), otherwise therapy for moderately emetogenic regimens.
- Commence H_2-antagonist or PPI.
- Oral systemic *P. jiroveci* prophylaxis according to local protocol recommended (generally co-trimoxazole 480mg bd three days per week) throughout treatment and for 8 weeks after completion.
- Oral systemic antifungal prophylaxis, e.g. fluconazole and aciclovir prophylaxis of HZV or HSV reactivation recommended.
- Daily aperient recommended to soften stool, e.g. docusate or senna.
- In patients with renal impairment, when creatinine clearance <60mL/min administer 80% mustine dose, 85% etoposide dose & 75% Bleomycin dose; <30mL/min omit mustine, administer 75% etoposide dose <60mL/min.
- In patients with hepatic dysfunction, if bilirubin 1–2 x ULN reduce doxorubicin, vinblastine, vincristine, & etoposide doses to 50%; 2–4 x ULN reduce doses to 25%; >4 x ULN omit doxorubicin, vinblastine, and etoposide.
- If neutrophils $0.5–1.0 \times 10^9$/L, administer 65% doses of doxorubicin, mustine, vincristine & etoposide but 100% dose of other drugs; if $<0.5 \times 10^9$/L delay doxorubicin, mustine, vincristine & etoposide by 1 week but no delay or dose reduction of other drugs.
- If dose reduction or delay is required, administer G-CSF SC on days 3–7 & 17–21 of each cycle.
- No dose reductions or delay if platelets $>10 \times 10^9$/L; if $<10 \times 10^9$/L, transfuse platelets to maintain count $>10 \times 10^9$/L.

1. Horning, S.J. *et al.* (2000). Assessment of the Stanford V regimen and consolidative radiotherapy for bulky and advanced Hodgkin's disease: Eastern Cooperative Group Pilot Study E1492. *J Clin Oncol*, **18**, 972–80.

VAPEC-B

Indication

HL stage IA or IIA without B symptoms or bulky disease.

Schedule: 6-week chemotherapy and radiotherapy regimen given once only (Table 15.32)

Table 15.32 VAPEC-B

Days	Drug	Dose	Route
1–28	Prednisolone	50mg/d	PO in a.m.with food; taper after d29–38
1 & 15	Doxorubicin	35mg/m^2	IV bolus or IVI in 100mL 0.9% saline over 15min
1	Cyclophosphamide	350mg/m^2	IVI in 250mL 0.9% saline over 15min
15–19	Etoposide	100mg/m^2/d for 5 days	PO 1h before food on empty stomach
8 & 22	Vincristine	1.4mg/m^2 (max 2mg)	IVI in 50ml 0.9% saline over 5–10min
8 & 22	Bleomycin†	10,000iu/m^2	IVI in 250mL 0.9% saline over 60min
36	IF radiotherapy	30-40Gy to initial volume of disease	

† Prescribe hydrocortisone 100mg IV before bleomycin.

Adminstration

- Involved field radiotherapy is given at a dose of 30–40Gy to the initial volume of the disease, during week 6, 2 weeks after the last dose of chemotherapy.
- Outpatient treatment.
- Consider sperm banking in ♂ (low risk of infertility).
- Oral systemic *P. jiroveci* prophylaxis according to local protocol (generally co-trimoxazole 480mg bd tiw) is recommended for the first 6 weeks.
- Oral systemic antifungal prophylaxis is optional.
- Antiemetic therapy for moderately emetogenic regimens on days 1 and 15.
- Add an H_2-antagonist or PPI
- Delay doxorubicin, cyclophosphamide, or etoposide by 1 week if platelets <100 × 10^9/L or neutrophils <1 × 10^9/L.
- Reduce cyclophosphamide to 75% dose if creatinine clearance 10–50mL/min, 50% dose if creatinine clearance <10mL/min.
- Reduce doxorubicin, vincristine, and etoposide to 50% dose if serum bilirubin 1.7–2.5 upper limit normal and 25% if 2.5–4 upper limit normal. Caution with cyclophosphamide in patients with hepatic impairment.
- All cellular blood components should be irradiated indefinitely.
- Total regimen 6 weeks treatment.

1. Radford, J.A. *et al.* (1996). Four weeks of neoadjuvant chemotherapy significantly reduces the progression rate in patients treated with limited field radiotherapyfor clinical stage IA/IIA Hodgkin's disease. *Ann Oncol*, **7**(suppl3), 21.

2. Radford, J.A. *et al.* (2002). Four weeks of VAPEC-B chemotherapy before involved field radiotherapy minimises the relapse rate in early stage, low risk Hodgkin's disease and is not associated with an excess of second malignancy. *Ann Oncol*, **13** (suppl 2), 25.

Chapter 16

Haematological investigations

Full blood count

Rapid analysis by the latest generation automated blood counters using either forward angle light scatter or impedance analysis provides enumeration of leucocytes, erythrocytes, and platelets and quantification of haemoglobin, MCV plus derived values for haematocrit, MCH, and MCHC red cell distribution width (a measure of cell size scatter), mean platelet volume and platelet distribution width, and a 5 parameter differential leucocyte count. The counter also flags samples which require direct morphological assessment by examination of a blood film.

Sample: peripheral blood EDTA; the sample should be analysed in the laboratory within 4h.

Blood film

Morphological assessment of red cells, leucocytes, and platelets should be performed by an experienced individual of all samples in which the FBC has revealed any result significantly outside the ↔ range, samples in which a flag has been indicated by the automated counter and if clinically indicated. A manual differential leucocyte count may be performed and may differ from that produced by the automated counter most notably in patients with haematological disease affecting the leucocytes.

Sample: peripheral blood EDTA; the sample should be analysed in the laboratory within 4h. May be made directly from drop of blood or EDTA sample, air-dried and fixed.

Plasma viscosity

This test is a sensitive but non-specific index of plasma protein changes which result from inflammation or tissue damage. The plasma viscosity is unchanged by haematocrit variations and delay in analysis up to 24h and is therefore more reliable than the ESR. It is not affected by sex but is affected by age, exercise, and pregnancy.

Sample: peripheral blood EDTA; the sample should be analysed in the laboratory within 24h.

ESR

This test is a sensitive but non-specific index of plasma protein changes which result from inflammation or tissue damage. The ESR is affected by haematocrit variations, red cell abnormalities (e.g. poikilocytosis, sickle cells), and delay in analysis and is therefore less reliable than measurement of the plasma viscosity. The ESR is affected by age, sex, menstrual cycle, pregnancy, and drugs (e.g. OCP, steroids).

Sample: peripheral blood EDTA; the sample should be analysed in the laboratory within 4h.

Haematinic assays

Measurement of the serum B_{12} and red cell folate are necessary in the investigation of macrocytic anaemia, and serum ferritin in the investigation of microcytic anaemia, in order to assess body stores of the relevant haematinic(s). Serum folate levels are an unreliable measurement of body stores of folate. The serum ferritin may be elevated as an acute phase protein in patients with underlying neoplasia or inflammatory disease (e.g. rheumatoid arthritis) and may give an erroneously ↔ level in an Fe deficient patient.

Sample: clotted blood sample and peripheral blood EDTA.

Haemoglobin electrophoresis

This test is performed in the diagnosis of abnormal haemoglobin produc-tion (haemoglobinopathies or thalassaemia). It is usually performed on cellulose acetate at alkaline pH (8.9) but may be performed on citrate agar gel at acid pH (6.0) to detect certain haemoglobins more clearly. Haemoglobin electrophoresis has been largely replaced by HPLC analysis.

Sample: peripheral blood EDTA.

Haptoglobin

The serum haptoglobin should be measured in patients with suspected haemolysis (extravascular or intravascular) and is frequently reduced in patients with haemolysis. Low concentrations of haptoglobin may be found in hepatocellular disease. It should generally be accompanied by estimation of the serum methaemalbumin, free plasma haemoglobin, and urinary haemosiderin.

Sample: clotted blood.

Schumm's test

This spectrophotometric test for methaemalbumin (which has a distinctive absorption band at 558nm) should be measured in patients with sus-pected intravascular haemolysis and may be abnormal in patients with significant extravascular (generally splenic) haemolysis. It should generally be accompanied by estimation of the serum haptoglobin level, free plasma haemoglobin, and urinary haemosiderin.

Sample: heparinized blood or clotted blood.

Kleihauer test

The Kleihauer test which exploits the resistance of fetal red cells to acid elution should be performed on all Rh(D) –ve women who deliver a Rh(D) +ve infant. Fetal cells appear as darkly staining cells against a background of ghosts. An estimate of the required dose of anti-D can be made from the number of fetal cells in a low power field.

Sample: maternal peripheral blood EDTA.

Reticulocytes

Definition

- Immature RBCs formed in marrow and found in normal peripheral blood.
- Represent an intermediate maturation stage in marrow between the nucleated red cell and the mature red cell.
- No nucleus but retain some nucleic acid.

Detection and measurement

- Demonstrated by staining with supravital dye for the nucleic acid.
- Appear on blood film as larger than mature RBCs with fine lacy blue staining strands or dots.
- Some modern automated blood counters using laser technology can measure levels of reticulocytes directly.
- Usually expressed as a % of total red cells e.g. 5%, though absolute numbers can be derived from this and total red cell count.

Causes of ↑ reticulocyte counts

Marrow stimulation due to:

- Bleeding.
- Haemolysis.
- Response to oral Fe therapy.
- Infection.
- Inflammation.
- Polycythaemia (any cause).
- MPDs.
- Marrow recovery following chemotherapy or radiotherapy.
- EPO administration.

Causes of ↓ reticulocyte counts

Marrow infiltration due to:

- Leukaemia.
- Myeloma.
- Lymphoma.
- Other malignancy.

Marrow underactivity (hypoplasia) due to:

- Fe, folate, or B_{12} deficiency. *Note*: return of reticulocytes is earliest sign of response to replacement therapy.
- Immediately post-chemotherapy or radiotherapy.
- Autoimmune disease especially rheumatoid arthritis.
- Malnutrition.
- Uraemia.
- Drugs.
- Aplastic anaemia (📖 see p.98).
- Red cell aplasia (📖 see p.102).

Urinary haemosiderin

Usage

The most widely used and reliable test for detection of chronic intravascular haemolysis.

Principle

Free Hb is released into the plasma during intravascular haemolysis. The haemoglobin binding proteins become saturated resulting in passage of haem-containing compounds into the urinary tract of which haemosiderin is the most readily detectable.

Method

- A clean catch sample of urine is obtained from the patient.
- Sample is spun down in a cytocentrifuge to obtain a cytospin preparation of urothelial cells.
- Staining and rinsing with Perl's reagent (Prussian blue) is performed on the glass slides.
- Examine under oil-immersion lens of microscope.
- Haemosiderin stains as blue dots within urothelial cells.
- Ignore all excess stain, staining outside cells or in debris all of which are common.
- True +ve is only when clear detection within urothelial squames is seen.

Cautions

An Fe-staining +ve control sample should be run alongside test cases to ensure stain has worked satisfactorily. Haemosiderinuria may not be detected for up to 72h after the initial onset of intravascular haemolysis so the test may miss haemolysis of very recent onset—repeat test in 3–7d if –ve. Conversely, haemosiderinuria may persist for some time after a haemolytic process has stopped. Repeat in 7d should confirm.

Causes

Table 16.1 Causes of haemosiderinuria

Common causes	• Red cell enzymopathies e.g. G6PD and PK deficiency but only during haemolytic episodes • Mycoplasma pneumonia with anti-I cold haemag-glutinin • Sepsis • Malaria • Cold haemagglutinin disease TTP/HUS • Severe extravascular haemolysis (may cause intravascular haemolysis)
Rarer causes	• PNH • Prosthetic heart valves • Red cell incompatible transfusion reactions • Unstable haemoglobins • March haemoglobinuria

Ham's test

Usage

Diagnostic test for paroxysmal nocturnal haemoglobinuria (PNH). Now replaced by immunophenotyping methods.

Principle

- Abnormal sensitivity of RBCs from patients with PNH to the haemolytic action of complement.
- Complement is activated by acidification of patient's serum to pH of 6.2 which induces lysis of PNH red cells but not ↔ controls.

Specificity: high—similar reaction is produced only in the rare syndrome HEMPAS (a form of congenital dyserythropoietic anaemia type II) which should be easily distinguished morphologically.

Sensitivity: low—as the reaction is crucially dependent on the concentration of magnesium in the serum.

It appears to be a technically difficult test in most laboratories. Patients with only a low % of PNH cells may be missed at an early stage of the disease. Markedly abnormal PNH cells are usually picked up in ~75% of patients. Less abnormal cells are detected in only ~25% of patients.

Alternative tests

- Sucrose lysis—an alternative method of complement activation is by mixing serum with a low ionic strength solution such as sucrose.
  - *Sensitivity* of this test is high but *specificity* is low—i.e. the opposite of Ham's test.
- Immunophenotypic detection of the deficiency of the PIG transmembrane protein anchors in PNH cells is becoming a more widely used alternative cf. PNH section. Monoclonal antibodies to CD59 or CD55 (DAF) are used in flow cytometric analysis. Major advantage is that test can be performed on neutrophils and platelets in PB which are more numerous than the PNH red cells.

Immunophenotyping

Definition

Identification of cell surface proteins by reactivity with monoclonal antibodies of known specificity.

Uses

- Aids diagnosis and classification of haematological malignancy. Assess cellular clonality.
- Identify prognostic groups.
- Monitor minimal residual disease (MRD).

Terminology and methodology

Cell surface proteins are denoted according to their cluster differentiation (CD) number. These are allocated after international workshops define individual cell surface proteins by reactivity to monoclonal antibodies. Most cells will express many such proteins and pattern of expression allows cellular characterization.

Monoclonal antibodies (MoAbs)

MoAbs are derived from single B-lymphocyte cell lines and have identical antigen binding domains known as **idiotypes**. It is easy to generate large quantities of MoAbs for diagnostic use.

- Cell populations from, e.g., PB or BM samples are incubated with a panel of MoAbs e.g. anti-CD4, anti-CD34 which are directly or indirectly bound to a fluorescent marker antibody e.g. FITC.
- Sample is passed through a fluorescence-activated cell sorter (FACS) machine.
- FACS instruments assign cells to a graphical plot by virtue of cell size and granularity detected as forward and side light scatter by the laser.
- Allows subpopulations of cells e.g. mononuclear cells in blood sample to be selected.
- The reactivity of this cell subpopulation to the MoAb panel can then be determined by fluorescence for each MoAb.
- A typical result for a CD4 T-lymphocyte population is shown: CD3, CD4 +ve; CD8, CD13, CD34, CD19 –ve.

Common diagnostic profiles 📖 pp.124, 158 and 159

- **AML** CD13+, CD33+, ± CD 34, ± CD14 +ve
- **cALL** CD10 and TdT +ve
- **T-ALL** CD3, CD7, TdT +ve.
- **B-ALL** CD10, CD19, surface Ig +ve
- **CLL** CD5, CD19, CD23, weak surface Ig +ve

Clonality assessment

Particularly useful in determining whether there is a monoclonal B cell or plasma cell population.

- ► Monoclonal B cells from e.g. NHL will have surface expression of κ ***or*** λ light chains ***but not both***.
- ► Polyclonal B cells from e.g. patient with infectious mononucleosis will have both κ ***and*** λ expression.

Cytogenetics

Acquired somatic chromosomal abnormalities are common in haematological malignancies. Determination of patterns of cytogenetic abnormali-ties is known as karyotyping. 📖 See Table 10.2 for examples.

Uses

- Aid diagnosis and classification of haematological malignancy.
- Assess clonality.
- Identify prognostic groups.
- Monitor MRD.
- Determine engraftment and chimerism post-allogeneic transplant.

Terminology

- Normal somatic cell has 46 chromosomes; 22 pairs plus XX or XY.
- Numbered 1–22 in decreasing size order.
- 2 arms meet at centromere —short arm denoted **p**, long arm denoted **q**.
- Usually only visible during condensation at metaphase.
- Stimulants and cell culture used —colchicine to arrest cells in metaphase.
- Stained to identify regions and bands e.g. p1, q3.

Common abnormalities

- Whole chromosome gain e.g. trisomy 8 (+8).
- Whole chromosome loss e.g. monosomy 7 (–7).
- Partial gain e.g. 9q+ or partial loss e.g. 5q– .
- Translocation—material repositioned to another chromosome; usually reciprocal e.g. t(9;22)—the Philadelphia (Ph) translocation.
- Inversion—part of chromosome runs in opposite direction e.g. inv(16) in M4Eo.
- Many translocations involve point mutations known as oncogenes, e.g. *BCR*, *ras*, *myc*, *bcl-2*.

Molecular cytogenetics

- Molecular revolution is further refining the specific abnormalities in the genesis of haematological malignancies.
- Techniques such as FISH and PCR can detect tiny amounts of abnormal genes.
- BCR-ABL probes are now used in diagnosis and monitoring of treat-ment response in CML.
- IgH and T-cell receptor (TCR) genes are useful in determining clonality of suspected B and T cell tumours respectively.
- Specific probes may be used in diagnosis and monitoring of subtypes of AML e.g. PML-RARA in AML M3.

Table 16.2 Common karyotypic abnormalities

CML	
t(9;22)	Ph chromosome translocation creates *BCR-ABL*
AML	
t(8;21)	AML M2, involves *AML-ETO* genes—has better prognosis.
t(15;17)	AML M3 involves *PML-RARA* genes—has better prognosis.
inv(16)	AML M4Eo—has better prognosis.
–5, –7	Complex abnormalities have poor prognosis.
MDS	
–7, +8, +11	Poor prognosis.
5q– syndrome	Associated with refractory anaemia and better prognosis.
MPD	
20q– and +8	Common associations.
ALL	
t(9;22)	Ph translocation, poor prognosis.
t(4;11)	Poor prognosis.
Hyperdiploidy	↑ total chromosome number—good prognosis.
Hypodiploidy	↓ total chromosome number—bad prognosis.
T-ALL	
t(1;14)	Involves *tal-1* oncogene.
t(8;14)	
B-ALL and Burkitt's lymphoma	
t(8;14)	Involves *myc* and IgH genes, poor prognosis.
CLL	
+12, t(11;14)	
ATLL	
14q11	
NHL	
t(14;18)	Follicular lymphoma, involves *bcl-2* oncogene.
t(11;14)	Small cell lymphocytic lymphoma, involves *bcl-1* oncogene.
t(8;14)	Burkitt's lymphoma, involves *myc* and IgH genes.

Human leucocyte antigen (HLA) typing

HLA system major histocompatibility complex (MHC) is the name given to the highly polymorphic gene cluster region on human chromosome 6 which codes for cell surface proteins involved in immune recognition.

Box 16.1 The gene complex is subdivided into 2 regions

Class 1	The A, B, and C loci. These proteins are found on most nucleated cells and interact with CD8+ T lymphocytes.
Class 2	Comprising of DR, DP, DQ loci present only on B lymphocytes, monocytes, macrophages and activated T lymphocytes. Interact with CD4+ T lymphocytes.

- Class 1 and 2 genes are closely linked so one set of gene loci is usually inherited from each parent though there is a small amount of crossover.
- There is ~1:4 chance of 2 siblings being HLA identical.
- There are other histocompatibility loci apart from the HLA system but these appear less important generally except during HLA matched SCT when even differences in these minor systems may cause GvHD.

Typing methods

Class 1 and 2 antigens were originally defined by serological reactivity with maternal antisera containing pregnancy-induced HLA antibodies. Many problems with technique and too insensitive to detect many polymorphisms. Molecular techniques are increasingly employed such as SSP. Molecular characterization is detecting vast class 2 polymorphism.

Importance of HLA typing

- Matching donor/recipient pairs for renal, cardiac, and marrow SCT.
- Degree of matching more critical for stem cell than solid organ trans-plants.
- Sibling HLA matched STC is now treatment of choice for many malignancies.
- Unrelated donor SCTs are increasingly performed but outcome is poorer due to HLA disparity. As molecular matching advances, improved accuracy will enable closer matches to be found and results should improve.
- Functional tests of donor/recipient compatibility.
- Mixed lymphocyte culture (MLC)—now rarely used.
- Cytotoxic T lymphocyte precursor assays (CTLp)—determine the frequency of CTLs in the donor directed against the recipient—provides an assessment of GvHD occurring.

HLA related transfusion issues

- HLA on WBC and platelets may cause immunization in recipients of blood and platelet transfusions.

- May cause refractoriness and/or febrile reactions to platelet transfusions.
- WBC depletion of products by filtration prevents this.
- Diagnosis of refractoriness confirmed by detection of HLA or platelet specific antibodies in patient's serum.
- Platelet transfusions matched to recipient HLA type may improve increments.

Chapter 17

Blood transfusion

Introduction

During the last 10 years transfusion-medicine has changed dramatically There is an increasing awareness of the risks involved with transfusior of blood components. It has become apparent that lower thresholds o transfusion provide equal or even improve outcomes for patients. More and more guidelines are available that help guide transfusion practice Use of transfusion guidelines has proven to improve safety of transfusior practice as well as decrease the use of blood products. There are limitec resources, as well as a rising demand for specific blood products and ar ever more lowering numbers of donors.

If there is any doubt about the use or appropriateness of blood components for individual patients contact the haematology team or blooc transfusion laboratory or *National Blood Service* for advice.

Using the blood transfusion laboratory

Requests for group & save (blood-grouping) or cross-matching (compatibility testing)

Transfusion samples are taken in an EDTA bottle (6mL) and must b signed by the person taking the sample thus vouching for the identity the patient. Both sample and request form must be clearly, legibly identi fied with 3 points of identification for the patient: ***name, date of birt*** and ***hospital number***. In emergencies where the identity and date of bir of the patient are not known, emergency numbers and wristbands can b used.

- In case of any discrepancies between sampling and request form the sample will be discarded.
- Clinical information including the indication for transfusion or time an date of surgery must be given.
- For major elective surgery where the need for transfusion is likely, the transfusion laboratory should receive a group & save sample 7d prior to surgery so appropriate blood can be made available (see MSBO p.782).
- In haemorrhagic emergencies, ABO Rh (D) group compatible blood ca be given without crossmatching as in these circumstances the risks are outweighed by the immediate risk of death from exsanguination. These situations will be very rare as initial clinical stabilization of the bleeding hypovolaemic patient will be by means of plasma-expanders, giving the transfusion laboratory time to perform an emergency crossmatch, which can be done in 15min.
- Unmatched O Rh (D) –ve blood should only be used in extreme emergencies. Rh (D) –ve blood should in case of an emergency, only be reserved for women of childbearing age.
- Electronic issuing of blood units has greatly improved the speed at which blood products are made available. Downside is that historical records for the patients are necessary.

Issue and administration of blood and blood products

Strictly laid down hospital protocols must be followed for administratio of blood and blood products. *Errors carry the potential for major morbidi or fatality.*

1. The prescription of blood must be made by a registered medical prac titioner and details of the product's administration must be recorded i the case record.
2. Units of blood are matched for an individual patient and are labelle accordingly. They must be collected from the transfusion laborator with a blood collection slip and taken to the clinical area where the will be used.
3. Before administering the recipient's identity must be checked. Labe details are rechecked by trained nursing staff at the bedside immediatel prior to the transfusion. Any discrepancies identified must be referre urgently to the blood bank and the clinician responsible for the patien Transfusion cannot proceed until any ambiguity about identity has bee resolved.

4. Blood products must be given within its expiry date.
5. Always check for damage to the pack, discoloration, or any other visible abnormality.
6. Administration of the unit must commence within 30min after leaving the blood bank and be completed within 4h of commencing infusion.
7. Administration of blood products must be recorded in the case notes as well as documented on a special blood transfusion chart (usually part of the IV fluid chart). The number of blood units or blood products given should be entered in the notes.
8. If given warm, ensure a safe approved warming procedure is used.
9. No drug or other infusion solution should be added to any blood component.
10. Blood can only be stored in specially designated, monitored refrigerators.
11. Platelets should be used immediately and can not be kept on the ward.
12. For safety reasons each unit transfused must have a 'papertrail'. Regular audits are mandatory.

Transfusion of red blood cells

Transfusion of red cells should be avoided if possible. Haematinic def ciency should be treated with replacement therapy rather then with tran fusion. Only if clinically indicated should a transfusion be given (i.e. cardia history or complaints, lung disease). An initial 2-unit transfusion shoul suffice.

As a general rule, most otherwise fit adults tolerate Hb levels of 8–1 g/dL without major problems. There is no universal transfusion trigge Comorbidities may determine a higher transfusion trigger. Transfusion ca precipitate severe cardiac failure.

Medication that interferes with platelet function or has a coagulation effe should be stopped prior to surgery to avoid unnecessary bloodloss. Th of course should be done in a safe manner with possibly continuation anticoagulation with unfractionated heparin or preferably LMWH.

Autologous blood transfusion, acute normovolaemic haemodilutio (ANH) and cell salvage during surgery can play a role in avoiding unnece sary or unwanted transfusions.

- Red cells have a shelf life of 35d at 4°C and are supplied as concentrated red cells with a PCV between 0.55 and 0.75. Most units in the UK are supplied in 'optimal additive solution', SAG-M*, which allows removal of all the plasma for preparation of other blood components and results in a less viscous product. The volume of a unit of concentrated cells is 280 ± 20mL.
- Acute blood loss should initially be stabilized by giving the hypovolaemic haemorrhagic patient plasma-expanders. Only use uncrossmatched in true emergencies. If RBC transfusion is required it can infused at the same time as other colloids.
- All blood in UK is leucodepleted at source since 1999.
- Irradiated RBCs are indicated in certain circumstances to stop transfusion transmitted graft versus host disease. Blood products are irradiated at 2500 cGy.
- CMV –ve blood products are indicated in certain circumstances. Cytomegalovirus is an important cause of morbidity and mortality following BMT/PBSC transplant and is important in premature neonates. 📖 See Table 17.1.
- Frozen RBCs are available in a few NBS centres around the country. They are expensive to process, store, and handle; they must be used within 24h after thawing. Clinical usage is restricted to patients with extremely rare blood groups or with highly problematic blood group allo-antibodies.
- In autoimmune haemolytic disorders transfusion can be lifesaving as a short term support pending response to immunosuppression.

Table 17.1 Indications for red cell transfusion

Blood loss	Massive/acute
Bone marrow failure	• Post-chemotherapy, leukaemias, etc. • Supportive therapy with concentrated cells
Inherited RBC disorders	• Homozygous β-thalassaemia • Red cell aplasia, etc. • Hb SS (some circumstances)
Acquired RBC disorders	• Myelofibrosis • Myelodysplasia • Some chronic disorder anaemias • Selected use in renal failure
Neonatal & and exchange transfusions	• Haemolytic disease of the newborn • Meningococcal septicaemia • Falciparum malaria

Monitoring

- Monitoring of the patient involves recording temperature, pulse, O_2-saturation and BP before transfusion, every 15 min for the first hour and hourly until transfusion is finished.
- Adverse events should be meticulously recorded.
- Major reactions require immediate cessation of the transfusion and instigation of a full investigative protocol (📖 see Transfusion reactions, p.634).
- Minor febrile reactions are not uncommon. Review by a registered medical practitioner is advised. Their occurrence should be recorded, simple measures such as slowing the rate of infusion or administration of an antihistamine may deal with the problem; if not, transfusion of the specific unit should be stopped.
- An RBC pack should be given within 30min of removal from the blood bank fridge.
- The target infusion time for an individual unit should be 4h.

Platelet transfusion

Platelets are giving to prevent or treat bleeding associated with thrombocytopaenia. They may also be given as prophylaxis against bleeding e.g. in patients undergoing intensive chemotherapy (📖 see Table 17.2). Platelets may be required to cover surgery and dentistry. Platelets have a shelf life of 5d. Irradiated or 'washed' platelets should be transfused within 24h.

Table 17.2 Indications for platelet transfusion

↓ production due to BM failure/ infiltration	• Acute and chronic leukaemias • Myelodysplasia • Myeloproliferative disorders and myelofibrosis • Marrow infiltration with other malignant tumours • Post-chemotherapy or TBI • Aplastic anaemia
↑ platelet destructionin peripheral circulation	• Hypersplenism 2° splenic infiltration or portal hypertension • Consumptive coagulopathies e.g. DIC • Avoid in TTP (📖 p.656) • Acute and chronic ITP (in emergencies only) • Alloimmune thrombocytopenias e.g. PTP and perinatal thrombocytopenia (need to be HPA typed) • Sepsis • Drug induced
Platelet function abnormalities	• Aspirin and NSAIDs • Myelodysplasia • Rare congenital disorders e.g. Bernard–Soulier
Dilutional	Massive blood transfusion—in practice not usually required unless some other haemostatic abnormality (e.g. consumption)
Cardiac bypass	Dilution and damage to platelets in extracorporeal circulation.

- Guidelines state a general threshold for procedures with regards to a patient's platelet count. A platelet count of $\geq 50 \times 10^9$/L is sufficient for minor surgery and procedures such as lumbar punctures, biopsies (including liver biopsy), insertion and removal of central lines.
- For major surgery as well as neurosurgery and eye surgery a platelet count of $\geq 100 \times 10^9$/L is recommended.
- Patients can tolerate low platelet counts very well and platelets should not be given if the patient is well with no signs of bleeding and a platelet count $>10 \times 10^9$/L.

- In certain conditions, such as MDS or ITP even platelet counts in single figures are acceptable as long as there are no clinical signs of bleeding.
- Where there is high consumption of platelets, i.e. bleeding, infection, or DIC, multiple repeated doses of platelets might be needed to achieve haemostasis.
- Even in immune-causes of thrombocytopaenia where routinely platelet transfusions are not indicated, platelet transfusions should be given in the acute event of a life-threatening bleed to try and achieve haemostasis.
- Platelet refractoriness is defined as failure to increment more than 10×10^9/L after 2 separate transfusions of random platelets. Very important to follow-up further transfusions with increments so the diagnosis can be confirmed and management optimized.
- Both immune and non-immune causes should be considered.
  - *Non-immune*: old low dose platelets, high consumption (DIC, bleeding), hepatosplenomegaly, drug-induced (amphotericin B, AmBisome®, vancomycin, heparin, and others).
  - *Immune*: class-I HLA antibodies or HPA-antibodies. HLA-matched should be given if HLA antibodies are suspected.
- Platelets are all leukodepleted at source since 1999.
- Group ABO matched platelets are preferred but not necessary. Do not give Group O platelets to group A, B, or AB patients, unless they have been tested –ve for high titre antibodies (HTO).
- Indications for irradiated and CMV –ve products are the same as for red cell transfusions.
- Currently under consideration is a bacterial screening and pathogen inactivation process/system which could increase the shelf life for platelets from 5 to 7d.
- 'Washed platelets': platelets in additive solution (plasma extracted and additive added). They only have a 24-h shelf life, but carry less risk of TRALI and a theoretical lower risk of vCJD transmission.

Fresh frozen plasma (FFP)

Plasma is prepared from donor red cell units within 8h of donation, snap frozen at –80°C, and maintained deep frozen until use. It has a shelf life of 2 years if frozen. FFP is ABO grouped. Rh (D) grouping is not needed. Irradiation is not required.

Table 17.3

Factor	II	VII	IX	X
Range (U/dL)	53–121	41–140	32–102	61–150
Median	82.5	92.0	61.0	90.5

Indications for use

- Warfarin overdose (see p.650).
- DIC (see p.642).
- Liver disease and biopsy. Routinely done but not evidence based.
- Massive blood transfusion. The use of FFP in these patients is not
- supported by documented clinical benefit. Generally it is accepted that after ≥1.5 total blood volume loss coagulation factor deficiency can be anticipated. FFP should be give as dictated by coagulation tests (PT ≥1.5 × the ↔ value). FFP is one of the components of the massive transfusion packs available from the transfusion laboratory in these cases.
- Isolated coagulation deficiencies where no specific concentrate is readily available.
- Treatment of thrombotic thrombocytopenia purpura/haemolytic uraemic syndrome (TTP/HUS) (see pp.534–536).
- Non-specific haemostatic failure in a bleeding patient, e.g. following surgery, in intensive care with disturbed coagulation tests where no definite diagnosis is made.

Contra-indications for use

- Hypovolaemic shock. Never use FFP as a plasma-expander!
- Plasma-exchange, except in TTP/HUS.

Instructions for use

- The average volume of 1U is 220–250mL.
- Defrost the bag in a water-bath (5min) or at room temperature (20min).
- FFP must be given as soon as possible and at least within an hour of thawing through a filter needle.
- Dose 10–15 ml/kg body weight.
- Usual starting dose in an adult = 2–4U depending on the PT.
- Check PT and APTT before and 5min after infusion to assess response.
- Response is monitored with the clinical response in a bleeding patient. FFP has a short half life (see table 17.4) and might have to be repeated.

Table 17.4 Half-life of infused coagulation factors in FFP

<12h	Factors V, VII, VIII, and protein C
>12 <24h	Factor IX and protein S
>24 <48h	Factor X
>48h	Fibrinogen, factors XI, XII, XIII, ATIII

What to give

- FFP ideally should be ABO group specific, but this is not essential. Group O FFP should only be given to Group O patients, due to the presence of high-titre antibodies.
- FFP in the UK is collected from ♂ donors and ♀ donors without previous pregnancies or transfusions (less risk of high titre antibodies).
- Only FFP from known donors is used (not from 1st time or lapsed donors).
- Everyone <16 years old receives FFP from ♂ volunteer USA donors and treated with methylene blue (MB-FFP). This is to reduce the risk of transmission of vCJD.
- Methylene blue is a form of pathogen inactivation.
- Octaplas: FFP treated with solvent detergent (SD-FFP). It virally inactivated FFP (only lipid coated viruses, so not parvovirus B19 and HAV). Octaplas as FFP, is ABO matched (not Rh (D)). There is a slight pro-thrombotic risk due to 50% loss of protein S.

1. Makris, M. *et al.* (1997). Emergency oral anticoagulant reversal: the relative efficacy of infusions of fresh frozen plasma and clotting factor concentrates on correction of coagulopathy. *Thrombosis Haemostasis*, **77**, 477–80.

Cryoprecipitate

Cryoprecipitate is prepared by slow thawing of FFP at 4–6°C. The precipitate formed is cryoprecipitate which is then stored at −30°C. It is rich in factors VIII, XIII, fibrinogen and von Willebrand's factor.

Per unit (bag):
- Factor VIII and vWF ~ 80–100IU.
- Fibrinogen ~ 250mg.
- Factor XIII and fibronectin.
- Does not contain other coagulation factors.
- May contain anti-A and anti-B blood group antibodies.

Indications for use

- Additional support for the clotting defects induced by massive transfusion. Hypofibrinogenaemia can be anticipated if there has been ≥1 TBV bloodloss
- DIC with fibrinogen <1g/dL.
- Hypo/dysfibrinogenaemia in liver disease/transplant to prevent and treat bleeding.
- Haemophilia A and vWD: not treatment of choice where virally inactivated concentrates are available. May still have a role in acquired vWD when purified factor VIII products are ineffective.
- Congenital dys/hypofibrinogenaemia.

Contra-indications

- Should never be given for plasma-expansion
- Cryoprecipitate should not be given if the fibrinogen is >1g/L
- Of no proven value as empirical treatment in post-op or uraemic bleeding.

Instructions for use

- Keep frozen until required.
- Thaw at room temperature (takes 5–10min). FFP must be used immediately
- ABO compatibility not required.
- Given through filter needle.
- Dose 1U per 5–10kg body weight (regular adult dose is 10U or 2 pools)
- 1 pool = 5 units of cryoprecipitate.
- Aim to keep fibrinogen >1g/L.

Intravenous immunoglobulin (IVIg)

IVIg is used as antibody replacement in 1° and 2° antibody deficiency state and as immune modulator (📖 see Table 17.5).

Preparations of IVIg

- Contain predominantly IgG (with small amounts of IgA and IgM).
- Prepared from large pool of normal donors e.g. >1000.
- Contain all subclasses of IgG encountered in normal population.
- In view of the risk of vCJD non-UK plasma is used for fractionation.

Mechanisms of action

The mechanism of action is not fully understood: natural anti-idiotypi antibodies suppress antibody production in patient; Fc receptor blockad on macrophages (thereby blocking RE function) and T/B lymphocyte (inhibits autoantibody production); suppression of production of inflam matory mediators (e.g. TNF-α, IL-1) produced by macrophages.

Administration

Usual dose 0.4g/kg/d for 5d or 1 g/kg/d for 2d for 1° immune-deficienc or immune-modulation or 0.2–0.4 g/d monthly for 2° immune deficienc (CLL, myeloma, etc).

Check the patient's observations pre-infusion. With the 1st infusio patient should be monitored closely and observations taken ½ hourly fo the first hour. Side effects are more likely at the start of an infusion and i the 1st hour. (📖 see pack insert and BNF for details).

Complications

- Fevers, chills.
- Backache.
- Myalgic symptoms.
- Flushing.
- Nausea ± vomiting.
- Severe allergic reactions in IgA-deficient patients (due to small amount of IgA in IVIg preparation).

Note: Department of Health Guidelines are being developed to promot good IVIg prescribing practice across all specialties that use IVIg. Thes guidelines have been written in response to the world shortage of IVI since it was felt that many patients were receiving IVIg where little evi dence exists for its beneficial effect.

Table 17.5 Uses for IVIg

Antibody replacement	
• 1° immune deficiency • Transient hypogammaglobulinaemia of infancy • Common variable immune deficiency • Sex-linked hypogammaglobulinaemia • Late-onset hypogammaglobulinaemia • Hypogammaglobulinaemia + thymoma	• 2° immune deficiency • CLL • Non-Hodgkin's lymphoma • Multiple myeloma • Post-BMT
Immune modulation	
• Autoimmune diseases • ITP • Autoimmune haemolytic anaemia • Autoimmune neutropenia • Red cell aplasia • Coagulation factor inhibitors • Post-transfusion purpura (PTP) • Neonatal platelet alloimmunization • Thrombocytopenia in pregnancy	• Prophylaxis/treatment of CMV in BMT patients • B19-induced red cell aplasia • Haemophagocytic syndromes (viral)

Data from Department of Health, *Clinical guidelines for immunoglobulin use (second edition)*, June, 2008.

Transfusion transmitted infections (TTI)

There is an increasing awareness of the risks involved with transfusion of blood-components (Table 17.6). Blood components can transmit infections. Screening of donations is mandatory. Every sample is routinely checked for syphilis, HBV, HIV, HCV, and HTLV. Tests have been added throughout the years depending on new discoveries and developments. Although the risk of a TTI is small, recipients should be informed about the possibility. The risk of a bacterial infection through platelet transfusion is the greatest and it is likely that in the (near) future routine screening will become a reality.

- The introduction of nucleic acid testing (NAT) for HIV and HCV has significantly reduced the window-periods for infections in donors. The window period for HCV with NAT is 9d, and 3–4d for HIV.
- The transfusion risk for HTLV is currently unknown. Up to 5% of patients infected with HTLV-1 develop ATLL. Endemic regions are the Caribbean, South America, Central Africa, and Japan.
- CMV testing in selected donors. Relevant to recipient.
- Variant Creutzfeldt–Jacob disease (vCJD) has been proven to be transmissible through blood transfusion. No screening method is available.

Bacterial infections

There are approximately 4 cases of transfusion-related bacterial infections per year in the UK with a mortality of 50%. They constitute approximately 11% of fatal transfusion reactions. The greatest risk is with pooled platelets, followed by apheresis platelets, and red cells. Visual inspection of the unit to be transfused is very important.

- Platelets are kept at room-temperature and pose the greatest risk. The shelf life for platelets is 5d. Platelet screening for infection at days 1 and 2 can increase the shelf life to 7d, but is currently not routinely done.
- Source: donors arm, silent bacteraemia in donor (recent dental treatment, infectious diarrhoea, chronic infections) or due to collection system or storage.
- Staphylococci (*Staph. epidermidis* and *Staph. aureus*), *Bacillus cereus*, *Clostridium perfringens*, *P. aeruginosa*, *Yersinia*, *Serratia*, *Salmonella*, and others.
- The collection equipment is a closed system to reduce infection risk.
- Clinically: fever, flushing, rigors, DIC, ARDS, shock.

Transmissible spongiform encephalopathies (TSE)

TSEs are prion diseases. Bovine spongiform encephalopathy (BSE) first diagnosed in cattle in the UK cattle in 1986. Ongoing epizoonosis amplified by feeding bovine offal and bone meal to cattle. An official specified offal ban has eradicated BSE with no new cases in cattle born since 1999 (last case in 1998).

- vCJD is the human form of BSE, initially transmitted from cows to humans through eating beef.
- Clinically: depression, anxiety, burning sensations on trunks and legs. vCJD has a median survival of 14 months
- The 4th case of transfusion transmitted vCJD in the UK was confirmed in January 2007.

Transmissible agent unknown. Various precautions for reducing vCJD transmission have been taken (see Table 17.7)
No testing available.

Table 17.6 Risks of transfusion-transmitted infections

TTI	Testing introduced	Risk
Syphilis	1940	Virtually absent due to antibody testing
HBV	1970	1 per 600.000 transfusions
HIV	1985	1 per 5.000.000 transfusions
HCV	1990	1 per 32.000.000 transfusions
HTLV	2002	Unknown
Bacterial infection—platelets	Future?	1 per 90.000 transfusions
Bacterial infection—red cells	Future?	1 per 5.000.000 transfusions

Table 17.7 Precautions for reducing vCJD transmission

- Exclusion of blood donors:
  - On pituitary hormones now or in the past
  - Neurosurgery or cataract surgery
  - Relatives with CJD (familial CJD)
  - Previous transfusion
  - Donors to vCJD cases
- Leukocyte depletion (since 1999)
- Plasma depletion ('washed' platelets and blood in SAGM)
- Non-UK plasma for fractionation
- Recombinant factors

TRALI and TA-GVHD

Transfusion related acute lung injury (TRALI)

TRALI is defined as acute dyspnoea and hypoxia with bilateral lung-infiltrates on chest X-ray within 24h of having a transfusion. The clinical picture is ARDS-like with raised temperature and hypotension.

- 1 per 5000 transfusions.
- 5–10% fatal.
- Mainly caused by HLA- or HNA-antibodies in transfused blood product (80%) or by biologically active lipids in stored blood products.
- Pooled platelets >FFP >red cells.
- Treatment is supportive with ventilatory support. Usually improves within 48–96 hours.
- 2-hit hypothesis:
  - → HLA/HNA antibodies or biologically active lipids in transfused products ***and***
  - → Predisposing clinical condition with ↑ levels of cytokines: ongoing infection, surgery (CABG), malignancy.
- Prevention: pheresis platelets from ♂ donors.

Transfusion associated GVHD (TA-GVHD)

Donor T lymphocytes in blood products engraft and clonally expand in the recipient. Activated donor lymphocytes produce cytokines, and cause general inflammation and tissue damage.

- Very rare.
- Related to the number of lymphocytes in donor blood products. Greatly reduced with lymphocyte depletion.
- High risk patients: defective inherited or acquired recipient cell mediated immunity, HLA matched transfusions or transfusions from relatives, transplant patients, patients who had purine analogues.
- Symptoms within 2–30d: fever, skin rash, diarrhoea, hepatitis, pancytopenia.
- 90% mortality.
- Prevention: leukocyte depleted, irradiated blood products (HLA matched products should ALWAYS be irradiated).

TA-GVHD is invariably fatal. Patients who are considered to be at risk of developing this condition as a result of exposure to donor T lymphocytes must receive irradiated blood products.

Irradiated and CMV-negative blood products

In an emergency and where CMV-–ve or irradiated blood components are not available, transfusion of leukodepleted components is acceptable if transfusion outweighs the associated risks.

Table 17.8 Indications for irradiated blood-products

Allogeneic and autologous BMT or PBSC recipients from 1 month before pre-transplant conditioning until at least 6 months post transplant
Allogeneic BM and stem cell donors
Hodgkin's disease
Those who have received purine analogue drugs (fludarabine, cladribine, 2-deoxycoformycin)
All donations from HLA matched donors or 1st or 2nd-degree relatives
Children with congenital immunodeficiency states
Intra-uterine transfusions and transfusions for infants who have had intra-uterine transfusions
Exchange transfusions in neonates

Table 17.9 Indications for CMV–ve blood-products

All newly diagnosed leukaemic and aplastic patients until CMV status known
Allogeneic BM and stem cell donors
Solid organ transplant recipients who are CMV-–ve
All CMV –ve patients who may proceed to BMT/PBSCT
CMV –ve allogeneic BMT or PBSCT recipients, even if the donor is CMV positive
CMV –ve BMT/PBSCT donors given allogeneic blood
CMV –ve haemoglobinopathy patients who may come to transplant.
CMV –ve autograft recipients of CD34+ stem cells from time of harvest
Premature and low birth weight babies (<1500g)
Neonatal exchange transfusion and infants <1 year old
CMV –ve patients with HIV infection
GvHD
1° immunodeficiency syndromes

Autologous blood transfusion

Allows patient to be transfused with his/her own red cells, avoiding (some problems associated with transfusion of allogeneic blood, such as immu nological incompatibility, risks of transmission of infection, and transfusior reactions. It is useful for patients who do not wish to receive allogenei blood or who have irregular antibodies that make cross-matching difficult

Pre-deposit system

Involves collection of 2–4U of blood: the first unit is collected ~2 week before the operation and the second is taken 7–10d prior to surgery. Fe replacement is usually given. Some pre-deposit programmes use EPC (enables a larger number of units to be collected, but is very expensive and not licensed).

Advantages

- Can store RBCs up to 5 weeks at 4°C.
- May donate 2–4U pre-op.
- Avoids many problems associated with allogeneic blood transfusion.

Disadvantages

- Generally requires Hb ≥11.0g/dL. Patients must be 'fit' for pre-donation programme and live near transfusion centre.
- Requires close coordination between surgeon, patient, and transfusion lab as well as a fixed date for surgery.
- Little/no reduction in workload. Blood must be treated in the same way as regular donor units (including microbiological screening, grouping, compatibility testing, etc).
- Cost is high.
- Transfusion should be to donor only.
- Bacterial contamination of blood units may still occur.
- Patient may still require additional allogeneic units.
- Blood may be wasted if operation cancelled.
- Patients with epilepsy excluded (risk of seizures).

Intra-operative blood salvage

Allows blood lost during surgery to be re-infused into patients using suction catheters and filtration systems. Its use is increasing in the UK Intra-operative blood salvage is useful in orthopaedic and cardiovascular surgery, but may be used for almost any surgical procedure (provided no faecal contamination or risk of tumour dissemination).

- Single-use disposable canisters (e.g. Solcotrans™). The patient is heparinized and anticoagulated blood is collected into ACD anticoagulant in the canister. Red cells are re-infused after filtration through a microaggregate filter.
- Automated or semi-automated salvage (e.g. Hemonetics Cell Saver™). Blood is collected, washed centrifugally, filtered, and red cells held for reinfusion.
- Labour intensive.

Pre-operative haemodilution

Involves reducing the Hb concentration prior to surgery. This reduces blood viscosity and red cell loss (through reduced haematocrit). It provides a bank of freshly collected autologous whole blood for return later.

- 2–3U of blood are collected with replacement using crystalloids or colloid solutions.
- Hb is reduced to ~10g/dL and haematocrit to 30% (0.3).
- O_2 transport improves (↑ cardiac output).
- Used mainly in younger patients and in those with no pre-existing cardiopulmonary disease.

Pharmacological methods of blood saving

- Any anticoagulation or anti-platelet drugs should be stopped prior to surgery to reduce the risk of bleeding.
- Desmopressin
- Platelet inhibitory drugs e.g. epoprosterol
- Aprotinin. Widely used in cardiovascular surgery, liver transplantation, and other surgical procedures.

Maximum surgical blood ordering schedule (MSBOS)

A system of tailoring blood requirements to particular elective surgical procedures, including—importantly—procedures which do not usually require blood cover.

- The ABO group and Rh (D) type of the patient is determined on duplicate samples, and the serum screened for significant RBC ('atypical') antibodies. If there are no antibodies, the serum is kept available ('saved') for a determined period (usually a week)—this is the 'Group, Screen, and Save' (G&S) procedure.
- If there are no atypical antibodies, and the planned surgery is likely to need peri-operative transfusion, the required number of red cell units are matched by routine tests, labeled, and set aside in an accessible refrigerator. Storage conditions must meet certain standards (continuous recording of appropriate temperature, alarms, etc.).
- If more blood is required than anticipated, extra units must be readily available. If the need is urgent, suitable arrangements—such as rapid matching (using the 'saved' serum) and despatch procedures—must enable the timely supply of blood.
- If there are atypical antibodies, which may occur in up to 10% patients, their specificity must be determined and, if clinically significant, sufficient (extra) red cell units lacking the relevant antigen provided and matched by detailed techniques. (These are often referred to as 'phenotyped red cells'.)
- If there is no 'MSBOS' more units must be matched than are usually required for transfusion, in order to give rapid access if extra blood is needed. Matched 'bespoke' blood is therefore unavailable for other patients for the 2–3d set aside.
- A good MSBOS gives better access to blood stocks and enables more efficient use, in particular of O Rh (D) –ve blood. There is no good reason for regarding O Rh (D) –ve blood as a 'universal' donation type. It can be antigenic; and it is a precious resource, being available from <8% of the population.
- The surgical team must be confident in the system, and the blood bank staff committed to 'minimal barriers'. The cross-match:transfusion ratio of a blood bank may well become lower than 2 (i.e. overall <2U matched for every unit transfused) which is an indication of efficient practices. It could even be nearer to 1 than to 2.
- MSBOS schedules will vary between hospitals—depending on demographic factors, general layout, access to the blood bank refrigerators, types of surgery etc.

Jehovah's Witnesses

- Religious sect numbering 120,000 in the UK.
- Pose ethical and management difficulties due to their refusal of blood transfusion, derived from a literal interpretation of a number of biblical passages (*Acts* 15:28–29).
- Jehovah's Witnesses still die during both elective and emergency surgery due to their beliefs.

Elective surgery—discuss

- Risks of surgery and the specific risk of refusing blood.
- Extent of religious belief (preferably alone to prevent any external pressure).
- What blood derived products they personally are willing to accept e.g. albumin, FFP, platelets, etc?

If the surgeon agrees to an operation, communication then becomes paramount and the Jehovah's Witness should be referred to both an anaesthetist and haematologist—preferably when the patient is placed on the waiting list to allow time for any optimization and for further counselling with their family.

Pre-operative considerations

- Timing (e.g. liver transplantation before clotting function deteriorates).
- Autologous blood transfusion—not permitted but may be acceptable to some.
- Morning list—to allow post-op observations during 'office hours'.
- Admission to ITU for invasive monitoring if required.
- Stop anticoagulants and NSAIDs.
- Optimize Hb—nutrition, B_{12}, folate, Fe, EPO.

Operative considerations

Surgeon

- Consultant.
- Positioning of patient—to prevent venous congestion.
- Tourniquets if possible.
- Speed.
- Meticulous haemostasis.

Anaesthetist

- Consultant.
- Regional blocks.
- Hypotensive anaesthesia.
- Hypothermia Isovolaemic haemodilution—permitted as long as blood remains linked to circulation.
- Hypervolaemic haemodilution.
- Intraoperative blood scavenging e.g. cellsavers.
- Blood substitutes (fluorocarbons).
- Pharmacological methods to improve clotting e.g. desmopression, tranexamic acid, aprotinin.

Post-operative considerations

- Observation for re-bleed—HDU, senior surgeon review.
- Optimize Hb—nutrition enteral or parenteral feeding, B_{12}, folate, Fe, EPO.
- Severe anaemia—IPPV to reduce O_2 demand.
- Reduce phlebotomy and use paediatric vials.
- Acid suppression to reduce GIT bleeding.

Emergency surgery

- Advanced directives.
- Early investigations CT, USS abdomen, pelvis.
- Low threshold to theatre.

Children

- Communication with parent.
- Judicial intervention if required.

Marsh, J.C. & Bevan, D.H. (2002). Haematological care of the Jehovah's Witness patient. *Br J Haematol*, **119**, 25–37.

Chapter 18

Phone numbers and addresses

American Society of Hematology

E-mail: ash@hematology.org
www.hematology.org

Birmingham Clinical Trials Unit (BCTU)

For randomization/entry of AML patients into MRC trials

BCTU
Division of Medical Sciences
Robert Aitken Institute
Edgbaston
Birmingham B15 2TT

Tel: 0121 415 9100
Fax: 0121 415 9135/6

E-mail: bctu@contacts.bham.ac.uk
www.bctu.bham.ac.uk

British Society for Haematology

BSH
100 White Lion Street
London N1 9PF

Tel/fax: 0207 713 0990

E-mail: info@b-s-h.org.uk
www.b-s-h.org.uk

CancerBACUP

A major European cancer information and support charity; aims to provide clear, accurate, up-to-date information as well as sensitive and confidential support for patients and their families. Also provides assistance to health care professionals with specific enquiries relating to patients in their care.

CancerBACUP services for patients and their families

- A national freephone cancer information service (tel: 0808 800 1234), staffed by specialist oncology nurses.
- Cancer counselling service offering people the chance to talk through their concerns face-to-face.
- CancerBACUP produces excellent written information e.g. booklets on specific cancers, treatments, and aspects of living with cancer and fact sheets on specific chemotherapy drugs, hormonal therapies, brain tumours, and rare tumours. Available from CancerBACUP's administration.

CancerBACUP services for health professionals

Medical Advisory Committee Statements produced by an expert panel on controversial or complex oncology issues including:

- Clinical trials.
- Cancer screening—cervical, breast, prostate, colorectal, and ovarian cancer.
- Breast cancer, the pill and hormone replacement therapy.
- Information on
- Support groups Sources of help
- Lists of booklets and factsheets.

www.cancerbackup.org.uk

CTSU

For randomization into: CLL4, CLL5, PT1, UKALL XII, and childhood ALL

CTSU
Richard Doll Building
Old Road Campus
Rosevelt Drive
Oxford OX3 7LF

Tel: 01865 743743
Fax: 01865 743985

www.ctsu.ox.ac.uk

European Hematology Association

EHA Office
Westblaak 71
3012 KE Rotterdam
The Netherlands

E-mail: info@ehaweb.org
www.ehaweb.org

Leukaemia Research Fund (LRF)

The LRF is one of the major UK based research charities in the field of leukaemia and related conditions. It supports leukaemia research in major academic institutions; work supported ranges from basic science relating to the molecular genetics of leukaemogenesis to extensive case controlled studies into epidemiology of leukaemia and related disorders.

In addition to funding major research it provides information booklets on a range of (mainly) malignant blood disorders which are suitable for patients, their relatives, and carers and also appropriate for non-specialist professional staff who become involved in specific aspects of the clinical care of the patient with leukaemia or a related disorder.

The stated aim of the fund is to improve treatments, find cures, and prevent all forms of leukaemia and related cancers through a programme of nationally funded, high calibre research activities.

Booklets are available on the acute and chronic leukaemias, lymphomas including Hodgkin's disease, myeloma, and related disorders, myelodysplasia myeloproliferative disorders, and aplastic anaemia. A revised series of booklets was produced in 1997. Availability of such information on the wards or in the clinic is very helpful to patients and their carers.

Leukaemia Rsearch Fund
43 Great Ormond Street
London WC1N 3JJ
Tel: 0207 405 0101
Fax: 0207 405 3139

E-mail: info@lrf.org.uk
www.lrf.org.uk

Medical Research Council

20 Park Crescent
London W1N 4AL
Tel: 0207 636 5422
Fax: 0207 436 6179

E-mail: corporate@headoffice.mrc.ac.uk
www.mrc.ac.uk

National Cancer Research Network

NRCN Coordinating Centre
Arthington House
Cookridge Hospital
Hospital Lane
Leeds LS16 6QB

E-mail: enquiries@ncrn.org.uk
www.ncrn.org.uk

Northern and Yorkshire Clinical Trials and Research Unit

NYCTRU
17 Springfield Mount
University of Leeds
LeedsLS2 9NG

www.ctruleeds.co.uk

Chapter 19

Haematology online

Haematology online

There are many Internet resources available for haematology, including organizations, journals, atlases, conference proceedings, and newsgroups. The main difficulty with Internet resources is that they change so frequently and they are constantly being updated and outdated. It would be impossible to list every known site, and we have provided only URLs for those we think are of most value.

General websites

Anaemiaweb
www.anaemiaweb.org

Bloodline
www.bloodline.net

BloodMed
www.bloodmed.com

Breaking Barriers
www.liv.ac.uk/breakingbarriers

Clinical Leaders of Thrombosis (C.L.O.T.)
www.clotuk.com

Congenital Dyserythropoietic Anaemia Research Initiative Oxford
www.imm.ox.ac.uk/groups/mrc_molhaem/cda/

DICsepsis
www.DICsepsis.org

Doctor Online
www.doctoronline.nhs.uk

Elimination of Leukaemia Fund
www.leukaemia-elf.org.uk/

Free Medline Searching
www.ncbi.nlm.nih.gov/PubMed/

Health News -The Media Medical Agency
www.health-news.co.uk/

Health Workforce Bulletin
www.health-workforce.com

Hematologic Diseases (CliniWeb: Oregon Health Sciences University)
www.ohsu.edu/cliniweb/C15/C15.378.html

Hematology Case Studies (UC Davis School of Medicine)
medocs.ucdavis.edu/IMD/420A/course.htm

Hospital Web
neuro-www.mgh.harvard.edu/hospitalweb.shtml

International Medical News
www.internationalmedicalnews.com

Lymphoma Forum
www.lymphoma.org.uk

lymphoma-net.org
www.lymphoma-net.org

MPD Support
www.mpd-support.co.uk

Medical Matrix
www.medmatrix.org/Index.asp

Meducation
www.meducation.com

Medweb
www.medweb.emory.edu/medweb

MRC Molecular Haematology Unit
www.imm.ox.ac.uk/groups/mrc_molhaem

Myeloma Forum
www.ukmf.org.uk/guidelines.shtml

National Library of Medicine
www.nlm.nih.gov

NIH Consensus Conferences
http://odp.od.nih.gov/consensus

Oncolink
www.oncolink.com

Oxford Haemophilia Centre
www.medicine.ox.ac.uk/ohc

Oxford Regional Blood Club
www.btinternet.com/~phm/BloodClub.html

Pharmaceutical Technology
www.pharmaceutical-technology.com

Reuters Health News
www.reutershealth.com

RD Direct
www.rddirect.org.uk

Sickle Hut
www.sicklehut.com

The Hematology Site
www.geocities.com/HotSprings/5340

Virtual Hospital
http://indy.radiology.uiowa.edu/VirtualHospital.html

WebPath
www-medlib.med.utah.edu/WebPath/webpath.html

Atlases

Atlas of Genetics and Cytogenetics in Oncology and Haematology
atlasgeneticsoncology.org

Atlas of Hematology
www.medic.bgu.ac.il/mirrors/pathy/Pictures/atoras.html

Atlas of Hematology (Nagoya)
pathy.med.nagoya-u.ac.jp/atlas/doc/atlas.html

Cells of the blood (University of Leicester: Department of Microbiology and Immunology)
www-micro.msb.le.ac.uk/MBChB/bloodmap/Blood.html

Digital Image Study Sets (UC Davis School of Medicine)
medocs.ucdavis.edu/IMD/420A/dib

Hematology Image Atlas
www.hms.medweb.harvard.edu/HSHeme/AtlasTOC.htm

Introduction to Blood Morphology
www.hslib.washington.edu/courses/blood/intro.html

The Crookston Collection, University of Toronto
www.thecrookstoncollection.com

Journals and books

ASH Education Book
www.asheducationbook.org

Blackwell Publishing
www.blackwellpublishing.com

Blood
www.thebloodjournal.org

Blood Book .Com
www.bloodbook.com

Blood Cells, Molecules and Disease
www.scripps.edu/bcmd

British Journal of Haematology
www.blackwellpublishing.com/journals/bjh

British Medical Journal
www.bmj.com

Cancer
caonline.amcancersoc.org

Haematologica
www.haematologica.org

Hematological Oncology
www.interscience.wiley.com/journal/hon

Journal of Clinical Investigation
www.jci.org

Journal of Clinical Oncology
www.jco.ascopubs.org

Lancet
www.thelancet.com

Leukemia
www.Nature.com/leu

Leukemia and Lymphoma
www.tandf.co.uk/journals/titles/10428194.html

Nature
www.nature.com

New England Journal of Medicine
www.nejm.org

Oxford University Press
www.oup.com

Science
www.sciencemag.org

Societies and organizations

American Association of Blood Banks (AABB)
www.aabb.org

American Association for Cancer Research (AACR)
www.aacr.org

American Cancer Society
www.cancer.org

Association of Clinical Scientists
www.assclinsci.org

American Medical Association
www.ama-assn.org

American Society of Clinical Oncology
www.asco.org

American Society of Hematology
www.hematology.org

American Society of Pediatric Hematology/Oncology (ASPHO)
www.aspho.org

Anticoagulation.org.uk
www.anticoagulation.org.uk

Aplastic Anemia Foundation of America
www.medic.uth.tmc.edu/ptnt/00001045.htm

Association of Pediatric Oncology Nurses (APON)
www.apon.org

Bloodline
www.bloodline.net

British Blood Transfusion Society (BBTS)
www.bbts.org.uk

British Committee for Standards in Haematology
www.bcshguidelines.com

British Society of Blood and Marrow Transplantation
www.bsbmt.org

British Society for Haematology
www.b-s-h.org.uk

British Society for Haemostasis & Thrombosis (BSHT)
www.bsht.bham.ac.uk

CancerBACUP
www.cancerbacup.org.uk

Centers for Disease Control (CDC), Atalanta
www.cdc.gov

European Bone Marrow Transplant Association
www.embt.org

European Society of Paediatric Haematology and Immunology
www.esphi.org/

European Hematology Association
www.ehaweb.org

Imperial Cancer Research Fund
www.cancerresearchuk.org

Institute of Biomedical Science
www.ibms.org

International Histiocytosis Organization (Histiocytosis Association of America)
www.histio.org

International Hospital Federation
www.hospitalmanagement.net/

International Myeloma Foundation UK
www.myeloma.org.uk

Irish Haemovigilance Association (IHA)
www.ihaonline.ie

Leukemia and Lymphoma Society
www.leukemia-lymphoma.org

Leukemia Research Fund
www.lrf.org.uk

Leukemia Society of America
www.leukemia.org

Medical Research Council
www.mrc.ac.uk

National Blood Service
www.blood.co.uk

National Cancer Institute
www.cancer.gov

National Children's Leukemia Foundation
www.leukemiafoundation.org

National Guidelines Clearinghouse
www.guidelines.gov

National Heart, Lung, and Blood Institute
www.nhlbi.nih.gov

National Institutes of Health
www.nih.gov

NHS Centre for Reviews and Dissemination
www.york.ac.uk/inst/crd

NHS Professionals
www.nhsprofessionals.nhs.uk

Royal College of Pathologists
www.rcpath.org

Royal College of Physicians
www.rcplondon.ac.uk

Royal Society of Medicine
www.roysocmed.ac.uk

Sickle Cell Information Centre Home
www.scinfo.org

Society for Hematopathology (Dartmouth College)
www.dartmouth.edu/~nlevy/wwwx.html

The Cochrane Library
www.update-software.com/cochrane

UK NEQAS Schemes
www.ukneqas.org.uk

UK CLL support association
www.cllsupport.org.uk

Wellcome Trust
www.wellcome.ac.uk

World Federation of Hemophilia
www.wfh.org

World Health Organization
www.who.int/en

Guidelines, trials, and evidence-based practice

British Committee for Standards in Haematology (BCSH)
www.bcshguidelines.com

Cochrane Library (The)
www.cochrane.org/reviews/en/topics/55.html

cancerTrials (National Cancer Institute)
www.cancertrials.nci.nih.gov

Clinical practice guidelines: hematology (Canadian Medical Association)
www.cma.ca/cpgs/hema.htm

Clinical trials: hematology (CenterWatch)
www.centerwatch.com

Comprehensive Sickle Cell Center at Grady Health System
www.scinfo.org

National Center for Biotechnology Information
www.ncbi.nlm.nih.gov

National Guideline Clearinghouse (Agency for Health Care Policy and Research (AHCPR))
www.guidelines.gov

National Library of Medicine
www.nlm.nih.gov

Patient-Reported Health Instruments
http://phi.uhce.ox.ac.uk

Transfusionguidelines.org.uk
www.transfusionguidelines.org.uk

Chapter 20

Charts and nomograms

Karnofsky performance status

Table 20.1 Karnofsky performance status

Normal, no complaints; no evidence of disease	100%
Able to carry on normal activity; minor signs or symptoms of disease	90%
Normal activity with effort; some signs or symptoms of disease	80%
Cares for self; unable to carry on normal activity or to do active work	70%
Requires occasional assistance but is able to care for most of his/her needs	60%
Requires considerable assistance and frequent medical care	50%
Disabled; requires special care and assistance	40%
Severely disabled; hospitalization is indicated although death not imminent	30%
Very sick; hospitalization necessary	20%
Moribund; fatal processes progressing rapidly	10%
Dead	0%

WHO/ECOG performance status

Table 20.2 WHO/ECOG performance status

0	Fully active; able to carry on all pre-disease performance without restriction.
1	Restricted in physically strenuous activity, but ambulatory and able to carry out work of a light or sedentary nature, e.g. light housework, office work.
2	Ambulatory and capable of all self-care but unable to carry out any work activities; up and about more than 50% of waking hours.
3	Capable of only limited self care, confined to bed or chair more than 50% of waking hours.
4	Completely disabled; cannot carry on any self care; totally confined to bed or chair.

1. Oken, M.M. *et al.* (1982). Toxicity and response criteria of the Eastern Cooperative Oncology Group *Am J Clin Oncol*, **5**, 649.

WHO haematological toxicity scale

Table 20.3 WHO haematological toxicity scale

Parameter	Grade 0	Grade 1	Grade 2	Grade 3	Grade 4
Haemoglobin (g/dL)	≥11.0	9.5–10.9	8.0–9.4	6.5–7.9	<6.5
Leucocytes (× 10^9/L)	≥4.0	3.0–3.9	2.0–2.9	1.0–1.9	<1.0
Granulocytes (× 10^9/L)	≥2.0	1.5–1.9	1.0–1.4	0.5–0.9	<0.5
Platelets (× 10^9/L)	≥100	75–99	50–74	25–49	<25
Haemorrhage	None	Petechiae	Mild blood loss	Gross blood loss	Debilitating blood loss

Body surface area nomogram

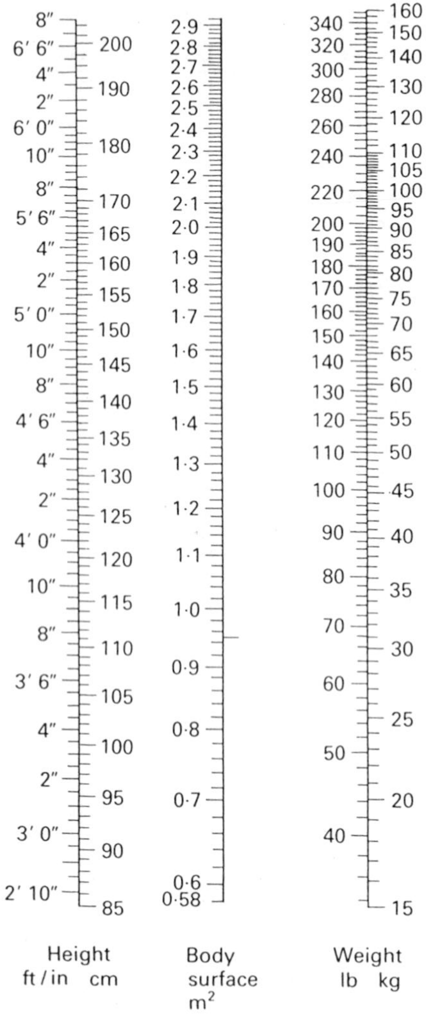

Fig. 20.1 Body surface area nomogram. Reproduced with permission from Ramrakha, P. and Moore, K. (1997) *Oxford Handbook of Acute Medicine* 2e. Oxford University Press, Oxford.

Gentamicin dosage nomogram

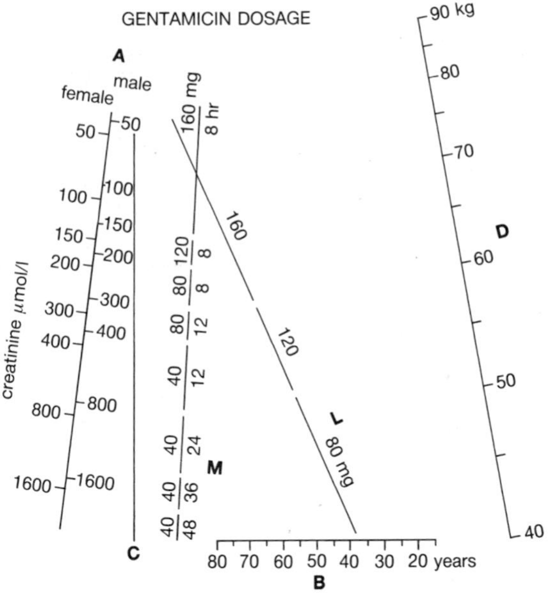

Fig. 20.2 Gentamicin dosage nomogram Reproduced with permission from Longmore *et al.* (2007) *Oxford Handbook of Clinical Medicine*, 7e. Oxford University Press, Oxford.

The Sokal Score for CML prognostic groups

Table 20.4 The Sokal Score for CML prognostic groups

Score	= Exp[0.0116 (age–43.4)] + 0.0345 (spleen size–7.51) + 0.188 ([platelets/700]^2–0.563) + 0.0887 (blasts%–2.1)
Low risk	<0.8
Intermediate risk	= 0.8–1.2
High risk	>1.2

Chapter 21

Normal ranges

Adult normal ranges

Table 21.1 Haematology

Haemoglobin	13.0–18.0g/dL	(♂)
	11.5–16.5g/dL	(♀)
Haematocrit	0.40–0.52	(♂)
	0.36–0.47	(♀)
RCC	$4.5–6.5 \times 10^{12}$/L	(♂)
	$3.8–5.8 \times 10^{12}$/L	(♀)
MCV	77–95fL	
MCH	27.0–32.0pg	
MCHC	32.0–36.0g/dL	
WBC	$4.0–11.0 \times 10^9$/L	
Neutrophils	$2.0–7.5 \times 10^9$/L	
Lymphocytes	$1.5–4.5 \times 10^9$/L	
Eosinophils	$0.04–0.4 \times 10^9$/L	
Basophils	$0.0–0.1 \times 10^9$/L	
Monocytes	$0.2–0.8 \times 10^9$/L	
Platelets	$150–400 \times 10^9$/L	
Reticulocytes	0.5–2.5% (or $50–100 \times 10^9$/L)	
ESR	2–12mm/1st hour (Westergren)	
Red cell mass	25–35mL/kg	(♂)
	20–30mL/kg	(♀)
Serum B12	150–700ng/L	
Serum folate	2.0–11.0mcg/L	
Red cell folate	150–700mcg/L	
Serum ferritin	15–300mcg/L (varies with sex and age)	
	14–200mcg/L (premenopausal ♀)	
INR	0.8–1.2	
PT	12.0–14.0sec	
APTT ratio	0.8–1.2	
APTT	26.0–33.5sec	
Fibrinogen	2.0–4.0g/L	
Thrombin time	± 3sec of control	
XDPs	<250mcg/L	
D-dimer	<500ng/mL	
Factors II, V, VII, VIII, IX, X, XI, XII	50–150IU/dL	
RiCoF	45–150IU/dL	
vWF: Ag	50–150IU/dL	
Protein C	80–135U/dL	
Protein S	80–135U/dL	
Antithrombin III	80–120U/dL	
APCR	2.12–4.0	
Bleeding time	3–9min	

Table 21.2 Biochemistry and immunology

Serum urea	3.0–6.5mmol/L	
	11.5–16.5g/dL	
Serum creatinine	60–125 micromol/L	
Serum sodium	135–145mmol/L	
Serum potassium	3.5–5.0mmol/v	
Serum albumin	32–50g/L	
Serum bilirubin	<17micromol/L	
Serum alk phos	100–300IU/L	
Serum calcium	2.15–2.55mmol/L	
Serum LDH	200–450IU/L	
Serum phosphate	0.7–1.5mmol/L	
Serum total protein	63–80g/L	
Serum urate	0.18–0.42mmol/L	
Serum γ-GT	10–46IU/L	
Serum iron	14–33mcmol/L	(♂)
	11–28mcmol/L	(♀)
Serum TIBC	45–75mcmol/L	
Serum ALT	5–42IU/L	
Serum AST	5–42IU/L	
Serum free T4	9–24pmol/L	
Serum TSH	0.35–5.5mU/L	
Immunology		
IgG	5.3–16.5g/L	
IgA	0.8–4.0g/L	
IgM	0.5–2.0g/L	
Complement:		
C3	0.89–2.09g/L	
C4	0.12–0.53g/L	
C1 esterase	0.11–0.36g/L	
CH50	80–120%	
C-reactive protein	<6mg/L	
Serum β_2-microglobulin	1.2–2.4mg/L	
CSF proteins:		
IgG	0.013–0.035g/l	
Albumin	0.170–0.238g/L	
Urine proteins:		
Total protein	<150mg/24h	
Albumin (24h)	<20mg/24h	

Paediatric normal ranges

Table 21.3 Full blood count

Age	Hb (g/dL)	MCV (fL)	Neuts	Lymph	Platelets
Birth	14.9–23.7	100–125	2.7–14.4	2–7.3	150–450
2 weeks	13.4–19.8	88–110	1.5–5.4	2.8–9.1	170–500
2 months	9.4–13.0	84–98	0.7–4.8	3.3–10.3	210–650
6 months	10.0–13.0	73–84	1–6	3.3–11.5	210–560
1 year	10.1–13.0	70–82	1–8	3.4–10.5	200–550
2–6 years	11.5–13.8	72–87	1.5–8.5	1.8–8.4	210–490
6–12 years	11.1–14.7	76–90	1.5–8	1.5–5	170–450
Adult ♂	12.1–16.6	77–92	1.5–6	1.5–4.5	180–430
Adult ♀	12.1–15.1	77–94	1.5–6	1.5–4.5	180–430

Neuts, neutrophils; lymph, lymphocytes and platelets (all × 10^9/L)

Table 21.4 Haemostasis

Parameter	Neonate	Adult level
Platelet count	150–400 × 10^9/L	As adult
Prothrombin time	Few sec longer than adult	Up to 1 week
APTT	Up to 25% increase	By 2–9 months
Thrombin time		As adult
Bleeding time	2–10 min	As adult
Fibrinogen	2.0–4.0g/L	As adult
Vit K factors:		
Factor II	30–50% adult level	Up to 6 months
Factor VII	30–50% adult level	By 1 month
Factor IX	20–50% adult level	Up to 6 months
Factor X	30–50% adult level	Up to 6 months
Factor V		As adult
Factor VIII	Variable: 50–200% adult level	
vW factor	Usually raised (up to 3 × adult level)	
Factor XI	20–50% adult level	6–12 months
Factor XII	20–50% adult level	3–6 months
Factor XIII	50–100% adult level	1 month
FDP/XDP	Up to twice adult level	by 7 days
AT	50–80% adult level	6–12 months
Protein C	30–50% adult level	Up to 24 months
Protein S	30–50% adult level	3–6 months
Plasminogen	30–80% adult level	2 weeks

Index

C

M

N

T

U

V